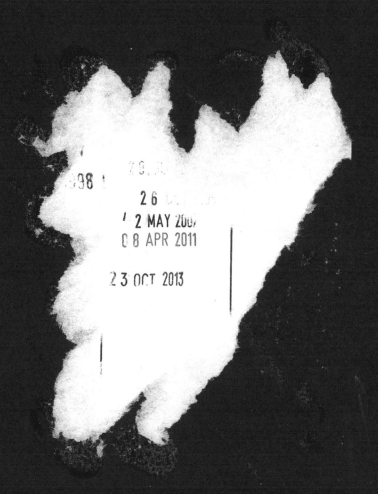

Ultrasound in Obstetrics and Gynaecology

This title is a self-contained work entitled *Ultrasound in Obstetrics and Gynaecology*. Additionally it forms an integral part of *CLINICAL ULTRASOUND a comprehensive text* together with its companion titles, *Abdominal and General Ultrasound* and *Cardiac Ultrasound*, each of which may also be purchased separately.

For Churchill Livingstone

Publisher: Simon Fathers
Project Editor: Clare Wood-Allum
Indexer: Michele Clarke
Production Control: Neil Dickson
Sales Promotion Executive: Caroline Boyd

For Longman Malaysia

Production Co-ordination: Shirley Kerk

CLINICAL ULTRASOUND a comprehensive text

Ultrasound in Obstetrics and Gynaecology

Edited by

Keith Dewbury BSc MB BS FRCR
Consultant Radiologist and Honorary Senior Lecturer,
Southampton University Hospitals, Southampton, UK

Hylton Meire FRCR
Consultant Radiologist, King's College Hospital, London, UK

David Cosgrove MA MSc FRCR FRCP
Consultant in Nuclear Medicine and Ultrasound, Royal
Marsden Hospital, London, UK

Associate Editor: **Pat Farrant** DCRR DMU
Superintendent Research Sonographer, King's College
Hospital, London, UK

Foreword by
Barry B. Goldberg MD
Professor of Radiology, Director, Division of Diagnostic
Ultrasound, Thomas Jefferson University Hospital,
Philadelphia, Pennsylvania, USA

CHURCHILL LIVINGSTONE
EDINBURGH LONDON MADRID MELBOURNE NEW YORK AND TOKYO 1993

CHURCHILL LIVINGSTONE
Medical Division of Longman Group UK Limited

Distributed in the United States of America by Churchill
Livingstone Inc., 650 Avenue of the Americas, New York,
N.Y. 10011, and by associated companies, branches and
representatives throughout the world.

First published 1993
   Reprinted 1993
   Reprinted 1994

ISBN 0-443-04279-9

British Library Cataloguing in Publication Data
A catalogue record for this book is available from the
British Library.

Library of Congress Cataloging in Publication Data
A catalog record for this book is available from the Library
of Congress.

The
publisher's
policy is to use
**paper manufactured
from sustainable forests**

Printed and bound in Great Britain by
William Clowes Limited, Beccles and London

Foreword

There has been rapid progress in the development of ultrasound almost since its beginnings in the late 1940s. However, it was not until the mid 1970s with the development of gray scale and real time ultrasound that it became an accepted clinical procedure. In the 1980s, with the development of color Doppler as well as the miniaturization of transducers allowing for the development of a variety of endoluminal transducers, its worldwide acceptance expanded exponentially.

In the past few years, the revenue generated from ultrasound equipment sales has exceeded that of all other imaging modalities, including magnetic resonance imaging. With this rapid expansion of ultrasound in a variety of areas throughout the world, the need for education has also expanded. No matter how good the equipment purchased and the number of transducers employed, the key for the success of ultrasound diagnosis and improved patient care depends on the abilities of the individual physicians and sonographers who use this technique. This series of books covering all of ultrasound, not only the major areas such as the abdomen, echocardiography, and obstetrics and gynecology, but also newly developed and more novel uses, makes an important contribution to raising the standards of knowledge in this field.

Chapters from a diverse group of contributors, recognized for their expertise, have been coordinated by the editors into a comprehensive text that meets the needs of those individuals wishing to have a complete knowledge of the current usefulness of ultrasound in medicine. Used as a complete compendium or as individual books on specific areas of interest, this work should become a standard in every ultrasound library throughout the world. It should prove of value not only to those experienced in ultrasound, both physicians and non-physicians, but also to students wishing to obtain an in-depth knowledge of the multiple uses of ultrasound. I extend my congratulations on this unique accomplishment to the editors as well as to the many contributors to this well illustrated and referenced text.

B.B.G.

Preface

Most textbooks, at least in the field of diagnostic imaging, stem from the wish of the authors or editors to make their special expertise more widely available. The origin of *Clinical Ultrasound* is rather unusual in that it is a response to a proposal by the publishers, Churchill Livingstone, that the time was right for a comprehensive ultrasound textbook with a strong clinical content.

At first approach, we have to confess to having been sceptical of the need for such a textbook and we were most reluctant to embark on such a monumental task but, as we began to review the field, it was possible to envisage it being broken down into more manageable components. It was also clear that there really was no comprehensive textbook on the market, all of the available books concentrating on a particular application or body region.

An initial hurdle was to secure the editorship of Dr Peter Wilde to oversee the cardiology section; initially Peter was as reluctant as the rest of us, having heavy commitments on his hands but, fired by the prospect of a comprehensive and strongly clinical reference work, he was persuaded. The Cardiology section has been completely under his editorship, though it adheres to the general format and goals of the entire book.

For the remaining large sections, a decisive influence in our agreeing to proceed was the fact that Pat Farrant was enthusiastic, something she may have come to regret as time went by! Pat agreed to take control of the massive task of handling all of the editing and advising that underlay the organising of the extensive text and innumerable figures together with their orientation diagrams,[1] keeping track of where alterations had to be entered, checking that tables referred to in the text were, in fact, contained in the chapter or appendix and generally managing the entire process of creation and collation which extended to double the 18 months that we had originally anticipated. However, that was not all for, as we got further into the project, Pat was also called upon to contribute large portions of chap-

ters that had somehow fallen by the wayside and her input into almost every section has been absolutely invaluable. It was in the knowledge that she would give this kind of support that we entered the 'battle'. None of us foresaw just how protracted a battle it would become nor how large Pat's contribution would turn out to be – 'siege' would have been a more apposite term!

We would also like to thank our families and friends who have borne with us during the past three stressful years. Special thanks are due to Christine Dewbury and Gill Meire for their continuing support and encouragement, and for hosting so many editorial meetings.

From this explanation, our intentions should be clear. We have aimed to provide an up-to-date textbook on clinical diagnostic ultrasound that would cover the entire gamut of its applications, both imaging and Doppler. Because of its clinical basis, the physics of ultrasound does not feature as a formal topic, though its important practical consequences and implications, especially in newer, less familiar areas such as Doppler, are covered.

Diagnostic ultrasound has become so extensive that, inevitably, this had to be a large book and a small team of specialists could not hope to cover the entire field. Therefore, we commissioned a large number of contributing authors from Europe and the Americas, most well known experts in their own areas. We stand to lose friends however, because we have exercised strong editing rights in the interests of maintaining a uniform style – we hope our loyal contributors will feel that our sometimes heavy alterations have contributed to the overall quality of the book and will not take offence that we have freely altered their prose and even sometimes substituted scans that seemed clearer or that made the intended point better.

With respect to the division of material through the book, the separation of Cardiology from the other applications already referred to, made it obvious that this should form a separate volume that is available on its own. Obstetrics and Gynaecology formed a second distinct section and so we have arranged that this also be a separate volume with its own page numbering and index. The other

---

[1] Actually there are approximately 3000 figures and 500 tables!

two volumes, which contain the remaining applications (abdominal, small parts, vascular, miscellaneous), are offered together as two sections of a single book: the pages are numbered through and they are indexed together in the expectation that few users will need only one of the pair.

We hope that *Clinical Ultrasound* will become a reference work for all who use ultrasound in their clinical practice and that users will find in it comprehensive answers to their everyday needs. It should provide critical information in a form that is easy to look up, as well as form the basis for specialist training.

1992

H.M.
D.C.
K.D.

Terminology and scan position indicators

The aim of this book is to serve both as a reference text and as an aid to education and teaching. During the editorial process it was clear to us that the terminology used to describe ultrasound appearances is extremely diverse, confusing and occasionally inaccurate. We have therefore unified the terminology in *Clinical Ultrasound*. In doing this we have considered the two main interactions between the ultrasound beam and the tissue; namely reflection and attenuation.

Meaningless terms such as 'sonolucent' and 'echo dense' have been eradicated. We also considered the use of the prefixes 'hyper-' and 'hypo-' a source of confusion and found several instances where the secretaries typing the manuscripts had confused the two.

Where backscattered amplitude is being discussed the ultrasound appearances are described as of reduced, normal or increased reflectivity (by inference compared with that which would normally be expected).

The above features of *Clinical Ultrasound* have been incorporated in an attempt to make these volumes more valuable and easier to understand, and it is hoped that the terminology we have used will encourage readers to consider more carefully the terminology they use to describe their own ultrasound findings.

The relatively small field of view of modern ultrasound scanners, and the infinitely variable planes of imaging, sometimes lead to difficulties in interpreting the anatomy and orientation of an ultrasound image. Rather than using extensive free narrative to describe the positions from which images have been obtained we have used a system of body markers on which the position of the scans has been indicated. When referring to these the reader should be aware that the scans indicating a lateral area of contact do not necessarily imply that the patient was moved into an oblique or decubitus position but simply that the transducer was located on the lateral aspect of the patient.

The orientation of the conventional extracavitory images included in this book has generally been adjusted such that longitudinal scans are viewed as if from the patient's right side and transverse scans as if from the patient's feet. Unfortunately there is no standardisation for the orientation of intracavitory images and, in general, these have been displayed with the orientation unaltered from that supplied by the individual authors. We have not attempted to identify the position of the transducer or the orientation of the image for intracavitory scans as these should be clear from the accompanying text in each case.

1992

H.M.
D.C.
K.D.

Contributors

Lindsey D. Allan MD FRCP
Professor of Fetal Echocardiology, Guy's Hospital, London, UK

Douglas G. Altman BSc
Head of the Medical Statistics Laboratory, Imperial Cancer Research Fund, London, UK

Heather S. Andrews MB BS DMRD MRCP FRCR
Consultant Radiologist, United Bristol Healthcare Trust, Bristol, UK

Tom Bourne MB BS MRCOG
Lecturer and Honorary Senior Registrar, Ovarian and Gynaecological Scanning Unit, Department of Obstetrics and Gynaecology, King's College Hospital, London, UK

Sarah Bower MRCOG
Former Research Fellow, Department of Obstetrics and Gynaecology, King's College Hospital, London, UK

Stuart Campbell FRCOG
Professor and Head, Department of Obstetrics and Gynaecology, King's College Hospital, London, UK

Lyn S. Chitty BSc PhD MRCOG
Senior Registrar in Genetics, Regional Genetics Centre, Guy's Hospital, London, UK

Glyn Constantine MRCP MRCOG
Consultant Obstetrician and Gynaecologist, Good Hope Hospital, Sutton Coldfield, UK

David O. Cosgrove MA MSc FRCR FRCP
Consultant in Nuclear Medicine and Ultrasound, Royal Marsden Hospital, Sutton, UK

Richard De Chazal MD MRCOG
Consultant Obstetrician, Leicester Royal Infirmary, Leicester, UK

Paul A. Dubbins MB BS BSc FRCR
Consultant Radiologist, Plymouth General Hospital, Plymouth, UK

Alison Fowlie FRCOG
Consultant Obstetrician and Gynaecologist with a Special Interest in Fetal Medicine, Derby City Hospital, Derby, UK

Andrew M. Fried MD FACR
Professor, Diagnostic Radiology; Director, Special Procedures Division; Chief, Ultrasound Division, University of Kentucky, Kentucky, USA

Rajat K. Goswamy MB BS MRCOG
Medical Director, Fertility and IVF Centre, Churchill Clinic, London; Senior Lecturer/Consultant, St Thomas' Hospital, London, UK

David R. Griffin MRCOG
Consultant Obstetrician and Gynaecologist, Watford General Hospital, Watford, UK

Eric Jauniaux MD PhD
Obstetrician and Gynaecologist, Department of Obstetrics and Gynaecology, University Hospital, Erasme, Brussels, Belgium

Josephine McHugo MRCP FRCR
Consultant Radiologist, Birmingham Maternity Hospital, Birmingham, UK

Hylton B. Meire FRCR
Consultant Radiologist, King's College Hospital, London, UK

Ian G. Parkin MB ChB
Senior Lecturer in Anatomy, University of Birmingham, Birmingham, UK

John H. Parsons MB ChB MRCOG DA
Senior Lecturer and Honorary Consultant, King's College School of Medicine and Dentistry, London, UK

J. Malcolm Pearce MD FRCS FRCOG
Consultant Perinatal Obstetrician, St George's Hospital, London, UK

Charles H. Rodeck BSc MB BS FRCOG DSc
Professor of Obstetrics and Gynaecology, University
College, London, UK

Christopher V. Steer MRCOG
Senior Registrar, Department of Obstetrics and
Gynaecology, Royal Free Hospital, London, UK

Janet I. Vaughan MBBS MRCOG FRACOG DDU
Senior Lecturer, Royal Postgraduate Medical School,
London, UK

Martin J. Whittle MD FRCOG FRCP(Glasg)
Professor of Fetal Medicine, Birmingham Maternity
Hospital, Birmingham, UK

Contents

Note: These plates are reproduced in black and white in the appropriate position within the text.

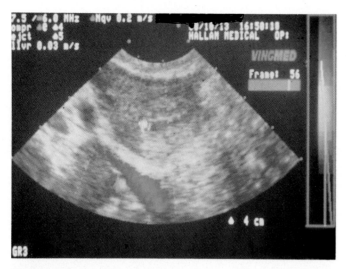

Ch. 5

Plate 1 **Vascularisation within a corpus luteum** visualised by trans-vaginal colour flow mapping.

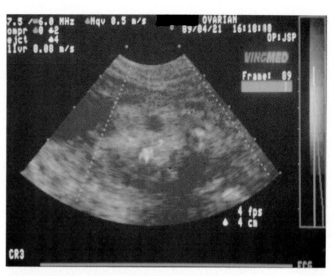

Ch. 5

Plate 3 **Vascularisation within a stage I ovarian cancer.**

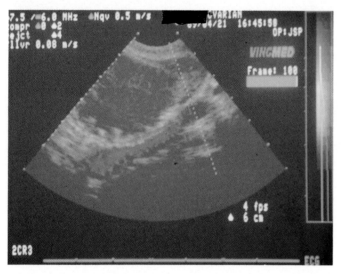

Ch. 5

Plate 2 **Colour flow mapping of a benign dermoid cyst.** Although the iliac vessels are defined by the colour Doppler, there are no areas of vascularisation within the cyst.

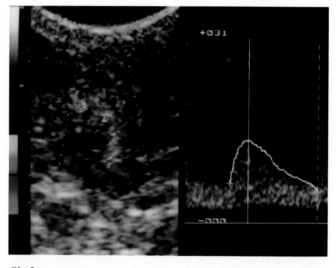

Ch. 5

Plate 4 **Vascularisation within the endometrium and flow velocity waveforms from the uterine arteries** in a case of endometrial carcinoma using trans-vaginal colour flow mapping.

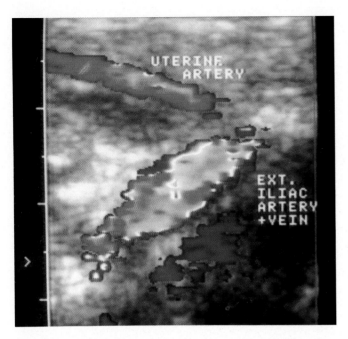

Plate 1 **The apparent 'cross-over' of the main uterine artery with the external iliac artery and vein.**

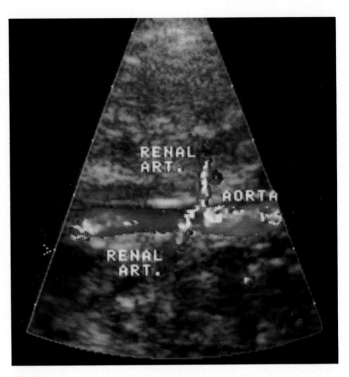

Plate 3 **Fetal aorta and renal artery** visualised by colour flow imaging.

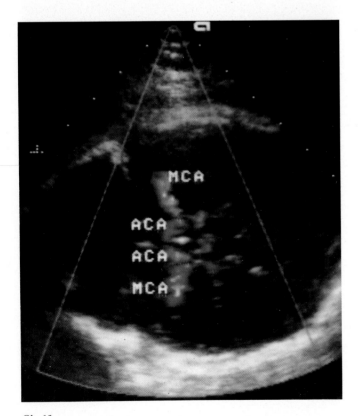

Plate 2 **Circle of Willis** visualised by colour flow imaging. MCA – middle cerebral artery, ACA – anterior communicating artery.

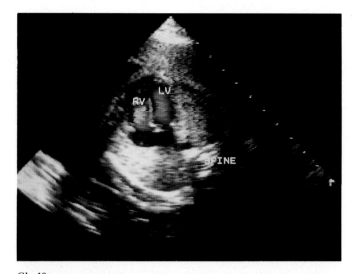

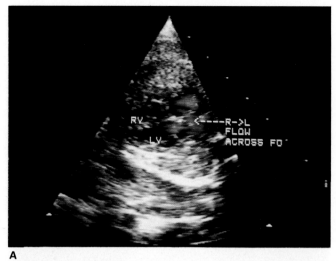

A

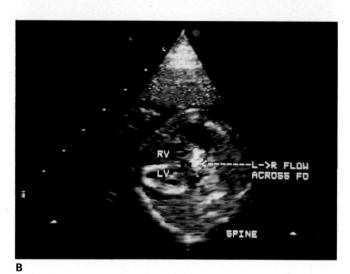

B

Ch. 19
Plate 1 The four chamber view. The apex of the heart is closest to the transducer. The colour flow map shows equal forward flow, coded in red, into both ventricles through the mitral and tricuspid valves. RV – right ventricle, LV – left ventricle.

Ch. 19
Plate 2 Flow through the foramen ovale. A: This shows a right to left jet coloured blue through the foramen ovale in a normal heart. **B:** Aortic stenosis. The left ventricle is thick walled and highly reflective due to aortic outflow obstruction. There is a left to right jet through the foramen ovale due to raised left atrial pressure.

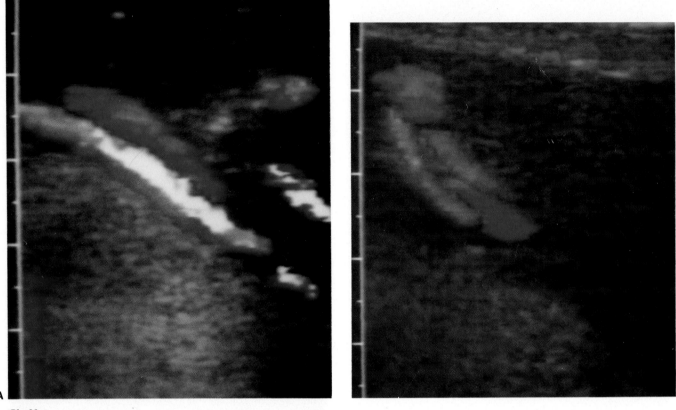

Ch. 23
Plate 1   Normal cord. A: Colour flow image of a normal cord at 21 weeks of gestation for comparison with Plate 1B. **B:** Single umbilical artery. Colour flow image of single umbilical artery cord at 18 weeks associated with multiple fetal malformations and oligohydramnios. (Reproduced with permission of the publisher from Jauniaux et al. Am J Obstet Gynecol 1989; 161: 1195.)

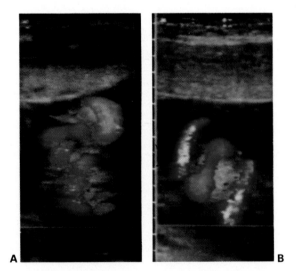

Ch. 23
Plate 2   Angiomyxoma of the cord. A: Colour flow image of the cord tumour described in Figures 35 and 36 showing an abnormal vascular pattern at the placental insertion. **B:** Colour flow image showing the three vessels separated by a reflective structure partially compressing the umbilical vein. (Reproduced with permission of the publisher from Jauniaux et al. Am J Obstet Gynecol 1989; 161: 1195.)

Choosing a scanner

Hylton B. Meire

INTRODUCTION

It is possible to obtain diagnostically adequate obstetric and gynaecological images using almost any available ultrasound equipment but the object of this chapter is to discuss the criteria which should be considered when selecting equipment primarily for obstetric and gynaecological use. In addition several important aspects concerning the conduct of an ultrasound examination are discussed including patient position, advice on transvaginal examinations and data recording systems.

Scanning systems

A range of different techniques has been developed for scanning the ultrasound beam through the patient. These different systems each have their own advantages and limitations which may influence their desirability for obstetric and gynaecological scanning.

Mechanical scanners

The majority of mechanical systems comprise a single ultrasound crystal which is rapidly oscillated through an angle of at least 90°. These have been given the generic name 'wobblers' (Fig. 1). An alternative mechanical approach is for several crystals, typically three or four, to be mounted on the circumference of a wheel which is rotated inside the scanner head. The crystals are brought into use

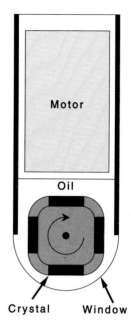

Fig. 2 The spinner mechanical ultrasound transducer. Several transducer crystals are mounted on a wheel. As the wheel rotates the transducers are selected in turn when they pass the window. In this example, four 90° sectors are scanned for each revolution of the wheel.

sequentially as they pass the acoustic window in the scanner assembly (Fig. 2). These systems are referred to as 'spinners'. Both wobblers and spinners are only capable of examining a 'sector' of the patient's anatomy via a small area of contact (the 'footprint'). A small footprint is particularly advantageous if the probe has to be angled down into the pelvis in very early pregnancy or to visualise the lower segment or cervix in the third trimester, and for gynaecological examinations.

The advantages of mechanical sector scanners lies in their small area of contact with a relatively wide field of view deep within the patient. In addition, the transmitting and receiving electronics are much simpler, and therefore potentially cheaper, than the more complex electronic systems. The main disadvantages are the inevitable wear and fatigue in the mechanical components with subsequent reduced life expectancy for the transducer. In addition the narrow field of view near the surface of the patient is sometimes a disadvantage, particularly in late pregnancy. A further minor disadvantage of the single crystal devices arises from the fact that the focal length of the transducer is fixed, giving rise to relatively poor resolution in the first few centimetres and in the distal portion of the field of view. It is possible to overcome this problem by dividing the transducer into a number of concentric rings to produce an 'annular array' transducer. With appropriate complex electronics this enables the operator to vary the depth of focus, but at the price of increased cost for both the transducer and associated electronics. In addition, in

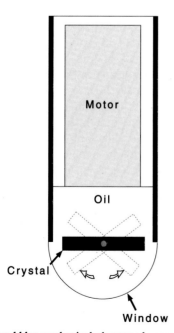

Fig. 1 The wobbler mechanical ultrasound scanner. The motor and associated mechanics oscillate the transducer crystal through an arc of about 90° thus scanning the ultrasound beam to and fro across the ultrasound window.

order to be effective, an annular array transducer must have a greater diameter (aperture) than a single crystal device so that the transducer assembly is larger.

Electronic scanners

All electronic scanning systems comprise transducers in which the active piezo-electric crystal is divided into small elements, numbering from 60 to 600 depending upon the design and application. The ultrasound beam is scanned through the patient by rapid sequential firing of groups of these elements. The earliest and simplest of these to be developed was the linear array (Fig. 3). This comprises a transducer with a flat surface within which are housed multiple small elements, typically 300 to 600 in number in current equipment. These elements are fired in groups to generate ultrasound pulses and receive the subsequent echoes. When one pulse echo sequence has been completed, the controlling electronics then excite the next group, sequentially stepping the active area along the length of the transducer face. The time taken for the transmission and reception of each group of pulses is extremely short thus permitting the ultrasound beam to be swept across the whole transducer surface in a time of typically 1/25th of a second.

These systems have the advantage that there are no moving parts and there is a wide field of view near the patient surface. In addition, using more sophisticated electronics, it is possible to enable the operator to vary the focusing characteristics of the ultrasound beam and thereby optimise resolution at selected depths within the patient. The major disadvantages are those of a large footprint and the fact that the width of the image area is determined by the length of the transducer. Since the transducer length is typically 8 to 10 cm this imposes considerable restrictions on the ability to image large portions of a fetus late in pregnancy; this may make assessment of the anatomy and measurement of the head and abdomen circumferences technically difficult or impossible.

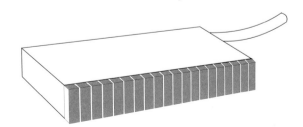

Fig. 3 The linear array ultrasound transducer. The active surface is divided into several hundred individual transducer elements. These are activated in groups in a rapid sequence so that the ultrasound beam is swept from one end of the probe surface to the other.

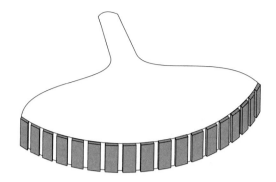

Fig. 4 The curvilinear ultrasound transducer. The principle is the same as the linear array but the curvature of the surface causes the ultrasound beam to sweep through an arc rather than a rectangle.

A development and refinement of the straight linear array is the curvilinear array (Fig. 4). The technology is essentially identical to the straight linear array but the array is generally shorter in length and has a slight curvature. These two features serve to overcome the two major difficulties, i.e. the large footprint and narrow field of view. The curvilinear array transducer geometry is an excellent compromise and, together with variable focusing on most modern machines, is the optimum configuration for both obstetric and gynaecological imaging, particularly if multiple transducers are not available.

A further alternative is the phased array transducer. This has many similarities to the linear array except that it is much shorter in length, typically 2 to 3 cm, and contains many fewer elements, normally 90 to 128 (Fig. 5). Using extremely complex electronics the individual elements of the transducer are excited in rapid sequence to produce a wavefront at an angle to the transducer face. The wavefront travels at right angles to itself and therefore at an angle to the transducer surface. The angle of propagation of the wavefront is determined by the delay interval between the firing of the individual elements. By varying this time interval it is therefore possible to sweep the ultrasound beam through an angle of approximately ± 45° thus giving rise to a 90° sector field of view.

The electronics of these devices is much more complex than the linear and curvilinear arrays and is therefore more expensive. The major single advantage is the production of a sector image with freedom from mechanical components. The advantages and disadvantages of the sector field of view are the same as for the mechanical transducers, except that the phased array does permit the operator to choose variable depths of focus.

Many electronic scanners permit multiple focal zones to be selected. It is only possible to focus the ultrasound at one depth range at a time and if multiple focal zones are selected these are implemented by the apparatus obtaining one image at one depth followed by separate images at each

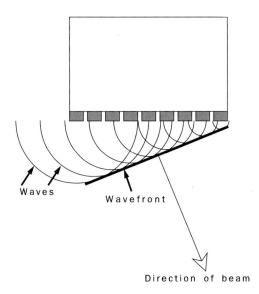

Waves

Wavefront

Direction of beam

Fig. 5 The phased array ultrasound transducer. This is like a small linear array but each element is activated separately. Each produces a small curved wave and these combine to form a wavefront. If there is a small delay between the firing of each element in sequence, the wavefront is directed at an angle to the transducer surface. As wavefronts travel at right angles to themselves the sound beam is thus steered through an angle. The angle is varied by varying the delays.

of the selected depth ranges. These images are then combined together to produce an apparently single image. Although the overall resolution throughout the image may be markedly improved a significant time penalty has been paid. Typically a single image is obtained in approximately $^1/_{25}$th of a second but if four focal zones are selected approximately $^1/_6$th of a second is required to obtain the entire image. The reduction in frame rate from 25 to 6 images per second is most noticeable to the operator and if either the fetus or transducer are not entirely stationary during the acquisition of each image, significant image blurring and degradation occurs and any potential advantage from the focusing is lost. As a general rule it is advisable to chose a single focal zone positioned in the centre of the field of interest. If greater resolution is required for assessment of fetal anatomy, the area of fetal anatomy should be identified first and the transducer held stationary while further focal zones are selected. An exception to this rule is fetal cardiac scanning. For this investigation the highest possible frame rate is essential and only one focal zone should be used in order to prevent severe image degradation.

Choice of equipment

Transabdominal scanning

Any general purpose ultrasound machine can be used with good effect for both obstetric and gynaecological investiga-

tions and, although different probe and equipment configurations may confer certain advantages for particular examinations, none of the types of equipment described above are incapable of performing diagnostic scans. The only possible exception to this generalisation is equipment designed specifically for adult echocardiography. Although such scanners can be used for imaging other organ systems, the signal processing within the equipment is usually optimised for cardiology and gives poor contrast resolution and an inferior ability to display low level echoes which may be important in both obstetric and gynaecological imaging.

As discussed above the curvilinear array transducers are the best compromise for transducer shape and field of view (Fig. 6) and are to be preferred for the majority of obstetric imaging. However, in the first trimester of pregnancy and for gynaecological examinations a sector scanner is often advantageous, particularly in view of its small footprint and the ability to angle the probe down into the pelvis from a suprapubic approach.

The nominal operating frequency of the transducer, together with its focusing characteristics, are of importance. Higher frequency transducers tend to give better resolution but are not able to penetrate to deeper structures adequately. These transducers are therefore generally constructed with a relatively superficial focal zone. Lower frequency transducers, for example 3.5 MHz, give better depth penetration, are usually able to focus at a greater depth and should be used where good resolution of deeper structures is important, for example third trimester pregnancy scans. As a general principle the user should always select a transducer with as high a frequency as possible consistent with obtaining penetration to the maximum required depth for each investigation. The sensitivity of more recent transducer materials is markedly greater than those which were available a decade ago and this has permitted an upward trend in transducer frequencies such that early to mid-pregnancy examinations can often be performed with a 5 MHz transducer and, with certain makes of equipment, even at 7.5 MHz.

Trans-vaginal scanning

The last few years has seen the development of a number of dedicated systems for trans-vaginal scanning. The advantage of this route is the proximity of the transducer to the structures of interest, permitting the use of higher frequency and shorter focus with consequent dramatic improvement in resolution.

The scanning mechanisms of these transducers incorporate either mechanical or electronic sector scanners and curvilinear arrays. There are no specific advantages or disadvantages to either of these scanning systems, except that the very small components with the mechanical systems may increase problems of mechanical reliability. Once

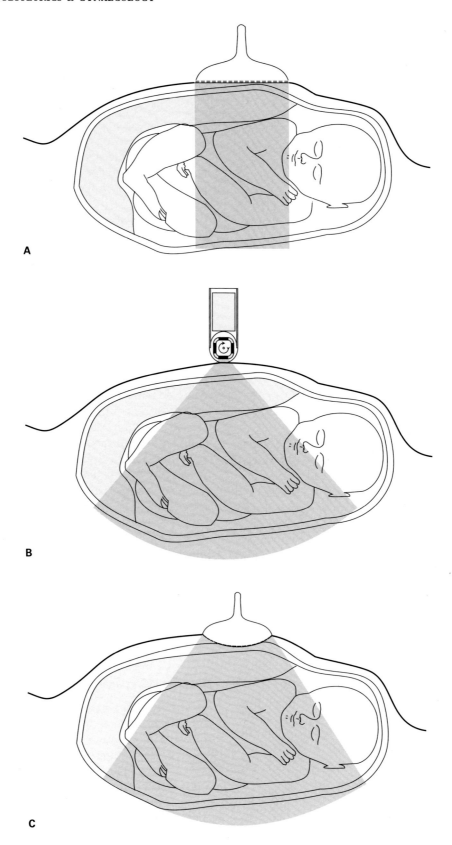

Fig. 6 Fields of view. A: The rectangular field of view of the linear array. **B:** The sector view of the mechanical and phased array sector scanners. **C:** The curvilinear array gives the best compromise of a not too large area of contact with a wide field of view.

again the curvilinear array seems to be the best compromise.

Of more importance than the scanning mechanism is the orientation of the field of view with respect to the probe shaft. For the majority of applications a long axis scanning plane off-set from the tip of the probe enables the operator to survey the majority of the pelvic contents merely by rotating the probe around its axis and by varying the depth to which it is inserted (Fig. 7). Some mechanical systems permit the operator to move the imaged sector throughout a much larger field of view (Fig. 8). In practice this facility is of value in only a limited number of examinations.

Some makes of equipment also permit the operator to image in a transverse plane. The array scanners achieve this by having a second array mounted at right angles to the first or possibly an entirely separate transducer. Some of the mechanical systems enable the operator to rotate the plane of oscillation of the scanning head such that images

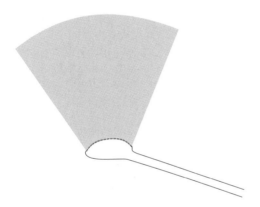

Fig. 7 The curvilinear trans-vaginal transducer. The proble can be made small and easy to use but has a limited field of view.

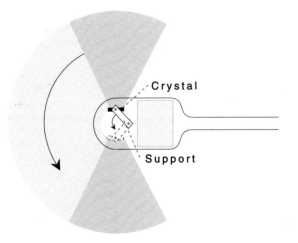

Fig. 8 A complex mechanical sector trans-vaginal scanner in which the scanning crystal is mounted on a support which can be moved through an arc to permit imaging of almost all the pelvis with very little change in probe position.

are obtained in the transverse axial plane. Transverse imaging may be helpful in a minority of investigations, particularly ovarian imaging, but is by no means essential, unless volume estimations of ovaries or gestation sacs are required.

Image orientation There is now universal acceptance of the orientation of transabdominal images. Longitudinal scans are viewed as if from the right side of the patient and transverse scans as if from the foot of the patient. There is as yet, however, no agreed orientation for the display of trans-vaginal images. Many equipment manufacturers permit the operator to rotate the image on the screen such that the transducer surface is no longer represented at the top of the screen. Many users choose to invert the image so that the apex of the sector is at the bottom of the screen and the longitudinal scans once again viewed as if from the patient's right side. This form of display seems logical as the display of the anatomy approximates to the orientation of structures within the patient.

The majority of trans-vaginal transducers have frequencies of either 5, 6 or 7.5 MHz. There is a significant difference in depth resolution between the 5 and 7.5 MHz transducers, for adequate imaging of a 12 week gestation or for a high lateral ovary a 5 MHz transducer may be found to be essential. If only one transducer is available the lower frequency is an adequate compromise, particularly if variable focusing is available.

Trans-rectal scanning

Trans-rectal scanning is seldom employed in obstetrics and gynaecology but there are a number of clinical situations in which it may be preferable to either the trans-vaginal or transabdominal approach. These include the investigation of threatened miscarriage, imaging of cervical pathology, including tumours and incompetence, and the assessment of vaginal malignant disease. Although dedicated trans-rectal scanners have been designed for urology, perfectly adequate images of these structures can be obtained with a conventional trans-vaginal transducer.

Doppler and colour flow imaging

The technical aspects of Doppler and colour flow imaging are covered in detail in *Abdominal and General Ultrasound*, Volume 1, Chapter 5; only those aspects pertinent to selection of equipment for obstetric and gynaecological examination are discussed here.

The simplest and least expensive form of Doppler equipment utilises a continuous transmission of ultrasound with simultaneous reception by a separate crystal, usually mounted within the same probe head. The commonest form of this equipment in obstetrics is that used for fetal heart monitoring in which an intentionally defocused ultrasound beam is used to detect fetal heart movements within a large insonated volume. Vascular surgeons use smaller versions of the same equipment in which the ultrasound is tightly focused and these systems can be used to detect and monitor the blood flow waveforms from the uterine, placental and fetal vessels. They do not incorporate any form of imaging and thus there is often an element of doubt about which vessel is actually being interrogated. Similarly, since the ultrasound is continuously transmitted, there is no mechanism by which the depth of a reflecting structure can be measured and therefore the position within the beam of any vessel cannot be determined and multiple vessels within the beam give rise to a composite Doppler signal. These continuous wave (CW) ultrasound systems have the advantage of being extremely inexpensive and also usually emit fairly low ultrasound powers. If depth and direction information is required to confirm the nature and position of a vessel giving rise to a Doppler signal, a pulsed echo system similar to that used for imaging must be used. The combination of imaging and pulsed Doppler ultrasound has been termed duplex scanning. The major advantage of these systems lies in the provision of a conventional ultrasound image to identify positively the target region or vessel for Doppler investigation and to interrogate closely adjacent vessels separately. The major disadvantages are a markedly increased ultrasound power level compared with CW and ultrasound imaging and an increase in equipment costs of 20% to 50% of a conventional imaging system. A further refinement of duplex Doppler uses a colour video facility to superimpose the Doppler flow information on a conventional image, giving a display commonly referred to as colour flow imaging (CFI). The major advantages of these systems lie in the ease with which vessels can be detected, even if they are too small to be seen on the conventional image. In obstetric and gynaecological diagnosis the mere identification of a vessel is seldom of any great value, the diagnostic information usually being produced by spectral analysis from a duplex system (see *Abdominal and General Ultrasound*, Vol. 1, Ch. 5). The major role of CFI is in the detection and correct identification of vessels and to act as a road map for placement of the range gate to obtain spectral Doppler information.

The major disadvantages of CFI are a further increase in machine cost, a significant increase in output power compared with conventional imaging, a markedly reduced frame rate and significantly worse resolution. The apparent dimensions of vessels are almost always greatly exaggerated on colour imaging systems and for this reason vessel dimensions must never be measured from a colour image.

Scanning techniques

Abdominal scanning

Transabdominal scanning is customarily performed with the patient lying supine on a suitable couch. For pelvic imaging and early pregnancy examinations it is necessary to have the patient's urinary bladder moderately filled to displace the small bowel out of the pelvis or to outline the lower half of the uterus. It is also necessary to use a sufficient quantity of scanning gel to ensure that the entire active surface of the transducer is adequately coupled to the patient's skin. This is particularly important for the array transducers. If the examination lasts for more than a few minutes it may be necessary to replenish the contact medium on the patient's abdomen. There is never any circumstance in which the transducer should be pressed upon the patient's abdomen. Adequate quantities of contact gel enable excellent imaging with only the very lightest of pressure of the transducer onto the patient's abdomen. Excessive pressure is not only uncomfortable for the patient, but distorts the fetal anatomy and corrupts abdominal circumference measurements and also serves to squeeze the gel out from between the transducer and the patient's skin.

Slight changes in patient position may occasionally be helpful in certain clinical situations. If difficulty is experienced in imaging the contents of the lower segment late in pregnancy it may be advantageous to tilt the operating couch head down by 15° to 20°. This manoeuvre, accompanied by a full urinary bladder, occasionally produces a significant improvement in image quality and may permit fetal head measurements which were not otherwise possible.

In late pregnancy pressure of the gravid uterus upon the vena cava may impair venous return and induce maternal hypotension. This should be relieved immediately by turning the patient into the left lateral decubitus position. In patients who are particularly susceptible to this problem it is possible to perform the entire examination with the patient in this position, or in the right lateral decubitus if they wish to observe the monitor during the examination. Patients with severe physical disabilities who present to the department in a wheelchair can readily be examined in the chair and thereby avoid the necessity for transferring them to the examination couch, although examination of the lower segment may be technically unsatisfactory.

Trans-vaginal scanning

The attitude of different operators to the performance of trans-vaginal scanning varies enormously. In view of the fact that there have already been a number of medicolegal cases arising from the apparently unsuspected introduction of trans-vaginal transducers, it now seems wise to advise all operators to ensure that the procedure is observed by a third party who is familiar with the examination and aware of normal practices.

The need for normal hygienic precautions and procedures to avoid transmission of infective agents from one patient to another are discussed in detail in the subsequent chapters.

The exact positioning of the patient for trans-vaginal examination is determined both by personal choice of the operator and the availability of an appropriate couch. Many users prefer the full lithotomy position with the patient's legs supported in stirrups or slings. Placing the patient in this position adds significantly to the duration of the examination and is less well accepted by patients. It is however necessary to attempt to move the perineum to the end of the examination couch to permit the handle of the transducer to be depressed below the level of the couch surface if it is necessary to manoeuvre the transducer into a more anterior position within the pelvis. This is obviously readily achieved with the patient in the lithotomy position but the same end can be realised with a conventional couch by placing a pillow under the buttocks or moving the patient to the end of the couch, bending the legs up and supporting the feet on a platform some 6 inches or so lower than the couch surface. A further alternative is to place the patient in the left lateral decubitus position with the legs fully flexed and the knees slightly separated. This position has the advantage of requiring no specialist apparatus and many patients prefer to have their back towards the operator during this investigation.

Image recording

The decision whether or not to make hard copy recordings of selected images from the examination depends upon a variety of factors including cost of recording materials, whether or not the examination is to be interpreted by a third party at a later time and by medicolegal considerations. In many clinics images from normal ultrasound examinations are not routinely recorded, only unusual or abnormal findings being documented. This policy has the advantage of reducing the cost of obtaining, storing, indexing and retrieving images but may be found wanting if a supposedly normal case subsequently becomes open to medicolegal litigation. There is no universal agreement concerning the medicolegal aspects of image recording in obstetrics and gynaecology. It is arguable that it might be advantageous to have good quality images to show that the examination was performed adequately by a competent operator and that no abnormality was detected. Conversely, if there are no images available, the operator may be given the benefit of the doubt. Certainly if any abnormality is detected it is essential to record sample images, firstly for comparison with subsequent examinations and secondly to support the reasons why the diagnosis was achieved. In many countries there is no legal requirement to take hard copies but if these have been taken there may be a requirement for them to be stored for a finite period; in the United Kingdom obstetric scans are supposed to be stored for at least 25 years and non-obstetric images for 7 years. This has serious cost and space consequences and is possibly a further disincentive to the recording of hard copy images.

Pelvic anatomy

David O. Cosgrove

INTRODUCTION

Since the skeleton forms the framework to which the viscera are attached, it determines the general anatomy of the pelvis and so needs to be understood although it is itself not well-visualised on ultrasound. In the following description the anatomy is described as viewed from within the pelvis, corresponding with the ultrasound point of view.[1-5]

The bony pelvis

The lateral elements, the paired hip bones or coxae (which bear the acetabula laterally) articulate with the wings of the sacrum posteriorly (Figs 1 and 2). Anteriorly each gives rise to two band-like bones, the superior and inferior pubic rami, which curve antero-medially to fuse in front as the pubic bones, the right and left articulating in the midline at the pubic symphysis. The spaces between the pubic rami, the obturator foramina, are covered by a fibrous membrane. Overall this complex forms a complete bony ring known as the true pelvis.

Superior to the true pelvis the iliac bones, arising from the hip bones, form the iliac fossae. They also articulate with the sacrum postero-medially but are unattached anteriorly and superiorly so that this upper part of the pelvis forms an incomplete bowl, known as the false pelvis – this space is actually the lowest part of the abdomen. The inlet to the true pelvis is marked by a prominent curved thickening of the hip bone, the arcuate line or ilio-pubic eminence. While the inlet to the true pelvis faces anteriorly, its outlet faces posteriorly, the change in direction of about 60° occurring because of the steep angulation of the sacrum on the lower lumbar vertebrae.

Pelvic muscles

All the muscles are paired; those in the true pelvis fall into two groups, lateral and medial. The obturator interni are the major lateral muscles; they arise from the membranes covering the obturator fossae and the surrounding bones, and form sheets a few millimetres thick that pass postero-inferiorly to leave the pelvis, their tendons angling laterally and attaching to the upper femora. They are seen on ultrasound as echo-poor strips forming the pelvic side walls (Fig. 3). Superior to the obturator internus lie the pyriformis muscles, forming transverse-lying strips that leave the pelvis laterally. They are pararectal in position and, being situated high in the pelvis, are difficult to image on ultrasound, requiring scans with a marked cephalad angulation.

The medial groups form the levator ani muscles (Fig. 3). Each is a curved sheet originating from the upper margin of the true pelvis and curving postero-medially to fuse with its opposite number in the midline to form a hammock-shaped muscular bowl (known as the 'pelvic sling') that closes the pelvic outlet. Midline perforations transmit the urethra, vagina and rectum. Each levator ani muscle is composed of two portions: one, the ilio-coccygeus, originating from the medial surface of the obturator internus muscle, has a mainly postero-medial lie while the other, pubo-coccygeus, taking origin from the inner surface of the pubic bone, passes posteriorly to the coccyx itself. This portion forms an antero-posterior lying band lying close to the midline; it is extremely variable, being rudimentary in some subjects and easily visualised in others.

The muscles of the false pelvis are iliacus, which arises from the entire iliac fossa, and psoas, which arises from the lumbar vertebrae and passes inferiorly to lie on the antero-medial surface of iliacus. Together the fused ilio-psoas muscles pass inferiorly immediately above and lateral to the brim of the true pelvis. Each passes under its respective inguinal ligament to attach to the lesser trochanter of the femora.

Vessels

The common iliac arteries, formed at the level of L5 by the division of the aorta, enter the false pelvis by crossing the ilio-psoas muscles as they diverge from the midline. At the level of the lower end of the sacro-iliac joints each divides into external and internal iliac branches. The former continue the inferior course, often swinging anteriorly also, to leave the pelvis by crossing under the inguinal ligament where they lie medial to the ilio-psoas muscles. They supply the leg and may be visualised by scanning across the pelvis using the filled bladder as a window (Fig. 4). All of the blood supply to the pelvic muscles and viscera comes from the internal iliac arteries. They form short trunks which soon divide into anterior and posterior main branches of equal size. These in turn rapidly break up into numerous smaller branches that supply the pelvic viscera. Important branches to note are the rectal and vesical arteries. In gynaecology the uterine branches are of major importance: they pass medially from the pelvic side walls and run to the lateral borders of the cervix. Here each divides into a descending vaginal branch and a larger, uterine branch that ascends along the lateral margin of the uterus, supplying it by curving branches known as arcuate arteries. The terminal portions of the main trunks continue along the uterine (fallopian) tubes, each ending in a small ovarian branch. By contrast, the main ovarian arteries are abdominal vessels, arising directly from the aorta at renal level; thus the ovaries have a dual supply.

Pelvic viscera

The pelvic viscera are cradled in the musculo-skeletal framework (Fig. 5). Anteriorly the bladder lies on the

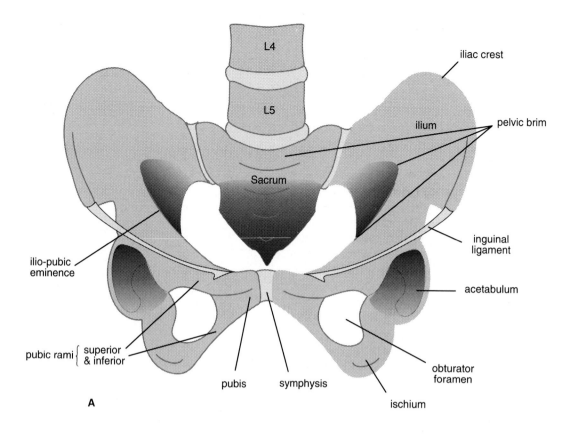

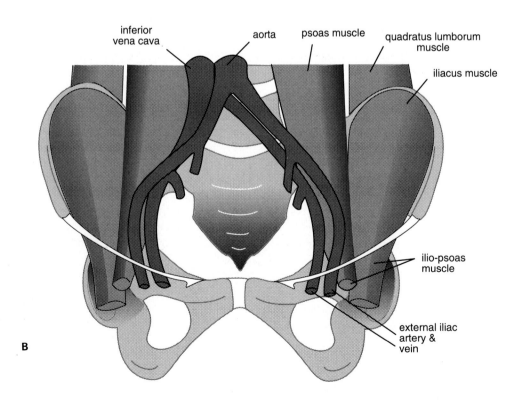

Fig. 1   The pelvic skeleton. Diagrams of the bony skeleton (**A**) to show the pelvic brim and (**B**) with the muscles of the false pelvis (ilio-psoas) as well as the major vessels added.

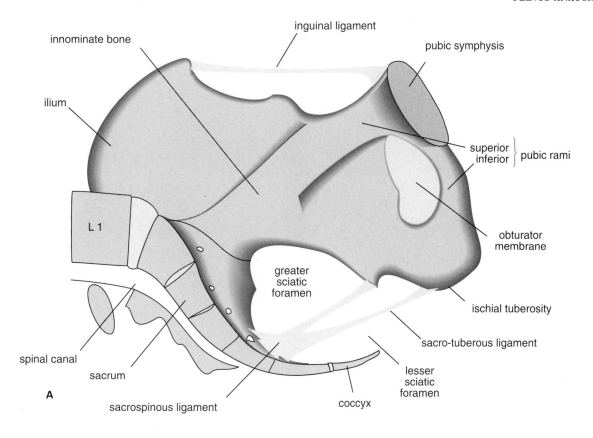

A

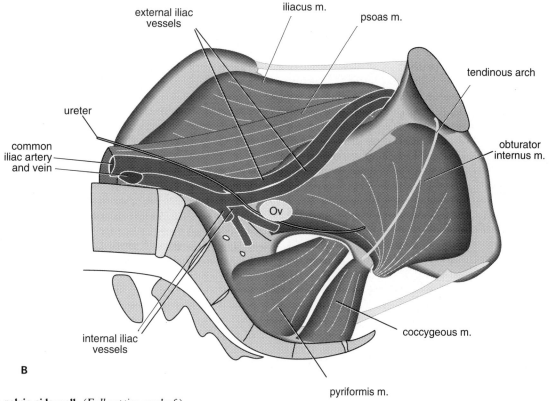

B

Fig. 2 The pelvic side wall. (*Full caption overleaf.*)

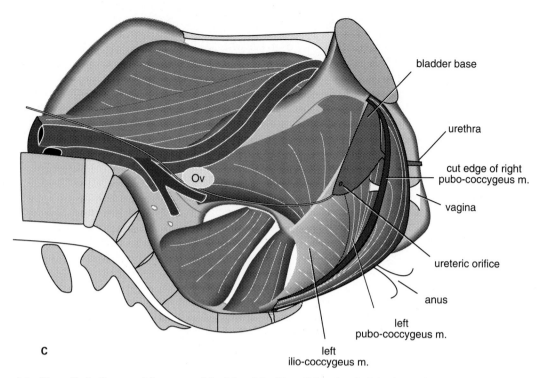

bladder base

urethra

cut edge of right
pubo-coccygeus m.

vagina

ureteric orifice

anus

left
pubo-coccygeus m.

left
ilio-coccygeus m.

Ov

C

Fig. 2 The pelvic side wall. A: Bones and ligaments of the left pelvic side wall in a hemipelvis viewed from the right. **B:** With side wall muscles and major blood vessels superimposed. Note the position of the ovary (Ov) in the fossa delineated by the external and internal iliac vessels; the ureter lies close by. **C:** With the ilio-coccygeus and pubo-coccygeus portions of the levator ani muscles added.

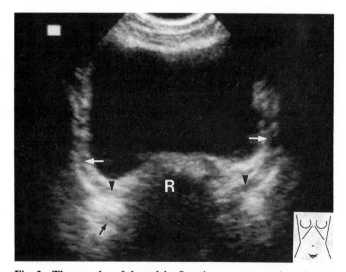

R

Fig. 3 The muscles of the pelvis. Seen in transverse section, the obturator internus muscles (white arrows) form echo-poor antero-posterior strips against the pelvic side walls. The ilio-coccygeus portions of the levator ani muscles (arrowheads) can often be discerned arising from their medial surfaces and passing posteriorly towards the midline. In this subject the right pyriformis muscle is also demonstrated (black arrow). R – rectum.

levator ani muscles, the urethra passing through a foramen between them. The ureters, having entered the pelvis by crossing medial to the common iliac artery and vein, curve inferiorly around the pelvic side wall and then pass medially to enter the bladder base. The undilated ureters are rarely visualised on ultrasound, but the position of the uretero-vesical junctions can be identified by the intermittent echoes from the jets of urine emptied into the bladder by ureteric peristalsis (Fig. 6). The uterus lies immediately posterior to the bladder, its anterior surface lying in contact with the bladder base and its posterior wall, while the rectum lies posteriorly. Gaps between the left and right levator ani muscles in the midline transmit the vagina and anus.

Uterus

The uterus, a pear-shaped muscular structure, is divided into the cervix inferiorly, and the body and domed fundus superiorly (Fig. 7). Since it is composed mainly of muscle, the uterus returns low level echoes, somewhat higher than those from the pelvic musculature (Fig. 8). The endometrium, with its complex tubular structure, on the

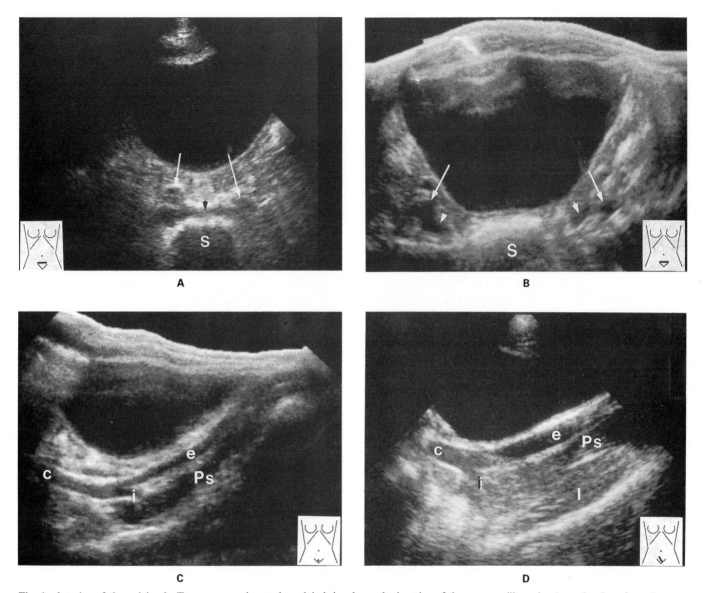

Fig. 4 Arteries of the pelvis. A: Transverse section at the pelvic brim shows the junction of the common iliac veins (arrowhead) to form the inferior vena cava. The common iliac arteries (arrows) lie antero-laterally. S – spine. **B:** Transverse section slightly further inferiorly shows the common iliac veins (arrowheads) and arteries (arrows). **C** and **D:** Oblique longitudinal sections in the iliac fossae along the line of the iliac artery show the division of the common (c) into internal (i) and external (e) arterial branches. The arteries lie on the psoas (Ps) and iliacus (I) muscles.

other hand, gives rise to higher amplitude echoes. Between the endometrium and the myometrium a fine echo-poor line is usually visible. It has been attributed to the more vascular, deepest layer of the myometrium; alternatively it may represent the outer layer of the endometrium, i.e. the non-deciduous portion.

The uterine cavity is usually empty and is seen only as a strong interface centrally positioned and straight or smoothly curved. A trace of endometrial fluid may be detected at the time of ovulation, perhaps representing secretions in response to hormone changes.[6] This fluid amounts to no more than a slight separation of the

endometrial layers and is transient, disappearing over the next 24 hours. During menstruation the shed endometrium may be visualised in the cavity as a fluid space a millimetre or so in thickness; there may also be menstrual fluid within the vagina, though this is often obscured by the intense echoes from a tampon. The menstrual fluid clears within a few days.

The uterus overall measures approximately 6 cm supero-inferiorly, by 4 cm antero-posteriorly and 5 cm transversely, but there are marked functional changes (Fig. 9). In the pre-pubertal child all dimensions are smaller while the cervix is disproportionately larger, occupying up to one

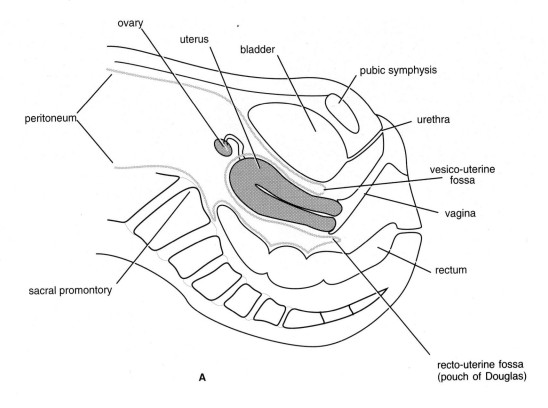

A

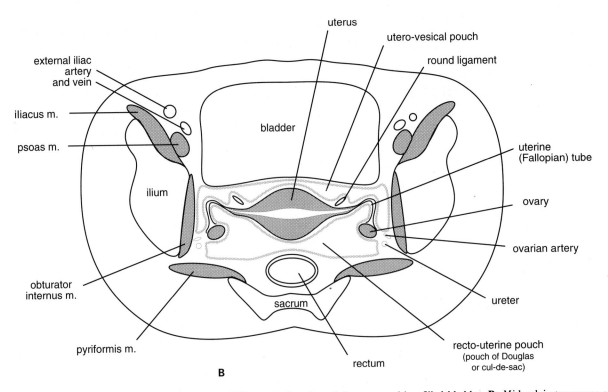

B

Fig. 5 Viscera of the pelvis – sectional anatomy. **A:** Midline sagittal section of the uterus with a filled bladder. **B:** Mid-pelvic transverse section. The peritoneum is indicated as a grey line.

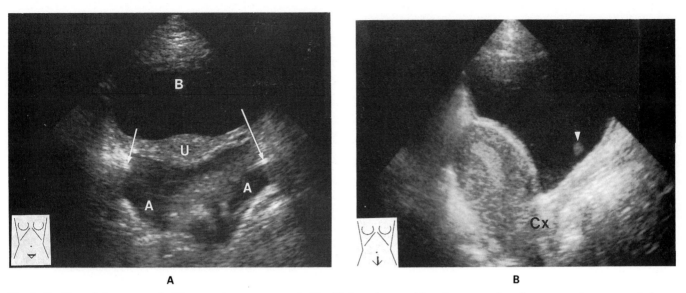

Fig. 6 Position of the ureters. A: The normal ureters are rarely identified on ultrasound but the strong echoes from a ureteric stent are obvious (arrows). This patient also had ascites (A). U – uterus, B – bladder. **B:** The jet in the bladder (arrowhead) indicates the position of the uretero-vesical junction; note that it lies close to the cervix (Cx), a fact that accounts for the high risk of ureteric obstruction in cervical carcinoma.

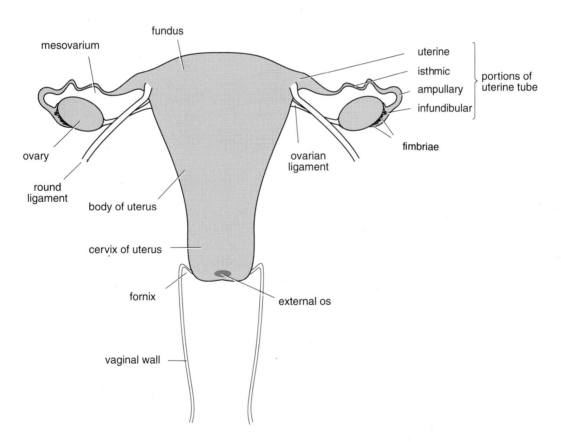

Fig. 7 The uterus and adnexae. The uterus and adnexae are illustrated viewed from in front with the uterus flattened, as by a full bladder for a transabdominal scan.

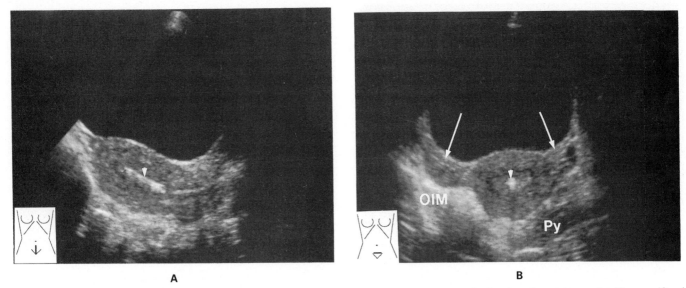

Fig. 8 The uterus. A: Longitudinal and **B:** transverse sections. The myometrium is a little more reflective than the pelvic muscles (Py – pyriformis muscle, OIM – obturator internus muscle) and about the same as the ovaries (arrows). The endometrial echo intensity depends on the stage of the menstrual cycle – in this subject, scanned towards the end of the follicular phase, the endometrium is thick and reflective. Note the very intense echoes from the intra-uterine contraceptive device (arrowhead).

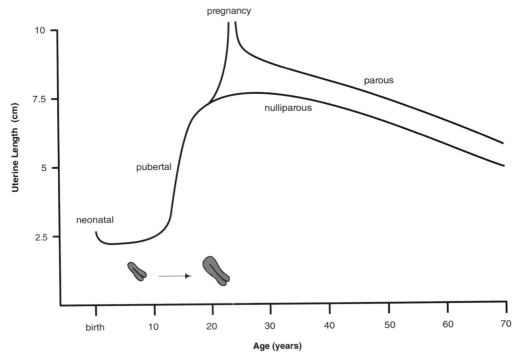

Fig. 9 Age changes in the uterus. The length of the uterus is plotted in relation to the changes with age and functional status. Note the relatively large cervix before puberty and the permanent increase in length following a pregnancy.

half the size of the uterus. (An exception is the neonate: the uterus may be large and have an active endometrium in response to the high maternal hormone levels of pregnancy.) At puberty the body and fundus enlarge more than the cervix to reach the adult proportions in which the cer-

vix occupies about one third of the uterus. The uterus never completely regresses from the dramatic changes in pregnancy, so that the parous uterus measures up to 7 cm in length. After the menopause it gradually atrophies while retaining the adult proportions.

The degree of bladder filling alters the lie of the uterus; when empty, as might be usual for trans-vaginal scanning, the uterus is angled forwards from the lie of the vagina, while with the bladder full, the uterus is straightened out. The body and fundus of the uterus very often lie to one side of the midline, sometimes markedly so, though the cervix always remains a midline structure.

Extending laterally from the cornua of the fundus of the uterus are the paired uterine ('fallopian') tubes; these fine tortuous structures with a lumen of about a millimetre in diameter are too small to be visualised reliably on trans-abdominal ultrasound, though they may be demonstrated with the superior resolution of trans-vaginal scanning. The lateral, fimbriated, end of each tube opens directly into the peritoneum in the immediate vicinity of its respective ovary, to which it is attached by one of the fimbria.

Ovaries

The ovaries are typically described as oval structures measuring some 4 × 2 × 1 cm (Fig. 8). In practice their shape varies widely from spherical to linear, in addition to the striking functional alterations associated with ovulation.[7] Because of this variation ovarian size is better evaluated as a volume, closely approximated in millilitres by taking one half of the product of the three diameters in centimetres.* For this measurement any cysts larger than 1 cm in diameter are excluded. The normal volume ranges up to 12 ml at or soon after puberty and then progressively decreases to about 2.5 ml at the menopause and 0.5 ml by 10 years post-menopause. The previously quoted upper limits of 6 ml have been found to be too conservative. The two ovaries should be approximately equal in volume, neither should be more than twice the volume of the other. Classically they lie against the pelvic side wall muscles in

---

* The volume of a sphere =

$$\frac{4}{3}\pi r^3 = \frac{4}{3}\pi\left(\frac{D}{2}\right)^3$$

For an ovoid, the product of the three radii is used, so the volume =

$$\frac{4}{3}\pi\left(\frac{D_1 \times D_2 \times D_3}{2 \times 2 \times 2}\right)$$

Within the accuracies possible with ultrasound, π may be taken as = 3; thus, cancelling, the volume becomes

$$\frac{D_1 \times D_2 \times D_3}{2}$$

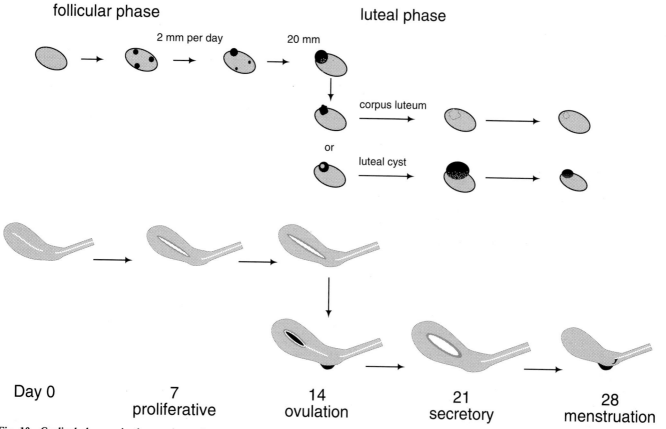

Fig. 10 Cyclical changes in the ovaries and uterus.

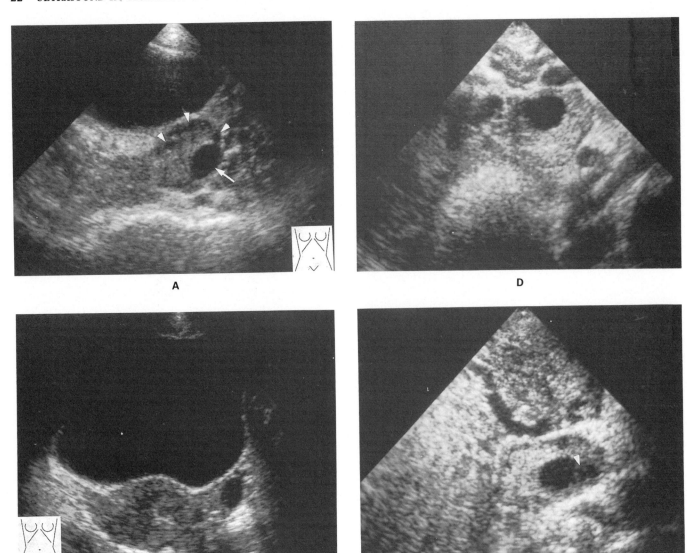

Fig. 11   Development of the ovarian follicle. A: Several small follicles (arrowheads) are seen alongside the dominant follicle (arrow) in the early stages of development. **B:** The dominant follicle has suppressed the others and **C:** continues to enlarge. **D:** The detailed features are better shown on a trans-vaginal scan. **E:** A mature follicle containing low level echoes (arrowhead) probably from the cumulus ovarii.

close proximity to the iliac vessels but their mobility leads to great variation in their positions. In longitudinal sections they indent the posterior surface of the bladder when this is well-filled.

The ovaries are uniform in texture at the beginning of the cycle (Fig. 8) but soon thereafter the developing follicles can be observed within them (Figs 10 and 11); initially there are several but, by about the end of the first week, one follicle dominates and enlarges progressively at approximately 1 mm per day to reach a mean diameter of

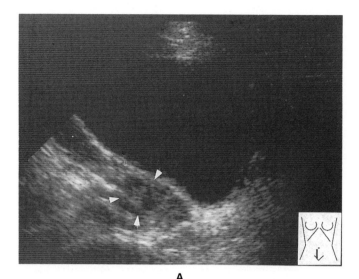

A

B

Fig. 12 Corpus luteum. A: Solid corpus luteum (arrowheads), with very similar echoes to the surrounding ovary. **B:** Part cystic corpus luteum (arrowhead). The ultrasound pattern is the same as a small complex cyst; the timing in the menstrual cycle will usually indicate its true nature but if there is doubt, a re-scan at another phase in the cycle will show that the 'cyst' has disappeared.

some 20 to 25 mm by mid-cycle. The follicles are echo-free apart from a few low level echoes representing the cumulus ovarii that are sometimes visualised with trans-vaginal probes shortly before ovulation. After ovulation a small amount of free fluid may be detectable in the pouch of Douglas.

The corpus luteum that develops from the follicle forms a mass of about a centimetre in diameter; usually its reflectivity is very similar to that of the normal ovary so that it may be inapparent (Fig. 12). However, when it forms as a cyst, it may be much larger and very obvious. Its irregular walls and its low level internal echoes (possibly due to

haemorrhage) may be a cause for concern and in addition, at this stage of the cycle, the Doppler signal from the ovary changes to a low impedance pattern with continuous diastolic flow. However, unless a pregnancy occurs, the corpus luteum involutes toward the end of the cycle so that, where there is real diagnostic difficulty, a repeat scan after 2 weeks will usually resolve any problem.

The scarred corpora lutea form corpora albicans which are usually not apparent on ultrasound, though on high resolution trans-vaginal studies they probably account for the small reflective foci commonly observed within the ovary. If a pregnancy ensues, the corpus luteum hypertrophies, producing sufficient progesterone to maintain the early pregnancy before atrophy by 15 weeks when the placenta takes over progesterone secretion.

The menopause occurs when the supply of ova is exhausted and the pituitary FSH can no longer stimulate an ovarian cycle. The ovaries subsequently atrophy so that the post-menopausal ovary usually measures 2.0 to 2.5 ml (upper limit 4 ml) in volume; their symmetry should be maintained.

Endometrium

The appearance of the endometrium also varies through the menstrual cycle,[8] acting as an indicator of the oestrogenic and progestogenic stimulation (Fig. 13). After menstruation, when the majority of the endometrium (the decidual inner layer) has been shed, no endometrial layer is visualised, only a fine cavitary line being demonstrable. As the endometrium thickens in the proliferative phase of the cycle, the endometrium becomes more prominent, though it remains relatively echo-poor. Through the second, secretory, phase the endometrium continues to thicken but also becomes more reflective; presumably the strong echoes are caused by the multiple tissue/fluid interfaces as the glands become tortuous and fill with mucin. At the end of the cycle the endometrium, measured as the double thickness of the echogenic layers, reaches up to 10 mm.[9] The endometrium may have a lower attenuation (probably because of its high fluid content) apparent on transverse sections as a band of enhancement on the deeper myometrium – it is not known why this is not as obvious on longitudinal sections. The margin between the endometrium and the myometrium may cast an edge shadow, again more obvious on transverse sections.

Following menopause, the endometrium is inactive, though it may remain as a thin layer (<5 mm) for a year or so after menstruation ceases. An inactive endometrium is also characteristic of any condition in which ovulation is suppressed, such as when the contraceptive pill is used and, contrariwise, the post-menopausal endometrium may be prominent in women using hormone replacement therapy.

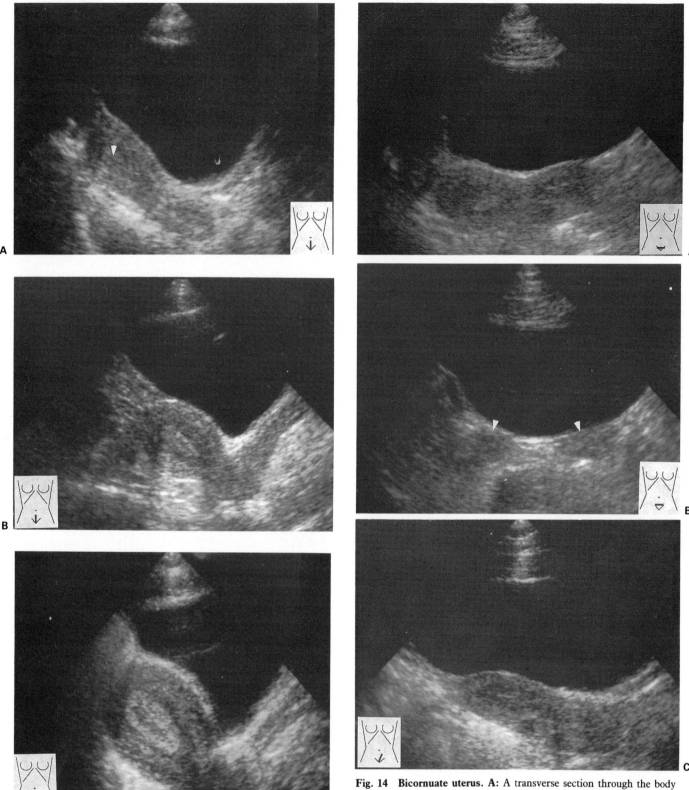

Fig. 13 Endometrial cyclical changes. A: After menstruation the endometrium is thin and seen only as a fine line (arrowhead). **B** and **C:** Hypertrophy through the proliferative and secretory phases of the cycle result in an increase in both thickness and reflectivity to a maximum double thickness of some 20 mm.

Fig. 14 Bicornuate uterus. A: A transverse section through the body of the uterus shows a dumb-bell configuration while **B:** a section further superiorly shows the two separate cornua (arrowheads). **C:** In longitudinal section a bicornuate uterus may be surprisingly difficult to detect, though the disproportion between the sizes of the cervix and fundus may suggest the anomaly. In this patient the left kidney was absent with compensatory hypertrophy on the right: anomalies of the renal tract are commonly associated with fusion failures of the uterus.

Anomalies

Apart from their variable positions the ovaries are not subject to anomalies. However, the uterus frequently reveals evidence of its complex embryology from fusion of the paired Müllerian ducts. Complete failure of fusion results in duplication of the uterus, cervix and occasionally even also of the vagina. This extreme form, the 'didelphic uterus', is rare but minor fusion failures are common, for example where the upper part of the fundus of the uterus has a notch or where a muscular septum extends inferiorly from the fundus, partially dividing the cavity. On ultrasound these may be evidenced by a widening in the transverse plane of the uterus and in particular of the endometrial line and, in the more marked variants, in the appearance of two endometrium lined cavities lying side by

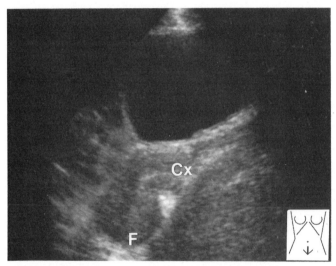

Fig. 15 Retropositioned uterus. The uterine fundus lies further posteriorly than normal and thus may be difficult to evaluate on transabdominal ultrasound. In this case the retropositioning can be seen to be the result of a sharp angulation at the body-cervix junction, a variant known as retroflexion. Cx – cervix, F – fundus.

side at the upper part of the uterus (Fig. 14). Full evaluation of these anomalies requires a salpingogram.

Minor variations in uterine position are so common as to be within the range of normal. For example, the fundus of the uterus may be tipped posteriorly, either by flexion at the lower segment of the uterus or by rotation around the vaginal vault (retroversion) (Fig. 15). Both produce confusing appearances, particularly on transabdominal scanning, where the deeper portions of the fundus are difficult to delineate and may appear to be abnormal because of shadowing from the intervening body and cervix. They are less confusing on trans-vaginal scanning. It is not usually possible with ultrasound to distinguish between retroversion and retroflexion so the general term 'retropositioned' is often used.

On trans-vaginal scans all these features are more easily observed because of the higher resolution obtained. However, the most immediately obvious difference from transabdominal scans is the position of the uterus: since trans-vaginal scanning is performed with the bladder empty (in order to keep the pelvic viscera as close as possible to the probe) the uterus is usually anteflexed so that the fundus comes to lie anterior to the cervix. When imaged from below, the cervix is encountered first, either in longitudinal or transverse section, depending on probe orientation. As the transducer is advanced into the posterior fornix of the vagina, the body and fundus of the uterus come into view. Commonly the entire length of the uterus can be imaged in one plane though, when it is sharply angled, the tomogram may pass through the upper part of the uterus alone or vice versa. Initially these relationships are confusing; together with the greater detail obtainable, the user may be disorientated but the true anatomical content is similar but superior to that on transabdominal scanning. A further confusing feature is the prominence of the pelvic veins which are compressed by the full bladder in transabdominal scans; they are seen as tortuous channels around the uterus and adnexae in which flowing 'particles' may be visualised, though often the flow velocity is too low for Doppler detection.

REFERENCES

1 Netter F H. The Ciba collection of medical illustrations. Volume 2: reproductive system, 1954. Volume 6: kidneys, ureters and urinary bladder, 1973. Ciba-Geigy, Summit, New Jersey
2 Schneck C D, Friedman A C, Peterson R O. Embryology, anatomy and histology. In: Friedman A C, Radecki P D, Lev-Toaff A S, Hilpert P L. eds. Clinical pelvic imaging. St Louis: Mosby. 1990: p 1–27
3 Schneck C D. The anatomical basis of abdomino-pelvic sectional imaging. Clin Diag Ultrasound 1983; 11: 13–41
4 Sanders R C, James A E. eds. The principles and practice of ultrasonography in obstetrics and gynaecology. (3rd Edition). Norwalk, Connecticut: Appleton-Century Crofts. 1990
5 Athey P A, Hadlock F P. Ultrasound in obstetrics and gynaecology

(2nd Edition) St Louis: Mosby. 1985
6 Hansmann M, Hackeloer B-J, Staudach A. Ultrasound diagnosis in obstetrics and gynaecology. Berlin: Springer Verlag. 1985
7 Fleischer A C, Wentz A C, Jones H W. Ultrasound evaluation of the ovary. In: Callen P W. ed. Ultrasonography in obstetrics and gynaecology. (2nd Edition) Philadelphia: WB Saunders. 1988
8 Forrest T S, Elyaderans M K, Muilenberg R I. Cyclical endometrial changes: US assessment with histological correlation. Radiology 1988; 167: 233–237
9 Malpani A, Singer J, Wolverson M K, Merenda G. Endometrial hyperplasia: value of endometrial thickness in ultrasonographic diagnosis and clinical significance. JCU 1990; 18: 173–177

Uterine pathology

Heather S. Andrews

Ultrasound is the imaging method of choice for the uterus and the more recent introduction of intracavity transducers has further refined the technique. CT and MRI are generally complementary techniques though, in certain situations, notably the staging of uterine malignancy, they are superior.

Trans-vaginal ultrasound scanning resolves many of the diagnostic problems encountered with transabdominal ultrasound as better visualisation of the pelvic structures is afforded by the close proximity of a high resolution transducer. Thus visualisation of the endometrium is improved and the retroverted uterus better assessed. The differentiation between uterine and adnexal masses is made easier and, where the uterine outline is blurred by the presence of pelvic inflammatory disease, better delineation is achieved.

Before beginning the examination knowledge of the patient's age, parity, menstrual history and presenting symptoms and signs is essential, thus allowing the examination to be tailored to that patient's needs. The commonest clinical presentation of gynaecological disease is abnormal menstrual bleeding whether pre- or post-menopausally.

Abnormal bleeding

The causes are very variable and are often age related. Apparent uterine bleeding may be caused by disease in other organs.

Uterus	– fibroids
	– endometrial hyperplasia
	– endometrial polyp
	– adenomyosis
	– endometrial carcinoma
	– oestrogen producing tumours of the ovary
	– chronic endometritis
	– salpingitis
	– pregnancy related problems
	– atrophic post-menopausal endometritis
Cervix	– chronic cervicitis
	– carcinoma
	– polyp
Vagina	– carcinoma
	– trauma
	– infection
	– foreign body
	– atrophic vaginitis
Other	– fallopian tubes
	– urinary tract
	– external genitalia
	– endocrinopathies
	– blood dyscrasias

Hormonal influences on the endometrium

The endometrium is a specialised form of mucous membrane, the appearance of which reliably reflects the hormonal status of the patient. During the menstrual years the endometrium is relatively thick, up to 14 mm, but is very thin prior to the menarche and post-menopausally. This hormonal stimulation is provided by naturally secreted oestrogen and progesterone, although exogenously administered hormones produce a similar effect. Oestrogen is responsible for the early proliferative phase of the menstrual cycle and progesterone for involution in the secretory phase. An imbalance between these hormones may alter the normal appearances. An inappropriate endometrial pattern not characteristic of either the proliferative or secretory phase of the cycle suggests ovarian dysfunction or hormonal imbalance. During the later menstrual years the uterus enlarges slightly, almost certainly due to the effect of oestrogen unopposed by progesterone and associated with anovulatory cycles. This slight increase in size should not be considered pathological.

Abnormal thickening of the endometrium

Dysfunctional uterine bleeding Endometrial thickening is often demonstrated in patients presenting with dysfunctional uterine bleeding although in many such patients the appearance of the uterus and endometrium is quite unremarkable. In 30% to 40% of women with dysfunctional uterine bleeding a histological diagnosis of endometrial hyperplasia is made. On ultrasound this is shown as endometrial thickening. Other patients may show evidence of adenomyosis and indeed the two conditions may be associated. In patients with dysfunctional uterine bleeding assessment of endometrial thickness may dictate the appropriate therapy: progesterone for those with thickened endometrium and combined oestrogen and progesterone for those with thinning of the endometrium.[1]

Hormone replacement therapy Hormone replacement therapy (HRT) is commonly used in post-menopausal women with a combination oestrogen and progestagen pill being administered cyclically. This produces cyclical changes in the endometrium which causes thickening and increased reflectivity of the endometrium (Fig. 1A). This change is of a secretory phase type and the thickness may exceed 10 mm. Occasionally fluid is seen in the endometrial cavity. When oestrogen alone is used there is a small but definite risk of endometrial carcinoma developing, but the addition of the progesterone greatly reduces this risk.[2]

Tamoxifen® This is an anti-oestrogenic drug which has been used in the treatment of breast carcinoma for many years. Long-term therapy leads to endometrial hyperplasia[3] (Fig. 1B) and polyp formation, and an

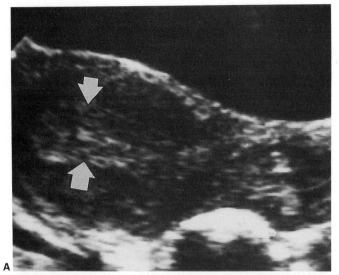

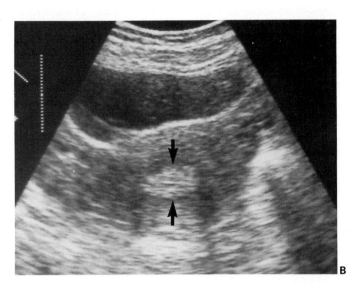

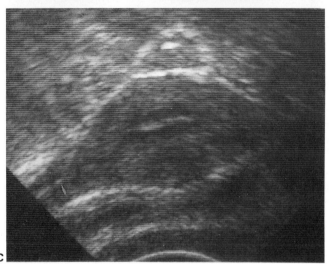

Fig. 1 **Endometrial hyperplasia. A:** Post-menopausal uterus in a woman on HRT. Thick reflective endometrium (arrows) (9 mm AP thickness). **B:** Post-menopausal woman with breast carcinoma receiving treatment with Tamoxifen®. Endometrial thickening (arrows) due to endometrial hyperplasia (15 mm AP thickness). **C:** Thin endometrium in normal post-menopausal woman for comparison (trans-vaginal scan).

association with endometrial carcinoma has been reported.[4] However, since there is a well-recognised association between endometrial and breast carcinoma, it is a matter of some conjecture as to whether the Tamoxifen® therapy itself is a cause of endometrial carcinoma. Tamoxifen® therapy is also associated with the development of reversible ovarian cysts in the premenopausal woman.

Thinning of the endometrium

Endometrial thinning is considered normal in the post-menopausal woman. This appearance has been described as 'single line' endometrium and is commonly seen when oestrogen levels are low, whatever the cause.

- Aetiology of 'single line endometrium'
  - post-menopause
  - perimenopause
  - oral contraceptive pill
  - oligomenorrhoea or amenorrhoea.

The persistent 'single line' appearance of the endo-metrium is very similar to that of the endometrium in the late menstrual phase of the cycle in normal women.

Oral contraceptive pill

This is generally a combined oestrogen and progesterone pill taken cyclically. The characteristic unstimulated endo-metrium appears as a 'single line' which is slightly thicker than that seen in post-menopausal women.[5] There may also be a slight overall increase in uterine size. Ovarian follicular development and ovulation may occur.

Post-menopausal uterus

The endometrium is thin and histologically atrophic with a normal total thickness of less than 6 mm (Fig. 1C). Significant thickening (greater than 10 mm total thick-ness) must be monitored and investigated, unless the patient is receiving HRT when cyclical changes may occur. In the perimenopausal woman a total endometrial thick-ness of 12 mm or more warrants investigation to exclude carcinoma.

Post-menopausal bleeding is defined as bleeding from the genital tract at least 1 year after the last menstrual period. The commonest causes are atrophic endometritis, endometrial hypoplasia, senile vaginitis and endometrial and cervical carcinomata. Trans-vaginal ultrasound can

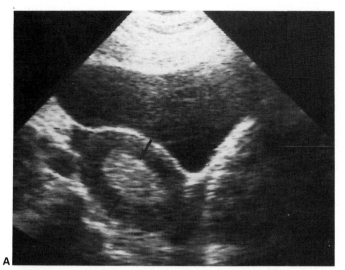

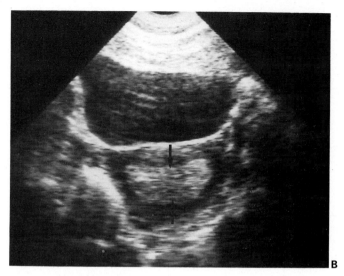

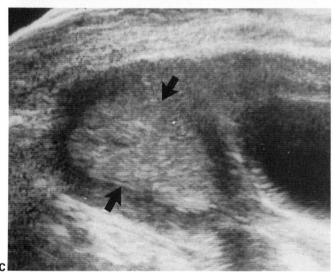

Fig. 2 Endometrial hyperplasia. A: Longitudinal and **B:** transverse scan showing marked symmetrical cystic endometrial hyperplasia (arrows). **C:** Longitudinal scan of severe cystic endometrial hyperplasia (arrows), enlarging the uterus to the size of a 12 week pregnancy.

provide a reliable assessment of endometrial thickening and cavity fluid and this allows selection of those patients requiring further investigation.[6]

Cystic endometrial hyperplasia

This common condition presents with abnormal uterine bleeding, generally in women in their late reproductive years, but it may present post-menopausally and may coexist with endometrial carcinoma. Endometrial hyperplasia results from excessive oestrogen stimulation unopposed by progesterone. It is invariably associated with anovulatory cycles in which the ovarian follicles fail to rupture and thus continue to produce oestrogen. Alternating periods of amenorrhoea and continuous uterine bleeding may occur. It is a common condition and is often discovered at diagnostic curettage where it has been noted to affect up to 10% of all patients. Pathologically, two types of endometrial hyperplasia may be identified, benign

and that with malignant potential. In the latter group it may be very difficult to separate markedly atypical hyperplasia from a well-differentiated endometrial carcinoma.[7]

Ultrasound appearances The central endometrial echo complex is thickened, measuring greater than 1 cm.[8] It is highly reflective and does not substantially change in appearance through the menstrual cycle (Figs 2A and B). In severe cases the endometrium may measure up to 5 cm in thickness and cause moderate generalised uterine enlargement (Fig. 2C). Associated functional ovarian cysts are common and are often multiple. Most importantly the differential diagnosis includes endometrial carcinoma. Endometrial polyps and hydatidiform mole are other diagnostic possibilities. It will not always be possible to differentiate between these conditions but it should be noted that trans-vaginal ultrasound scanning is considerably more helpful than transabdominal scanning in their differentiation.

Causes of increased uterine reflectivity

Endometrium
 – secretory phase of normal menstrual cycle
 – HRT in the post-menopausal patient
 – endometrial carcinoma
 – endometrial polyp
 – endometrial hyperplasia

Endometrial cavity contents
 – haematometra/pyometra
 – retained products of conception
 – trophoblastic disease

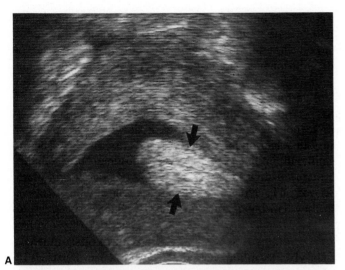

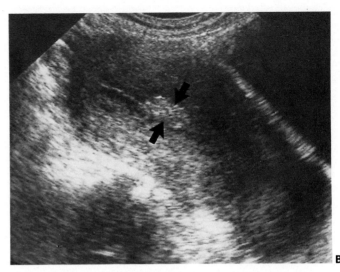

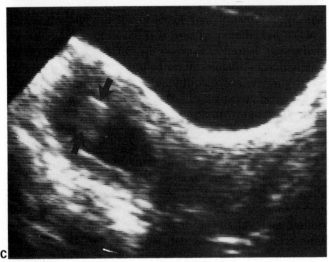

Fig. 3 Endometrial polyp. A: Highly reflective endometrial polyp (arrows) within fluid distended uterine cavity (trans-vaginal scan). **B:** Longitudinal scan shows moderately reflective 20 mm polyp (arrows) in uterine cavity. **C:** Longitudinal scan of relatively echo-poor 15 mm polyp (arrows) in fluid filled uterine cavity.

within the endometrial cavity (Fig. 3A). The reflectivity is variable but they are generally echo- poor (Fig. 3B). Polyps may be particularly well-demonstrated when surrounded by cavity fluid (Fig. 3C). The polyp may secrete serous fluid or may bleed. On occasion it may be possible to demonstrate mobility of the polyp. If the polyp is very large there may be generalised uterine enlargement. The differential diagnosis includes a pedunculated submucosal fibroid, polypoid endometrial carcinoma or other uterine tumour and retained products of conception.

Carcinoma of the endometrium

Endometrial carcinoma is the fourth commonest female malignancy. Due to the efficacy of the cervical carcinoma screening programme it has become the commonest gynaecological tumour with 4000 new cases per year in the UK. Most patients are post-menopausal with a peak age incidence of 55 to 65 years. The majority present with post-menopausal bleeding or with other menstrual irregularities. Histologically 90% to 95% are adenocarcinomata with very few squamous cell or stromal tumours.

Exfoliative cytology only identifies 67% of cases and thus a definitive diagnosis is made by endometrial biopsy obtained at dilatation and curettage or hysteroscopy. However, as only 10% of the women presenting with post-menopausal bleeding actually have a diagnosis of endometrial carcinoma other methods of diagnosis are being sought in order to reduce the number of unnecessary

Endometrial polyps

Polyps are focal areas of adenomatous or hyperplastic endometrial tissue which range in size from 0.5 to 5.0 cm in diameter but are rarely larger than 1 cm.[7] They may be single or multiple and may lie anywhere in the uterine cavity. Although generally sessile they may be pedunculated and may extrude into the cervical canal or upper vagina. Polyps generally develop in the peri- or post-menopausal patient and are usually asymptomatic although when large may occasionally present with abnormal uterine bleeding. The true incidence is unknown as the polyps are often unrecognised at curettage. Uterine polyps are usually benign, particularly in pre-menopausal women. In 10% to 15% of patients with endometrial malignancy endometrial polyps are associated but only 1% undergo malignant change.[9]

Ultrasound appearances As may be expected polyps are better visualised on trans- vaginal scanning and are demonstrated as small, generally well-defined masses

anaesthetics. Ultrasonic endometrial assessment is proving useful in this clinical context.

Aetiology Very many predisposing factors have been identified but a common link is the effect of unopposed oestrogen stimulation on the endometrium.

- family history
- late menarche/early menopause
- nulliparity/low parity
- obesity
- anovulatory conditions, e.g. polycystic ovary syndrome whereby reduced progesterone levels resulting from the lack of a corpus luteum allow relatively high oestrogen levels
- exogenous oestrogen therapy
  - oral contraceptive pill
  - hormone replacement therapy (HRT)
- Tamoxifen® therapy for breast carcinoma
- feminising tumours, e.g. granulosa-theca cell tumour of the ovary
- endometrial hyperplasia and endometrial polyps may be present in association with endometrial carcinoma but may not necessarily be tumour precursors.

As described above, carcinoma of the endometrium has been shown to develop in patients with high oestrogen levels but this would appear to contradict the higher incidence in post-menopausal patients who would be expected to have relatively low oestrogen levels. The explanation seems to relate to the even lower levels of progesterone produced post-menopausally which allows relative unopposed oestrogenic activity.[10]

Ultrasound appearances The diagnosis is essentially clinical (Table 1). The ultrasound appearances are variable, depending on the stage at presentation. Generally there is no uterine enlargement at the time of diagnosis but changes in the endometrium and inner myometrium may be apparent. Endometrial thickening is always pathological but no morphological features specific to malignancy have been identified.[11] Initially the endometrium thickens and there is irregularity of the cavity interface (Fig. 4). Small

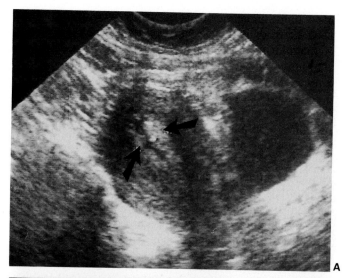
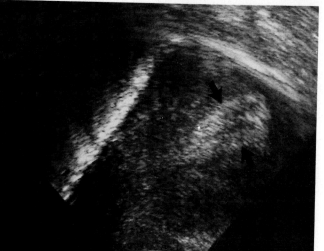

Fig. 4 Endometrial carcinoma. A: Transabdominal and **B:** trans-vaginal scans show thickened irregular reflective endometrium (arrows) with cavity fluid.

Table 1 FIGO staging of endometrial carcinoma

Stage		
	I	– Carcinoma confined to the corpus
	IA	– The length of the uterine cavity is 8 cm or less
	IB	– The length of the uterine cavity is greater than 8 cm
Stage	II	– Carcinoma has involved corpus and cervix but has not extended outside the uterus
Stage	III	– Carcinoma has extended outside the uterus but not outside the true pelvis
Stage	IV	– Carcinoma has extended outside the true pelvis or has obviously involved the mucosa of the bladder or rectum
	IVA	– Carcinoma has spread to adjacent organs
	IVB	– Carcinoma has spread to distant organs

cystic areas may be identified within the endometrium. Asymptomatic endometrial carcinoma can be detected on ultrasound.[11]

The endometrial reflectivity is variable, less differentiated tumours tending to be relatively echo-poor and, conversely, more differentiated tumours tending to be highly reflective.[12] There may be fluid in the endometrial cavity, either blood or mucin, produced by the hyperplastic glandular elements of the endometrium. Large exophytic or polypoid tumours may be apparent within the cavity (Fig. 5). Invasion of the myometrium by the tumour leads to disruption of the subendometrial/myometrial interface. It may be difficult to distinguish between exophytic tumours associated with myometrial thinning and a truly invasive tumour. Trans-vaginal ultrasound is superior to the abdominal approach for the assessment of both the endometrium and the degree of myometrial invasion. In

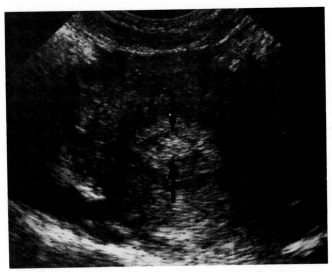

Fig. 5 Endometrial carcinoma. Polypoid mass (straight arrows) and generalised endometrial thickening (angled arrows) (trans-vaginal scan).

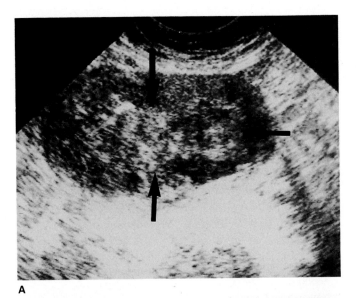

A

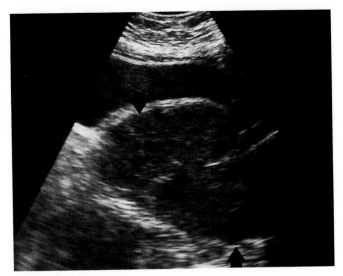

Fig. 6 Endometrial carcinoma. A large ill-defined lobulated mass (arrows) involving the whole uterine body due to endometrial carcinoma.

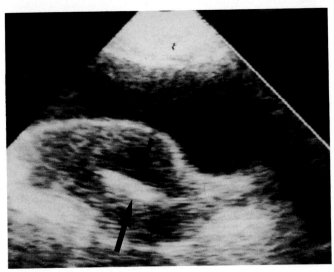

B

Fig. 7 Pyometra. A: Transverse scan shows generalised uterine enlargement with distension of the uterine cavity. Cavity contents exhibit mixed reflectivity due to coexistent tumour and pyometra (arrows). **B:** Longitudinal scan of pyometra with intracavity gas (arrows).

more advanced disease the appearances are variable. The uterus enlarges sometimes with an irregular or lobulated outline and may appear fixed (Fig. 6). There may be marked distension of the endometrial cavity with a haemato- or pyometra due to cervical stenosis (Fig. 7). In advanced tumours the uterine mass may be very large indeed with a generally heterogeneous echo texture (Fig. 8). Local invasion of the para-uterine structures, bladder and rectum may be apparent. Distant spread may be manifest by regional lymphadenopathy, ascites and liver metastases.

A reduction in the number of unfruitful investigations involving general anaesthesia performed in patients with post-menopausal bleeding is desirable. A number of studies have recently been undertaken to determine whether ultrasound assessment of the endometrium alone is sufficiently accurate to determine whether the patient requires further investigation. In one study 283 normal post-menopausal women and 103 women presenting with post-menopausal bleeding were scanned trans-vaginally. All women with single layer endometrial thickness greater than 4 mm underwent endometrial curettage and biopsy. 12.6% of the women with post-menopausal bleeding and 3.5% of the asymptomatic women had histologically proven endometrial carcinoma.[11]

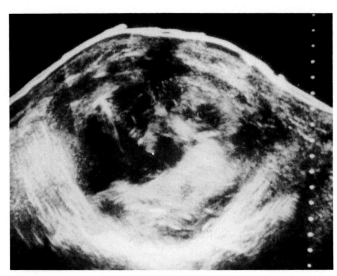

Fig. 8 Endometrial carcinoma. Huge mass of mixed reflectivity causing abdominal distension.

In another study ultrasonic measurements of endometrial thickness in prehysterectomy patients were found to be within 1 mm of the actual endometrial thickness in the pathological specimens, confirming the accuracy of the technique.[12] An ultrasound measured endometrial thickness of 4 mm is a suitable threshold for screening post-menopausal women with or without atypical bleeding for endometrial carcinoma.[11] It should be noted that other studies quote an upper limit of normal as 8 to 10 mm, but the figure refers to the combined thickness of both endometrial layers, not including the cavity or any fluid contained therein. In practice it is generally simpler to measure the total double layer endometrial thickness.

In another study, using 10 mm as the upper limit of normal for total endometrial thickness, 99% of endometrial carcinomas were detected, but there was a false positive rate of 41%.[13] Thus endometrial thickening has been shown to be a somewhat non-specific sign of endometrial malignancy. In an attempt to refine this diagnosis trans-vaginal colour flow Doppler scanning has been used to assess the uterine artery blood flow with some favourable initial results. In one study 108 patients were studied, of whom 54 were asymptomatic post-menopausal women, 20 had histologically proven normal endometrium prior to HRT therapy and 34 had presented with post-menopausal bleeding. In the latter group 17 were subsequently proven to have endometrial carcinoma. The pulsatility indices (PI) of the uterine arteries were assessed. The values in asymptomatic women and those with non-malignant post-menopausal bleeding were similar. The PI values in the group with endometrial carcinoma were consistently lower. There may also be value in measuring the PI within the tumour itself (see Ch. 5).[13] This work is in the early stages but shows potential for further reducing the number of patients undergoing endometrial biopsy in the search for endometrial carcinoma.

The prognosis depends on the patients' age, tumour stage, tumour location, uterine size, depth of myometrial penetration and lymph node involvement. Staging is problematic. Over the last 20 years the cure rate has not improved and thus methods have been sought for more accurately assessing the depth of myometrial invasion and adnexal spread, in order to plan treatment more accurately. Trans-vaginal sonography, CT and MRI are complementary techniques but all with relative weaknesses. With MRI carcinoma limited to the endometrium cannot be differentiated from endometrial hyperplasia and cavity blood. However, it provides an overall accuracy of 82% in assessing depth of myometrial invasion and 92% overall accuracy in staging.[14] CT is useful in determining lymphatic spread but it cannot differentiate endometrial tumour from either cervical or para-uterine tumour; neither can it reliably demonstrate myometrial or vaginal invasion. Trans-vaginal ultrasound has been shown to be moderately accurate in staging myometrial penetration. In 14 out of 20 patients (70%) with histologically proven endometrial carcinoma the ultrasound estimation of the depth of myometrial invasion was within 10% of the actual measurement on the pathological specimen. However, with an exophytic or polypoid tumour lying within the endometrial cavity the depth of invasion might be overestimated. Demonstration of the sub-endometrial echo-poor halo usually indicated superficial invasion, whereas absence of the halo was frequently associated with deep invasion.[15] Intra-luminal uterine scanning may also be of value in demonstrating integrity of the subendometrial halo, but has the disadvantage of requiring general anaesthesia. Where less than one third of the myometrial depth has been invaded by tumour lymph node metastases are rare. This information may allow a definite treatment plan to be made pre-operatively, although some centres rely on clinical assessment at surgery.

MRI and CT are best at showing lymph node involvement and distant spread; with trans-vaginal ultrasound and MRI being used to assess myometrial invasion. As with cervical carcinoma, early disease is treated with radical surgery and later disease with radiation therapy. Whether a screening programme for the early diagnosis of endometrial carcinoma with trans-vaginal ultrasound and/or colour Doppler will be of value has not as yet been fully established.

Haematometra and similar conditions

Obstruction of the female genital tract may occur at differing levels – usually distally at the introitus, but also at various levels in the vagina, or more proximally at the level of the cervix. In the child or adolescent, obstruction results from an intact hymen or vaginal obstruction which may be due to atresia, stenosis or the presence of an obstructing membrane (see *Abdominal and General Ultrasound*, Vol. 2, Ch. 56). In the adult, the obstruction is usually at the cervical level, whatever the cause. Obstruction leads to an accumulation of fluid which may be serous, due to mucus secretion by cervical or vaginal glands, menstrual blood or pus. The most usual content is blood. Fluid accumulation produces distension of the organs above the level of the obstruction. Coexistent urinary tract anomalies are common in these patients and must always be sought (Fig. 9A).[16] In the neonate and infant, the fluid in the distended uterus and vagina may be menstrual blood due to the effect of maternal hormones on the endometrium.

The terminology used for these conditions depends on the organ involved and the nature of the contents:

– vaginal distension – haematocolpos
– vaginal and uterine distension – haematometrocolpos
– uterine distension alone – haematometra

– distension of the fallopian tubes – haematosalpinx. Depending on the nature of the contained fluid, whether blood, serous fluid or pus, the appropriate prefix is applied, i.e. haemato-, hydro- or pyo-.

Some or all of the following symptoms and signs may be present – abdominal pain, pelvic mass, amenorrhoea and urinary obstruction. .

Ultrasound appearances A central cystic lower abdominal mass of varying shape, size and reflectivity is apparent. It is often impossible to determine the nature of the fluid but internal echoes indicate the presence of blood or pus. Multiple, almost confluent, fine low level echoes similar to those seen with an endometriotic cyst suggest the presence of altered blood. Occasionally this may be highly reflective and layering of the fluid may be seen. When no internal echoes are present and there is good transmission of sound, the fluid is likely to be serous (Fig. 9B). There may be associated ascites (Fig. 9B).

Vaginal distension

A large tubular cystic, fluid-filled structure lies low and centrally in the pelvis (Fig. 10A). A normal vagina cannot be separately identified. The uterus, whether distended or not, can be identified in continuity with the cephalad aspect of the mass (Fig. 10B). In patients with vaginal atresia, abdominal ultrasound allows the diagnosis of vaginal obstruction to be made, but does not determine the nature and precise level of the lesion. The level of the obstruction is usually at the junction of the middle and lower thirds of the vagina. In order to plan reconstructive

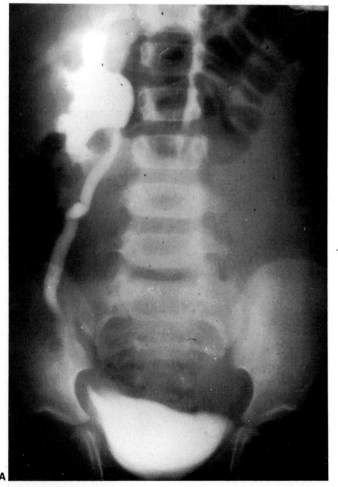

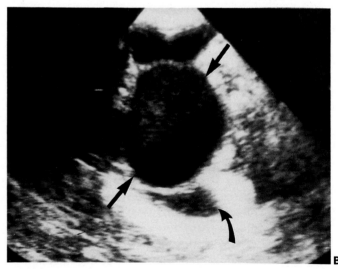

Fig. 9 Haematometra. A: Abdominal radiograph in a 1-year-old, showing an abdominal mass arising out of the pelvis causing right urinary obstruction. There is left renal agenesis. **B:** Transverse scan of the same child, showing uterine cavity distended with blood (straight arrows). The bladder lies anteriorly and ascitic fluid is seen posteriorly (curved arrow).

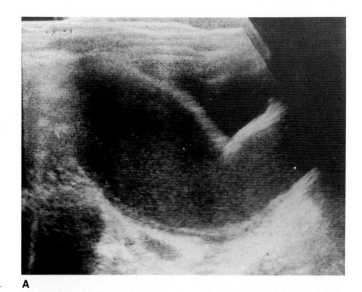

A

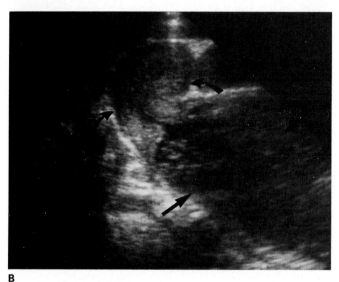

B

Fig. 10   Haematocolpos and haematometra. A: Longitudinal midline scan of blood filled vaginal and uterine distension (haematometrocolpos) in a 16-year-old girl, presenting with primary amenorrhoea. **B:** A normal uterus (curved arrows) is seen at the apex of the distended vagina (haematocolpos) (straight arrows).

surgery it is essential to know not only the level of the obstruction, but also its cause. Trans-perineal ultrasound, using a stand-off, produces very satisfactory images and can be used to evaluate the length of the stenotic segment (usually 1 to 4 cm), and demonstrates any solid tissue septum extending from the caudal aspect of the distended vagina to the perineum.[17]

Uterine distension

The normal uterus cannot be separately differentiated from the mass, and there may or may not be associated dis-

tension of the vagina and fallopian tubes. To distinguish between a haematocolpos and a haematometrocolpos the cervix should be identified. Due to its relatively fibrous nature, it is not very distensible and may appear as an 'hourglass' constriction between the dilated and distensible uterus above and the vagina below. The contents of the fluid-distended uterine cavity can be mistaken for retained products of conception.

Haematotrachelos

Haematotrachelos or distension of the cervix with blood is rare; it may be associated with congenital cervical atresia or may develop as a complication of cervical cone biopsy. The congenital type is usually associated with vaginal atresia, and the differential diagnosis is from a high vaginal septum. On ultrasound examination the normal cervix cannot be identified, and the relatively thick walled cervical canal is distended with blood.[18]

Aetiology of adult cervical obstruction:

- tumour   – cervical carcinoma
               – endometrial carcinoma
               – vaginal carcinoma
- radiation therapy (external or intracavity)
- trauma   – obstetric
               – post-instrumentation
               – cervical cone biopsy
               – senile atrophy.

Distension of the fallopian tubes

This is always associated with uterine distension and may be unilateral or bilateral, depending on the nature of the obstruction. Problems with the diagnosis may be encountered where only one moiety of a uterus didelphys is obstructed and the unobstructed moiety is assumed to be a normal uterus and the obstructed moiety mistaken for a cystic adnexal mass.

Endometritis

Endometritis is an infective process involving the endometrium, which is generally chronic but when acute it is commonly associated with an infection elsewhere. It may be regarded as a part of generalised pelvic inflammatory disease (PID), but may also be associated with IUCD's, uterine instrumentation or may develop after abortion or in the puerperium. When associated with PID endometritis develops as a result of an ascending venereal infection, passing from the vagina to the fallopian tubes and adnexae via the uterine cavity.[19] However, the cervical mucus often prevents ascent of the infection and limits it to the vagina. In general terms the endometrium is relatively resistant to infection due to the cyclical shedding of the endometrium and consequent drainage of infected material. Myometritis may be associated with endometritis and it may be impossible to distinguish between the two conditions. The common causal agents are the venereal organisms *Chlamydia trichomatis*, *Neisseria gonorrhoea* and *mycoplasmata* although less commonly *coliforms* and *Staphylococci* may be implicated.[20] As a result of the infection the endometrium becomes oedematous and hyperaemic, sometimes with secondary inflammation of the myometrium. The clinical presentation is very variable depending on the chronicity of the lesion. Abnormal bleeding is rare, but occasionally there may be hypomenorrhoea or amenorrhoea. A vaginal discharge may be associated

with lower abdominal pain and pyrexia. Diagnosis is made by endometrial biopsy and culture of the organisms.[21] In the long-term there may be infertility and, rarely, Asherman's syndrome may develop. The ultrasound is often normal, or may be non-specifically abnormal with an echo-poor and moderately enlarged uterus with an indistinct outline (Fig. 11). Loss of differentiation between the endometrium and myometrium is common and, when myometritis develops, the myometrium may also appear echo-poor. The endometrium thickens and later becomes highly reflective, with a small amount of reactive fluid in the endometrial cavity.[7] If the cavity fluid is purulent it may appear highly reflective or there may be multiple internal echoes. If anaerobic organisms are responsible for the infection, gas may form in the uterine cavity (Fig. 12A). There is rarely much distension of the uterine cavity as the fluid readily drains through the cervical canal (Fig. 12B). Fluid in the pouch of Douglas, tubo-ovarian abscesses and other signs of adnexal PID are commonly seen (see Ch. 4).

Uterine cavity fluid collections

The aetiology of uterine fluid collections depends on the patient's age:

Infancy and childhood (pre-menarche)
  – hydro/haematocolpos
  – hydro/haematometra
Menstrual years
  – normal or complicated pregnancy
  – menstruation
  – endometritis/PID
  – post-instrumentation
  – endometrial hyperplasia
  – endometrial polyp
  – uterine, cervical and fallopian tube tumours
Post-menopausal
  – endometrial carcinoma
  – cervical carcinoma
  – endometrial hyperplasia
  – endometrial polyp.

In one series 94% of post-menopausal women with uterine fluid collections had endometrial or cervical carcinomas.[22]

The uterine fibroid

The fibroid, leiomyoma or myoma is the commonest uterine tumour, affecting 40% of women older than 35 years.[23] Fibroids are common in black women in whom they tend to develop at a relatively early age.[24] It is a benign tumour, composed mainly of smooth muscle fibres very similar to normal myometrium, with a variable fibrous tissue element. The fibrous tissue is arranged in concentric

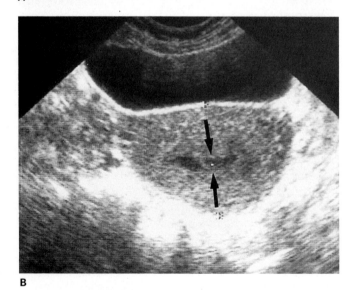

A

B

Fig. 11 Uterine infection. A: Longitudinal and **B:** transverse scan of the uterus showing enlargement, indistinctness of the endometrial/myometrial interface with a small amount of cavity fluid (arrows) in a patient with coexistent endometritis and myometritis.

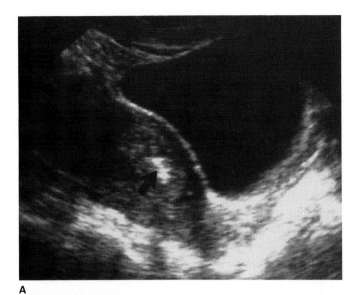

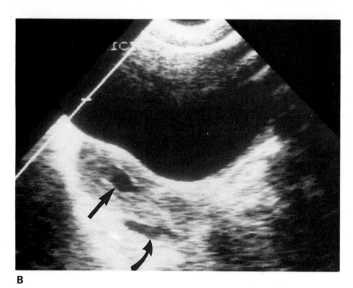

Fig. 12 Endometritis. A: Longitudinal scan in a patient with postabortal endometritis, with gas (arrow) in the uterine cavity. **B:** Longitudinal scan showing fluid in the uterine cavity (straight arrow) and fluid in the pouch of Douglas (curved arrow).

stimulation uninterrupted by pregnancy and lactation. Accordingly the risk is reduced with increasing parity. The oral contraceptive pill and smoking reduce the risk of developing fibroids, although obesity increases the risk. In essence the risk factors are very similar to those of endometrial carcinoma i.e. high and unopposed oestrogen levels.[25]

Characteristically fibroids only develop after puberty, enlarge during the reproductive years and decrease in size after menopause. Presentation is very variable and does not always relate to size; indeed very large fibroids may be asymptomatic, whereas small lesions may present with serious menstrual difficulties. Menstrual irregularity,

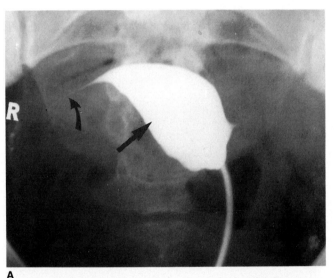

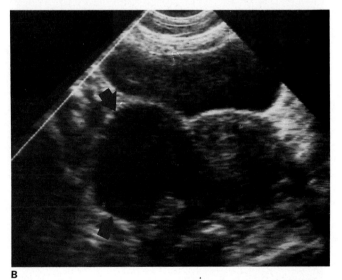

Fig. 13 Subserosal fibroid. A: Hysterosalpingogram performed in subfertile patient shows deviation and deformity of the uterine cavity (straight arrow) with associated stretching of the right fallopian tube (curved arrow). **B:** Transverse scan shows echo-poor right adnexal mass (arrows), which at operation was confirmed as a subserosal fibroid.

whorls which may account for some of the ultrasound appearances. The fibroid is smooth in outline, with only a thin layer of connective tissue separating it from the normal myometrium. As fibroids enlarge they tend to outgrow their blood supply and areas of central necrosis and cystic degeneration appear. A very small number may undergo malignant sarcomatous change but no reliable figures as regards to the incidence are available.

Aetiology The exact aetiology is unknown but there is a causal relationship with oestrogen which also stimulates fibroid growth. Fibroids are associated with nulliparity, which suggests an association with continuous oestrogen

menorrhagia and dysmenorrhoea are common presenting features.[26] A pelvic mass may be palpable and this may produce urinary symptoms due to its pressure effect.

Fibroids are multiple in 98% of patients.[27] The vast majority arise in the uterine body, and only 5% in the cervix. Their position within the myometrium is variable, the majority being intramural or subserosal (Fig. 13). Only 5% are submucosal (Fig. 14) but, due to their situation, these cause disproportionate symptoms since the increased endometrial surface area may cause menorrhagia. Submucosal fibroids may also become polypoid and enlarge the uterine cavity.[24] Intramural and subserosal fibroids may project anteriorly, posteriorly or laterally from the uterine surface. Laterally projecting fibroids may lie within the layers of the broad ligament and simulate an adnexal mass. Some very superficial subserosal fibroids may become pendulated and mobile, and may indeed lie at some distance from the uterine body, which causes diagnostic difficulties.

Ultrasound appearances   The description of the structure and situations of fibroids indicates the likelihood of a very variable ultrasound appearance, which is indeed the case. Focal or generalised uterine enlargement is common and often massive (Fig. 15). Depending on the position of the fibroids the uterine outline may be smooth or lobulated and there may be some distortion or displacement of the endometrial echo complex. Most fibroids are poorly reflective with relatively poor through-transmission of sound. Some fibroids produce focal areas of attenuation, the so-called 'venetian blind' sign of diverging linear bands of acoustic shadowing (Fig. 16A). Calcification within the fibroid, which is most usually of a speckled punctate nature, may develop as a result of internal degeneration, necrosis or haemorrhage (Fig. 16B). Occasionally this calcification is of a circumferential rim-like nature. Whatever the type of calcification acoustic shadowing may occur. These appearances may be confirmed with a plain abdominal radiograph where dense calcification (Fig. 16C), unlike the fine amorphous calcification rarely associated with ovarian carcinoma, may be demonstrated. Calcification is most marked in the older age groups. Occasionally central cystic areas may develop which may be smooth or irregular in outline with occasional septa, fluid/fluid levels and solid inclusions, usually resulting from internal necrosis or haemorrhage (Fig. 17).[28] Trans-vaginal scanning is generally superior in demonstrating the internal architecture unless the mass is very large or very attenuating. Where the mass is large external compression of the distal ureters may lead to reversible bilateral or unilateral hydroureter or hydronephrosis.

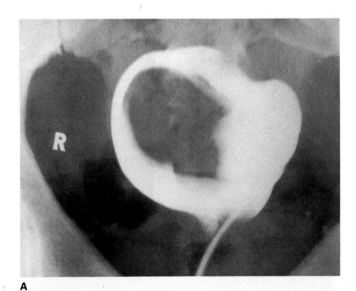

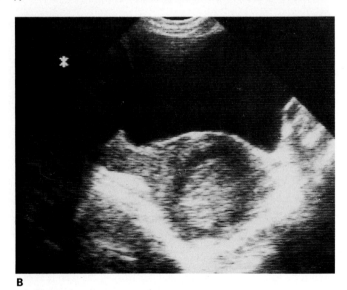

Fig. 14 Submucosal fibroid. A: Hysterosalpingogram shows enlargement of the uterine cavity and a large intracavity mass which was confirmed on **B:** as a central reflective intra-uterine mass.

Highly reflective intra-uterine foci with acoustic shadowing:

- calcification — fibroid (punctate or circumferential)
  - tumour — metastatic
    - lymphoma
  - vascular — uterine arteries
- pregnancy — retained fetal parts
  - lithopoedian — calcified mummified fetal remains
- gas (endometrial cavity/myometrium)
  - infection
  - post-instrumentation, D & C, hysterotomy
  - necrotic tumour
- foreign body — IUCD
  - suture material
  - radiation implant
- intra-uterine osseous metaplasia

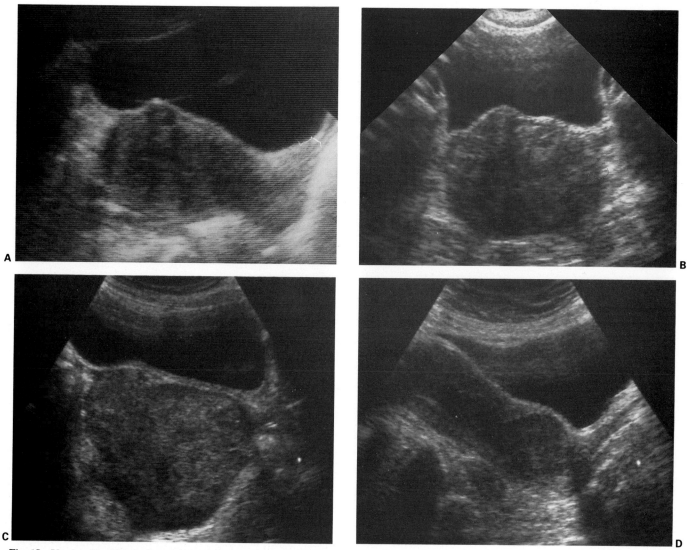

Fig. 15 Uterine fibroids. A: Longitudinal scan of moderately enlarged fibroid uterus with a lobulated outline produced by a small focal anterior fibroid. **B:** Transverse scan of enlarged fibroid uterus, with irregular outline and poor through-transmission of sound posteriorly. **C:** Transverse scan of large typical uterine fibroid mass. The heterogeneity of the enlarged uterus is typical of multiple small fibroids. **D:** Fibroid in the cervix. Fibroids in this site, although uncommon, may cause problems during pregnancy.

Without acoustic shadowing:
– abnormally reflective endometrium
– some fibroids
– IUCD
– intra-uterine adhesions (Asherman's syndrome).

Diagnostic pitfalls

The organ of origin of a large pelvic mass may be difficult to determine, particularly as it is often impossible to obtain adequate filling of the bladder. If the mass is continuous with the vagina, then it may be considered uterine in origin. Trans-vaginal ultrasound scanning is often helpful in this situation.

When a fibroid is highly attenuating it may be difficult to visualise the posterior wall of the uterus and the gain settings must be adjusted. This particularly applies to posteriorly situated fibroids.

Subserous and broad ligament fibroids may be mistaken for ovarian or other adnexal masses. In this case trans-vaginal ultrasound scanning is particularly useful in demonstrating continuity with the body of the uterus. Ovarian fibromas may be particularly confusing as their reflectivity is very similar to that of uterine fibroids. Similarly cystic uterine fibroids may mimic ovarian cysts and other cystic adnexal masses.[29]

A bicornuate uterus may give the impression of a normal uterine body with an adjacent fibroid, but the presence of two central endometrial echo complexes allows a differentiation.

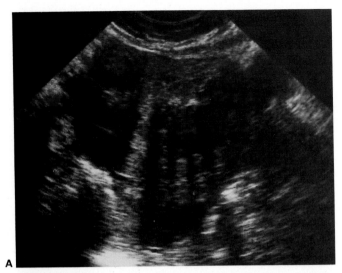

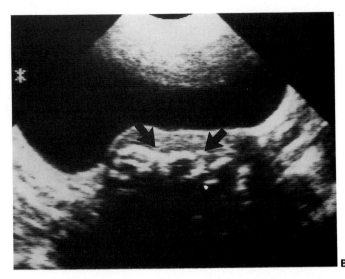

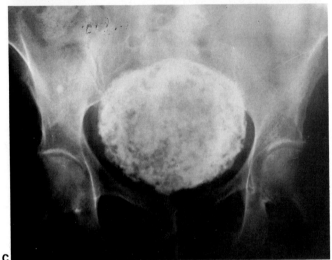

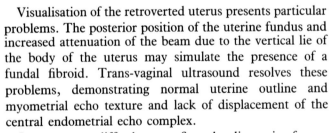

Fig. 16 Calcified fibroids. A: Large fibroid mass with linear bands of attenuation. **B:** Large fibroid mass with extensive calcification (arrows) producing marked attenuation. **C:** Pelvic radiograph shows typical dense calcification in post-menopausal fibroid uterus.

Visualisation of the retroverted uterus presents particular problems. The posterior position of the uterine fundus and increased attenuation of the beam due to the vertical lie of the body of the uterus may simulate the presence of a fundal fibroid. Trans-vaginal ultrasound resolves these problems, demonstrating normal uterine outline and myometrial echo texture and lack of displacement of the central endometrial echo complex.

It may prove difficult to confirm the diagnosis of a pedunculated fibroid, which may appear entirely separate from the uterine body. Depending on the length of the pedicle the fibroid may be mobile, lie outside the pelvis above the uterine fundus and, if it degenerates, may be cystic and tender. Ovarian fibroma is an important differential diagnosis.

Trans-vaginal ultrasound scanning usually gives superior images and provides significant additional information, particularly with regard to the internal architecture of masses, unless the fibroid is large or far from the transducer.

Ultrasound fails to demonstrate 22% of uterine fibroids,

particularly those smaller than 2 mm.[30] MRI has proved more accurate in the diagnosis of fibroids and clearly demonstrates tumour size, number, location and details of internal architecture.[31,32] It detects 92% of fibroids, including those as small as 5 mm. When myomectomy is being considered in the sub-fertile patient very precise knowledge of the size, number and situation of the fibroids, particularly if submucosal, is required. Trans-vaginal ultrasound is more accurate than transabdominal scanning in this context and MRI is superior to both.[31]

Treatment

Previously surgery was the only form of treatment, whether by hysterectomy or myomectomy, but the introduction of LHRH analogues offers the possibility of medical treatment. These drugs are derivatives of the hypothalamic hormone LHRH. Continuous administration leads to suppression of the pituitary-ovarian axis inducing a pseudo-menopause. Typically the volume of the fibroid reduces by 50%, and this can be monitored by ultrasound. However, once treatment is stopped they usually regrow, 80% of patients becoming symptomatic once again.[25]

Differential diagnosis of uterine enlargement:

- pregnancy
- trophoblastic disease
- fibroids
- cystic endometrial hyperplasia
- tumour   – carcinoma of the endometrium

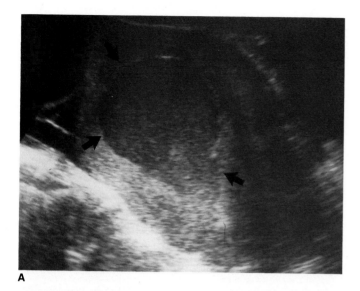

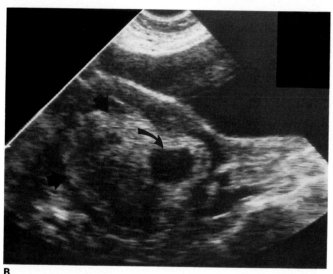

Fig. 17 Degenerating fibroids. A: Large smooth walled cystic cavity within fibroid. Blood and fluid within the cavity (arrows) is shown. **B:** Longitudinal scan shows complex fibroid mass of mixed reflectivity (straight arrows), with a small area of cystic degeneration within the mass (curved arrow).

- carcinoma of the cervix
- sarcoma
- hydro/haemato/pyometra.

Fibroids and pregnancy

Several recent series have contradicted the traditional teaching that fibroids increase in size during pregnancy. Indeed 78% are unchanged or even decrease in size.[33] Fibroids may be a contributory factor in many complicated pregnancies but, conversely, pregnancy may adversely affect a pre-existing fibroid. There is no doubt that changes in the uterine blood supply may render a fibroid ischaemic and produce painful acute necrosis and cystic degeneration, the 'red degeneration' of pregnancy.

Complications of pregnancy relating to fibroids

The majority of problems are related to submucosal fibroids.

a) Subfertility: fibroids may block the tubal ostia or prevent implantation of the embryo due to distortion of the uterine cavity. However, a review of 670 patients undergoing major operations for preservation or enhancement of fertility revealed that in only 2% undergoing myomectomy could no other cause for infertility be found.[26]

b) Spontaneous abortion: is more likely to occur in the first or second trimester, due to abnormal placentation. There is also an increased risk of ectopic pregnancy. .

c) Compression effects: mainly occur in the third trimester, leading to fetal malpresentation and fetal compression deformities. This may be particularly important with cervical fibroids.

d) Cavity distortion: in the third trimester leads to an increased incidence of placental abruption, antepartum haemorrhage, retained placenta, post-partum haemorrhage and premature rupture of the membranes. When a fibroid lies in the lower uterine segment or cervix, normal vaginal delivery may be impossible. All these problems are likely to be exacerbated if there are multiple fibroids.[34,35]

Ultrasound appearances For the most part these are very similar to those in the non-pregnant uterus (Fig. 18A). In pregnancy the majority of fibroids are echo-poor (Fig. 18B); some are heterogeneous and a few have a highly reflective rim, in part due to calcification. This circumferential calcification may simulate the appearance of a fetal head or, if incomplete, fetal parts (Fig. 19A).[24] As previously mentioned cystic degeneration may also be a feature (Fig. 19B). Braxton Hicks uterine contractions can be mistaken for fibroids by their typically transient alteration in the myometrial contour with normal reflectivity (Fig. 20).

Uterine sarcoma

This is a rare form of uterine tumour, accounting for less than 3% of all uterine malignant disease. The histology is variable but all forms are aggressive. Uterine leiomyosarcoma is the commonest form of genital tract sarcoma and accounts for half to three quarters of all uterine sarcomas. Although uterine sarcomas may arise de novo they generally develop from pre-existing fibroids, typically in the fourth, fifth and sixth decades. These tumours often present with minimal symptoms but may present with a pelvic mass or abnormal uterine bleeding. The sonographer should be alerted to the diagnosis by rapid growth of a

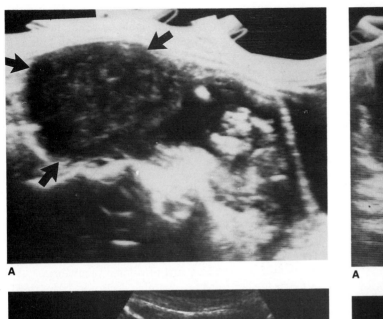

A

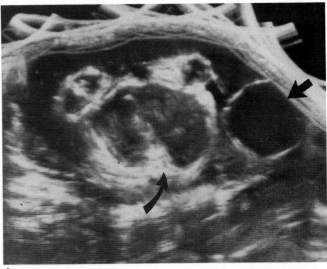

A

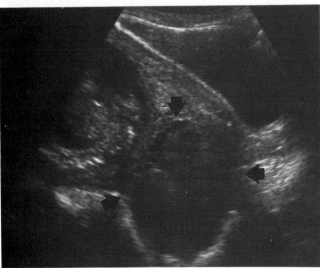

B

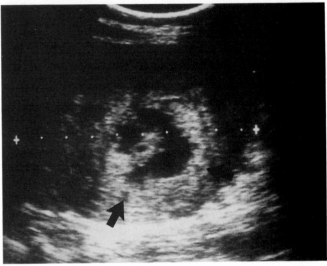

B

Fig. 18 Fibroids in pregnancy. A: Longitudinal scan showing large fundal fibroid (arrows) at 20 weeks gestation. **B:** 70 mm posterior cervical fibroid (arrows) in 20 week gestation.

Fig. 19 Complicated fibroids in pregnancy. A: A rim of calcification in a fibroid (arrow) mimicking a fetal head in this 35 week pregnancy. A cross-section of the fetal trunk (curved arrow) is shown in the same image. **B:** Degenerating fibroid (arrows) in pregnancy with an irregular central cavity.

pre-existing 'fibroid' in a post-menopausal woman. A large uterine mass with or without evidence of fibroids is found. The texture is generally heterogeneous, often with areas of cystic change. This appearance is indistinguishable from a large non-malignant fibroid or a large endometrial carcinoma. The diagnosis can only be made histologically. There may be ultrasound evidence of urinary tract obstruction and of local or distant tumour spread.[36]

Other malignant uterine tumours

Uterine metastases

Metastases to the uterus are rare, most originating in the breast or stomach. Krukenberg tumours of the ovaries may be associated. The endometrium is more commonly involved than the myometrium. Presentation is generally with abnormal bleeding and pain and ultrasound shows single or multiple masses of varying reflectivity. Dystrophic calcification may be present.[37]

Lymphoma

Lymphoma may infiltrate the uterine corpus and cervix and is usually a part of generalised disease. Primary lymphoma of the genital tract represents less than 1% of

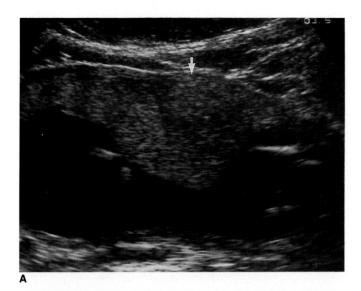

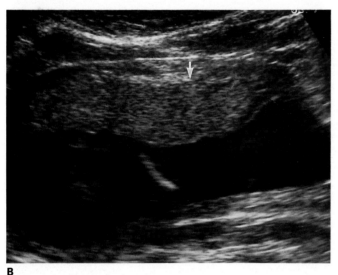

Fig. 20 Braxton Hicks contraction. Longitudinal uterine scans in pregnancy showing **A:** Braxton Hicks contraction (arrow). **B:** Relaxation of uterine wall 10 minutes later (arrow).

extranodal involvement. Ultrasound shows a focal echo-poor mass which may rarely be calcified.[38]

Mixed Müllerian carcinoma

These rare uterine tumours are part carcinoma and part sarcoma on histology. They arise from pluripotential primordial cells in the Müllerian duct system, from which the uterus develops. These aggressive, often rapidly invasive, endometrial tumours generally show deep myometrial penetration. The prognosis is poor.[39]

Primary uterine osteosarcoma

A very rare uterine tumour presenting as a calcified mass,

the differential diagnosis of which is fibroid, leiomyosarcoma, metastases or lymphoma.[40]

All these tumours are rare and usually present with postmenopausal bleeding. Ultrasound confirms the uterine mass or other abnormalities, but further investigation with CT and MRI are generally required. Even so the diagnosis is usually only made by biopsy.

Carcinoma of the fallopian tube

These rare cystadenocarcinomata may present with postmenopausal bleeding but characteristically also with a copious watery vaginal discharge. The discharge occurs as a result of fluid secretion by tumour within the affected tube. Ultrasound often demonstrates a cylindrically shaped cystic adnexal mass, separate from the uterus. Multiple small polypoid, moderately reflective tumours may be shown projecting into the cystic structure. The cystic mass is a fallopian tube distended with the fluid secretions of multiple tumours. It may be observed to change in shape and size periodically, as fluid is discharged into the uterine cavity. The cystic mass can be mistaken for a simple hydrosalpinx or ovarian cyst and the diagnosis is rarely made pre-operatively but should be considered in a postmenopausal women presenting with a watery vaginal discharge.[41]

Choriocarcinoma

Trophoblastic disease ranges from the benign hydatidiform mole through invasive mole to the highly malignant choriocarcinoma (see Chs 8 and 23). The incidence of hydatidiform mole is 1:1500 pregnancies in the UK but is much more common in South East Asia, with approximately 8% developing the malignant form. Diagnosis is made histologically. β-HCG may be a valuable tumour marker.

Choriocarcinoma is a very fast growing aggressive tumour which characteristically metastasises to the lungs early in the course of the disease, and occasionally to the liver and, less commonly, to the brain. Chemotherapy is highly effective, with a cure rate better than 90%. The tumour produces a serological marker, human chorionic gonadotrophin (HCG), which is useful to monitor progress of the disease. Although HCG is a sensitive indicator of disease activity, complementary imaging methods to assess residual and recurrent disease have been employed. In the pelvis, both ultrasound and MRI are useful with distant spread most reliably assessed by CT or MRI.

Ultrasound appearances No common ultrasound pattern has been described, either before or after chemotherapy. Prior to chemotherapy uterine enlargement is a common finding. Changes in uterine morphology are variable, ranging from well-defined reflective myometrial areas to complex heterogeneous masses causing marked uterine enlargement. These large lesions may extend into the parametrium. In general the extent of the ultrasound appearances reflects HCG levels and those with gross ultrasound changes are more likely to have distant spread.[42]

Following successful chemotherapy (as judged by falling HCG levels) the ultrasound appearance of the uterus has been studied to ascertain whether ultrasound is of any value in predicting residual or recurrent disease. 50% of patients have normal uterine appearances. The remainder have varying abnormalities, ranging from increased uterine volume to intra-uterine foci of mixed reflectivity due to necrotic tumour tissue or blood clot. In approximately one fifth of patients there are associated ovarian luteal cysts.

These variable ultrasound patterns do not offer any specific prognostic markers to indicate recurrence of disease.[43] Characteristically the myometrial spiral arteries and the uterine arteries are enlarged and may be imaged or detected on Doppler. The low pulsatility index of the uterine artery indicates a decrease in arteriolar resistance.[44] The role of ultrasound and Doppler in the management of choriocarcinoma has yet to be clearly defined. At present treatment is monitored by serology.

Uterine adenomyosis

Adenomyosis is a variation of endometriosis in which ectopic endometrial tissue invades the myometrium producing diffuse uterine enlargement. The typical patient with endometriosis is nulliparous and in her 20's or 30's with subfertility. Conversely, with adenomyosis a multiparous woman in her 40's is most likely to be affected. The aetiology is unknown but the disease is probably related to elevated oestrogen levels. The true incidence is variously reported to involve between 5% and 60% of all surgically removed uteri. This variation in incidence depends on how thoroughly the histological examination is performed.[45]

The disease is usually generalised though a localised focus may be termed an adenomyoma. Generalised adenomyosis involves the inner two thirds of the myometrium of the body of the uterus; it is very rare in the cervix. It is said that caesarean section may predispose to adenomyosis, due to ectopic implantation of endometrium in the myometrium at the time of operation. Patients usually present with menorrhagia and dysmenorrhoea. The differential diagnosis includes dysfunctional uterine bleeding and fibroids, which often cannot be differentiated either clinically or on ultrasound.[46]

Ultrasound appearances Moderate symmetrical uterine enlargement is present in three quarters of patients. The uterus is smooth in outline, with a normal myometrial and endometrial echo texture (Fig. 21A). Occasionally small cystic areas, measuring 2 to 4 mm, are apparent (Fig. 21B). These represent distended endometrial stromal glands containing menstrual products. A focal adeno-

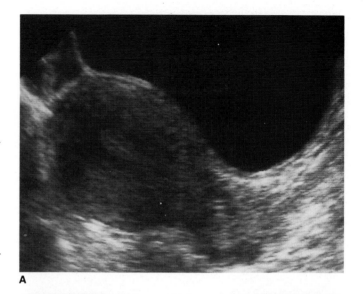

A

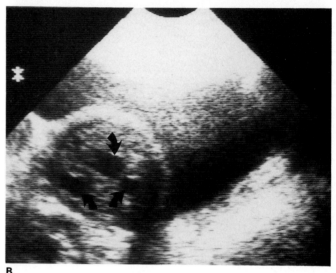

B

Fig. 21 Adenomyosis. A: Longitudinal scan shows moderate globular uterine enlargement with a normal echo texture. **B:** Longitudinal scan of globular uterus with small intra-uterine cystic foci (arrows) due to adenomyosis.

myoma may occasionally be recognised as a small bulge on the uterine surface but with no associated change in echo texture, as would be expected with a fibroid.

Adenomyosis may coexist with fibroids (Fig. 22) and with cystic endometrial hyperplasia in which case a precise diagnosis is impossible. Trans-vaginal ultrasound may be helpful in distinguishing these conditions and can demonstrate small echo-poor myometrial masses when abdominal ultrasound has been unremarkable. In a retrospective study the ultrasound scans of eight patients with histologically proven generalised adenomyosis were evaluated. Diffuse uterine enlargement with normal myometrial echo texture, normal contour and endometrial

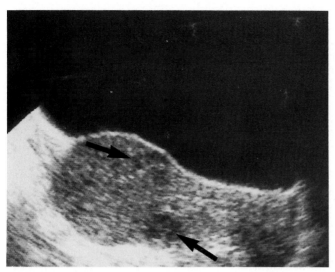

Fig. 22 Coexistent adenomyosis and fibroids. Longitudinal scan shows generalised uterine enlargement with two small fibroids (arrows).

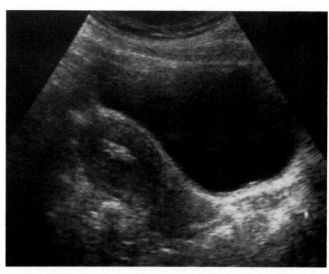

Fig. 23 Asherman's syndrome. Longitudinal scan shows highly reflective foci within the uterine cavity.

cavity echoes were shown to be reliable indicators of the disease.[45] Ultrasound may also show evidence of more generalised extra-uterine endometriosis.

Excellent evaluation of the zonal architecture of the uterus by MRI has been shown to be of value in distinguishing adenomyosis from fibroids.[47] In most patients the diagnosis is made histologically after hysterectomy.

Asherman's syndrome

Intra-uterine adhesions (or synechiae) develop as a result of over-zealous curettage of the uterus after miscarriage, post-partum or after termination. The adhesions develop less commonly following myomectomy or caesarean section and also occasionally as a result of endometritis. In pregnancy the myometrium is softer than normal so that deeper layers of the endometrium are removed at curettage. Trauma to the basal layer of the endometrium produces scarring. As healing occurs fibrinous bands develop between the two opposing endometrial walls. Symptoms and signs are variable but include amenorrhoea, hypomenorrhoea and dysmenorrhoea. Infertility may result from tubal occlusions and from implantation problems. Should pregnancy ensue, there is an increased risk of early miscarriage and, later, of post-partum haemorrhage and placental retention.

Ultrasound appearances Single or multiple highly reflective foci in the endometrial cavity mark the sites of the adhesions which are usually asymmetrically located (Fig. 23). The foci measure only a few millimetres across and do not produce acoustic shadowing.[48] As the lesions are small they are best demonstrated on trans-vaginal ultrasound. Adhesions straddling the amniotic cavity may be demonstrated in the second and third trimester as

thick membranes producing two communicating intra-amniotic cavities.[49] The diagnosis may be suspected on ultrasound but needs confirmation at hysterosalpingogram or hysteroscopy. Treatment is by division of the adhesions at hysteroscopy.

Uterine surgery

Hysterectomy

This is the commonest major surgical procedure in women and is generally performed pre-menopausally for non-malignant disease. Generally a simple hysterectomy is performed, either abdominally or vaginally and involves removal of the uterus and cervix with conservation of the ovaries provided they are normal. Post-operative ultrasound demonstrates the residual vagina as a blind-ending midline tubular structure (Fig. 24). Occasionally small retention cysts are demonstrated in the upper vagina in the region of the vault scar, but these are of no clinical significance. It should be cautioned that a small post-menopausal uterus, particularly when retroverted, may be difficult to identify on ultrasound: questioning of the patient should ensure that this is not mistaken for absence of the uterus after hysterectomy. Sub-total hysterectomy with preservation of the cervix is now rarely performed. On ultrasound the cervix is demonstrated as a rounded soft tissue structure in continuity with the upper vagina. Retention cysts may develop in the cervical stump and, when supracervical hysterectomy has been performed for cervical carcinoma, recurrence may occur in the stump.

Radical hysterectomy is performed for malignant uterine, cervical or ovarian disease. This involves a more extensive pelvic clearance, depending on the primary

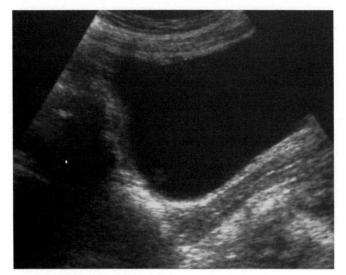

Fig. 24 Post-hysterectomy vagina. Longitudinal scan of blind-ending vagina post-hysterectomy.

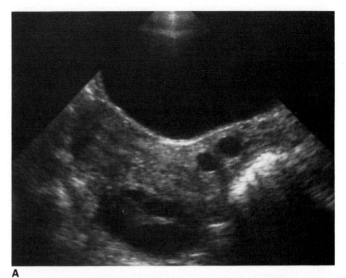

A

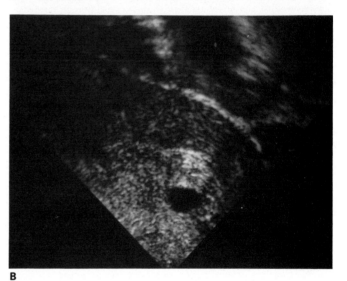

B

Fig. 25 Nabothian cysts. A: Longitudinal scan shows two Nabothian cysts in the cervix. Note the hyperstimulated ovary in the pouch of Douglas. **B:** Trans-vaginal scan demonstrating a single 6 mm Nabothian cyst.

lesion, and may be combined with pelvic lymphadenectomy.

Significant post-operative complications following hysterectomy are uncommon but are more likely when there has been radical surgery. Small pelvic fluid collections may be considered normal immediately post-operatively. Larger or loculated pelvic fluid collections may represent haematomata or abscesses, which may need drainage under ultrasound control. In the long-term, lower abdominal or pelvic lymphoceles may develop, particularly when there has been lymph node clearance. They are simple thin walled, unilocular cysts of varying sizes, whose content can be confirmed on aspiration.

Nabothian cysts

These are small endocervical cysts which develop as a result of chronic cervitis and are of no clinical significance.[50] Cervical inflammation leads to the formation of erosions and once these heal, residual islands of columnar epithelium covered with squamous epithelium continue to secrete mucus. Thus mucus retention cysts are formed.

Ultrasound appearances These cysts are fairly common and easily identified by their position in the cervix. The cysts are 0.5 to 4 cm in size and echo-free generally with only a narrow interface with normal cervical tissue (Fig. 25). Care should be taken not to confuse them with a small low lying gestation sac in the cervical canal.

Cervical incompetence

The diagnosis of cervical incompetence is initially clinical, from repeated painless, bloodless, miscarriages in the second trimester. Premature dilatation of the cervical canal

leads to expulsion of an intact sac with its contents early in the second trimester. The incidence is less than 2 per 1000 pregnancies. Although often idiopathic, predisposing factors include previous obstetric and gynaecological trauma with cone biopsy of the cervix and dilatation and curettage commonly implicated. Congenital genital tract anomalies may also be contributory. Although precautionary cervical cerclage may be performed at 12 to 14 weeks gestation, it may be preferable to monitor the appearance of the cervix with serial ultrasound examinations. In the non-pregnant patient hysterosalpingography has been of value in the assessment of the cervix.

Ultrasound assessment of the cervix has been shown to be superior to digital examination. Ultrasonic evaluation of the cervix and lower uterine segment is adequate in 76%

with the transabdominal technique compared to 83% with the trans-vaginal approach.[51] The diagnosis is based on the interdependent observation of cervical shortening together with dilatation of the internal os. Transabdominally the cervix is examined in the long axis and in the transverse plane at the level of the internal os, the level of which is determined by the transverse course of the uterine arteries.[52]

A similar approach is made trans-vaginally. The mean length of the pregnant cervix at 12 to 16 weeks gestation in primigravid women is 42 mm, compared to 40 mm in parous women.[52] The relationship of the normal lower uterine segment to the normal cervix may be described as Y-shaped (Fig. 26) whereas, with cervical incompetence, the lower segment may balloon or funnel into a shortened cervix (Fig. 27). The dilated cervix may contain membranes, liquor and, occasionally, fetal parts. In very severe cases these may be seen bulging through the external os into the upper vagina. In that situation the differentiation between cervical incompetence and inevitable abortion may be impossible. It should be noted that a small amount of fluid or mucus in the cervical canal visualised as a thin echo-poor line within the cavity is a normal finding and is of no significance when the cervix is of normal length. If the cervix is less than 3 cm in length and the transverse diameter of the canal is greater than 1 cm then a diagnosis of cervical incompetence is likely.[53]

Following the diagnosis cervical cerclage will normally be performed. This involves trans-vaginal suturing of the ectocervix in order to prevent dilatation of the cervical canal. The suture material is very highly reflective and is clearly visible in both transverse and sagittal scan planes (Fig. 28).[54] Cervical cerclage does not alter the configuration of the internal os as no suture is placed closer

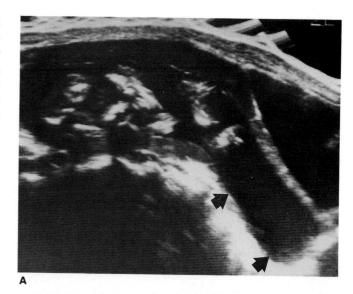

A

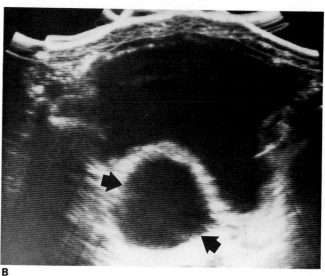

B

Fig. 27 Cervical incompetence. A: Longitudinal scan shows ballooning of membranes and liquor into the cervix (arrows). B: Transverse scan shows dilated cervical canal (arrows).

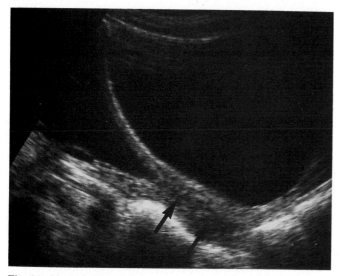

Fig. 26 Normal cervix in pregnancy. Longitudinal scan in an 18 week gestation shows the normal Y-shaped relationship of the lower uterine segment to the cervix (arrows).

than 1 cm to the internal os, the average distance being 2 cm. Cervical cerclage allows 85% of patients to deliver normally at full term following removal of the suture.

Carcinoma of the cervix

Carcinoma of the cervix is the second commonest gynaecological tumour with approximately 4000 new cases per year in the UK. It is the sixth commonest female tumour. National screening programmes are steadily reducing the incidence of invasive disease as early micro-invasive disease is diagnosed by exfoliative cytology. In more advanced disease menstrual irregularities, vaginal discharge and postmenopausal bleeding are the usual modes of presentation.

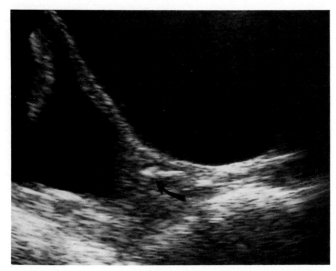

Fig. 28 Shirodkar suture. Cervical cerclage performed for cervical incompetence. Longitudinal scan shows sutures (curved arrow) and ballooning membranes.

Table 2 FIGO staging of carcinoma of cervix

Stage	0	– Carcinoma in situ
Stage	I	– Carcinoma confined to cervix
	IA	– Micro-invasive (only diagnosed histologically)
	IB	– Clinically invasive carcinoma confined to cervix
Stage	II	– Carcinoma extends beyond the cervix but has not extended to the pelvic side wall. The carcinoma involves the vagina but not the lower third
	IIA	– No obvious parametrial involvement
	IIB	– Obvious parametrial involvement
Stage	III	– Carcinoma has extended to the pelvic side wall and/or the lower third of the vagina
	IIIA	– Lower third of the vagina involved
	IIIB	– Extension to pelvic side wall and/or hydronephrosis
Stage	IV	– Carcinoma has extended beyond the true pelvis and/or has clinically involved the bladder or rectum
	IVA	– Biopsy proves bladder or rectal tumour
	IVB	– Distant metastases beyond the pelvis

The peak incidence is 40 to 45 years, although many patients now present in their twenties as a result of changing sexual mores. The disease is rare in the sexually inactive and there is a well-established relationship with frequent coitus at an early age, promiscuity and venereal disease. Low socio-economic class and high parity are also related factors. The diagnosis is clinical, either with local or cone biopsy of the cervix. On histology 90% of cervical carcinomas are squamous cell, arising from the squamous epithelium of the ectocervix. 10% are adenocarcinomata which arise from the columnar epithelium of the endocervical canal. About 20% of the tumours lie in the cervical canal and may not be clinically apparent, only being diagnosed at cone biopsy. Other rare tumours include sarcomata, melanoma, lymphoma and metastases.[55] The prognosis is determined by the stage of the disease and tumour volume at presentation and falls steeply and progressively. FIGO staging is based on a clinical assessment made at examination under anaesthetic (Table 2).

Ultrasound appearances Early tumours cannot be detected by ultrasound imaging. Cervical enlargement may be the first visible feature, the differential diagnosis being fibroid, lymphoma or sarcoma. Cervical tumours are relatively echo-poor when compared with normal cervix and small cystic areas may be apparent if tumour necrosis occurs (Fig. 29). Irregularity of the cervical outline is a common feature, that suggests tumour spread into the parametrium or invasion of the bladder (Fig. 30). (The parametrium is the tissue lying below the level of the uterine arteries, between the cervix and the pelvic side wall.) The endometrium generally appears normal. If tumour extends to the cervical canal the endometrial cavity may be distended with blood or pus. Cervical stenosis developing after cone biopsy or radiation therapy may also

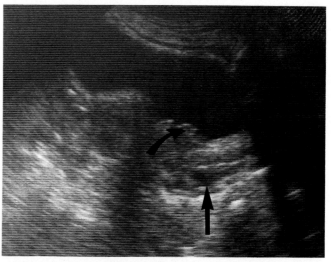

Fig. 29 Cervical carcinoma. Longitudinal scan post-partial hysterectomy shows cystic necrosis within tumour (straight arrow) and bladder invasion (curved arrow).

lead to the development of hydrometra, haematometra or pyometra (Fig. 31). Hydroureter and hydronephrosis result from ureteral invasion. Regional lymphadenopathy and evidence of distant spread may occasionally be apparent in advanced disease. Vaginal ultrasound demonstrates the tumour and this may be facilitated by introduction of saline into the vaginal vault. The role of trans-rectal ultrasound (TRUS) is evolving. In the axial plane the normal parametrium appears as a sharply defined relatively echo-poor crescent interrupted by the centrally placed cervix (Fig. 32A). It may be difficult to distinguish between the cervix and the medial aspects of the parametrium and thus assessment of the parametrial width can be difficult. The parametrial width should not exceed 1 cm at its mid-

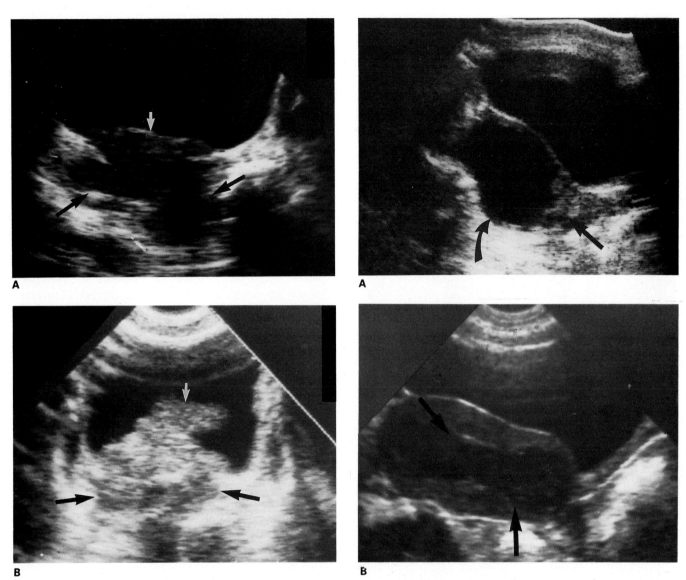

Fig. 30 Cervical carcinoma. A and **B:** Transverse scans show parametrial (black arrows) and bladder invasion (white arrow).

Fig. 31 Hydrometra. A: Longitudinal scan shows cervical tumour (straight arrow) and hydrometra (curved arrow). **B:** Longitudinal scan shows distended cervical canal and uterine body due to scarring following cervical biopsy.

point.[56] Variation in parametrial width with varying parity and changes in appearance in inflammatory disease may cause problems with interpretation of the image. Parametrial invasion by cervical tumour leads to loss or irregularity of the crescentic outline and mass formation may be seen within the parametrium (Fig. 32B). Inflammatory changes in the parametrium associated with PID or developing as a result of cone biopsy may produce a very similar appearance to the parametrial spread of cervical carcinoma and, indeed, the two may be associated. This leads to diagnostic confusion as the inflammatory changes and tumour may not be distinguishable. Unfortunately this problem is not resolved by other imaging methods. Paracervical lymph nodes are identified as well-defined separate echo-poor structures adjacent to the cervix.[56]

Changes in cervical or parametrial reflectivity have not been shown to be reliable indicators of malignancy.[57] Combined radial and sagittal rectal sector scanning (TRUS) allows calculation of tumour volume and thus treatment planning.[57]

Before planning therapy accurate staging is essential. Traditionally this has been done at examination under anaesthetic, but has been notoriously inaccurate; particularly resulting in under-staging of tumours. Thus the newer imaging modalities are now regularly employed. Endosonography, CT and MRI will all diagnose advanced disease, but as already stated, the diagnosis of early disease is made clinically. Generally, stage I and IIA disease is

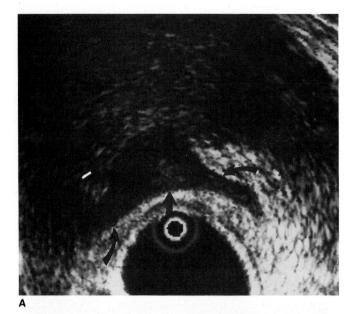

A

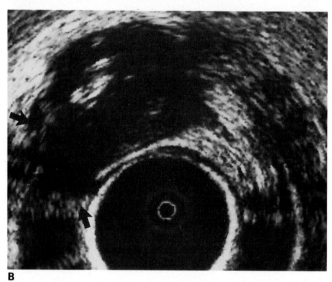

B

Fig. 32 Carcinoma of the cervix. A: TRUS shows normal cervix (straight arrow) and normal crescentic parametra (curved arrows). **B:** TRUS shows cervical carcinoma (arrows) invading the right parametrium with loss of crescentic outline.

treated with radical surgery, and more advanced disease with radiation therapy. In practical terms it is essential to distinguish between IIA and IIB disease in order to make this crucial management decision.

Abdominal ultrasound has no place in the diagnosis of early disease, and is only of value in demonstrating the gross effects of advanced disease, i.e. hydronephrosis. Endosonography, CT and MRI are all being used for assessment of tumour extension. The principal mode of spread of cervical carcinoma is by direct local invasion via the lymphatic system. Haematological spread occurs rarely and late. Absence of a defining membrane around the cervix allows local spread to occur early. Tumour spreads laterally into the parametrium and postero-laterally to the uterosacral ligaments. Regional lymph node spread occurs early. Anterior extension to the bladder occurs later and posterior extension to the rectum even later. Tumour spread to the uterine body and vagina is relatively uncommon but, when it does occur, differentiation from primary tumours of those organs may be impossible. Lateral extension of the tumour to involve one or both ureters is of particular importance as uraemia due to the resultant obstructive uropathy is the commonest cause of death in these patients.

Until recently, CT was the imaging method of choice for staging cervical carcinoma. However, CT is unable to distinguish between normal and abnormal cervical tissue; nor can it reliably distinguish between stage IIA and IIB disease i.e. whether there is evidence of parametrial disease. However, tumour spread to the pelvic side walls and regional lymphadenopathy can be clearly demonstrated.[58] MRI has been used to stage cervical carcinoma with good results.[59] Direct multiplanar imaging has great advantages. The cervix, vagina and uterus are well-demonstrated. Tumour can be easily differentiated from normal cervical tissue and tumour volume can be assessed. Parametrial invasion, vaginal wall extension and lymphadenopathy can all be demonstrated. However, as with other modalities, MRI is unable to distinguish between inflammatory and malignant disease of the parametrium.

Recently, there has been some interest in using TRUS to assess local spread of the disease. Studies comparing this with EUA, CT and MRI have been carried out, with some conflicting results being reported. In one study, 39 women with cervical tumour were assessed using EUA, TRUS and MRI, with concordance in tumour staging in less than one third of patients. TRUS assessment was at variance when compared with other modalities, more frequently than EUA or MRI. Conversely, however, another recent study[57] compared endosonography (trans-vaginal and trans-rectal), CT and MRI and found endosonography and MRI to be of comparable accuracy. CT was shown to be the least accurate in staging early disease and in distinguishing between IIA and IIB tumour. Results for combined trans-vaginal ultrasound and TRUS and MRI were very similar, although regional lymphadenopathy was better demonstrated by both CT and MRI. In essence cervical carcinoma is diagnosed and staged clinically, but combined TRUS and trans-vaginal ultrasound best show the degree of local spread, while CT and MRI demonstrate spread to local lymph nodes.

Vaginal pathology

The diagnosis of vaginal pathology is usually made at clinical examination but, on occasion, vaginal abnormalities are incidentally diagnosed at pelvic ultrasound.[60]

Vaginal fluid collections

Transient small collections of fluid may be readily identified in the vagina, and are most commonly due to menstrual blood. Larger collections of vaginal blood may be seen after abortion (Fig. 33) and with vaginal obstruction resulting in haematocolpos (Fig. 10A). Urine may be present in the vagina in the young child as a result of vaginal reflux during micturition. Larger pathological collections of urine may be found in the vagina in those suffering from urinary incontinence, or due to continuous leakage of urine into the vagina through a urinary fistula; or via an ectopic ureter.[61] Although it is uncommon, extra-vaginal fluid collections such as urethral cysts and para-vaginal haematomata may compress the normal vagina, giving the erroneous impression of a vaginal mass.

Gartner's duct cyst

These cysts arise from vestigial remnants of the mesonephric or Wolffian duct systems which, as the 'so-called' Gartner's ducts, course along the anterior outer aspects of the vaginal canal.[62]

These are the commonest vaginal cysts and are invariably asymptomatic with no treatment being required. Gartner's duct cysts are usually incidental findings at ultrasound.[63] The cysts may be single or multiple, and although generally small they may measure up to 5 cm in diameter. Occasionally the cysts communicate with the cervix or may be large enough to bulge through the introitus. On ultrasound examination the cysts may be shown to distend the upper vagina and may outline the ectocervix (Fig. 34). When large, the cyst may mimic a hydrocolpos. There is an association with ipsilateral renal agenesis and

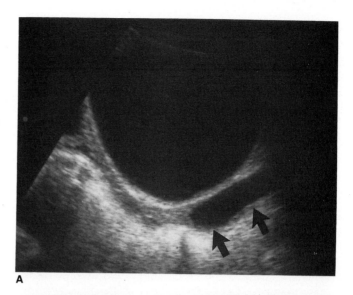

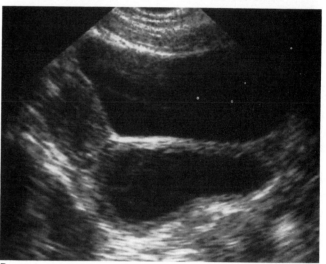

Fig. 34 Gartner's cysts. A: Longitudinal scan of sausage-shaped Gartner's cyst (arrows), distending upper vagina in pregnancy. **B:** Similar finding of a larger cyst in a non-pregnant patient.

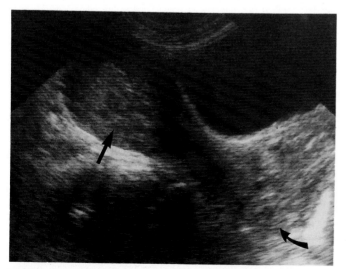

Fig. 33 Incomplete abortion. Longitudinal scan shows retained products of conception in the uterine cavity (straight arrow) and markedly distending the vaginal vault (curved arrow).

thus the urinary tract should always be examined when this diagnosis is made.

Vaginal foreign bodies

The presence of a foreign body, expected or otherwise, may cause vaginitis presenting with a persistent bloody or serous vaginal discharge. Abdominal ultrasound generally demonstrates the presence of such a structure often with an associated fluid collection. A pelvic radiograph will confirm the observation and may give more precise information as to the exact nature of the foreign body.

A tampon may be clearly visualised due to its well-defined highly reflective rectilinear shape. It is seen to lie centrally in the vaginal cavity and produces strong acoustic

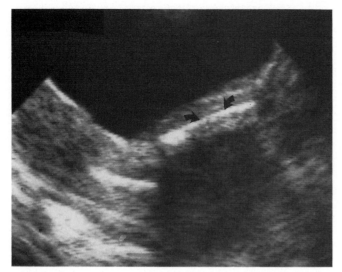

Fig. 35 Vaginal tampon. Longitudinal scan of vagina, showing characteristic appearance of tampon (arrows) with acoustic shadowing.

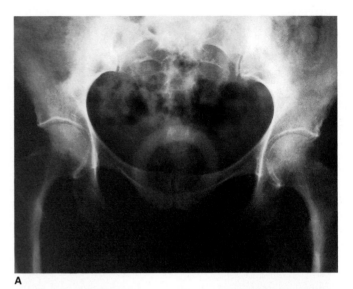

A

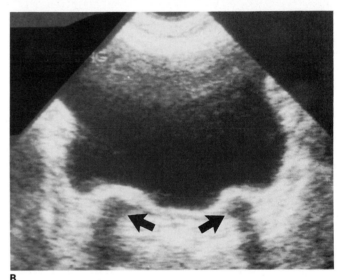

B

Fig. 36 Vaginal ring pessary. A: Pelvic radiograph shows typical appearance of vaginal ring pessary. **B:** Transverse scan shows lateral margins of the ring (arrows).

shadowing (Fig. 35). A retained tampon commonly causes vaginitis.

Uterine prolapse may be treated conservatively with a vaginal pessary placed high in the vaginal vault. The pessary produces intense acoustic shadowing high in the vagina, both on transverse and sagittal scans (Fig. 36).

Vaginal calculi are rare. They may occur as a result of ulceration of a bladder stone through the vesico-vaginal septum. Both congenital and acquired vaginal strictures are said to predispose to the formation of vaginal calculi as does urinary incontinence.[61] These calculi often calcify and become radio-opaque.

Gas may be visible in the vagina, especially after instrumentation or other manipulation. A tampon contains air in the cotton wool, which explains its strongly reflective appearance. Emphysematous vaginitis is an unusual condition in which gas filled blebs develop in the submucous layer of the upper vagina. The aetiology is unknown and the condition may occur in association with pregnancy.[64]

Vaginal tumours

Primary tumours of the vagina are rare, accounting for only 1% to 2% of all gynaecological malignancy. Squamous cell carcinomas account for 80% to 90% with adenocarcinomas and melanoma being very rare. The very rare sarcomas almost always present in childhood.

Secondary tumours are also rare, almost all spreading by local invasion, e.g. from the cervix, bladder, colon and rectum. Primary tumours usually present with vaginal bleeding and discharge and are clinically obvious with the diagnosis being made at biopsy. Examination under anaesthetic, endoscopic ultrasound (trans-vaginal and trans-rectal), CT and MRI are used for local staging and

monitoring tumour recurrence and have been shown to have similar efficacy.

Reported predisposing factors in the development of vaginal tumours include radiation therapy for carcinoma of the cervix, the use of a ring pessary and maternal treatment, for recurrent miscarriage, with diethylstilbestrol in early pregnancy. The daughters of those women, treated some 40 to 50 years ago, have a predisposition to develop an unusual, very aggressive clear cell adenocarcinoma of the upper vagina. Unlike the squamous cell carcinoma, which develops in the sixth and seventh decades of life, the clear cell carcinoma develops in the late teens.[65]

Ultrasound, whether abdominal, vaginal, or rectal demonstrates the tumour as a solid mass with low amplitude echoes. 50% develop in the upper third of the vagina

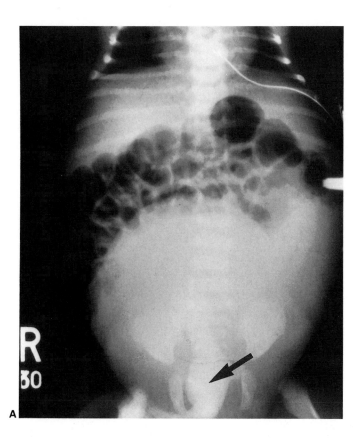

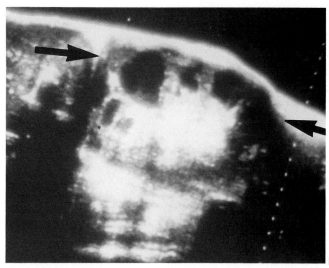

Fig. 37 Uterine rhabdomyosarcoma in infant. A: Abdominal radiograph shows large mass arising from pelvis. Contrast shows compression of an otherwise normal bladder (arrows). **B:** Longitudinal abdominal scan shows complex tumour mass (arrows). (Courtesy of Dr A W Duncan, Bristol Royal Hospital for Sick Children.)

and spread by a very similar pattern to that of carcinoma of the cervix. Stage I tumours are confined to the vagina. Stage II tumours extend beyond the vagina but not to the pelvic side walls. Stage III tumours reach the pelvic side walls, and stage IV tumours have distant spread. These tumours are difficult to treat as they usually present late. When accurate staging shows a stage I or II tumour radical surgery may be appropriate, but generally radiotherapy is used palliatively and the prognosis is poor.

Rhabdomyosarcoma Also known as embryonal sarcoma or sarcoma botryoides, this is the commonest soft tissue sarcoma in childhood. It is occasionally present at birth but usually presents before the age of 2 years and always before the age of 5. Embryonal sarcomas account for 4% to 8% of all malignant disease in children under 15 years of age; 18% affect the genitourinary tract.[66] The bladder and prostate are involved in the male; in the female

most are vaginal in origin, less commonly arising from the uterus.

A large red polypoid mass develops in the vagina, generally attached to the upper vaginal vault or cervix. Protrusion of the mass through the introitus may be the presenting feature. Alternatively a lower abdominal mass with vaginal bleeding or discharge may alert the clinician to the diagnosis. The tumour may grow very rapidly with invasion of the paravaginal tissues, uterus, bladder and other pelvic organs. Lymph node and pulmonary metastases are common.

The ultrasound appearances are variable but, in general, a large complex pelvic mass of variable reflectivity is apparent (Fig. 37). Multiple irregular cystic areas within the mass are common. Secondary features, such as hydroureter and hydronephrosis should be sought, together with evidence of distant spread. Staging by CT and MRI is preferable to ultrasound, although the reduction in tumour mass following chemotherapy may be monitored with ultrasound.

REFERENCES

1 Lewit N, Thaler I, Rottem S. The uterus: a new look with transvaginal sonography. JCU 1990; 18: 331–336
2 Schoenfeld A, Levavi H, Hirsh M, Pardo J, Ovadia J. Transvaginal sonography in postmenopausal women. JCU 1990; 18: 350–358
3 Cross S S, Ismail S M. Endometrial hyperplasia in an oopherectomized woman receiving tamoxifen therapy. Case report. Br J Obstet Gynaecol 1990; 97: 190–192
4 Killackey M A, Hakes T B, Pierce V K. Endometrial adenocarcinoma in breast cancer patients receiving antiestrogens. Cancer Treat Rep 1985; 69: 237–238
5 Dodson M L. Transvaginal ultrasound. Edinburgh: Churchill Livingstone. 1991: p 83
6 McCarthy K A, Hall D A, Kopans D B, Swann C A. Postmenopausal endometrial fluid collections: always an indicator of malignancy? J Ultrasound Med 1986; 5: 647

7 Fleischer A C, Gordon A N, Entman S S, Kepple D M. Transvaginal scanning of the endometrium. JCU 1990; 18: 337–349

8 Malpani A, Singer J, Wolverson M K, Merenda G. Endometrial hyperplasia: value of endometrial thickness in ultrasonographic diagnosis and clinical significance. JCU 1990; 18: 173–177

9 Novak's textbook of gynaecology. 11th edition. Baltimore: Williams and Wilkins. 1988: p 726

10 Novak's textbook of gynaecology. 11th edition. Baltimore: Williams and Wilkins. 1988: p 728–738

11 Osmers R, Volksen M, Schauer A. Vaginosonography for early detection of endometrial carcinoma? Lancet 1990; 335: 1569–1571

12 Nasri M N, Coast G J. Correlation of ultrasound findings and endometrial histopathology in post-menopausal women. Br J Obstet Gynaecol 1989; 96: 1333–1338

13 Bourne T H, Campbell S, Whitehead M I, Royston P, Steer C V, Collins W P. Detection of endometrial carcinoma in post-menopausal women by transvaginal ultrasonography and colour flow imaging. BMJ 1990; 301: 369

14 Hricak H, Stern J L, Fisher M R, Shapeero L G, Winkler M L, Lacey C G. Endometrial carcinoma staging by MR imaging. Radiology 1987; 162: 297–305

15 Fleisher A C, Dudley B S, Entman S S, Baxter J W, Kalemeris G C, James A E. Myometrial invasion by endometrial carcinoma: sonographic assessment. Radiology 1987; 162: 307–310

16 Hahn-Pedersen J, Kvist N, Mielson O H. Hydrometrocolpos: current views on pathogenesis and management. J Urol 1984; 132: 537

17 Scanlon K A, Pozniak M A, Fagerholm M, Shapiro S. Value of transperineal sonography in the assessment of vaginal atresia. AJR 1990; 154: 545–548

18 Sherer D M, Beyth Y. Ultrasonic diagnosis and assisted surgical management of haematotrachelos and haematometra due to uterine cervical atresia with associated vaginal agenesis. J Ultrasound Med 1989; 8: 321–323

19 Novak's textbook of gynaeocology. 11th edition. Baltimore: Williams and Wilkins. 1988: p 508

20 Novak's textbook of gynaeocology. 11th edition. Baltimore: Williams and Wilkins. 1988: p 512

21 Novak's textbook of gynaeocology. 11th edition. Baltimore: Williams and Wilkins. 1988: p 383

22 Breckenridge J W, Kurtz A B, Ritchie W G M, Macht E L. Postmenopausal uterine fluid collection: indicator of carcinoma. AJR 1982; 139: 529–534

23 Gompel C, Silverberg S G. Pathology, gynaecology and obstetrics. 2nd edition. Philadelphia: J B Lippincott. 1977

24 Ross R K, Pike M C, Vessey M P, Bull D, Yeates D, Casagrande J T. Risk factors for uterine fibroids: reduced risk associated with oral contraceptives. BMJ 1986; 293: 359–363

25 Vollenhoven B J, Lawrence A S, Healy D L. Uterine fibroids: a clinical review. Br J Obstet Gynaecol 1990; 97: 285–298

26 Buttram V C, Reiter R C. Uterine leiomyomata: etiology, symptomatology and management. Fertil Steril 1981; 36: 433–445

27 Sanders R C, James A E. Principles and practice of ultrasonography in obstetrics and gynecology. 3rd edition. Norfolk Connecticut: Appleton Centuary Croft. 1985: p 540–542

28 Borgstein R L, Shaw J J, Pearson R H. Uterine leiomyomata: sonographic mimicry. Br J Radiol 1989; 62: 1021–1023

29 Baltarowich O H, Kurtz A B, Pennell R G, Needleman L, Vilaro M M, Goldberg B. Pitfalls in the sonographic diagnosis of uterine fibroids. AJR 1988; 151: 728

30 Gross B H, Silver T M, Jaffe M H. Sonographic features of uterine leiomyomas. J Ultrasound Med 1983; 2: 401–406

31 Hricak H, Tscholakoff D, Heinrichs L, et al. Uterine leiomyomas: correlation of MR, histopathologic findings and symptoms. Radiology 1986; 158: 385–391

32 Weinreb J C, Barkoff N D, Megibow A, Demopoulos R. The value of MR imaging in distinguishing leiomyomas from other solid pelvic masses when sonography is indeterminate. AJR 1990; 154; 295–299

33 Aharoni A, Reiter A, Golan D, Paltiely Y, Sharf M. Patterns of growth of uterine leiomyomas during pregnancy: a prospective longitudinal study. Br J Obstet Gynaecol 1988; 95: 510–513

34 Lev-Toaff A S, Coleman B G, Arger P H, Mintz M C, Arenson R L, Toaff M E. Leiomyomas in pregnancy: sonographic study. Radiology 1987; 164: 375–380

35 Muram D, Gillieson M, Walters J H. Myomas of the uterus in pregnancy: ultrasonographic follow-up. Am J Obstet Gynecol 1980; 138: 16–19

36 Hannigan E V, Gomez L G. Uterine leiomyosarcoma: a review of prognostic, clinical and pathologic features. Am J Obstet Gynecol 1979; 134: 557–564

37 Kim S H, Hwang H Y, Choi B I. Case report: uterine metastasis from stomach cancer: radiological findings. Clin Radiol 1990; 42: 285–286

38 Malatsky A, Reuter K L, Woda B. Sonographic findings in primary uterine cervical lymphoma. JCU 1991; 19: 62–64

39 Shapeero L G, Hrick H. Mixed Müllerian sarcoma of the uterus: MR imaging findings. AJR 1989; 153: 317–319

40 Caputo M G, Reuter K L, Reale F. Primary osteosarcoma of the uterus. Br J Radiol 1990; 63: 578–580

41 Ajjimakorn S, Bhamarapravati Y. Transvaginal ultrasound and the diagnosis of fallopian tubal carcinoma. JCU 1991; 19: 116–119

42 Woo J S K, Wong L C, Ma H K. Sonographic patterns of pelvic and hepatic lesions in persistent trophoblastic disease. J Ultrasound Med 1985; 4: 189–198

43 Long M G, Boultbee J E, Begent R H J, Bagshawe K D. Ultrasonic morphology of the uterus and ovaries after treatment of invasive mole and gestational choriocarcinoma. Br J Radiol 1990; 63: 942–945

44 Long M G, Boultbee J E, Begent R H J. Doppler ultrasound of the uterine artery and uterus in invasive mole and choriocarcinoma. Br J Radiol 1987; 60: 621

45 Seidler D, Laing F C, Brooke Jeffrey R, Wing V W. Uterine adenomyosis. A difficult sonographic diagnosis. J Ultrasound Med 1987; 6: 345–349

46 Novak's textbook of gynaecology. 11th edition. Baltimore: Wilkins and Williams. 1988: p 450–453

47 Togashi K, Nishimura K, Itoh K, et al. Adenomyosis: diagnosis with MR imaging. Radiology 1988; 166: 111–114

48 Confino E, Friberg J, Giglia R V, Fleicher N. Sonographic imaging of intrauterine adhesions. Obstet Gynecol 1985; 66: 596–598

49 Smeele B, Wamsteker K, Sarstadt T, Exalto N. Ultrasonic appearance of Asherman's syndrome in the third trimester of pregnancy. JCU 1989; 17: 602–606

50 Vogel S T, Slaskyn B S. Sonography of Nabothian cysts. AJR 1980; 138: 927

51 Brown J, Theime G, Shah D, Fleicher A, Boehm F. Transabdominal and transvaginal endosonography: evaluation of the cervix and lower uterine segment in pregnancy. Am J Obstet Gynecol 1986; 155: 721–726

52 Quinn M J, Farnsworth B, Bisson D, Stirrat G M. Vaginal endosonography: a new method of the objective assessment of the pregnant cervix. Br J Radiol 1989; 62: 662

53 Bernstine R L, Lee S H, Crawford N L. Sonographic evaluation of the incompetent cervix. JCU 1981; 9: 417

54 Parulekar S G, Kiwi R. Ultrasound evaluation of sutures following cervical cerclage for incompetent cervix. J Ultrasound Med 1982; 1: 223–228

55 Novak's textbook of gynaecology. 11th edition. Baltimore: Wilkins and Williams. 1988: p 682–688

56 Yuhara A, Akamatsu N, Sekiba K. Use of transrectal radial scan ultrasonography in evaluating the extent of uterine cervical cancer. JCU 1987; 15: 507–517

57 Cobby M, Browning J, Jones A, Whipp E, Goddard P. Magnetic resonance imaging, computed tomography and endosonography in the local staging of carcinoma of the cervix. Br J Radiol 1990; 63: 673–679

58 Vick C W, Walsh J W, Wheelock J B, Brewer W H. CT of the normal and abnormal parametria in cervical cancer. AJR 1984; 143: 597–603

59 Togashi K, Nishimurak K, Sagoh T, et al. Carcinoma of the cervix: staging with MR imaging. Radiology 1989; 171: 245–251

60 McCarthy S, Taylor K J W. Sonography of vaginal masses. AJR 1983; 140: 1005–1008

61 Whitehouse G H. Gynaecological radiology. Blackwell Scientific Publications. 1981: p 135

62 Novak's textbook of gynaecology. 11th edition. Baltimore: Wilkins and Williams. 1988: p 567

63 Sheible F W. Ultrasonic features of Gartner's duct cysts. JCU 1987; 6: 438–439

64 Novak's textbook of gynaecology. 11th edition. Baltimore: Wilkins and Williams. 1988: p 567

65 In utero exposure to Diethylstilbestrol. Ch. 25. In: Novak's textbook of gynaecology. 11th edition. Baltimore: Wilkins and Williams. 1988

66 McLeod A J, Lewis E. Sonographic evaluation of pediatric rhabdomyosarcomas. J Ultrasound Med 1984; 3: 69–73

4

Ovaries

Andrew M. Fried

Normal appearances

The ovary varies in size and morphology with both the age and physiological status of the patient. Full evaluation of the ovary is best achieved by the combined use of trans-abdominal and trans-vaginal scanning. The transabdominal route utilises the filled urinary bladder as an acoustic window and provides an overview of both normal structures and pathological processes. When large masses or fluid collections are present this may be particularly important to define the full extent of the abnormality. The trans-vaginal probe can be used in almost all patients who are sexually active or using tampons and produces excellent detail of pelvic structures close to the transducer.

Technique of examination

Transabdominal scanning The ingestion of 1 litre of fluid one hour prior to the examination will generally provide adequate filling of the urinary bladder which serves both as a window into the pelvis and displaces bowel. A systematic study of the pelvis is then carried out in both sagittal and transverse planes. The sagittal scans begin in the midline and proceed to the pelvic side wall to include visualisation of the iliopsoas muscle group and/or the bony pelvis. The margin of the bony pelvis is identified as a highly reflective line with no through transmission of sound.

The variable position of the ovaries makes a complete survey of the pelvis necessary as they may lie anywhere from immediately posterior to the uterus in the cul-de-sac to laterally against the pelvic side wall.

The transverse scans should proceed from the level of the vagina to above the uterine fundus to ensure complete coverage. Again, the pelvic side walls should be reached by lateral angulation of the transducer. It is often useful to place the transducer in a paramedian position and angle through the filled bladder to image the contralateral adnexa; this technique tends to make maximum use of the bladder as an acoustic window and can be used in both sagittal and transverse scanning.

The overdistended urinary bladder is not only extremely uncomfortable but can displace pelvic masses out of the pelvis. Sizeable masses may be overlooked by not scanning sufficiently cephalad.

Trans-vaginal scanning For the trans-vaginal approach the patient should empty her bladder a little while before the examination. A small amount of urine still present in the bladder helps to maximise patient comfort and the range of angulation of the trans-vaginal probe.

Scanning gel is applied to the probe which is then covered by a protective sheath, usually a condom.

Elevating the patient's pelvis on a cushion provides increased latitude for motion of the probe. In the absence of a gynaecological examination table equipped with stirrups,

the patient merely places her heels together and lets her knees fall apart (see Ch. 9).

Scans are again performed in a systematic fashion in both sagittal and what is now the coronal plane extending as far toward each pelvic side wall, the sacral hollow and the retropubic space as can comfortably be managed by moving the handle of the probe. The uterus serves as a useful landmark, as do the internal iliac vessels, as the ovary is usually positioned immediately anterior to these vessels.

Size and morphology

The size of the ovary is generally calculated as an approximate volume (of an ellipse) with the formula: length × width × height × 0.5. The ovary tends to be of slightly lower reflectivity than the uterus with low level echoes surrounding the follicles of varying sizes that are also often seen.

In the child under 5 years old, the volume of the ovary is generally less than 1 ml, frequently making it difficult to identify. No lower limit of normal has been offered in the literature but failure to identify the ovary does not necessarily imply agenesis or dysgenesis (see *Abdominal and General Ultrasound*, Vol. 2, Ch. 56).[1,2] In the premenarchal child from approximately 5 to 9 years of age, the ovary averages 3.0 ml and, at menarche when the average volume is 4.0 ml the maximum can reach 6.5 ml (Fig. 1).

The previously established maximum normal volume of 6.0 ml for the ovary of a menstruating female is now considered too low. In teenagers and young adults, the ovary may reach 14 ml in volume and should still be considered

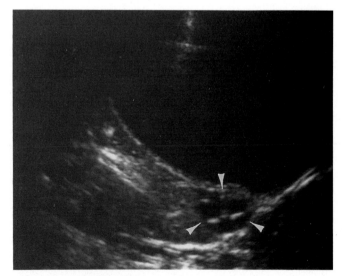

Fig. 1 Normal prepubertal ovary. Transabdominal scan of a normal ovary (arrowheads) in a 7-year-old girl. Multiple small follicles are recognisable as echo-free areas without a single dominant developing follicle in this premenarchal subject.

normal.[3-5] A recent study noted an average volume of 9.8 ml for an ovary of a woman in the childbearing years.[6]

In the post-menopausal patient, the average volume of a normal ovary has been estimated at 5.8 ml superseding the previous limit of 2.5 ml.[6,7] It is, however, not uncommon and not necessarily pathological to be unable to image the ovaries in a post-menopausal patient; this failure to visualise an ovary occurred in more than a quarter of clinically normal subjects of this age in one study.[8]

Cyclical variations

Although it is possible to detect small follicles in the ovary of a young child, they are not commonly seen until at or shortly before menarche. Subsequently throughout the childbearing years small, round, well-circumscribed 'cysts' are identified within the ovaries; these are follicles at varying stages of development (Figs 2 and 3). They measure 4 to 5 mm in diameter and commonly remain below 10 mm.

In patients of childbearing age several follicles may be discerned in each ovary at any given time, though there is usually only a single dominant follicle which enlarges over the course of the first half of the menstrual cycle to reach 20 to 22 mm in diameter (Figs 4 and 5). Ovulation generally occurs when the follicle has reached this size and timing of planned insemination oocyte retrieval for in-vitro fertilisation is carried out after daily monitoring of follicle size commencing at about the ninth day of the cycle.[9-11] Identification of the cumulus oophorus as a crescentic reflective focus with an echo-poor centre within the dominant follicle is taken to be a sign of imminent ovulation.[12] Failure to visualise the cumulus was encountered in 50% of women with primary or secondary infertility.

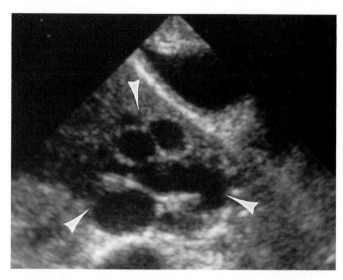

Fig. 3 Normal ovary – trans-vaginal scan. Multiple follicles are seen in great detail via the trans-vaginal route in this scan of a normal adult ovary (arrowheads).

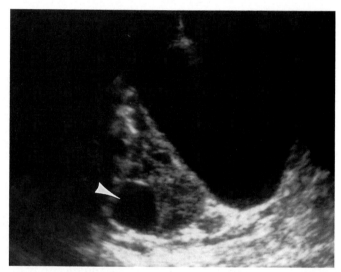

Fig. 4 A dominant follicle. In this transabdominal view, a dominant follicle (arrowhead) is developing and measures approximately 18 mm in maximum diameter. This is within the range of size (17 to 24 mm) at which ovulation will occur.

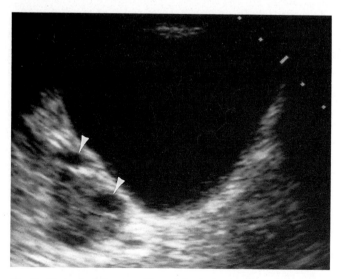

Fig. 2 Normal adult ovary. Transabdominal scan of an adult ovary early in the menstrual cycle demonstrates small follicles (arrowheads) none of which are dominant.

Following ovulation, the follicle shrinks to form a small highly reflective structure representing the corpus luteum. This forms initially with haemorrhage at the time of extrusion of the ovum and later by deposition of lipid-containing luteal cells.[13] Persistence of the corpus luteum as a recognisable cyst within the post-ovulatory period is not uncommon, particularly when fertilisation has occurred. The cyst normally regresses spontaneously. The greater anatomical detail that can be achieved using the trans-vaginal approach has led to this becoming the standard method for monitoring patients in infertility programmes. Cyclical changes cease after the menopause

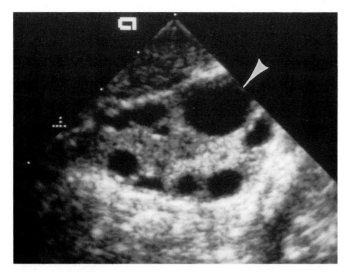

Fig. 5 Dominant follicle – trans-vaginal scan. In this trans-vaginal view, multiple follicles ranging in size from 3 to 8 mm in diameter are seen with one follicle (arrowhead) measuring 14 mm and destined to be the dominant follicle.

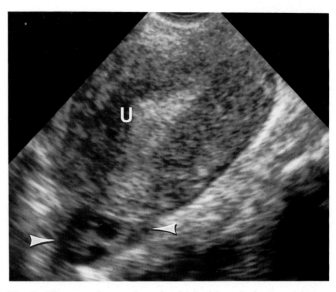

Fig. 7 The normal ovary (arrowheads) in this sagittal trans-vaginal scan lies posterior to the fundus of the uterus (U). This represents only one of many normal variants.

and the appearance of cystic enlargement of the ovary in the post-menopausal patient should be viewed with suspicion.

Position

The ovaries most commonly lie lateral to the uterus (usually within a few centimetres) at about the level of the cornua (Fig. 6). They are enveloped in the two layers of peritoneum which constitute the broad ligament. Variations are, however, frequent and of no clinical significance. It is, for example, not uncommon to find an ovary in the

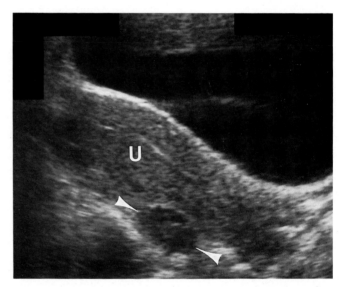

Fig. 8 Normal ovary. This ovary (arrowheads) is found in the cul-de-sac posterior to the uterus (U), another common location.

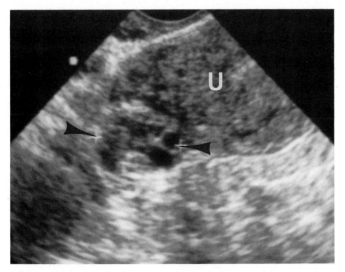

Fig. 6 Normal ovary. Transverse trans-vaginal scan displays the right ovary (arrowheads) in its most common location immediately adjacent to the lateral aspect of the uterus (U).

pouch of Douglas or lying laterally, near the pelvic side wall (this latter situation occurs particularly in multipara in whom the ligamentous structures may be relatively lax) (Figs 7 and 8). Ovarian masses, both benign and malignant, may displace the ovary out of the pelvis, as may the enlarging uterus in the pregnant patient.

A relatively constant relationship of the ovaries is their situation anterior to the internal iliac vessels. These vessels serve as particularly useful landmarks for location of the ovaries during trans-vaginal scanning, when orientation of the scan plane can sometimes be confusing (Fig. 9).

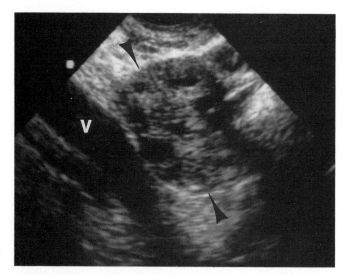

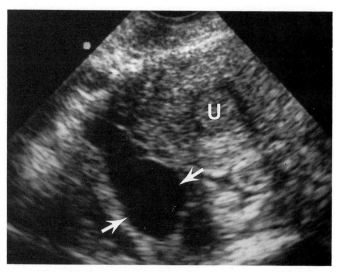

Fig. 9 Normal ovary. In this sagittal trans-vaginal scan the ovary (arrowheads) was located by first identifying the internal iliac vessels. The ovary is seen to lie immediately anterior to the internal iliac vein (v).

Fig. 10 Follicular cyst. Thin-walled cyst (arrows) seen in the right adnexa on trans-vaginal scan in all likelihood represents a follicular cyst in the right ovary and will regress spontaneously. U – uterus.

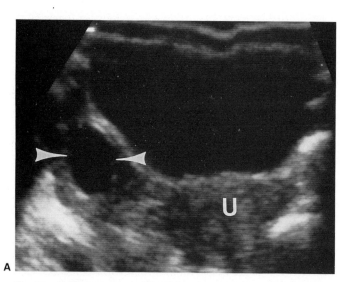

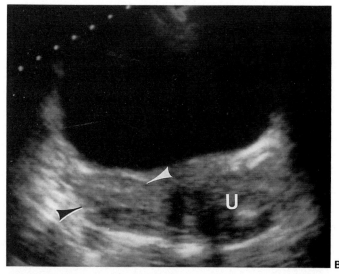

Fig. 11 Follicular cyst. A: The right ovary contains a well-marginated simple cyst (arrowheads), probably a follicular cyst. U – uterus. **B:** A follow up study several months later confirms spontaneous regression of the cyst leaving a normal sized ovary (arrowheads). U – uterus.

Pathological changes

Absence

In patients with Turner's syndrome (45 XO karyotype) ultrasound usually fails to demonstrate the ovaries, in keeping with the pathological descriptions of absent or fibrous streak ovaries. In genetic mosaicism, however, small or near-normal ovaries may be identified. As a consequence of this, the demonstration of ovarian tissue does not exclude Turner's syndrome.[14] Absence of the ovaries is also a feature of pure gonadal dysgenesis (Swyer's syndrome), but the patients are of normal stature.[15]

Some form of renal anomaly has been identified in a significant proportion of patients with Turner's syndrome (39% in one study); it is important therefore to examine the kidneys at the time of the pelvic examination. Horseshoe kidney is a particularly common morphological variant encountered in Turner's syndrome.[16]

Functional cysts

Follicular cyst The normal follicle typically reaches a maximum diameter of approximately 22 to 25 mm at ovulation and either shrinks dramatically or disappears en-

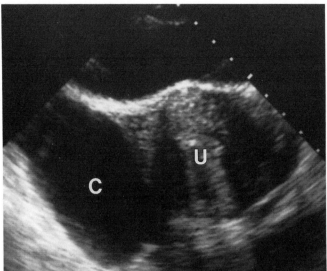
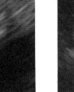

A

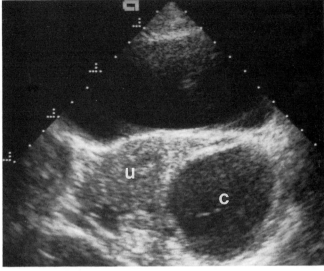

Fig. 13 Cyst with internal echoes. A large, thin-walled cyst (c) is seen in the left adnexa. The cyst contains low level echoes throughout representing internal haemorrhage. u – uterus.

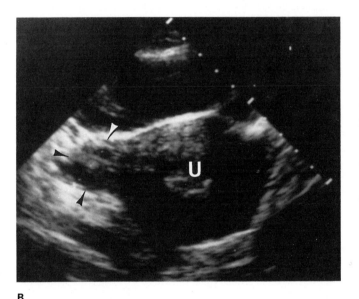

B

Fig. 12 Right adnexal cyst. A: A large, 4 × 7 cm right adnexal cyst (C) is seen adjacent to the uterus (U). **B:** 1 month later the cyst has spontaneously resolved leaving a normal ovary (arrowheads).

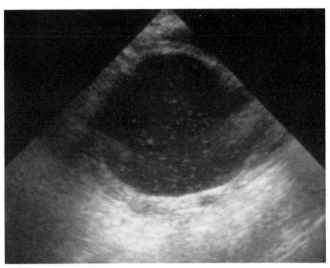

Fig. 14 Haemorrhagic functional cyst. A trans-vaginal view of a haemorrhagic functional cyst demonstrates the particulate matter representing breakdown products of clot.

tirely following extrusion of the ovum. Failure of the follicle to rupture or involute may result in a follicular cyst. Morphologically this remains a simple, sharply marginated cyst with very thin walls which may reach 4 cm in diameter (Fig. 10). Spontaneous regression is usual and repeating the study in 6 to 8 weeks will confirm this (Figs 11 and 12). Haemorrhage into a follicular cyst may occur resulting in internal echoes in the form of septa or gravity-dependent particulate debris (Figs 13 to 15). This should not alter the ultimate outcome.[17,18]

Corpus luteum cyst Failure of involution of the corpus luteum following ovulation may result in the formation of a corpus luteum cyst instead of the small highly reflective focus within the ovary, which represents the usual residuum. A corpus luteum cyst usually has a thicker wall than a follicular cyst and may grow to 5 to 10 cm in diameter. It is more likely to produce clinical symptoms. Here too haemorrhage may produce internal echoes in the form of debris or septation (Figs 16 and 17). Serial scans should document spontaneous regression of the cyst; this is of particular significance when the corpus luteum cyst coincides with pregnancy, as failure to regress by about 18 to 20 weeks gestation may be an indication for surgical intervention (Fig. 18). Torsion, spontaneous rupture and

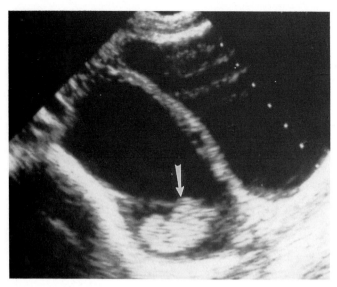

Fig. 15 Haemorrhagic cyst. In this haemorrhagic cyst, the clot (arrow) lies in the most dependent position. The clot moved on repositioning the patient.

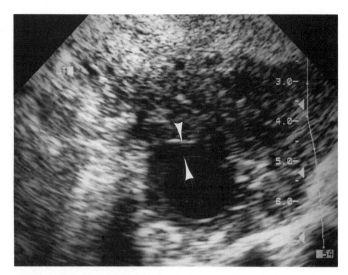

Fig. 17 Functional cyst. The relatively thick wall (arrowheads) of this functional cyst suggests a corpus luteum cyst rather than a follicular cyst which characteristically has a thin wall. Distinction is frequently difficult and histological proof is often lacking as both tend to regress spontaneously.

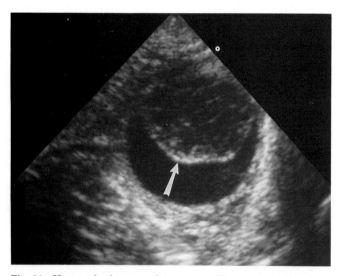

Fig. 16 Haemorrhagic corpus luteum cyst. Trans-vaginal view of a haemorrhagic corpus luteum cyst in which a clot of intermediate reflectivity (arrow) is seen to be retracting within the cyst. This cyst was discovered in association with an ectopic pregnancy.

mechanical obstruction of delivery are problems associated with the persistence of a sizeable corpus luteum cyst. The functional role of the corpus luteum in early pregnancy is the production of progesterone, which supports the secretory endometrium.

Congenital ovarian cyst

Congenital ovarian cysts can reach quite large sizes and occasionally contain internal septations or debris. There have been an increasing number of these detected during ante-natal ultrasound examination. They are almost invariably benign but when very large can produce significant compression of the abdominal viscera (and even elevation of the diaphragm) requiring surgical intervention.[19,20] Growth of such cysts is presumed to result, at least in part, from the influence of maternal hormones (Figs 19 and 20).

Polycystic ovaries

The clinical triad of hirsutism, obesity and oligomenorrhoea constitutes the Stein-Leventhal syndrome.[21] The classic appearance of polycystic ovaries at ultrasound is that of enlarged, spherical ovaries (the ovary is normally ovoid) with multiple small peripheral cysts (Figs 21 and 22).[22] More than 10 cysts of greater than 5 mm diameter in an ovary whose volume exceeds the expected 14 ml is considered typical. Since the patients are often obese trans-vaginal scanning may be particularly useful for full evaluation. The characteristic morphology of polycystic ovaries is seen in less than half the patients with clinical and biochemical evidence of the syndrome.[23,24] 30% of patients have normal ovarian volumes at ultrasound and, in an additional 25%, echo-poor ovaries will be seen without demonstrable follicles.[4,25]

Increased levels of luteinising hormone or elevated ratios of luteinising hormone to follicle stimulating hormone (LH/FSH) or direct pathological examination of the ovaries is definitive.[26] Decrease in the volume of the ovaries in response to LHRH analogue therapy for polycystic ovaries can be documented by ultrasound.[27]

The epidemiology of polycystic ovaries merits some consideration. The condition has been identified in 21% of all

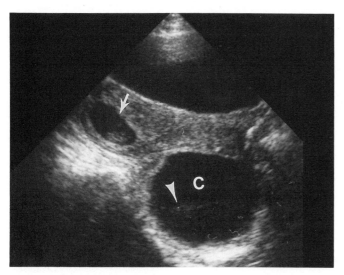

Fig. 18 Normal pregnancy and corpus luteum cyst. In association with a normal intra-uterine pregnancy of approximately 8 weeks gestation (arrow) is seen a 7.5 cm corpus luteum cyst (C) with some low level internal echoes (arrowhead). Most often, these cysts can be followed to spontaneous resolution.

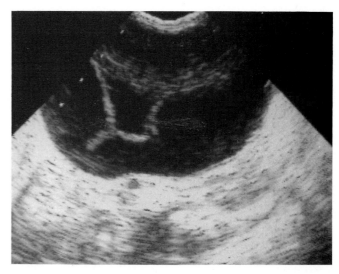

Fig. 20 Congenital ovarian cyst. Congenital ovarian cysts may display a variety of internal echo patterns beyond the simple fluid filled cyst. Note the multiple internal septations in this congenital ovarian cyst.

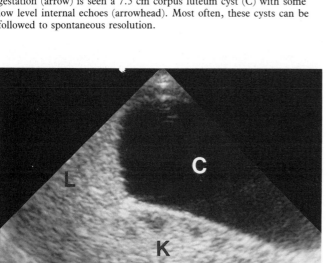

Fig. 19 Congenital ovarian cyst. A very large congenital ovarian cyst (C) rises out of the pelvis of this newborn infant to lie immediately below the liver (L) and anterior to the right kidney (K). Note the high reflectivity of the normal neonatal kidney.

Hyperstimulated ovaries

Increased circulating levels of human chorionic gonadotrophin (HCG) can produce cystic enlargement of both ovaries. Two situations are commonly responsible for this phenomenon, trophoblastic disease and exogenous administration in cases of infertility.

Trophoblastic disease produces extremely high levels of HCG irrespective of the histology of the disease (i.e. hydatidiform mole, chorioadenoma destruens or invasive mole, or choriocarcinoma). Large, multiseptated ovaries are encountered in some 20% to 50% of cases and are bilateral in as many as 50% (Fig. 23). These theca lutein cysts regress spontaneously following evacuation of the trophoblastic tissue from the uterus but the ovaries may take several months to return to normal size and morphology.[8,32]

Therapeutic administration of HCG to stimulate ovulation in the infertile patient can produce similar multiloculated cystic enlargement of the ovaries (Fig. 24). A broad spectrum of hyperstimulated ovaries has been observed in this setting, ranging from several small cysts to ovaries which reach and exceed 10 cm in diameter (Figs 25 and 26). The presence of ascites and severe electrolyte imbalances which accompany the full-blown hyperstimulation syndrome may signal a life-threatening condition.[8,33] Even with simple bilateral cystic enlargement of the ovaries resulting from iatrogenic overstimulation, pursuit of pregnancy during that cycle is considered inadvisable because of the increased risk of multiple gestations.[34,35] A decrease in the fraction of mature follicles and an increase in the number of very small follicles cor-

presentations to infertility clinics and, in fact, in 22% of the general population.[28,29] A strong familial tendency was documented in that same study in which polycystic ovaries were identified in 92% of pedigrees studied.[28] A significant association of polycystic ovaries has also been identified in patients with congenital adrenal hyperplasia; more than 80% of adults and 40% of post-pubertal girls with adrenal hyperplasia were found to have polycystic ovaries as well.[30,31]

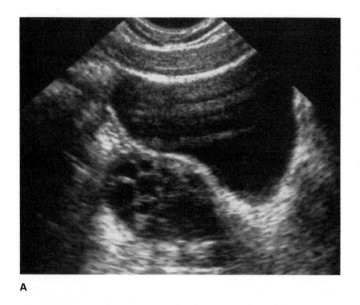

A

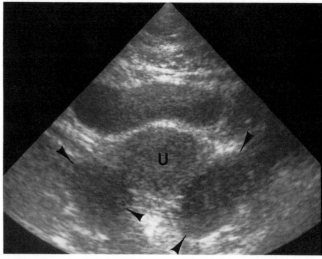

A

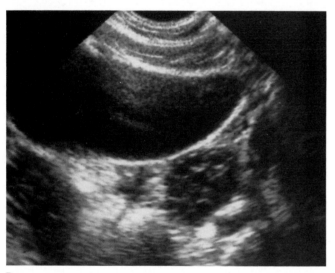

B

Fig. 21 Polycystic ovary syndrome. A: Longitudinal and **B:** transverse scans. The ovary is enlarged with scattered follicles in this patient with polycystic ovary syndrome. The ovaries were symmetrically enlarged.

B

Fig. 22 Polycystic ovaries. A: Bilateral ovarian enlargement is evident in this transverse transabdominal scan of a patient with polycystic ovaries (arrowheads). The ovarian volumes were 15.4 and 21.4 ml. U – uterus. Visualisation is often compromised because of the patient's obesity. **B:** Trans-vaginal view of the ovary in the same patient demonstrates a number of follicles of different sizes (arrowheads). U – uterus.

relates with the risk for development of the ovarian hyperstimulation syndrome.[36]

The incidence of ovarian hyperstimulation syndrome in all degrees of severity has been reported as high as 23% and varies from a mild, essentially asymptomatic condition identifiable only by ultrasound recognition of ovarian enlargement with an increase in the number and size of the follicles to a condition in which massive shifts of fluid out of the vascular space produce ascites, hydrothorax and renal failure.[37,38] Classification of the severity of the syndrome is based on a combination of clinical, laboratory and ultrasound findings. In general, ovarian size is less than 5 cm in the mild form, 5 to 12 cm in the moderate,

and greater than 12 cm in severe cases. The syndrome is more common in patients with polycystic ovary disease who are treated with gonadotrophins (see Ch. 6).

Ovarian remnant syndrome

If even a small amount of functioning ovarian tissue is left behind at oophorectomy, cyst formation may occur producing confusion in the face of a history of prior surgical removal of both ovaries (Fig. 27). Both simple and haemorrhagic cysts have been reported in this context, and the possibility must be considered.[39]

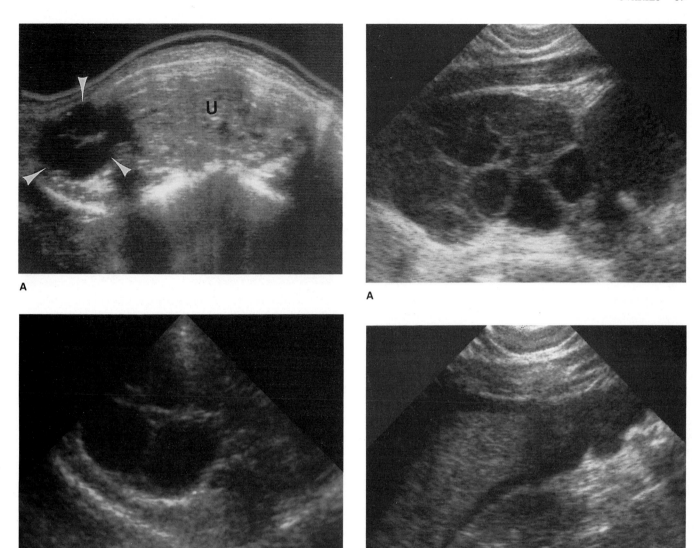

Fig. 23 Hydatidiform mole and theca lutein cyst. A: A transverse static image includes the uterus (U) markedly enlarged by the presence of trophoblastic tissue in this patient with a hydatidiform mole along with the right ovary enlarged by theca lutein cysts (arrowheads). Such cysts are frequently bilateral. **B:** A sector scan better demonstrates the multilocular nature of the right theca lutein cyst.

Fig. 24 Hyperstimulated ovaries. A: Longitudinal scan in the midline showing a massively enlarged ovary superior to the bladder. Under the influence of fertility drugs, such as clomiphene citrate, the ovaries may grow large with multiseptated cysts, as in this patient with hyperstimulated ovaries. Pregnancy is to be avoided during such a hyperstimulated cycle. **B:** A scan in the right upper quadrant showing ascites which is a complication of this condition.

Torsion

Torsion of the ovary is seen most commonly in teenagers and young adults; the presence of an ovarian mass, such as a functional cyst or dermoid, as well as inflammatory processes, are thought to predispose to this condition.[40] Such underlying pathology is reported to occur in as many as 70% of cases. Pain, fever and nausea and vomiting may constitute the presenting clinical picture; leukocytosis frequently accompanies torsion which may therefore simulate a wide variety of clinical conditions including gastroenteritis, appendicitis and urinary tract infection.[41]

The ultrasound appearance of the torted ovary is highly variable. Enlargement to 4 to 10 cm in diameter is common, the texture varies from largely solid to nearly cystic and good through transmission of sound is generally preserved in either case (Fig. 28).[42] Free fluid is frequently found in the pelvis.

The position of the torted ovary is quite variable with the midline being a common location; identification of the ovary superior to the uterus has also been reported.[43] The

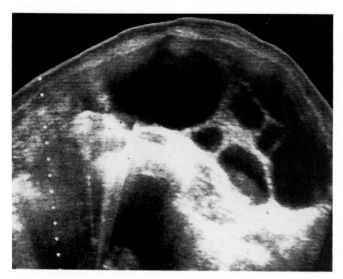

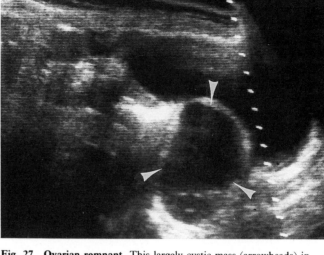

Fig. 25   Hyperstimulated ovaries. The static scan in this patient with hyperstimulated ovaries outlines a left ovary which measures more than 16 cm in diameter. No ascites is in evidence, however, and the patient did not display all the features of the hyperstimulation syndrome.

Fig. 27   Ovarian remnant. This largely cystic mass (arrowheads) in this patient with a history of prior oophorectomy is most worrisome for malignancy. At operation, however, this was found to be an ovarian remnant. Only a small amount of functioning tissue is required to produce such a phenomenon.

torsion may also involve portions of the tube which becomes dilated.[44]

Both duplex and colour flow Doppler techniques may be helpful; some observers have noted a cluster of dilated vessels in the periphery of a torted ovary.

Epithelial neoplasms

Serous cystadenoma – cystadenocarcinoma The most common neoplasms of the ovary are of epithelial origin.

Serous cystadenoma, which constitutes approximately 20% of all benign neoplasms of the ovary, appears as a unilocular or multilocular cystic mass with thin septations, few or no internal echoes and sharply defined walls (Figs 29 and 30). The septa are sufficiently diaphanous to undulate when gently palpated with the transducer, a phenomenon easily identified at real time examination. These septa are generally 2 to 3 mm thick without nodularity or mural nodules of solid tissue. Although papillary projections may sometimes be encountered in the

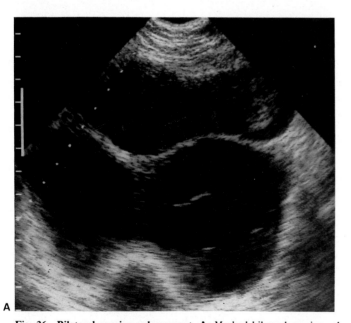

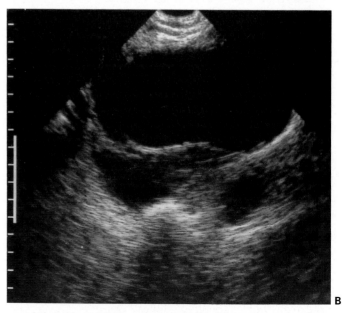

Fig. 26   Bilateral ovarian enlargement. A: Marked bilateral ovarian enlargement is in evidence in this patient on fertility drugs. **B:** 3 weeks after cessation of therapy the ovaries have returned to near-normal size.

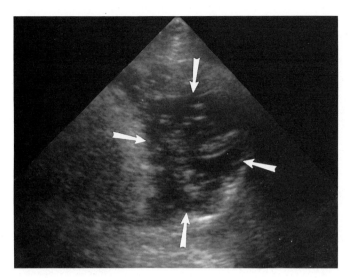

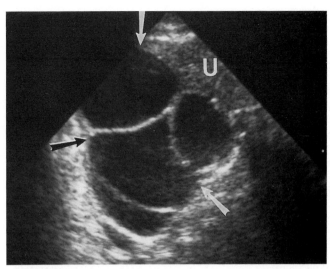

Fig. 28 Torsion of the ovary. The enlarged, echo-poor, disorganised appearance of this ovary (arrows) is the result of torsion.

Fig. 30 Serous cystadenoma. A trans-vaginal scan demonstrates a small benign serous cystadenoma of the right ovary (arrows) with multiple thin septa. U – uterus.

benign form, the greater the amount of solid tissue present, the greater is the concern for borderline or malignant histology (Fig. 31).[45]

About 15% of epithelial malignancies of the ovary are of borderline histology; the ultrasound distinction between benign and malignant, always difficult, is nearly impossible in this situation.[46] Features suggesting the malignant histology of serous cystadenocarcinoma include thickening of the septa, increased number and size of mural nodules, foci of solid tissue and the presence of ascites (Figs 32 and 33). Ascites has been reported with a frequency of greater than 50% in malignant epithelial neoplasms of the ovary (and is always associated with peritoneal spread of the tumour)

whereas it is said never to occur with benign disease.[47] Malignant ovarian tumours may be bilateral in as many as 62.5% of cases.[47,48] Ultrasound is relatively insensitive in the recognition of peritoneal spread of tumour (as is computed tomography). Serous cystadenocarcinoma accounts for approximately 40% of malignant tumours of the ovary.

Mucinous cystadenoma – adenocarcinoma Like their serous counterpart, mucinous tumours of the ovary display multiple septa dividing fluid-containing loculations. Septa in mucinous disease tend to be more numerous than in serous neoplasms and fine, low-level internal echoes are more common. These are thought to represent the viscid mucin and can often form fluid/debris levels (Fig. 34). Al-

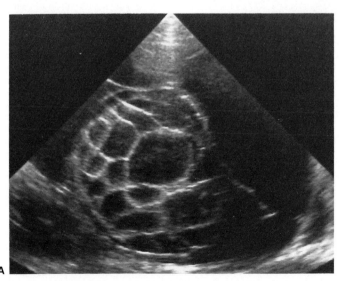

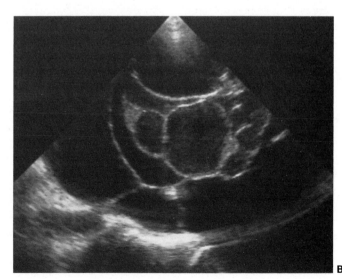

Fig. 29 Benign serous cystadenoma. A: Longitudinal and **B:** transverse scans. This very large benign serous cystadenoma has very thin septa, a characteristic finding in benign lesions. A few low level echoes are present in some of the cysts.

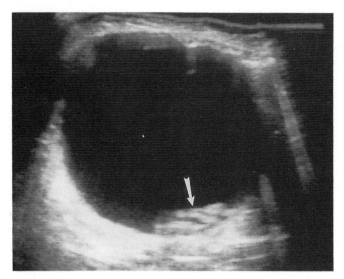

Fig. 31 Serous cystadenoma. This benign serous cystadenoma contains some gravity-dependent debris (arrow).

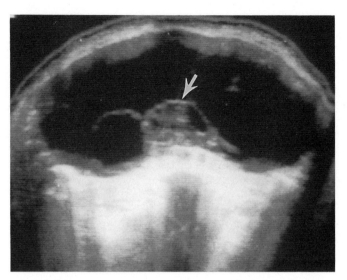

Fig. 33 Borderline mucinous cystadenoma. Although there cannot be said to be a one-to-one correlation, increasing proportions of solid tissue within ovarian masses raise suspicions of malignancy. A mural nidus of solid tissue (arrow) is seen in this borderline mucinous cystadenoma.

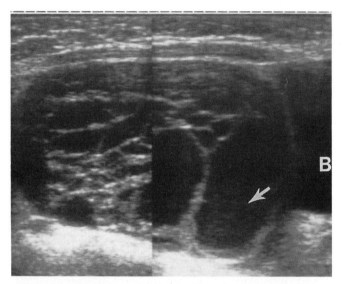

Fig. 32 Borderline mucinous cystadenoma. Increasing number of soft tissue septa are seen in this histologically borderline mucinous cystadenoma. The low level echoes of contained mucin (arrow) are characteristic. B – bladder.

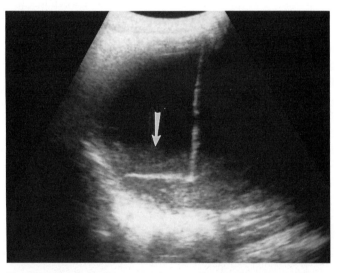

Fig. 34 Benign mucinous cystadenoma. Gravity-dependent low level echoes (arrow) are seen in this benign mucinous cystadenoma. The septa are quite thin.

though most mucinous neoplasms are in the range of 15 to 30 cm in diameter, they can grow considerably larger and have been reported to reach 50 cm.[45] Mucinous neoplasms represent some 20% of ovarian masses and are more likely to be benign than malignant (Figs 35 to 38).

The larger a mass becomes the more difficult it is to identify its organ of origin with certainty. Large necrotic uterine leiomyomata could, for example, be a problem in differential diagnosis from ovarian neoplasm. Identification of the ovary as separable from the mass is often extremely difficult, but if achieved helps to make this distinction.

Conversely, failure to separate such a mass from the ovary strengthens the likelihood of an ovarian origin.

Germ cell tumours

Dermoid (teratoma) Few other pathological processes or neoplasms display the broad spectrum of ultrasound appearances of which ovarian dermoid tumours are capable. Comprised of mixtures of fat, hair, sebum, calcium, epithelial tissue, neural elements and debris in varying proportions, dermoids may be cystic, complex, or solid and

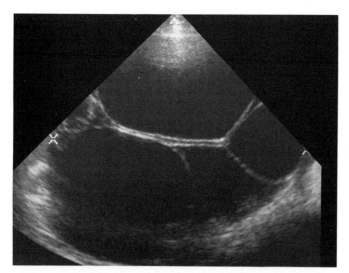

Fig. 35 **Mucinous cystadenocarcinoma**. With its thin septa and minimal soft tissue components, there is little to distinguish this well-differentiated grade I mucinous cystadenocarcinoma from its benign counterpart.

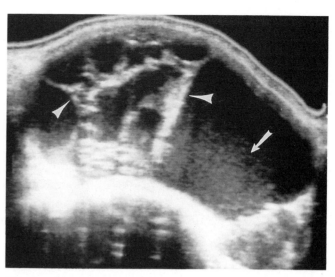

Fig. 37 **Mucinous cystadenocarcinoma**. Irregularly thickened septa (arrowheads) are seen in this mucinous cystadenocarcinoma along with the low level echoes of mucin (arrow).

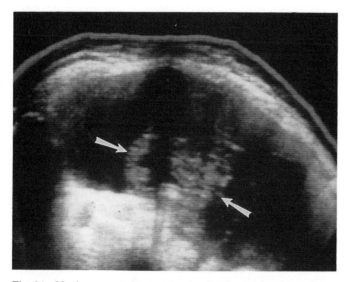

Fig. 36 **Mucinous cystadenocarcinoma**. A substantial amount of solid tissue (arrows) is seen in this otherwise cystic well-differentiated mucinous cystadenocarcinoma of the ovary. Low level echoes anteriorly represent reverberation artefact.

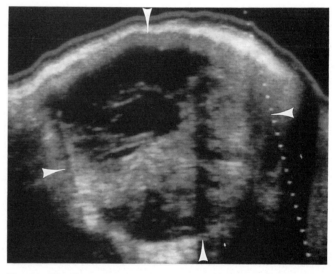

Fig. 38 **Mucinous cystadenocarcinoma**. A predominantly solid lesion with some areas of cyst formation is produced by this mucinous cystadenocarcinoma in combination with anaplastic carcinoid (arrowheads).

any combination of these, depending upon which component predominates.[41]

The classic and almost pathognomonic appearance of an ovarian dermoid is a relatively well-circumscribed mass containing a fluid/debris level with an internal focus of highly reflective material, which may produce an acoustic shadow. The fluid/debris level represents the interface between hair and sebum or sebum and cellular debris and the reflective focus either fat (no acoustic shadow) or calcification (shadowing) (Fig. 39). A mural nodule of solid tissue, the 'dermoid plug', has also been described as strongly suggestive of the diagnosis (Fig. 40);[49] it may also produce an acoustic shadow. Identification of a mural nodule or shadowing component in these tumours is found much more often after puberty.[50]

Hair floating on sebum is strongly reflective and may produce shadowing distally which obscures the tissues deep to it. In this case only the anterior margin of the dermoid will be visualised giving rise to the 'tip of the iceberg' sign in which most of the volume of the mass is not seen.[51] It should be noted here that the stool filled rectosigmoid colon can produce a similar appearance, at least in the

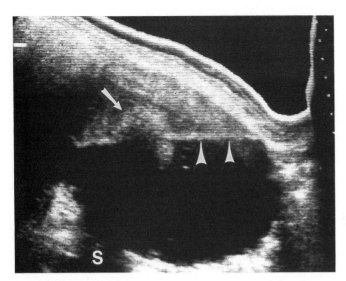

Fig. 39 **Dermoid.** This classic dermoid displays a fluid/debris level (arrowheads) probably representing hair floating on sebum with a highly reflective focus of calcium (arrow) which produces an acoustic shadow (S).

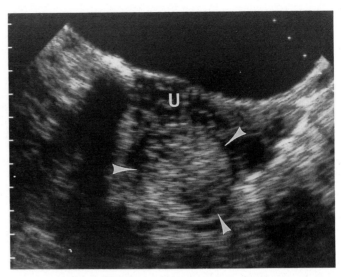

Fig. 41 **Dermoid.** When a dermoid is comprised almost entirely of solid soft tissue, a moderately reflective mass (arrowheads) such as this results. U – uterus.

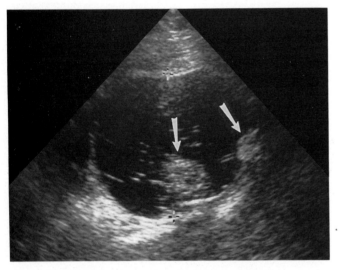

Fig. 40 **Cystic dermoid.** Two foci of solid tissue (arrows) are seen in the periphery of this largely cystic dermoid. These represent the so-called 'dermoid plug' phenomenon.

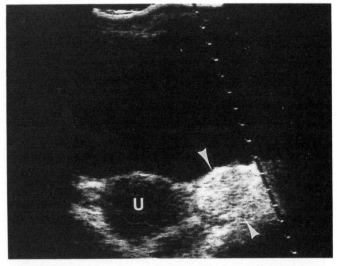

Fig. 42 **Dermoid.** A markedly reflective pattern without acoustic shadowing is produced by a dermoid which is mostly composed of fat (arrowheads). Compare this echo pattern to that of the muscle of the uterus (U).

transverse plane. Sagittal views should demonstrate the linear pattern of the colon thus distinguishing it from a dermoid.

By virtue of the broad range of appearances of ovarian dermoids the differential diagnosis includes haemorrhagic ovarian cyst, epithelial neoplasm, tubo-ovarian abscess, pedunculated leiomyoma, ectopic gestation and endometrioma to list only the more common conditions (Figs 41 to 43).[52] Sacrococcygeal teratoma is a mass of equally heterogeneous composition and, particularly when large, can simulate an ovarian dermoid.

Malignant changes in ovarian dermoids are not common and tend to occur mainly in post-menopausal patients with a reported frequency of 2% to 4%. Unfortunately there are no specific ultrasound signs which allow differentiation between benign and malignant teratomas (Fig. 44), unless liver metastases and ascites can be demonstrated (Figs 45 to 47).[45]

Sex cord – stromal tumours The hormonally active tumours constitute approximately 10% of all ovarian tumours and 2% of malignant neoplasms.[53] With one exception (the thecoma), these tumours of the ovary show no distinguishing ultrasound features to allow definitive identification.

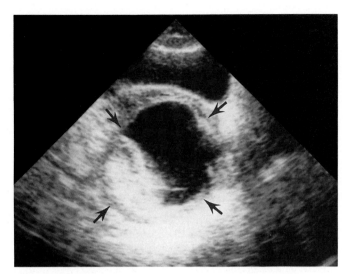

Fig. 43 Dermoid. The echo-free portion of this dermoid was sanguinous fluid and the reflective component a mixture of hair and caseous material. The arrows indicate the outline of the mass.

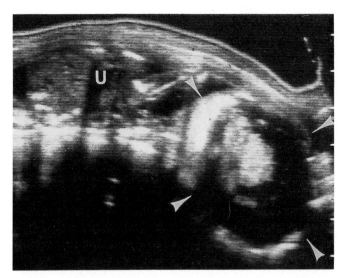

Fig. 45 Complex dermoid. This large complex dermoid (arrowheads) was initially thought to represent a bulging amniotic sac with fetal small parts in this patient who was 23 weeks pregnant. Gentle pressure demonstrated that the dermoid moved independently of the uterus (U).

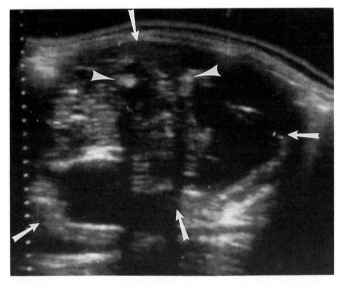

Fig. 44 Teratoma. This large teratoma (arrows) in a 13-year-old was a teratocarcinoma grade I. It contains a mixture of heterogeneous cystic and solid elements including foci of calcification (arrowheads).

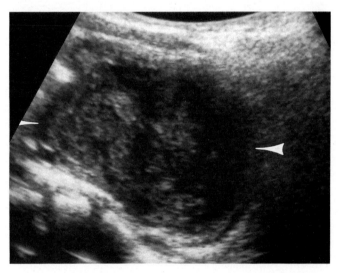

Fig. 46 Embryonal cell sarcoma. Neoplasms other than ovarian may be indistinguishable from those arising from the ovary. This embryonal cell sarcoma (arrowheads) was of indeterminate origin in the pelvis; the mixed texture is similar to that of many ovarian tumours.

Thecomas, which occur in the post-menopausal age group, are reported to produce extensive acoustic shadowing involving the entire extent of the tumour. No obvious explanation has been offered for this phenomenon. Thecomas are unilateral and are histologically benign.[54,55]

Granulosa cell tumours produce oestrogen in post-menopausal patients; although solid when small, they may become cystic and septated when larger and be difficult to distinguish by ultrasound from epithelial neoplasms of the ovary, or even pedunculated fibroids of the uterus.[56]

Masculinisation is produced by Sertoli-Leydig cell tumours of the ovary; they account for less than 0.5% of ovarian neoplasms and display a non-specific ultrasound appearance.

Fibromas of the ovary may occur in both pre- and post-menopausal patients; they constitute about 5% of ovarian neoplasms. Although they are generally echo-poor fibromas attenuate the sound beam quite markedly (Fig. 48). Enlarging to 5 to 10 cm and beyond, they can be associated with ascites and pleural effusion (Meig's syndrome) in a small percent of cases (1% to 3%).[57,58] Although Brenner tumours are histologically classified as

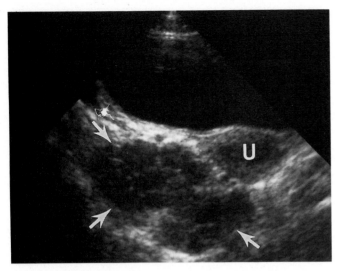

Fig. 47   Neurofibromas. Underscoring the wide variety of tumourous conditions which may present as adnexal masses is this lobular, echo-poor mass in the right adnexal region (arrows) which are neurofibromas. U – uterus.

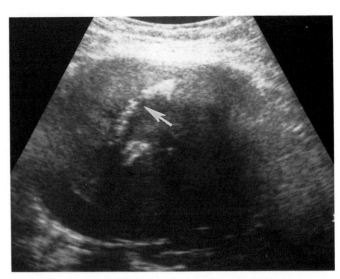

Fig. 49   Brenner tumour. The solid, echo-poor but attenuating character of this large Brenner tumour is indistinguishable from that of an ovarian fibroma. As here, Brenner tumours occasionally contain peripheral calcification (arrow).

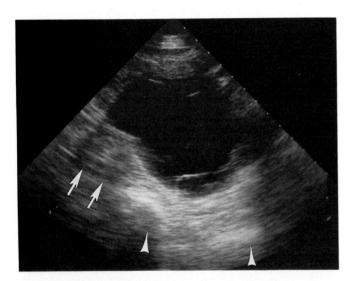

Fig. 48   Cystadenofibroma. This mass proved to be a serous cystadenofibroma at histological examination. Note that some areas demonstrate enhanced through transmission (arrowheads) while others, despite an echo-poor texture, attenuate most of the beam (arrows).

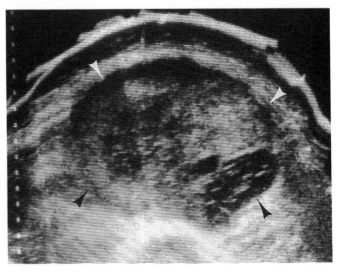

Fig. 50   Endometrioid carcinoma. Although it may have large areas of cyst formation, endometrioid carcinoma is characteristically solid as in this case (arrowheads).

epithelial neoplasms they are ultrasonically indistinguishable from fibromas, being solid, echo-poor and with good transmission. They occasionally contain peripheral calcifications (Fig. 49).[59]

Endometrioid carcinoma   Accounting for approximately 20% of ovarian malignancies, endometrioid carcinoma usually shows a solid appearance with areas of necrosis and/or haemorrhage in a significant number of cases (Fig. 50). This pattern is unlike that of the epithelial tumours of the ovary and should raise the possibility of endometrioid histology. It has been suggested that long-standing endometriosis predisposes to this malignancy but

this concept is not universally accepted.[60,61] It is true, however, that the histology of endometrioid carcinoma is quite similar to that of endometrial carcinoma of the uterus.[62]

Secondary ovarian neoplasms

The original description of the Krukenberg tumour was of metastases to the ovary from signet ring cell mucin-producing malignancies of the gastrointestinal tract, chiefly the stomach. Over the years the term 'Krukenberg tumour' has come to be applied to a variety of malignancies which metastasise to the ovary, notably breast, lung, endometrium and the gastrointestinal tract. Metastatic deposits to the ovary account for approximately 10% of malignancies of the ovary.[63,64]

The ultrasound appearance of ovaries enlarged by metastatic tumours is variable, but a predominant solid component is generally sufficient to direct the diagnosis away from the more common cystadenomatous disease with its predominantly fluid structure and multiple septations (Fig. 51). No specific appearance of the ovaries at ultrasound enables identification of the primary malignancy.

The lymphoproliferative disorders, lymphoma and leukaemia, can also involve the ovary. Echo-poor enlargement of one or both ovaries is occasionally seen in leukaemia but more often in lymphoma, chiefly non-Hodgkin's and Burkitt's, as opposed to Hodgkin's disease (Fig. 52).[65,66] Lymphadenopathy elsewhere such as the retroperitoneum may serve to suggest this possibility. Involvement of the uterus may blend together with enlarged ovaries to form a lobular echo-poor mass with indistinct borders between the individual organs. Computed tomography is the method most often employed for monitoring regression of disease with chemotherapy but ultrasound can also be used to monitor shrinkage of the tumour.

Adnexal pathology

Pelvic inflammatory disease

A number of factors predispose to the development of pelvic inflammatory disease. Sexually transmitted infections, foreign bodies (e.g. intra-uterine contraceptive devices), and non-sterile instrumentation (e.g. septic abortion) are among the most common factors. Neisseria, chlamydia and streptococcal infections are frequently implicated and clini-

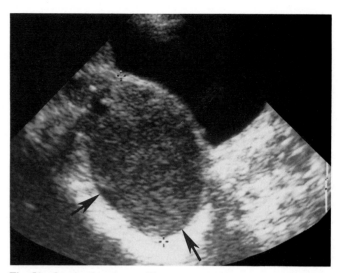

Fig. 52 Ovarian lymphoma. Homogeneous echo-poor enlargement of the ovary (arrows) is a typical pattern of involvement by leukaemia and lymphoma. This 8-year-old girl was found to have non-Hodgkin's lymphoma.

cal findings include pelvic pain, vaginal discharge, pyrexia, gastrointestinal symptoms and leukocytosis.

The ultrasound findings of early pelvic inflammatory disease (PID) may be minimal. Beginning as an endometritis from an ascending infection, PID may be manifest as mild uterine enlargement with or without a small fluid collection within the endometrial canal.[67] However, since a small amount of free fluid is a frequent normal finding in the pelvis of a female of childbearing age, this observation is of little diagnostic significance. Enlargement of the ovaries and thickening of the adnexal tissues has been described in PID but is difficult to identify with confidence.

With a clinical picture of PID but without demonstrable findings at ultrasound, antibiotic treatment should not be delayed. The role of ultrasound will have been of value in excluding a frank abscess.[68]

With progression of the disease, ultrasound will demonstrate irregularly marginated fluid collections or complex masses in the adnexae and/or cul-de-sac representing abscess formation (Fig. 53). Internal echoes are frequent within the fluid collections as a result of highly proteinaceous material or cellular debris (Fig. 54). It is frequently difficult or impossible to identify the ovaries separately from the inflammatory mass as they, along with the fallopian tubes, have been engulfed in the formation of what is now a tubo-ovarian abscess. The outlines of the uterus are commonly also obscured (Figs 55 and 56).

The occluded tube frequently produces a characteristic picture of a figure eight-shaped fluid collection, often with internal echoes which may be gravity-dependent (Figs 57 and 58). This represents a pyosalpinx and requires surgical drainage as does any other definable adnexal fluid collection. Some investigators have reported good results with

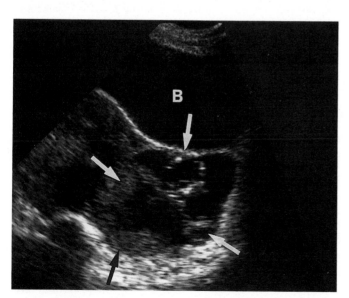

Fig. 51 Krukenberg tumour. Irregular, heterogenous enlargement of the ovary (arrows) by metastatic adenocarcinoma.

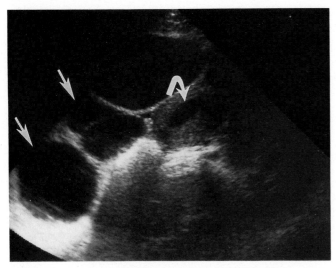

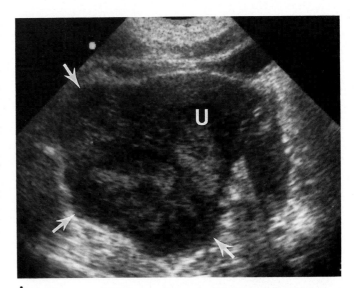

A

Fig. 53 Tubo-ovarian abscesses. Multilocular fluid collections (arrows) are seen in the right adnexa representing tubo-ovarian abscesses. The uterus contains an empty fluid filled sac (curved arrow) due to a missed abortion secondary to the inflammatory process.

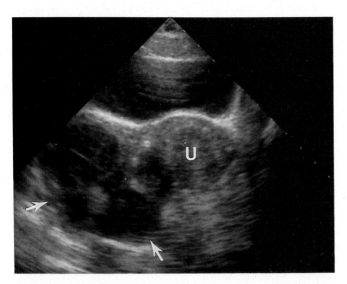

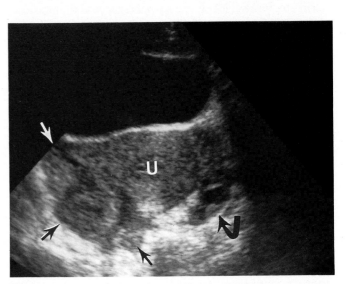

B

Fig. 55 Tubo-ovarian abscess. A: Large, poorly marginated complex mass in the right adnexa (arrows) represents a tubo-ovarian abscess obscuring the border of the uterus (U). **B:** After 5 days of intensive intravenous antibiotic therapy the inflammatory mass (arrows) is much diminished. Curved arrow – left ovary, U – uterus.

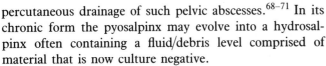

Fig. 54 Inflammatory mass. A large complex mass occupies the right adnexa (arrows), with the inflammatory process engulfing the tube, ovary, and broad ligament. U – uterus.

percutaneous drainage of such pelvic abscesses.[68–71] In its chronic form the pyosalpinx may evolve into a hydrosalpinx often containing a fluid/debris level comprised of material that is now culture negative.

The ultrasound finding of a complex pelvic mass most often defies interpretation in the absence of clinical information as such a picture can be produced by a wide variety of markedly different pathological processes. Epithelial neoplasms of the ovary (benign or malignant), haemorrhagic ovarian cysts, necrotic uterine leiomyomata, endometriomas, haematomata and ovarian dermoids repre-

sent some of the more common differential diagnostic considerations (Fig. 59).

Chronic pelvic inflammatory disease may cause a loss of the normal mobility of bowel and other pelvic structures because of peritoneal and mesenteric adhesions (Fig. 60). Gentle compression with the transducer may prove useful in demonstrating the lack of normal motion. A major contributing factor to infertility, PID is apparently on the increase. Its effects upon tubal patency and motility are significant and difficult to overcome.

It must also be remembered that not all inflammatory

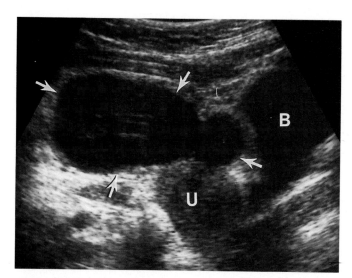

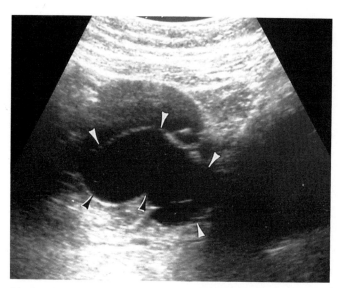

Fig. 56 Multilocular tubo-ovarian abscess. With the passage of several days and continuation of antibiotic therapy this multilocular tubo-ovarian abscess (arrows) became more sharply marginated. U – uterus, B – bladder.

Fig. 58 Hydrosalpinx, particularly when chronic, may assume a figure eight configuration, as in this patient (arrowheads).

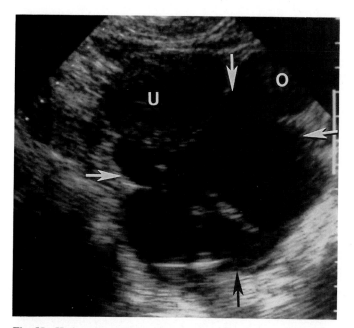

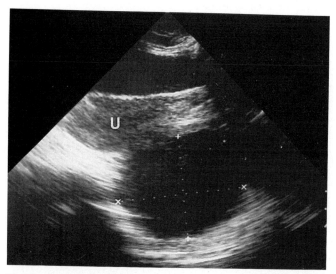

Fig. 57 Hydrosalpinx. The multilocular cystic mass (arrows) in the left adnexa and cul-de-sac represents a hydrosalpinx, the ultrasound appearance being produced by multiple folds of the distended fallopian tube. U – uterus, O – left ovary.

Fig. 59 Haematoma. Within the differential diagnosis of cystic or complex pelvic masses haematomas are ubiquitous. This largely cystic haematoma (cursors) resulted from continued bleeding following caesarean section.

processes found in the pelvis are of gynaecological origin. Inflammatory bowel disease such as Crohn's disease, ruptured appendicitis and diverticulitis may all produce complex pelvic masses indistinguishable from those found in PID.

Endometriosis

Endometriosis is primarily a condition of young Caucasian women estimated to occur in 5% to 20% of women of childbearing age. It is implicated as a major causative factor in 40% of women presenting with infertility. Endometriosis has been reported in 10% to 25% of laparotomies in patients of menstrual age.[72–74] The presenting clinical picture of endometriosis includes infertility (defined as failure to conceive after 1 year of unprotected intercourse), dysmenorrhoea, abdominal pain, and an abdominal mass. Since implants of endometrial tissue can be found in a wide range of locations, reports of dysuria, bowel symptoms and even haemoptysis and pneumothorax are extant indicating involvement of these organ systems.[75–77]

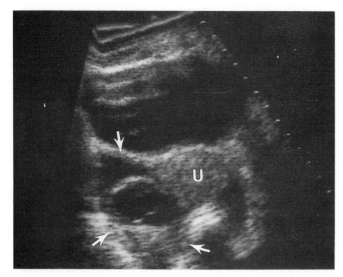

Fig. 60 Multiple adherent bowel loops. Occasionally, the appearance of a complex pelvic mass may be produced by post-inflammatory or post-surgical adhesion of multiple bowel loops, as in this case. The apparent right adnexal mass (arrows) was produced by multiple adherent bowel loops; the appearance persisted unchanged over 3 days. At operation, no focal mass was identified. U – uterus.

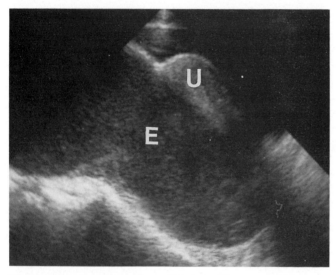

Fig. 61 Bilocular endometrioma. This large bilocular endometrioma (E) is filled with low level echoes representing small fragments of clot breakdown. Note the excellent through transmission of sound characteristic of any blood filled structure. U – uterus.

Two general morphological types of endometriosis are recognised, a diffuse form and a tumefactive pattern. By far the more common is the diffuse variety which consists of small, discrete implants of endometrial tissue on the serosal surfaces of both abdominal and pelvic viscera and peritoneum. These foci are described at laparoscopy as 'powder burns' on the normally smooth and glistening surfaces; they are readily identified under laparoscopy but are invisible to ultrasound. Reports of a diffuse increase in the

reflectivity of the pelvis and increased arterial pulsations in the region as indicators of the diffuse form of endometriosis have not been widely reproducible and it is generally considered that ultrasound is of minimal value in this context.[60] Since ultrasound is of such limited value in the common diffuse form of endometriosis, screening without a clinically palpable mass has a low yield.[73]

Endometriotic cysts, or endometriomas, result from cyclical haemorrhage of functioning endometrial tissue into a confined space. Varying in size from only a centimetre to large, relatively well-circumscribed masses of 10 to 15 cm, endometriomas are most often complex with low level internal echoes, sometimes gravity-dependent but occasionally in the form of internal septations (Fig. 61). The proportion of internal echoes tends to decrease over time. Throughout their course, endometriomas display enhanced through transmission of sound despite the extensive internal echoes (Fig. 62).[78–80]

Because of the cyclical nature of the process, multiple endometriomas may exhibit differing ultrasonic characteristics as they are at different stages of resolution of the contained fluid (Figs 63 and 64). This variegated appearance places endometriomas in the rather lengthy differential diagnosis of complex pelvic masses which includes epithelial ovarian neoplasms, tubo-ovarian abscesses, dermoids and necrotic uterine leiomyomata among the more common pathologies. Endometriosis, focal or diffuse, can also occur in the patient who has undergone hysterectomy.

Para-ovarian cyst

The para-ovarian cyst represents a remnant of Gartner's duct and appears in the adnexa as a simple, smooth-walled

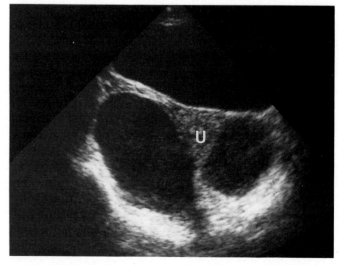

Fig. 62 Bilateral endometriomas. This transverse scan demonstrates bilateral endometriomas, both with low level internal echoes. U – uterus.

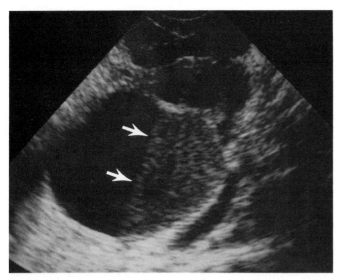

Fig. 63 Endometrioma. On this trans-vaginal view of an endometrioma, the particulate portions of the clot have settled out to form a fluid/debris level (arrows).

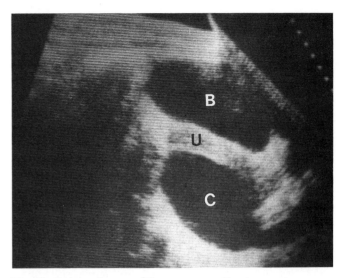

Fig. 65 Para-ovarian cyst. There are no specific ultrasound characteristics to distinguish this para-ovarian cyst (C) located in the cul-de-sac from a simple or functional cyst of the ovary. Its persistence will generally require surgery. U – uterus, B – urinary bladder.

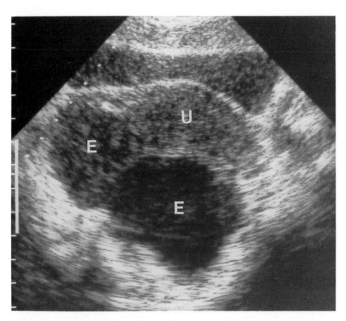

Fig. 64 Endometriomas. The endometriomas in this patient (E) are at different stages in their natural history with considerably more echoes still remaining in the mass on the right as compared with that occupying the cul-de-sac. Again, however, note that through transmission of sound is excellent for both. U – uterus.

cyst which may be indistinguishable from a functional cyst of the ovary (Fig. 65). As with functional ovarian cysts, haemorrhage will produce low level internal echoes. Use of the trans-vaginal probe may allow recognition of a para-ovarian cyst as separable from the ovary, thus indicating the true diagnosis. Para-ovarian cysts are most commonly 3 to 5 cm in diameter and do not change with the menstrual cycle, as do functional cysts.[81,82] Failure of spontaneous regression of such a cyst will most often lead to surgical removal to ensure that it is not an epithelial neoplasm, particularly in the older premenopausal patient. In the post-menopausal age group, in which functional cysts should not occur, adnexal masses, cystic or solid, should be investigated further. Para-ovarian cysts are histologically benign.

Ectopic pregnancy

The incidence of ectopic pregnancy continues to rise in developed countries secondary to the use of intra-uterine contraceptive devices, the increased incidence of pelvic inflammatory disease and the more common use of tubal surgery for infertility or reversal of sterilisation.[83,84] It is, paradoxically, the successful treatment of pelvic infections with the newer antibiotic regimens which contributes to the frequency of ectopic pregnancies by preserving tubal patency in the presence of adhesions which render tubal mobility abnormal. Endometriosis, with the induction of fibrosis and adhesions, is also thought to be a predisposing factor for ectopic pregnancy.

The current incidence is reported to be 1.4% of all pregnancies; of the women who conceive following treatment for an ectopic pregnancy (60%), 10% will have another ectopic gestation, a fact which requires early ultrasound confirmation of the intra-uterine location of a subsequent pregnancy in such an individual.

Confirmation of the presence of an intra-uterine gestation with the trans-vaginal probe should be possible at about 32 days menstrual age (i.e. from the first day of the last menstrual period) or a serum beta HCG of 1000 mIU (Second International Standard).[85] Visualisation of either an embryo or yolk sac (which is of fetal origin) is proof of an intra-uterine pregnancy; the so-called 'double decidual sac sign' is also excellent, if not absolute, evidence for an intra-uterine location of the pregnancy (see Chs 8 and 9). Identification of an intra-uterine pregnancy is the most useful function of ultrasound as it rules out, for all practical purposes, the presence of an ectopic gestation. The incidence of an intra-uterine pregnancy with an extra-uterine twin is now estimated to be 1 in 7000 at most; it would, therefore, be impractical and unrealistic to manage every possible ectopic pregnancy on the expectation of such a scenario.

The ultrasound findings in ectopic pregnancy are widely variable and, unless an intra-uterine gestation is identified, cannot be excluded by ultrasound. The differential diagnosis, without consideration of the clinical setting, includes endometriosis, tubo-ovarian abscess, haemorrhagic ovarian cyst and ovarian torsion.[86] Some 20% of ectopic gestations present with no ultrasound findings whatever; that is to say that the images are those of a normal, non-pregnant pelvis with no evidence of masses, fluid collections or other adnexal abnormalities.

Correlation with the serum beta HCG is of particular importance in such a situation as a pregnancy, normal or ectopic, at less than 4 weeks menstrual age may not be visualised. If, then, the HCG level is commensurate with a 3 week gestation, observation may be the appropriate course of action.[87]

The trans-vaginal transducer has made it possible to detect a living embryo in 17% of ectopic pregnancies (Fig. 66).[88] A 'tubal ring', representing the reflective chorion can be identified on trans-vaginal scanning in as many as 68% of patients.[89] It has been further observed that identification of this sac-like adnexal ring indicates

functioning trophoblasts and an intact fallopian tube (Fig. 67). The finding of an adnexal mass of complex texture raises the suspicion of tubal haematoma or frank rupture.[90] Free fluid is also more easily detected. A small amount of fluid in the cul-de-sac or adnexa may be a normal finding in the non-pregnant pelvis; however, moderate to large amounts of fluid are indicative of abnormality.[91,92] The presence of recognisable echoes within the fluid suggests a haemoperitoneum with a high risk for ectopic gestation. Echogenic fluid was identified in 56% of patients with proved ectopic pregnancies in a recent study.[93]

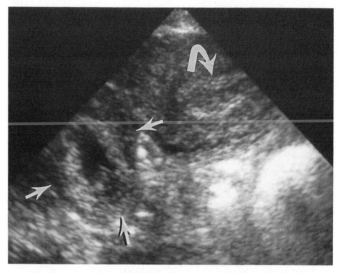

Fig. 67   Ectopic. Curved arrow indicates a poorly formed intra-uterine sac-like structure representing a reactive endometrium felt to result from sloughing of hypertrophied endometrium. The unruptured ectopic gestation (arrows) is seen in the right posterior adnexa.

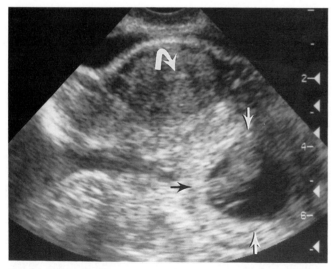

Fig. 66   Unruptured ectopic gestation. A living, unruptured ectopic gestation is identified in the left posterior adnexa (arrows). The endometrial echo (curved arrow) is seen confirming an empty uterus.

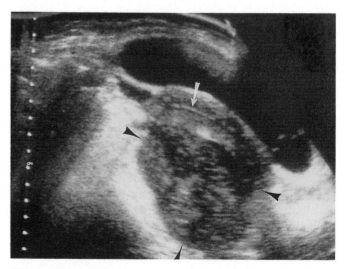

Fig. 68   Ruptured ectopic gestation. In this sagittal transabdominal scan a complex mass (arrowheads) is seen occupying the cul-de-sac and is haemorrhage from a ruptured ectopic gestation. The endometrial echo (arrow) confirms an empty uterus.

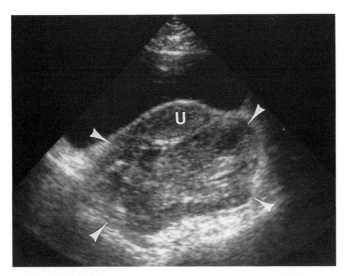

Fig. 69 Complex mass. A ruptured interstitial pregnancy has resulted in a complex mass (arrowheads) filling the cul-de-sac. The small empty uterus (U) is identified.

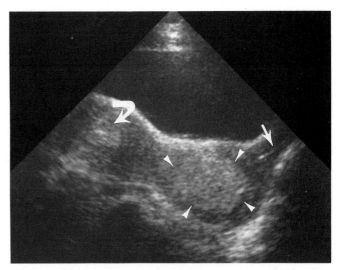

Fig. 71 Haemorrhage in a cervical ectopic gestation. A reflective mass (arrowheads) occupies the region of the endocervical canal and represents haemorrhage in a cervical ectopic gestation lying between the vaginal canal (arrow) and the empty endometrial canal (curved arrow).

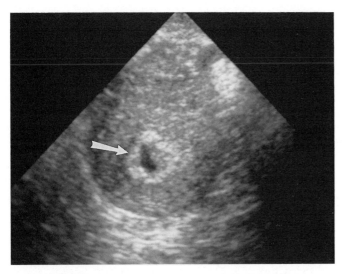

Fig. 70 Intra-uterine pseudosac. The intra-uterine pseudosac (arrow) accompanying an ectopic pregnancy can be quite confusing in its appearance as in this case. However, the double decidual sign is absent with a pseudosac.

gestation sac is identified less frequently by the trans-vaginal route than by abdominal scanning, reaching only 8.8% in one study.[98] Doppler evaluation of the intra-uterine sac has shown some promise in the differentiation between true sacs and pseudosacs.[99]

The vast majority of ectopic pregnancies occur in the ampullary portion of the tube. Approximately 1% to 2% may be situated in the interstitial segment of the tube (i.e. the intramural portion) and the cervical canal (Fig. 71). In both of these sites growth can persist for longer so that when the ectopic ruptures, haemorrhage is more catastrophic. Abdominal ectopics are quite rare (and unsuspected in 60% of cases) and can grow to surprisingly large sizes. They are characterised by the absence of amniotic fluid, extension of fetal parts that often lie close to the maternal abdominal wall, extra-uterine placenta and an empty uterus. Abdominal pregnancy is uncommon but well-documented.[100–103]

Leakage of blood from the fimbriated end of the fallopian tube is thought to account for the haemoperitoneum in most women, though frank tubal rupture occurs in only 10% to 15% of cases (Figs 68 and 69).[94,95]

In some 20% of patients with ectopic gestations a ring-like structure is identified within the endometrial cavity (Fig. 70).[96] Mimicking a true gestation sac in some respects, this 'pseudosac' is thought to represent the hyperplastic endometrium responding to the increased hormone levels of the ectopic. Lack of a double decidual reaction will generally distinguish the pseudosac from a true gestation sac.[97] It has been suggested that a pseudo-

Infertility

Infertility is estimated to affect one in six couples with ovarian dysfunction accounting for some 15% to 25% of female infertility.[104] Ultrasound and, in particular, trans-vaginal scanning, has become a corner-stone in the approach to infertility with its ability to identify hydrosalpinges, endometriomas and other mechanical impediments to conception. Ultrasound assessment of tubal patency by monitoring intra-uterine fluid injection, with documentation of peritoneal spillage, constitutes an ultrasound hysterosalpingogram.[105]

Monitoring of follicular development for timed insemination or oocyte retrieval in an in-vitro fertilisation programme is easily and precisely accomplished with ultrasound.[106] Trans-vaginal ultrasound guided oocyte retrieval has been shown to be as effective as its laparoscopic counterpart with less discomfort, expense and time.[107,108] Maximum efficiency with minimum interobserver error is achieved by having the same sonographer scan a patient on each visit. In general, daily monitoring is begun on or about the ninth day of the cycle and carried through until ovulation has occurred. Sudden shrinkage or

disappearance of the follicle, sometimes accompanied by the appearance of internal echoes representing haemorrhage, marks ovulation.

The follicle grows at about 2 to 3 mm per day from the ninth day of the menstrual cycle to reach a mature diameter of 17 to 24 mm at ovulation.[109,110] Identification of the precise time of ovulation is somewhat difficult, even with current techniques.[111] Oocyte retrieval, either via transvesical or trans-vaginal routes, is best accomplished under ultrasound guidance (see Ch. 6).[10]

REFERENCES

1 Ivarsson S A, Nilsson K O, Persson P H. Ultrasonography of the pelvic organs in prepubertal and postpubertal girls. Arch Dis Child 1983; 58: 352

2 Orsini L F, Salardi S, Pilu G, et al. Pelvic organs in premenarcheal girls: real-time ultrasonography. Radiology 1984; 153: 113

3 Munn C S, Kiser L C, Wetzner S M, Baer J E. Ovary volume in young and premenopausal adults: US determination. Radiology 1986; 159: 731

4 Nicolini U, Ferrazzi E, Bellotti M, et al. The contribution of sonographic evaluation of ovarian size in patients with polycystic ovarian disease. J Ultrasound Med 1985; 4: 347–351

5 Sample W F, Lippe B M, Gyepes M T. Gray-scale ultrasonography of the normal female pelvis. Radiology 1977; 125: 477

6 Cohen H L, Tice H M, Mandel F S. Ovarian volumes measured by US: bigger than we think. Radiology 1990; 177: 189–192

7 Hall D A, McCarthy K A, Kopans D B. Sonographic visualization of the normal postmenopausal ovary. J Ultrasound Med 1986; 5: 9

8 Rankin R N, Hutton L C. Ultrasound in the ovarian hyperstimulation syndrome. JCU 1981; 9: 473

9 Hackeloer B. The role of ultrasound in female infertility management. Ultrasound Med Biol 1984; 10: 35

10 Bonilla-Musoles F, Pardo G, Perez-Gil M, Serra V, Pellicer A. Abdominal ultrasonography versus transvaginal scanning: accuracy in follicular development. Evaluation and prediction for oocyte retrieval in stimulated cycles. JCU 1989; 17: 469–473

11 Andreotti R F, Thompson G H, Janowitz W, et al. Endovaginal and transabdominal sonography of ovarian follicles. J Ultrasound Med 1989; 8: 555–560

12 Hilgers T W, Dvorak A D, Tamisiea D F, Ellis R L, Yaksich PJ. Sonographic definition of the empty follicle syndrome. J Ultrasound Med 1989; 8: 411–416

13 Ganong W F. The gonads: development and function of the reproductive system. Review of medical physiology. 7th edition. Los Altos CA: Lange. 1975: p 310–341

14 Shawker T H, Garra B S, Loriaux D L, Cutler G B, Ross J L. Ultrasonography of Turner's syndrome. J Ultrasound Med 1986; 5: 125–129

15 Sohval A R. The syndrome of pure gonadal dysgenesis. Am J Med 1965; 38: 615

16 Lippe B M. Primary ovarian failure. In: Kaplan S A. ed. Clinical pediatric and adolescent endocrinology. Philadelphia: WB Saunders. 1982: p 286–287

17 Reynolds T, Hill M C, Glassman L M. Sonography of hemorrhagic ovarian cysts. JCU 1986; 14: 449

18 Baltarowich O H, Kurtz A B, Pasto M E, et al. The spectrum of sonographic findings in hemorrhagic ovarian cysts. AJR 1987; 148: 901–905

19 Suita S, Ikeda K, Koyamagi T, et al. Neonatal ovarian cyst diagnosed antenatally: report of two patients. JCU 1984; 12: 517

20 Nussbaum A R, Sanders R C, Hartman D S, et al. Neonatal ovarian cysts: sonographic-pathologic correlation. Radiology 1988; 168: 817–821

21 Stein I F, Leventhal M L. Amenorrhea associated with bilateral polycystic ovaries. Am J Obstet Gynecol 1935; 29: 181–191

22 Rottem S, Levit N, Thaler I, et al. Classification of ovarian lesions by high-frequency transvaginal sonography. JCU 1990; 18: 359–363

23 Yeh H C, Futterweit W, Thornton J C. Polycystic ovarian disease: US features in 104 patients. Radiology 1987; 163: 111

24 Orsini L F, Venturoli S, Lorusso R, et al. Ultrasonic findings in polycystic ovarian disease. Fertil Steril 1985; 43: 709

25 Hann L E, Hall D A, McArdle C R, Seibel M. Polycystic ovarian disease: sonographic spectrum. Radiology 1984; 150: 531

26 Hall D A. Sonographic appearance of the normal ovary, of polycystic ovary disease, and of functional ovarian cysts. Semin Ultrasound 1983; 4: 149–165

27 Jaffe R, Abramowicz J, Eckstein N, et al. Sonographic monitoring of ovarian volume during LHRH analogue therapy in women with polycystic ovarian syndrome. J Ultrasound Med 1988; 7: 203–206 7: 203–206

28 Hague W M, Adams J, Reeders S T, Peto T E A, Jacobs H S. Familial polycystic ovaries: a genetic disease? Clin Endocrinol 1988; 29: 593–605

29 Polson D W, Wadsworth J, Adams J, Franks S. Polycystic ovaries – a common finding in normal women. Lancet 1988; 1: 870–872

30 Adams J, Polson D W, Franks S. Prevalence of polycystic ovaries in women with anovulation and idiopathic hirsutism. BMJ 1986; 293: 355–359

31 Hague W M, Adams J, Rodda C, et al. The prevalence of polycystic ovaries in patients with congenital adrenal hyperplasia and their close relatives. Clin Endocrinol 1990; 33: 501–510

32 Goldstein D P, Berkowitz R J, Cohen S M. The current management of molar pregnancy. Curr Probl Obstet Gynecol 1979; 3: 1

33 Geishovel F, Skubsch U, Zabel G, et al. Ultrasonographic and hormonal studies in physiologic and insufficient menstrual cycles. Fertil Steril 1983; 39: 277

34 Queenan J T, O'Brien J D, Bains L M, et al. Ultrasound scanning of ovaries to detect ovulation in women. Fertil Steril 1980; 34: 99

35 Ritchie W G M. Sonographic evaluation of normal and induced ovulation. Radiology 1986; 161: 1

36 Blankstein J, Shalev J, Saadon T, et al. Ovarian hyperstimulation syndrome: prediction by number and size of preovulatory follicles. Fertil Steril 1986; 47: 597–602

37 Polishuk W Z, Schenker J G. Ovarian hyperstimulation syndrome. Fertil Steril 1969; 20: 443

38 Golan A, Ron-El R, Herman A, et al. Ovarian hyperstimulation syndrome: an update review. Obstet Gynecol Surv 198; 44: 430–440

39 Phillips H E, McGahan J P. Ovarian remnant syndrome. Radiology 1982; 142: 487

40 Warner M, Fleischer A, Edell S, et al. Uterine adnexal torsion: sonographic findings. Radiology 1985; 154: 773–775

41 Haller J O, Friedman A P, Schaffer R, Lebensart D P. The normal and abnormal ovary in childhood and adolescence. Semin Ultrasound 1983; 4: 213

42 Graif M, Itzchak Y. Sonographic evaluation of ovarian torsion in childhoood and adolescence. AJR 1988; 150: 647–649
43 Helvie M A, Silver T M. Ovarian torsion: sonographic evaluation. JCU 1989; 17: 327–332
44 Farrell T P, Boal D K, Teele R L, et al. Acute torsion of the normal uterine adnexa in children: sonographic demonstration. AJR 1982; 139: 1223–1225
45 Williams A G, Mettler F A, Wicks J D. Cystic and solid ovarian neoplasms. Semin Ultrasound 1983; 4: 166
46 Kliman L, Rome R M, Fortune D W. Low malignant potential tumors of the ovary; a study of 76 cases. Obstet Gynecol 1986; 68: 338–344
47 Buy J-N, Ghossain M A, Sciot C, Bazot M, Guinet C, et al. Epithelial tumors of the ovary: CT findings and correlation with US. Radiology 1991; 178: 811–818
48 Czernobilsky B. Common epithelial tumors of the ovary. In: Kurman R J. ed. Blaustein's pathology of the female genital tract. 3rd ed. New York: Springer-Verlag. 1987: p 560–606
49 Quinn S F, Erickson S, Black W C. Cystic ovarian teratomas: the sonographic appearance of the dermoid plug. Radiology 1985; 155: 477
50 Sisler C L, Siegel M J. Ovarian teratomas: a comparison of the sonographic appearance in prepubertal and postpubertal girls. AJR 1990; 154: 139–141
51 Gutman P H Jnr. In search of the elusive benign cystic ovarian teratoma: application of the ultrasound 'tip of the iceberg' sign. JCU 1977; 5: 403
52 Sheth S, Fishman E K, Buck J L, et al. The variable sonographic appearance of ovarian teratomas: correlation with CT. AJR 1988; 151: 331–334
53 Robbins S L, Cotran R S, Kumar V. eds. Female genital tract. In: Pathologic basis of disease. 3rd edition. Philadelphia: WB Saunders. 1984
54 Diakoumakis E, Vieux U, Seife B. Sonographic demonstration of thecoma: report of two cases. Am J Obstet Gynecol 1984; 150: 787
55 Yaghoobian J, Pinck R L. Ultrasound findings in thecoma of the ovary. JCU 1983; 11: 91
56 Novak E R, Woodruff J D. Novak's gynecologic and obstetrical pathology. 8th edition. Philadelphia: WB Saunders. 1979
57 Stephenson W M, Laing F C. Sonography of ovarian fibromas. AJR 1985; 144: 1239
58 Athey P A, Malone R S. Sonography of ovarian fibromas/thecomas. J Ultrasound Med 1987; 6: 431–436
59 Athey P A, Siegel M F. Sonographic features of Brenner tumor of the ovary. J Ultrasound Med 1987; 6: 367–372
60 Birnholz J C. Endometriosis and inflammatory disease. Semin Ultrasound 1983; 4: 184–192
61 Scully R E, Richardson C S, Barlow J F. The development of malignancies in endometriosis. Clin Obstet Gynecol 1966; 9: 384
62 Robbins S L, Cotran R S, Kumar V. Female genital tract. In: Pathologic basis of disease. 3rd edition. Philadelphia: WB Saunders. 1984: p 1142–1155
63 Peel K R. Benign and malignant tumors of the ovary. In: Whitfield C R. ed. Dewhurst's textbook of obstetrics and gynecology for postgraduates. Oxford: Blackwell Scientific Publications. 1986: p 733–754
64 Griffiths C T, Berkowitz R. The ovary. In: Kistner R W. ed. Gynecology: principles and practice. Chicago: Year Book Medical Publishers. 1986: p 289–377
65 Talerman A. Mesenchymal tumors and malignant lymphoma of the ovary. In: Blaustein. ed. Pathology of the female genital tract. 2nd edition. New York: Springer-Verlag. 1982: p 705–715
66 Bickers G H, Siebert J J, Anderson J C. Sonography of ovarian involvement in childhood acute lymphocytic leukemia. AJR 1981; 137: 399–401
67 Swayne L C, Love M B, Karasich S R. Pelvic inflammatory disease: sonographic-pathologic correlation. Radiology 1984; 151: 751–755
68 Nosher J L, Winchman H K, Needell G S. Transvaginal pelvic abscess drainage with ultrasound guidance. Radiology 1987; 165: 872
69 Tyrrel R T, Murphy F B, Bernardino M E. Tubo-ovarian abscesses: CT-guided percutaneous drainage. Radiology 1990;

175: 87–89
70 Worthen N J, Gunning J E. Percutaneous drainage of pelvic abscesses: management of the tubo-ovarian abscess. J Ultrasound Med 1986; 5: 551–556
71 Nosher J L, Needell G S, Amorosa J K, Krasna I H. Transrectal pelvic abscess drainage with sonographic guidance. AJR 1986; 146: 1047–1048
72 Dawood M Y. Endometriosis. In: Gold J F, Josimovich J B. eds. Gynecologic endocrinology. 4th edition. New York: Plenum Press. 1987: p 387
73 Friedman H, Vogelzang R L, Mendelson E B, Neiman H L, Cohen M. Endometriosis detection by ultrasound with laparoscopic correlation. Radiology 1985; 157: 217–220
74 Sample W F. Pelvic inflammatory disease and endometriosis. In: Sanders R C, James A E Jnr. eds. The principles and practice of ultrasonography in obstetrics and gynecology. 2nd edition. New York: Appleton-Century Crofts. 1979: 322–333
75 Gorell H A, Cyr D R, Wang K Y, Greer B E. Rectosigmoid endometriosis. Diagnosis using endovaginal sonography. J Ultrasound Med 1989; 8: 459–461
76 Kumar R, Haque A K, Cohen M S. Endometriosis of the urinary bladder: demonstration by sonography. JCU 1984; 12: 363–365
77 Im J-G, Kang H S, Choi B I, et al. Pleural endometriosis: CT and sonographic findings. AJR 1987; 148: 523–524
78 Athey P A, Diment D D. The spectrum of sonographic findings in endometrioma. J Ultrasound Med 1989; 8: 487
79 Deutsch A L, Gosink B B. Nonneoplastic gynecologic disorders. Semin Roentgenol 1982; 14: 269
80 Goldman S M, Minkin S I. Diagnosing endometriosis with ultrasound. Accuracy and specificity. J Reprod Med 1980; 25: 178
81 Alpern M, Sandler M, Madrazo B. Sonographic features of parovarian cysts and their complications. AJR 1984; 143: 157
82 Athey P, Cooper N. Sonographic features of parovarian cysts. AJR 1985; 144: 83
83 Loffer F D. The increasing problem of ectopic pregnancies and its impact on patients and physicians. J Reprod Med 1986; 31: 74–77
84 Filly R A. Ectopic pregnancy: the role of sonography. Radiology 1987; 162: 661–668
85 Nyberg D A, Mack L A, Laing F C, Jeffrey R B. Early pregnancy complications: endovaginal sonographic findings correlated with human chorionic gonadotrophin levels. Radiology 1988; 167: 619–622
86 Manor W F, Zweibel W J, Hanning R V, Raymond H W. Ectopic pregnancy and other causes of acute pelvic pain. Semin Ultrasound CT MR 1985; 6: 181–206
87 Peisner D B, Timor-Tritsch I E. The discriminatory zone of beta-hCG for vaginal probes. JCU 1990; 18: 280–285
88 Dashefsky S M, Lyons E A, Levi C S, Lindsay D J. Suspected ectopic pregnancy: endovaginal and transvescical US. Radiology 1988; 169: 181–184
89 Fleischer A C, Pennell R G, McKee M S, et al. Ectopic pregnancy: features at transvaginal sonography. Radiology 1990; 174: 375–378
90 Cacciatore B. Can the status of tubal pregnancy be predicted with transvaginal sonography. A prospective comparison of sonographic, surgical, and serum hCG findings. Radiology 1990; 177: 481–484
91 Romero R, Kadar N, Castro D, et al. The value of adnexal sonographic findings in the diagnosis of ectopic pregnancy. Am J Obstet Gynecol 1988; 158: 52–55
92 Mahony B S, Filly R A, Nyberg D A, et al. Sonographic evaluation of ectopic pregnancy. J Ultrasound Med 1985; 4: 221–228
93 Nyberg D A, Hughes M P, Mack L A, Wang K Y. Extrauterine findings of ectopic pregnancy at transvaginal US: importance of echogenic fluid. Radiology 1991; 178: 823–826
94 Cacciatore B, Stenman U-H, Ylostalo P. Comparison of abdominal and vaginal sonography in suspected ectopic pregnancy. Obstet Gynecol 1989; 73: 770–774
95 Bateman B G, Nunley W C, Kolp L A, Kitchin J D III, Felder R. Vaginal sonography findings and hCG dynamics of early intrauterine and tubal pregnancies. Obstet Gynecol 1990; 75: 421–427

96 Marks W M, Filly R A, Callen P W, Laing F C. The decidual cast of ectopic pregnancy: a confusing ultrasonographic appearance. Radiology 1979; 133: 341–344

97 Nyberg D A, Laing F C, Filly R A, et al. Ultrasonographic differentiation of the gestational sac of early intrauterine pregnancy from the pseudogestational sac of ectopic pregnancy. Radiology 1983; 146: 755–759

98 Hill L M, Kislak S, Martin J G. Transvaginal sonographic detection of the pseudogestational sac associated with ectopic pregnancy. Obstet Gynecol 1990; 75: 986–988

99 Dillon E H, Feyock A L, Taylor K J W. Pseudogestational sacs: Doppler US differentiation from normal or abnormal intrauterine pregnancies. Radiology 1990; 176: 359–364

100 Rahman M S, Al-Suleiman S A, Rahman J, Al-Sibai M H. Advanced abdominal pregnancy: observations in 10 cases. Obstet Gynecol 1981; 59(3): 366–372

101 Beacham W D, Hernquist W C, Beacham D W, et al. Abdominal pregnancy at Charity Hospital in New Orleans. Am J Obstet Gynecol 1962; 84: 1257–1270

102 Strafford J C, Ragan W D. Abdominal pregnancy: review of current management. Obstet Gynecol 1977; 50(5): 548–552

103 Stanley J H, Horger E O III, Fagan C J, Andriole J G, Fleischer A C. Sonographic findings in abdominal pregnancy. AJR 1986; 147: 1043–1046

104 Fleischer A C, Pittaway D, Wentz A, et al. The uses of sonography for monitoring ovarian follicular development. In: Ultrasound annual 1983. New York: Raven Press. 1983

105 Richman T S, Viscomi G N, deCherney A, et al. Fallopian tubal patency assessed by ultrasound following fluid injection. Radiology 1984; 152: 507–510

106 Feldberg D, Goldman J A, Ashkenazi J, et al. Transvaginal oocyte retrieval controlled by vaginal probe for in vitro fertilization: a comparative study. J Ultrasound Med 1988; 7: 339–343

107 Gonen Y, Blanker J, Casper R F. Transvaginal ultrasonically guided follicular aspiration: a comparative study with laparoscopically guided follicular aspiration. JCU 1990; 18: 257–261

108 Wiseman D A, Short W B, Pattinson H A, et al. Oocyte retrieval in an in-vitro fertilization – embryo transfer program: comparison of four methods. Radiology 1989; 173: 99–102

109 Mendelson E B, Friedman J, Neiman H L, et al. The role of imaging in infertility management. AJR 1985; 144: 415

110 Hull M E, Moghissi K S, Magyar D M, et al. Correlation of serum estradiol levels and ultrasound monitoring to assess follicular maturation. Fertil Steril 1986; 46: 42

111 Zandt-Stastny D, Thorsen M K, Middleton W D, et al. Inability of sonography to detect imminent ovulation. AJR 1989; 152: 91–95

Screening for ovarian and uterine cancer

Tom Bourne and Stuart Campbell

INTRODUCTION

Ovarian cancer is an insidious and intractable disease. The incidence in the UK increases with age to about 60 cases per 100 000 women per year, the cumulative risk up to 75 years being 1.3%.[1,2] The disease is responsible for 4.5% of deaths in women below the age of 60. The relationship between 5 year survival and disease stage, at the time of diagnosis, is well-known. At stage IV survival is less than 5% whilst at stage I it may be greater than 90%, even without chemotherapy.[3] The overall survival rate of the order of 20% reflects the fact that most women present with clinical signs at stages III and IV when often all that can be achieved is palliation. Over the past two decades these survival data have changed very little despite the introduction of new treatment regimens. Whilst it is possible that a breakthrough may be made in treatment, early diagnosis of ovarian cancer is probably the best approach to achieve a reduction in mortality and morbidity.

Ovarian cancer was responsible for more than 12 000 cancer deaths in the USA and over 4000 in the UK during 1990. This is more than for uterine and cervical cancer combined; this fact has, until recently, received limited media cover.

A questionnaire given to members of the British College of Obstetricians and Gynaecologists showed that at the time of hysterectomy only 50% of members would remove the ovaries from women aged over 50 years. Around half would not be influenced in their decision by a family history of gynaecological cancer.[4] This indicates a degree of ignorance about this disease even amongst professionals.

Screening principles

Screening has been described by Wald and Cuckle[5] as 'the identification amongst apparently healthy individuals of those who are sufficiently at risk of a specific disorder to justify a subsequent diagnostic test or procedure, or in certain circumstances, direct preventative action.' This description makes two fundamental points about the nature of screening. First that it is carried out on a seemingly healthy population, and second that it does not necessarily aim to make a diagnosis; rather it tries to identify a group that merits further investigation.

Any screening technique must be judged using standard indices of test performance:

a) the sensitivity or the detection rate of the disease, and the specificity, which is the ability of the test to identify the disease free state correctly;
b) the positive predictive value, which expresses the chances of an individual with a positive test result actually having the disease in question, and the negative predictive value; which gives the chance of a negative test predicting a disease free state;
c) the same data may be expressed as an odds ratio which is the chance in favour or against the presence of ovarian cancer at surgery in women with a positive screen result.

Sensitivity and specificity are by their nature related, and should not be considered in isolation. Because of the poor prognosis for ovarian cancer when detected late, any screening procedure must have a high pick up for early disease if any impact on the mortality and morbidity of the disease is to be achieved.

If we refer to the WHO criteria for screening[6] for a disease, the present situation as regards ovarian cancer leaves many questions unanswered.

Principles of screening (WHO[6])

a) The condition sought should pose an important public health problem.
b) The natural history of the disease should be well-understood.
c) There should be a recognisable early stage.
d) The treatment of the disease at an early stage should be of more benefit than treatment started at a later stage.
e) There should be a suitable test.
f) The test should be acceptable to the population.
g) There should be adequate facilities for the diagnosis and treatment of abnormalities detected.
h) For diagnosis of insidious onset, screening should be repeated at intervals determined by the natural history of the disease.
i) The chance of physical or psychological harm to those screened should be less than the likelihood of benefit.
j) The cost of a screening programme should be balanced against the benefit it provides.

Clearly one of the most difficult problems with ovarian cancer is the lack of knowledge regarding pathogenesis. It is not clear whether benign lesions have malignant potential, or indeed what the initial stages of ovarian cancer involve.

The possibility that detecting the disease at an earlier stage may not change prognosis has also to be considered. Survival from the time of diagnosis at stage I is greater than for more advanced disease, regardless of intervention. This is called the 'lead time' and represents the extra time during which the disease is observable from the time of diagnosis.

Thus early detection may seem to prolong survival, whilst in fact the time of death remains unchanged. This 'lead time bias' is an important factor. However it is considered that for ovarian cancer, the improved prognosis for women in whom intervention has been possible at an earlier stage[3] is a true reflection of altered outcome. Another factor to consider when interpreting the results of screening is that those cancers detected at stage I may be inherently less aggressive, and so the outcome may have been good regardless of the earlier intervention.

Possible screening techniques

Radio-immunoscintigraphy This technique relies on the presence of surface antigens on the tumour reflecting qualitative differences between cancer cells and normal cells. Monoclonal antibodies directed towards one of these proteins is labelled with a radioactive isotope and given to the patient intravenously. The binding sites of the isotope are monitored using a gamma camera. There is little data on the use of this method in a healthy population. Exposure to ionising radiation makes its use as a first stage screening test undesirable. It is, however, finding a role in directing the treatment of tumour recurrence and assessing residual tumour after first line therapy.[7]

Tumour markers These are antigens expressed by tumours. The most useful in ovarian cancer is Ca 125, an antigen expressed by coelomic epithelium detected by the murine derived antibody OC125. Blood levels of this marker are raised in 85% of patients with ovarian carcinoma at presentation,[8] 50% at stage I and 90% in more advanced cases. There is little information available regarding Ca 125 levels in apparently healthy individuals who are screened for ovarian cancer.

The sensitivity for stage I disease is unlikely to be better than the 50% achieved at presentation with stage I disease. In a prospective study, based on a Ca 125 cut-off level of 35 to 65 iu/ml, a sensitivity of 33% was achieved for stage I disease.[9] The odds ratio for Ca 125 in this study was one to 30, despite a very low cut-off level. This means that for every 30 women with a positive test, only one will actually have ovarian cancer though a sustained increase in Ca 125 may improve the specificity without reducing the sensitivity.[10] Clearly larger scale trials are needed. Other tumour markers are also being investigated: a urinary gonadotrophin fragment has been reported that appears to be complementary to Ca 125 with a low false positive rate. However there are no data for early stage disease.[11]

Thus whilst the concept of a simple blood test to identify a tumour associated antigen is attractive, those available at present do not have the sensitivity required for screening. Indeed given the histological heterogeneity of ovarian tumours, the development of a highly sensitive tumour associated antigen with wide application is unlikely. By using a rising level of a marker as an index of malignancy, specificity may be increased, and even if sensitivity for early disease is relatively low, some reduction in mortality may still be achieved.

Vaginal examination Vaginal examination is part of the overall assessment in many 'well women' clinics, yet it is accepted that its sensitivity for detecting small ovarian tumours is poor.[12] In another study vaginal examination was normal in 31 of 39 ovarian cysts.[13] The inclusion of vaginal examination in the London Hospital Study[14] was not thought to improve screening performance. Vaginal examination for screening therefore seems unjustified when compared to any of the other techniques available.

Ultrasonography

Since 1983 the group at King's College Hospital have been investigating the possible use of ultrasound for the early diagnosis of ovarian cancer. The ease with which ovarian follicles could be observed and measured led to the belief that changes in the ovary representing ovarian cancer in its earliest stages could be detected in the same way.

In a preliminary investigation[15] ovarian volume and morphology as recorded by ultrasound were compared to measurements made at laparotomy. 31 women were studied and a very close correlation (r = 0.97) was found between ultrasound determined ovarian volumes and those obtained by direct measurement. Having validated the technique in this way, an ovarian screening clinic was set up in order to evaluate its use on a population basis.

Transabdominal ultrasound The only large scale prospective study on a representative normal population of women has been carried out at King's College Hospital. The objective of this trial was to study the ovaries of 5000 self-referred asymptomatic women of age greater than 45 years on an annual basis for 3 years.[16,17]

By referring to changes in volume between initial scans and any subsequent rescan, the screening strategy was subsequently refined further. Those with an abnormal scan were recalled for a repeat scan 3 to 6 weeks later to rule out physiological changes in the ovary. In cases with a persisting lesion, laparotomy was performed, histological diagnosis and surgical staging being the end-point of the study.[18,19] By using a prolonged period of follow up it was possible, within the limits of the study design, to determine the sensitivity of the technique.

Technique of abdominal ultrasound The ultrasound scans were performed using the full bladder technique at first described by Donald in 1963.[20] The patients were scanned in the supine position, serial scans being performed both in the longitudinal and transverse planes. The pelvic vasculature is the most useful landmark in identifying the site of the ovary (Fig. 1), the vessels having characteristic bright walls and echo-free lumens. The normal ovary is often described as an ovoid structure. Before the menopause cyclical changes make it easy to visualise the ovary but the ultrasound findings may be difficult to interpret. The detection of a cyst on the ovary must therefore be related to a woman's menstrual dates and endometrial thickness to determine whether the cyst is appropriate for the phase of the cycle. Often with such a patient the safe course of action is to scan her at another stage in her menstrual cycle, when luteal or follicular cysts should have resolved.

After the menopause there is normally little variation in ovarian morphology, hence a cystic area is more likely to be significant. Although the post-menopausal ovary should be uniform in texture and have a smooth outline, transient morphological changes may continue for some years after the cessation of periods. Though the significance of this is

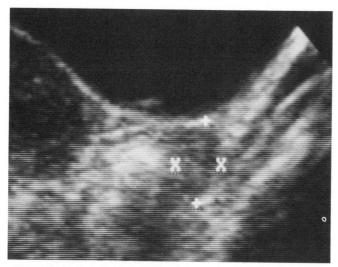

Fig. 1 Normal ovary. Transabdominal scan showing the relationship of the normal ovary to the iliac vessels.

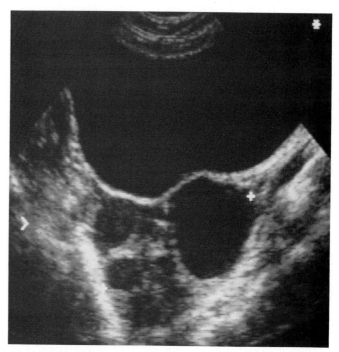

Fig. 2 Endometrioid carcinoma. Transabdominal scan of a complex endometrioid carcinoma.

unclear, it emphasises the need to reassess ovarian morphology at a rescan to allow for such physiological changes.

The normal ovary may vary in configuration, hence ovarian volume is a better representation of ovarian size. It is calculated using the well-known formula for an ellipsoid:

$$Vol = D_1 \times D_2 \times D_3 \times 0.5$$

If D_1, D_2 and D_3 are the diameters in the three axes in cm, the volume is given in ml.[21]

It is important to view the ovary in all three planes: often veins or hydrosalpinges may look cystic in one plane, but will open out into tubular structures when the transducer is rotated. The time taken to perform such a scan is around 5 to 10 minutes.

Results of the King's study The median time interval between screen 1 and screen 2 of the study was 614 days (range 289–1134), between screen 2 and 3 it was 564 days (range 214–1029). Overall 10.5% of women had an abnormal scan at the first study that had resolved by the time of rescan. Cysts in post-menopausal women seldom resolved spontaneously, emphasising the point that a cyst in a post-menopausal woman is more likely to represent significant pathology. 5.9% of women had persistently positive scans that required surgery.

At surgery primary cancers were found within six ovaries (five patients), metastatic cancer being found in a further six ovaries. Thus five women were diagnosed with primary ovarian cancer (Fig. 2), giving a prevalence of 0.09% or approximately 1:1000. It is significant that all the cancers were detected at stage I, demonstrating that ultrasound can pick up ovarian cancer at an early stage, but the dominance of early disease is surprising in a prevalence study when one might have expected more late stage tumours in the population. This may reflect the probability that the population of women likely to volunteer for screening are also likely to present early with disease.

Four out of the five cancers were found in post-menopausal women. Two were found at screen 1 and three at screen 2. There were no cancers and very little other significant pathology found at screen 3. The time intervals between screens 1 and 2 for the three cancers detected at screen 2 were 16, 18 and 22 months indicating the lead time which ultrasound may give.

Histologically three were borderline tumours, one serous papillary cystadenocarcinoma, and one a clear cell carcinoma (Table 1). Of the other lesions found 37% were benign epithelial tumours and 50% tumour-like conditions (Table 2). There were no morphological features on ultrasound that would have enabled a prediction to be made as to whether a lesion would be benign or malignant.

Table 1 Abdominal ultrasound trial: histology of primary ovarian cancers

Case no.	Screen no.	Age yrs	Menopausal state	Stage FIGO	Histological diagnosis
1	2	59	post	Ia	mucinous cystadenoma borderline
2	1	53	post	Ib	serous cystadenoma borderline
3	2	46	pre	Ia	endometrioid borderline
4	2	61	post	Ia	serous papillary cystadenoma
5	1	60	post	Ia	clear cell carcinoma

Table 2 Abdominal ultrasound trial: summary of histological classification of all masses

Classification	Screen			Totals
	1	2	3	
Epithelial				
benign	72	19	4	95
malignant	3	3	0	6
Sex-cord stromal	4	3	1	8
Germ cell	10	3	3	16
Metastatic tumours	5	1	0	6
Tumour-like	69	39	26	134
Unclassified	17	14	12	43
False positive on ultrasound	39	22	10	71
Totals	219	104	56	379

Further refinement of the screening strategy is necessary to improve specificity, perhaps using high resolution vaginal probes.

Conclusions from the study Although a negative screen result was not corroborated by any other test, within the limits of the study design a 100% sensitivity was achieved. The false positive rate for all the screens combined was between 2% and 3%. As one might have predicted, the false positive rate was lower in post-menopausal women, in whom a cystic lesion was more likely to persist and be of significance. This should be borne in mind when making comparisons with other studies, where often the study population is limited to the post-menopausal age group.

Perhaps a more meaningful way to examine the results is with the odds ratio. Using transabdominal ultrasonography the odds of a positive result being associated with an ovarian tumour was 1 in 3, for any ovarian cancer 1 in 37 and for primary ovarian cancer 1 in 67. If the data are then re-examined on the basis of volume change between initial scan and rescan for a persisting lesion, the odds ratio of a primary ovarian cancer being found at surgery is reduced to 1 in 50. In Andolf's study[22] of 805 women who were at increased risk in that they were attending the outpatient clinic with gynaecological symptoms, 83 women underwent rescan and 39 of these finally underwent surgery. Three primary ovarian cancers were found, giving an odds ratio of 1:13. This reduced odds ratio partly reflects the high disease prevalence in this study population.

The reason for the false positives is the difficulty encountered in characterising tissues on the basis of their ultrasound appearances. One of the issues that needs to be addressed is the risk of malignancy within a unilocular cystic lesion. To emphasise this problem it is worth noting that four out of 12 malignant lesions in our study were simple unilocular echo-free cysts. Meire et al found two malignant tumours out of a total of 42 unilocular simple cysts,[23] whereas a study by Granberg revealed only one malignancy out of 296 similar masses.[24] In this case papillary processes were visible macroscopically on the cyst wall,

it is quite possible that these small solid areas would have been recognised using vaginal sonography.

In another study size as well as morphology were considered, of 111 cysts surgically explored, 17 were found to be malignant. No cancer was found in any simple echo-free cyst less than 5 cm in diameter. In those of similar structure but with a diameter greater than 5 cm there were three malignancies, all at least 10 cm in diameter.[25] How these results are interpreted clearly depends on whether it is believed that benign epithelial and endometriotic cystic lesions of the ovary have malignant potential, if that is the case, characterisation of these cysts may not be important.[26]

An interesting point in this study was that only one interval cancer presented amongst the group of women studied during follow up, suggesting that by removing benign cysts it may be possible to reduce the incidence of ovarian cancer. This question can only be answered by large population studies using mortality as an end-point.

The literature suggests that abdominal ultrasound is a sensitive technique for recognising changes within the ovary indicative of ovarian cancer, however there remains a significant false positive rate. In an attempt to reduce this, and to achieve earlier detection, a trans-vaginal approach combining imaging and Doppler is being assessed.

Trans-vaginal ultrasonography Using a vaginal probe the ultrasound transducer is placed closer to the area of interest allowing the use of ultrasound frequencies of 5.0 to 7.5 MHz and so improving resolution. Trans-vaginal scanning has found applications in many areas of gynaecological practice.[27–29] It has shown potential in detecting subtle changes in morphology and size in the post-menopausal ovary,[30,31] as well as reliably monitoring small variations in the ovary during the menstrual cycle.[32,33] Trans-vaginal ultrasonography has the great practical advantage that a full bladder is not required, and so delays and discomfort caused by bladder filling are obviated.

Vaginal ultrasound is usually well-tolerated, 75% of post-menopausal women in our clinic expressing a preference for vaginal as opposed to abdominal scanning. There was slightly more embarrassment but less discomfort than an abdominal scan. In order to assess vaginal sonography in the context of a larger trial, a further screening study has been set up at King's involving over 1000 women with a positive family history of ovarian cancer.[34]

Screening women with a positive family history Many studies have been carried out to try to identify an 'at risk' group for ovarian cancer. Two factors have been implicated, reproductive history and family history.[35–37] Although such familial ovarian cancer is thought to contribute perhaps only 5% to 10% of cases, it offers a discrete target group. The OPCS study[38] has indicated that those women with one first degree relative with ovarian cancer have a six to eightfold increased risk of developing the disease. However, there is a subgroup with two or more affected relatives, who are at very high risk. This is thought to be due to the presence of an autosomal dominant gene with high penetrance, hence risk has been estimated to be 40% for women in this category.

These families provide a valuable study group in whom it might be possible to isolate the gene responsible for ovarian oncogenesis. By studying a group of women with a high prevalence of the disease the higher yield of tumours in this population may be utilised to assess new methods of detection.

Study design Women are recruited to the study using media advertising. Applicants have to provide evidence of a close relative with ovarian cancer as an inclusion criteria.

All those involved in this work must be aware of the possible anxiety engendered by screening.[39] All undergo a psychological assessment at the time of screening, and will be followed up.

Patients have a medical and family history taken. Blood is taken for the study of a panel of tumour markers as well as chromosome analysis. Both vaginal and abdominal ultrasonography are performed on each subject in order to compare the two techniques. A screen is called 'positive' on the basis of abnormal morphology or increased ovarian volume.[40,41] In this case a repeat screen is carried out 3 to 6 weeks later to rule out physiological changes. Based on the previous study at King's[42] a volume reduction to less than 68% of that recorded at the initial scan usually means that the initial changes are insignificant. Surgery is advised for persistent abnormalities.

Histological diagnosis is the end-point of the study. At the time of surgery blood and cyst fluid are taken for further tumour marker studies, and tissue is taken for genetic analysis. Clinical staging is based on the surgical findings, and combined with the histology report to evaluate the lesions accurately.[18,19]

Vaginal scanning technique Patients have an empty bladder, and are placed in the lithotomy position with slight reverse Trendelenberg tilt. The probe is covered with coupling gel and a condom.[43]

Two anatomical landmarks are of particular use when examining the ovary: the internal iliac vessels and the uterus (Fig. 3). The uterus is assessed first. The endometrium is best viewed in the longitudinal plane when it can be seen in its entirety. Doppler studies of the uterine artery can be carried out at this time with an optimal angle of insonation. These vessels can be sampled either in the transverse plane or longitudinally adjacent to the cervix. If there are difficulties differentiating between uterine and adnexal structures, the movement in relation to the uterus can be observed when displaced by the transducer. Adnexal structures slide over the uterus, a finding known as the 'sliding organ' sign, which is accentuated by the presence of free fluid in the pelvis. Whilst still in the longitudinal plane the probe is then turned towards the lateral

pelvic wall. The internal iliac vessels appear as echo-free tubular structures. The ovaries are almost always found adjacent to these vessels; a relationship that is of particular use following hysterectomy when the anatomy is often distorted.

Premenopausal ovaries are easy to locate because they contain follicles. After menopause they become more difficult to find.

Location of the post-menopausal ovary requires experience, the most difficult being in women who have undergone hysterectomy, for bowel often slides down into the space left by the uterus, obscuring the ovary (Fig. 4).

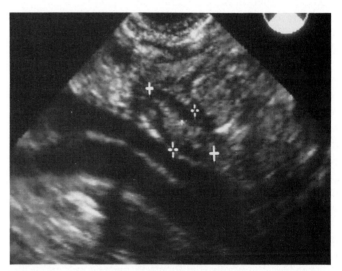

Fig. 3 Normal post-menopausal ovary visualised by trans-vaginal sonography.

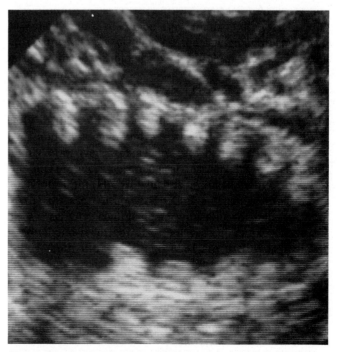

Fig. 4 Bowel obscuring the ovary (trans-vaginal scan).

In these cases if the operator's left hand is placed on the abdomen, the probe can be pushed towards it in the same way as performing a bimanual examination. Tilting the patient to one side or the other may also help.

Initially with abdominal sonography we were able to locate the ovaries in 85% of patients; with time this has risen to 99%, consistent with the study by Andolf.[22] The same sequence is developing with vaginal sonography, at present 85% of ovaries being visualised initially. If the ovaries are not seen clearly the woman is asked to fill her bladder for an abdominal scan, or an appointment is given for a separate abdominal scan.

The presence of solid or cystic areas, septa, as well as regularity of outline is recorded. The ovarian volume is determined from the formula for an ellipsoid as described above.[21]

Preliminary results and discussion   To date 776 'high-risk' women have been scanned in this study and already a statistically significant increased prevalence of ovarian cancer has emerged. 10.2% have had an abnormal ovary requiring a repeat scan to be performed. In 6.1% of cases the abnormality has persisted and the ovary has been removed, compared to 3.29% in the first scan of the general population trial. Three cases of stage Ia primary ovarian cancer have been detected. In Table 3 the pathology found in the current high-risk group is compared to the population study. There is a significant increase in the prevalence of ovarian cancer in those women with a family history of ovarian cancer. The increase in the number of tumour-like conditions is difficult to understand: possibly these lesions are a marker of increased risk of malignancy. As a result of this increase in pathology in general, the false positive rate for ovarian cancer is increased slightly to 5% compared to 3.5% in the general population at first screening. However, due to the increased prevalence of cancer, the predictive value of a positive test result is improved such that the probability of finding a cancer at surgery in a woman with a positive result is 1 in 14 compared to 1 in 99 in the general population at first screening. This figure may well be acceptable to many clinicians.

A further observation in this group has been the marked increase in women who have bilateral masses, and in women with masses who have had an hysterectomy. Though these are preliminary data, these results indicate a remarkably high prevalence of ovarian pathology in this group.

It would appear at this early stage of the King's 'family history' study, as well as from other data,[44] that vaginal ultrasound is able to detect small morphological changes within the ovary suggestive of malignancy. This may lead to a diagnosis being made at an earlier stage than has previously been possible, with a greater lead time being achieved (Fig. 5).

The fact that vaginal ultrasound can offer unique diagnostic information is supported by other authors. Fleischer, in a study of 34 patients with pelvic masses comparing trans-vaginal to transabdominal sonography, found that the vaginal route added unique diagnostic information in 70% of cases.[45] Mendelson, in another comparative study, found vaginal sonography superior in 37% of cases of ovarian pathology (Fig. 6).[46]

This ability to resolve very small cystic lesions such as inclusion cysts within the ovary (Fig. 7) suggests that the earliest structural changes that occur with ovarian oncogenesis are being demonstrated.[47]

It is too early to summarise effects of trans-vaginal scanning on sensitivity and specificity. The data so far suggest that sensitivity for early small tumours is enhanced. It is important to point out that one out of three of the malignant tumours found to date was detected in an ovary of

Table 3 Histological findings in the family history study compared to that in the general population

Classification	At risk family (%)	General population (%)*
Epithelial		
benign	1.66	1.30
malignant	0.39	0.05
Sex-cord stromal	0.13	0.07
Germ cell	0.39	0.18
Metastatic	0.00	0.09
Tumour-like	3.22	1.26
Unclassified	0.26	0.31
All	6.05	3.26

* first screening

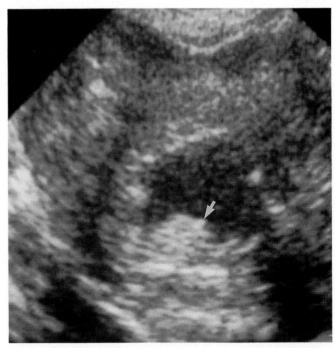

Fig. 5 Stage I serous cystadenocarcinoma. Note the irregular solid area protruding into the cyst cavity (arrow).

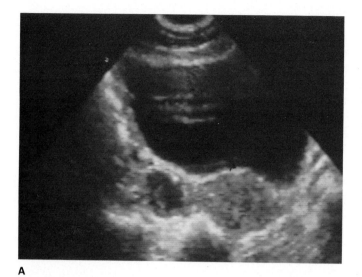

A

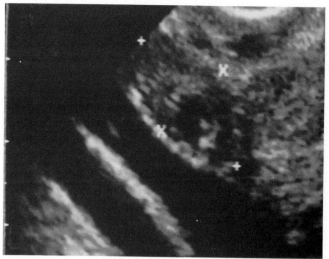

Fig. 7 An inclusion cyst within a post-menopausal ovary, note the close relationship of the iliac vessels.

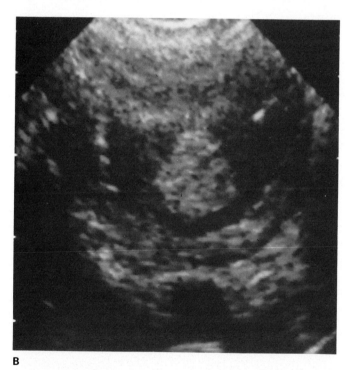

B

Fig. 6 Serous cystadenocarcinoma. A: Stage I borderline serous cystadenocarcinoma seen using transabdominal sonography.
B: The same tumour using trans-vaginal sonography. The more complex cystic nature of the lesion can be defined.

normal volume and only questionable morphological abnormality on abdominal scanning. All of the cancers have had an irregular cystic structure when scanned with the high resolution vaginal probe (Fig. 5), whilst no unilocular, simple cystic lesions less than 5 cm have harboured a malignancy. It may be that the cancer in Granberg's study[24] would not have been called a simple cyst had vaginal sonography been used. If morphological criteria for malignancy were to be applied to the cysts detected in this

screening population, the false positive rate would be markedly reduced.

Screening seems to be indicated for women with a family history of ovarian cancer. The development of a score for assessing ovarian cancer risk based on a family history of ovarian, breast, and colorectal cancer is therefore a priority.

Studies of ovarian blood flow

It is well-known that the growth of malignant lesions is dependent on angiogenesis and consequent vascularisation. That angiogenesis occurs in the period between hyperplasia and true neoplasia has been shown with nude mice.[48] A platelet derived growth factor that stimulates endothelial growth and chemotaxis in vitro and angiogenesis in vivo has been cloned.[49] This process of vascularisation also occurs during the formation of the corpus luteum in the normal menstrual cycle, a decreased impedance to flow through the ovary at this time has been described.[50]

The feasibility of measuring uterine and ovarian artery blood flow impedance was shown by Taylor in 1985: each artery has a particular flow velocity waveform permitting its recognition.[51] The investigation of small vascular areas is facilitated by colour flow mapping (Plate 1).[52]

The pulsatility index (PI) is a better index of impedance to flow, as in cases of absent diastolic flow the A/B ratio and resistance index (RI) becomes infinite or approaches unity respectively.[53] In a pilot study three groups of volunteers were assessed: (1) 10 healthy women with regular menstrual cycles and normal pelvic anatomy, (2) 10 patients from the gynaecology clinic with symptoms suggestive of ovarian cancer and (3) 36 asymptomatic women from the ovarian screening clinic. Ovarian morphology and volume were recorded as described above and

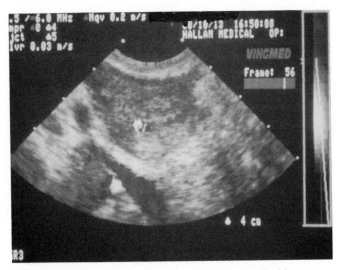

Plate 1   Vascularisation within a corpus luteum visualised by trans-vaginal colour flow mapping. This figure is reproduced in colour in the colour plate section at the front of this volume.

the impedance to blood flow within the ovary and any lesions was measured.

Results   The 10 women in group 2 were subsequently found to be suffering from stage III or IV primary ovarian cancer. Of the asymptomatic women recruited from the screening clinic 12/16 with a positive result had benign tumours, whilst 4/16 had stage Ia primary ovarian cancer. From this data the ovarian PI can be defined in the various groups of subjects and patients.

Healthy ovaries: ovarian PI was measured in 30 subjects, 10 pre- and 20 post-menopausal. Figure 8 shows a typical flow velocity waveform from a post-menopausal ovary, there is low diastolic flow indicative of high impedance. The mean PI was 5.1, with a range of 3.5 to 9.4.

Benign tumours (Fig. 9): all benign tumours had PI values within the normal range (Plate 2), with one exception. In this case the areas of vascularisation coincided exactly with areas of ectopic thyroid tissue in bilateral dermoid cysts, suggesting that this represents a local response to an angiogenic factor released by thyroid tissue.

Symptomatic malignant tumours (Fig. 9): the mean PI in cases of invasive cancer was 0.49. Blood vessels could be demonstrated in all 10 cases of late stage tumours with colour flow imaging (Plate 3). There is a sixfold difference in PI between this mean value and the lowest value in the range for healthy ovaries.

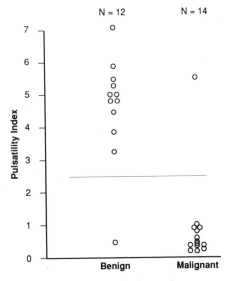

Fig. 9   Intra-ovarian pulsatility index in ovarian tumours.

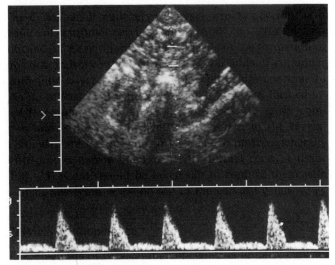

Fig. 8   Flow velocity waveforms demonstrating high impedance to flow within the ovary. Note the low diastolic flow.

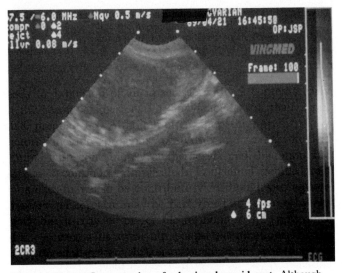

Plate 2   Colour flow mapping of a benign dermoid cyst. Although the iliac vessels are defined by the colour Doppler, there are no areas of vascularisation within the cyst. This figure is reproduced in colour in the colour plate section at the front of this volume.

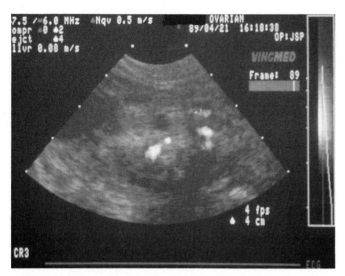

Plate 3 Vascularisation within a stage I ovarian cancer. This figure is reproduced in colour in the colour plate section at the front of this volume.

Figure 10 shows the flow velocity waveform obtained from vessels within an invasive cancer, in contrast with Figure 8 there is a highly significant degree of diastolic flow.

Asymptomatic malignant tumours: the four cancers in this group were all stage Ia. Vessels were visualised in all three cases of invasive carcinoma on colour Doppler and the PI values were 1.0 or less. The one borderline tumour had a normal PI value and no demonstrable vessels on colour Doppler. This is as one would expect since borderline malignancy does not have invasive characteristics and

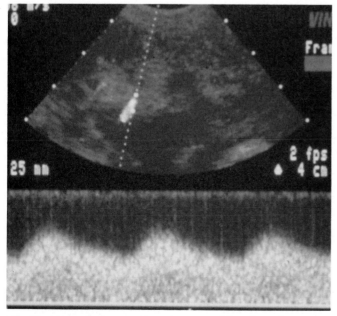

Fig. 10 Flow velocity waveforms in cancer. There is continuous flow throughout diastole.

neovascularisation is thought to occur during the transition to malignancy (Fig. 9).

Discussion Visible vascularisation on colour flow mapping within these cysts was sufficient to characterise them. However when the pulsed Doppler range gate was placed across such a vascularised area the flow velocity waveforms obtained were instantly recognisable, and were typical in all the invasive cancers.[54] We have seen the same waveforms in cases of uterine cancer,[55] as well as in the corpus luteum, emphasising the importance of not carrying out Doppler assessment for ovarian cancer during the luteal phase of the menstrual cycle. Scans should be scheduled on days 3 to 11 to avoid the vascular events occurring in the peri-ovulatory follicle as well as in the corpus luteum. Since 80% of ovarian cancer occurs in post-menopausal women, this is not a common practical problem.

When no vessels can be visualised on colour Doppler it is difficult to pick up a signal from the ovary. This may be because the flow velocity to the ovary is low, or because the angle between the ovarian artery and the probe approaches 90° leading to very small Doppler frequency shifts.

Assessing the flow velocity waveform to derive an index of impedance yields numerical data for comparison, but may not be necessary to make a diagnosis. As advocated by Goswamy in his studies of the uterine artery, visual analysis of these waveforms may be a better approach.[56] The preliminary results are consistent with other data[57] reporting low resistance flow within five primary ovarian malignancies.

These initial results suggest that the absence of vessels on colour Doppler and a high PI value exclude invasive cancers. 56 benign masses have been studied with this technique (Table 4). Vascularisation on colour Doppler has only been seen in four benign tumours (two luteal and two dermoid cysts). If the presence or absence of vessels on colour Doppler is added to morphological changes as a test for invasive ovarian cancer the false positive rate is reduced

Table 4 Ovarian colour flow signals in benign cystic ovarian lesions on trans-vaginal ultrasound

Classification	Absent	Present
Epithelial		
Serous	14	0
Mucinous	2	0
Sex-cord stromal	1	0
Germ cell	4	2
Tumour-like		
Follicular cyst	6	0
Simple cyst	10	0
Corpus luteum cyst	1	2
Inclusion cyst	2	0
Endometriosis	8	0
False positive		
Hydrosalpinges	4	0
Total	52	4

to 7% while the sensitivity remains at 100%. As a result the odds ratio in favour of finding cancer at surgery becomes 3 to 1.

Screening for uterine cancer

Around 3700 new cases of uterine cancer are reported in the United Kingdom each year.[1] Uterine bleeding is a common symptom, the diagnosis being established from histology of tissue obtained by curettage or hysteroscopy.

Trans-vaginal sonography offers a much clearer view of the myometrial-endometrial interface than transabdominal.[58] In a study of 93 known cases of endometrial cancer endometrial echoes were identified in 93% of cases scanned by the transabdominal route pre-operatively, with accurate staging of the cancers in 91% of cases.[59] More recently in a study of 63 symptomatic and 27 asymptomatic post-menopausal women, the finding of an endometrium greater than 5 mm in thickness was highly suggestive of underlying pathology (Fig. 11).[60,61]

Thus vaginal ultrasound with colour flow mapping might be useful to obviate the need for endometrial biopsy in some women, whilst screening for endometrial pathology at the same time as the ovarian scans (Plate 4). In a study to assess uterine morphology, endometrial thickness was defined as the maximum distance between the two endometrial–myometrial interfaces in the longitudinal plane, any free fluid in the cavity being excluded. Blood flow in the uterine arteries and the endometrium was measured in 134 women: 14 patients with proven

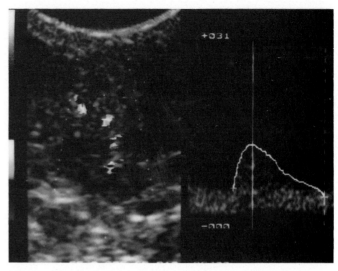

Plate 4 Vascularisation within the endometrium and flow velocity waveforms from the uterine arteries in a case of endometrial carcinoma using trans-vaginal colour flow mapping. This figure is reproduced in colour in the colour plate section at the front of this volume.

endometrial cancer (10 stage Ia, 1 stage II and 3 stage III), 17 with post-menopausal bleeding whose biopsy had failed to produce sufficient tissue for diagnosis, 35 women taking hormone replacement therapy, and 68 apparently healthy women.

All the women with uterine cancer had a thickened endometrium (2.2 cm ± 0.8–4.1 cm). However, as can be seen in Figure 12, there was overlap with the patients without cancer, particularly those with post-menopausal bleeding or on HRT. Even for a cut-off value of 1 cm, there is a significant false positive rate of 17%. The mean PI value, however, was always lower in patients with endometrial cancer than in the other groups (Fig. 13), such that clear cut-off values could be obtained. The PI values were inversely proportional to the stage of the cancer.

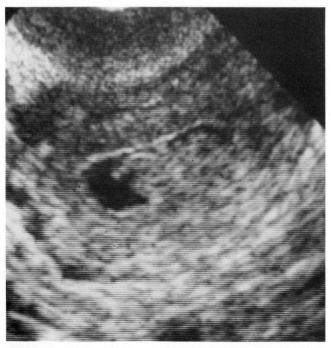

Fig. 11 Polypoid carcinoma. Transverse section of the uterus showing a polypoid carcinoma protruding into the uterine cavity.

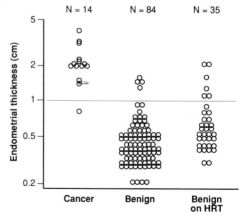

Fig. 12 Endometrial thickness in women with and without endometrial cancer.

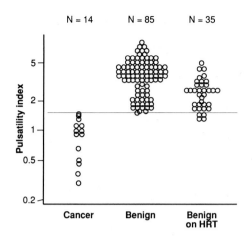

N = 14   N = 85   N = 35

Fig. 13 Pulsatility index in the uterine arteries in women with and without endometrial cancer.

Thus using the pulsatility index with a lower limit of normal of 1.6 as an indicator of the presence or absence of cancer, the predictive value of a positive result in this study was 100% with a false positive rate of 1% for women not taking HRT, but 11% for patients who do receive it. That HRT causes a decrease in impedance to arterial flow is in itself an important finding as this may contribute to the cardioprotective effect of oestrogens in these preparations.[62]

Our PI values within the endometrial tumours themselves were much lower than in the uterine arteries.

Doppler may have the potential to detect vessels within endometrial cancers in the same way as in the ovary. Further studies are needed to determine if this is a sensitive criterion of uterine malignancy. The marked differences in endometrial thickness found in women with endometrial cancer suggest that a value of greater than 1.0 cm indicates significant endometrial pathology. This value is greater than that based on abdominal sonography data,[60] but is consistent with a recommendation that the post-menopausal endometrium should be less than or equal to 0.8 cm.[63,64] The increase in impedance to blood flow between non-malignant changes and endometrial cancers indicates that a PI of 1.6 might be a useful discriminatory value.

These preliminary results indicate a potential for uterine cancer screening. The introduction of trans-vaginal colour flow mapping facilitates the recognition of changes in flow within the uterine artery, as well as detection of small areas of soft tissue vascularisation suggestive of malignancy.

ACKNOWLEDGEMENTS

We are grateful to the Imperial Cancer Research Fund (ICRF) and the Cancer Research Campaign (CRC) for financial support, and to Aloka Ltd., Japan, for the use of their ultrasound equipment.

REFERENCES

1 Cramer D W. Epidemiologic and statistical aspects of gynecologic oncology. In: Knapp R C, Berkowitz R S. eds. Gynecologic oncology. New York: Macmillan. 1986: 201–222
2 Beral V. The epidemiology of ovarian cancer. In: Sharp F, Soutter W P. eds. Ovarian cancer – the way ahead. Chichester: Wiley. 1987: 21–31
3 Young R C, Walton L A, Ellenberg S S, et al. Adjuvant therapy in stage I and stage II epithelial ovarian cancer – results of two prospective randomized trials. N Engl J Med 1990; 322: 1021–1027
4 Jacobs I, Oram D. Prevention of ovarian cancer: a survey of the practice of prophylactic oophorectomy by fellows and members of the Royal College of Obstetricians and Gynaecologists. Br J Obstet Gynaecol 1989; 96: 510–515
5 Cuckle H S, Wald N J. Principles of screening. In: Wald N J. ed. Antenatal and neonatal screening. Oxford: Oxford University Press. 1984
6 Wilson J M G, Jungner G. In: Principles and practice of screening for disease. (Public Health Papers 34). World Health Organisation. Geneva: 1968
7 Symonds E M, Perkins A C, Pimm M V, Baldwin R W, Hardy J G, Williams D A. Clinical implications for immunoscintigraphy in patients with ovarian malignancy: a preliminary study using monoclonal antibody 791T/36. Br J Obstet Gynaecol 1985; 92: 270–276
8 Jacobs I, Bast R C. The CA 125 tumour-associated antigen: a review of the literature. Hum Reprod 1989; 4: 1–12
9 Zurawski V R, Orjaseter H, Anderson A, Jellum E. Elevated serum CA–125 levels prior to diagnosis of ovarian neoplasia: relevance for the early detection of ovarian cancer. Int J Cancer 1988; 42: 677–680
10 Zurawski V R, Sjovall K, Schoenfeld D A, et al. Prospective evaluation of serum Ca 125 levels in a normal population, phase 1: the specificities of single and serial determinations in testing for ovarian cancer. Gynecol Oncol 1990; 36: 391–394
11 Cole L A, Joo-Hyun N, Chambers J T, Schwartz P E. Urinary gonadotrophin fragment, a new tumor marker. II. Differentiating a benign from a malignant pelvic mass. Gynecol Oncol 1990; 36: 391–394
12 Lundberg W I, Wall J E, Mathers J E. Laparoscopy in the evaluation of pelvic pain. Obstet Gynecol 1973; 42: 872–876
13 Andolf E, Jorgensen C. A prospective comparison of clinical ultrasound and operative examination of the female pelvis. J Ultrasound Med 1988; 7: 617–629
14 Jacobs I, Bridges J, Reynolds C, et al. Multimodal approach to screening for ovarian cancer. Lancet 1988; i: 268–271
15 Campbell S, Goessons L, Goswamy R, Whitehead M I. Real-time ultrasonography for the determination of ovarian morphology and volume. A possible new screening test for ovarian cancer. Lancet 1982; i: 425–426
16 Campbell S, Bhan V, Royston P, Whitehead M I, Collins W P. Transabdominal ultrasound screening for early ovarian cancer. BMJ 1989; 299: 1363–1367
17 Campbell S, Bourne T H, Collins W P. Detecting early ovarian cancer. Lancet 1990; ii: 436
18 Serov S F, Scully R E, Sobin L H. International histological classification of tumours. No 9. Histological typing of ovarian tumours. Geneva: World Health Organisation. 1973

19 Shepherd J H. Revised FIGO staging for gynaecological cancer. Br J Obstet Gynaecol 1989; 96: 889–892

20 Donald I. Use of ultrasonics in the diagnosis of abdominal swellings. BMJ 1963; ii: 1154–1155

21 Ivarsson S A, Nilsson K O, Persson P H. Ultrasonography of the pelvic organs in prepubertal and postpubertal girls. Arch Dis Child 1983; 58: 352–354

22 Andolf E, Svalenius E, Astedt B. Ultrasonography for early detection of ovarian carcinoma. Br J Obstet Gynaecol 1986; 93: 1286–1289

23 Meire H B, Farrant P, Guha T. Distinction of benign from malignant ovarian cysts by ultrasound. Br J Obstet Gynaecol 1978; 85: 893–899

24 Granberg S, Wikland M, Jansson. Macroscopic characterisation of ovarian tumours and the relation to the histological diagnosis: criteria to be used for ultrasound evaluation. Gynecol Oncol 1990; in press

25 Andolf E. Cystic lesions in elderly women, diagnosed by ultrasound. In: Sonography of the female pelvis with emphasis on ovarian tumours. Thesis, Lund University. Department of Obstetric and Gynecology. Lund, Sweden. 1989; paper VII p 2–14

26 Scully R E. Minimal cancer of the ovary. Clin Oncol 1982; 1: 379–387

27 Editorial. Transvaginal scanning. Lancet. 1989; i: 19–20

28 Timor-Tritsch I E, Farine D, Rosen M G. A close look at early embryonic development with the high frequency vaginal transducer. Am J Obstet Gynecol 1989; 159: 676–681

29 Quinn M J, Beynon N J, McMortenson N J, Smith P J B. Transvaginal endosonography: a new method to study the anatomy of the lower urinary tract in urinary stress incontinence. Br J Urol 1988; 62: 414–418

30 Higgins R V, Van Nagell Jnr J R, Donaldson E S, et al. Transvaginal sonography as a screening method for ovarian cancer. Gynecol Oncol 1989; 34: 402–406

31 Rodriguez M H, Lawrence L D, Medearis A L, Lacarra R N, Lobo R A. The use of transvaginal sonography for evaluation of postmenopausal ovarian size and morphology. Am J Obstet Gynecol 1988; 159: 810–814

32 Bonilla-Musoles F, Pardo G, Perez-Gil M, Serra V, Pellicer A. Abdominal ultrasonography versus transvaginal scanning: accuracy in follicular development evaluation and prediction for oocyte retrieval in stimulated cycles. JCU 1989; 17: 469–473

33 Gonzalez C J, Curson R, Parsons J. Transabdominal versus transvaginal ultrasound scanning of ovarian follicles: are they comparable? Fertil Steril 1988; 50: 657–659

34 Bourne T H, Whitehead M I, Campbell S, Royston P, Bhan V, Collins W P. Ultrasound screening for familial ovarian cancer. N Engl J Med. Submitted for publication

35 Schildkraut J M, Thompson W D. Familial ovarian cancer: a population based case–control study. Am J Epidemiol 1988; 128: 456–466

36 Cramer D W, Hutchison G B, Welch W R, Scully R E, Ryan K J. Determinants of ovarian cancer risk. 1. Reproductive experiences and family history. J Natl Cancer Inst 1983; 71: 711–716

37 Hartge P, Schiffman M H, Hoover R, McGowan L, Lesher L, Norris H J. A case–control study of epithelial ovarian cancer. Am J Obstet Gynecol 1989; 161: 10–16

38 Ponder B A J, Easton D F, Peto. Risk of ovarian cancer associated with a family history: preliminary report of the OPCS study. In: Sharp F, Mason W P, Leake R E. eds. Ovarian cancer, biological and therapeutic challenges. Chapman and Hall. 1990: p 3–6

39 Ellman R, Angeli N, Christians A, Moss S, Chamberlain J, Maguire P. Psychiatric morbidity associated with screening for breast cancer. Br J Cancer 1989; 60: 781–784

40 Andolf E, Jorgensen C, Svalenius E, Sunden B. Ultrasound measurement of the ovarian volume. Acta Obstet Gynecol Scand 1987; 66: 387–389

41 Goswamy R K, Campbell S, Royston J P, et al. Ovarian size in postmenopausal women. Br J Obstet Gynaecol 1988; 95: 795–801

42 Campbell S, Royston P, Bhan V, Whitehead M I, Collins W P. Novel screening strategies for early ovarian cancer by transabdominal ultrasonography. Br J Obstet Gynaecol 1990; 97: 304–311

43 Timor-Tritsch I E, Bar-Yam Y, Elgali S, Rottem S. The technique of transvaginal sonography with the use of a 6.5 MHz probe. Am J Obstet Gynecol 1988; 158: 1019–1024

44 Van Nagell J R, Higgins R V, Donaldson E S, et al. Transvaginal sonography as a screening method for ovarian cancer – a report of the first 1000 cases screened. Cancer 1990; 65: 573–577

45 Fleischer A C, Gordon A N, Entman S S. Transabdominal and transvaginal sonography of pelvic masses. Ultrasound Med Biol 1989; 15: 529–533

46 Mendelson E B, Bohm-Velez M, Joseph N, Neiman H L. Gynecologic imaging: comparison of transabdominal and transvaginal sonography. Radiology 1988; 166: 321–324

47 Cramer D W, Welch W R. Determinants of ovarian cancer risk. II. Inferences regarding pathogenesis. J Natl Cancer Inst 1983; 71: 717

48 Folkman J, Watson K, Ingber D, Hanahan D. Induction of angiogenesis during the transition from hyperplasia to neoplasia. Nature 1989; 339: 58–61

49 Ishikawa F, Miyazono K, Hellman U, et al. Identification of angiogenic activity and the cloning and expression of platelet derived endothelial growth factor. Nature 1989; 338: 557–561

50 Baber R J, McSweeney M B, Gill R W, et al. Transvaginal pulsed Doppler ultrasound assessment of blood flow to the corpus luteum in IVF patients following embryo transfer. Br J Obstet Gynaecol 1988; 95: 1226–1230

51 Taylor K J W, Burns P N, Wells P N T, Conway D I, Hull M G R. Ultrasound Doppler flow studies of the ovarian and uterine arteries. Br J Obstet Gynaecol 1985; 92: 240–246

52 Merritt C R B. Doppler blood flow imaging: integrating flow with tissue data. Diagnostic Imaging 1986; November: 146–155

53 Thompson R S, Trudinger B J, Cook C M. Doppler ultrasound waveform indices: A/B ratio, pulsatility index, and Pourcelot ratio. Br J Obstet Gynaecol 1988; 95: 581–588

54 Bourne T H, Campbell S, Steer C V, Whitehead M I, Collins W P. Transvaginal colour flow imaging: a possible new screening test for ovarian cancer. BMJ 1989; 68: 1367–1370

55 Bourne T H, Campbell S, Whitehead M I, Royston P, Steer C V, Collins W P. The detection of endometrial cancer in postmenopausal women by transvaginal ultrasonography and colour flow imaging. BMJ 1990; 301: 369

56 Goswamy R K, Williams G, Steptoe P V. Decreased uterine perfusion – a cause of infertility. Hum Reprod 1988; 3: 955–959

57 Kurjak A, Zalud I, Jurkovic D, Altirevic Z, Miljan M. Transvaginal colour flow Doppler for the assessment of pelvic circulation. Acta Obstet Gynecol 1989; 68: 131–135

58 Mendelson E D, Bohm-Velez, Joseph N, Neiman H L. Endometrial abnormalities: evaluation with transvaginal sonography. AJR 1988; 150: 139–142

59 Cacciatore B, Lehtovirta, Walstrom T, Ylostalo P. Preoperative sonographic evaluation of endometrial cancer. Am J Obstet Gynecol 1989; 160: 133–137

60 Nasri M N, Coast G J. Correlation of ultrasound findings and endometrial histopathology in postmenopausal women. Br J Obstet Gynaecol 1989; 96: 1333–1338

61 Granberg S, Friberg L–G, Norstrom A, et al. Endovaginal ultrasound scanning of women with postmenopausal bleeding. J Ultrasound Med 1988; 7: 256

62 Bourne T H, Hillard T, Whitehead M I, Crook D, Campbell S. Evidence for a direct vascular effect of oestrogens on human arteries. Lancet 1990; 335: 1470–1471

63 Fleischer A C, Mendelson E B, Bohm-Velez, Entman S S. Transvaginal and transabdominal sonography of the endometrium. Semin Ultrasound CT MR 1988; 9: 81–101

64 Osmers R, Volksen M, Shauer A. Vaginosonography for the early detection of endometrial cancer. Lancet 1990; i: 1569–1571

6

Infertility

John H. Parsons and Christopher V. Steer

INTRODUCTION

Ultrasound was first used to demonstrate the pelvic organs in 1966.[1] In 1972 Kratochwil[2] demonstrated that follicles may be seen in the preovulatory stage of the cycle. The early work[3-9] was laborious as it was done using static scanners and a full bladder. The development of real time equipment in the late seventies[10] and the vaginal probe in the early eighties[11] transformed pelvic ultrasonography into a technique that is simple to learn and use.

The incorporation of spectral Doppler, and more recently colour flow mapping, into ultrasound equipment has allowed changes in the uterine and ovarian blood supply to be studied during health and disease. The full potential of this is still being explored and looks likely to enhance the diagnostic yield significantly.

The importance of pelvic ultrasound in the investigation and treatment of infertility is demonstrated by the wide range of applications described in this chapter.

Technique and equipment

The pelvic organs may be scanned either transabdominally or trans-vaginally. The former requires a full bladder to displace the gas containing bowel and to provide an 'acoustic window' through to the pelvic organs.

In most infertility units trans-vaginal ultrasound has become the routine method. However, when the ovaries are high in the abdomen or when the uterus is enlarged, abdominal ultrasonography may be necessary for adequate visualisation.

During trans-vaginal ultrasound with the probe in the lateral and anterior fornices of the vagina only a few centimetres separate it from the uterus and ovaries with no intervening bowel gas. The elasticity of the vaginal vault allows these structures to be approached individually. Because there is no need for a full bladder the patient is comfortable and appointment times may be fixed. The proximity of the probe to the structures being examined allows the use of high frequency probes with a short focal length, giving enhanced resolution in comparison to transabdominal scanning.

The size of the trans-vaginal probe varies between manufacturers; the slimmer, round ended probes being the least uncomfortable. Patients who have not had intercourse but who have used tampons will tolerate such a vaginal probe. Cooperative patients who are virgo intacta may, if the probe is slim, be scanned rectally with minimal discomfort. Patients bleeding heavily at the time of the examination are best advised to leave a tampon in the vagina; the probe may be positioned beside it. Great care must be taken whilst performing vaginal ultrasonography to minimise the patients' natural embarrassment at being exposed in the lithotomy position.

Whichever gynaecological organ is being examined it is good practice to review the whole pelvis routinely using a standard sequence. To obtain the maximum amount of information it is preferable to carry out serial examinations. This is particularly important when assessing ovarian morphology and function.

Potential dangers of ultrasonography

There is no evidence that diagnostic ultrasound by either the transabdominal or the trans-vaginal route has any adverse effect on either the oocyte, the pre-embryo or the early developing pregnancy.[12]

It is not practical to sterilise the trans-vaginal probe between procedures so it is covered by either an especially designed sheath or by an ordinary contraceptive condom, though in infertility studies condoms lubricated with spermicidal gel must be avoided. Cross-infection remains a cause for concern, as occasionally the protective sheaths break. Furthermore, the British Standard to which condoms should conform in the United Kingdom (BS 3704/1989; British Standards Institution, London W1) means only that there are holes in less than four condoms per thousand.

Ovarian ultrasound

Identification

The ovaries are usually identified lying lateral to the uterus adjacent to the side wall of the pelvis. A useful landmark is their close relationship to the internal iliac vessels which are usually easily identified (Figs 1 and 2).

The stroma has a characteristic appearance and is outlined by loops of bowel in which peristalsis may be seen.

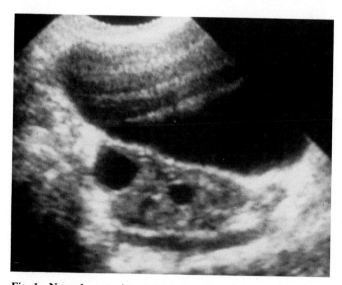

Fig. 1 Normal ovary. A transabdominal ultrasound scan of an unstimulated ovary. The internal iliac vein is seen immediately beneath the ovary.

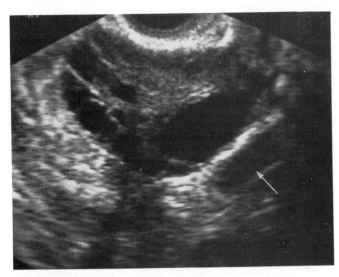

Fig. 2 Normal ovary. A trans-vaginal ultrasound scan of an ovary showing the close proximity to the internal iliac vein (arrow).

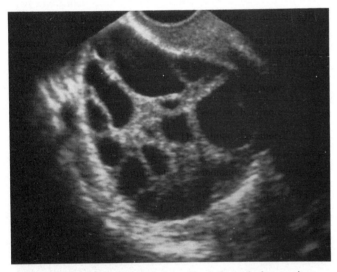

Fig. 3 A stimulated ovary seen immediately beneath the anterior abdominal wall with a 7 MHz probe.

Identification is made easier by the presence of follicles or cysts. It is occasionally necessary to search more widely for the ovary: it may be found behind or above the uterus or under the anterior abdominal wall. These unusual sites may be due to excessive mobility but are often due to adhesions (see Ch. 9).

A high ovary may sometimes be brought into the field of view of a trans-vaginal probe by pressing firmly on the lower abdomen. When the ovary will not descend in this manner a clear picture may sometimes be obtained by either a high frequency (5 to 7.5 MHz) abdominal or trans-vaginal probe scanning transabdominally, without a full bladder (Fig. 3).

The normal ovary is ellipsoid in shape. Its volume (in ml when measuring in cm) may be estimated using the approximate formula for an ellipsoid: length × breadth × depth × 0.5.[5]

Ovarian morphology

The unstimulated ovary in women with regular cycles contains a small number of cystic structures (Fig. 1) and has a mean volume of 5.4 ml.[13] However, 23% of women have ovaries which contain 10 or more such structures (2 to 8 mm in diameter) often distributed peripherally round a central core of stroma (Fig. 4). Such ovaries have been termed polycystic ovaries and are associated with menstrual irregularity, raised luteinising hormone concentrations, hirsutism, anovulation and an increased incidence of miscarriage. 87% of women with oligomenorrhoea and anovulation have polycystic ovaries.[14,15]

Ovaries with a polycystic morphology have a mean volume greater than the non-polycystic ovary (11.1 ml) but there is a considerable overlap in size between the two types of ovary. The presence of polycystic ovaries is more likely to be associated with infertility if the woman has a raised body mass index (BMI).[16]

The ovaries of women with a low BMI, those approaching their menarche and those suffering from anorexia nervosa, pass through characteristic changes as their BMI increases. Initially the ovaries are small and featureless but as the woman's weight rises the ovarian volume increases and small cysts appear. These cysts are associated, unlike the cysts in polycystic ovaries, with a normal amount of ovarian stroma, low or normal gonadotrophins and a small uterine volume. With further weight gain one of the cysts becomes dominant and the rest regress so that the mor-

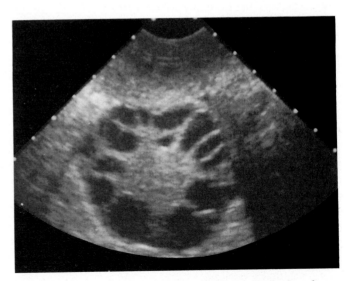

Fig. 4 A polycystic ovary showing the peripheral distribution of follicles and a central core of stroma (trans-vaginal).

phology returns to normal. This type of cystic ovary has been termed multifollicular[17] (Fig. 5) and its presence is suggestive of less than optimum weight in patients recovering from anorexia nervosa. If they conceive, these fetuses have an increased risk of fetal intra-uterine growth retardation.[18]

Functional ovarian cysts Ovaries commonly contain follicular or luteal cysts. These (Fig. 6) are characterised by their echo-free contents, failure to grow and disappear over the normal 2 week time span of a follicle, and a tendency to resolve spontaneously. They are usually less than 5 cm in diameter but may reach 10 cm, as long as their outline is sharp and smooth, the woman may be reassured.[19]

There is conflicting evidence as to whether ovarian cysts found prior to superovulation therapy in an assisted conception cycle affect ovarian response.[20,21] Such cysts may be aspirated but, although this may increase the number of follicles and eggs collected, the overall pregnancy rate is not improved.[22]

An irregular margin in a persistent cyst is an indication for ovarian cystectomy though this is very rarely necessary in women seeking treatment for infertility. The blood flow to such cysts may be assessed with colour flow Doppler. In a study of 50 women Bourne et al[23] found that the seven patients with primary ovarian cancer (two at stage 1a) had pulsatility indices (0.3 to 1.0) which clearly differentiated them from the patients with normal ovaries (3.2 to 7.0).

Blood filled ovarian cysts may be identified by their reflective contents.

Endometriosis Endometriomata contain thick syrupy altered blood which typically generates numerous low level echoes filling the space (Fig. 7). Endometriomata not adjacent to clear fluid containing cystic structures may be difficult to differentiate from ovarian stroma. The presence of ovarian endometriomata indicates a very significant degree of endometriosis which may have an important bearing on the patients' response to treatment.[24]

Other benign ovarian cysts and tumours Dermoid cysts and fibromata may occasionally be identified in the ovaries of women of reproductive age. These tumours may interfere with normal ovarian function, particularly if they are large.

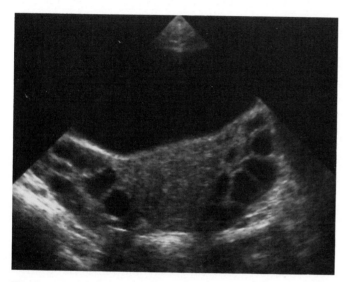

Fig. 5 Prepubertal ovary. Transabdominal ultrasound of an ovary 3 months before the menarche showing the multifollicular appearance.

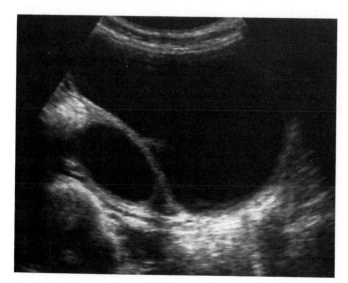

Fig. 6 A follicular cyst showing the echo-free contents and sharp outline.

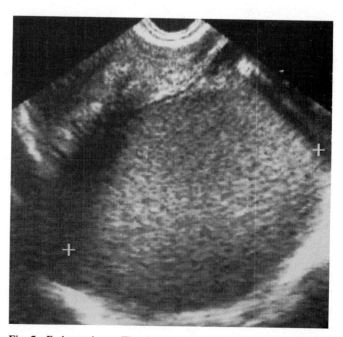

Fig. 7 Endometrioma. The characteristic ground glass appearance of an endometrioma (trans-vaginal).

Ovarian follicular monitoring

Serial monitoring of follicular development may be useful in both the natural and stimulated ovarian cycle. Observation of a developing follicle, the prediction of impending ovulation and the detection of ovulation allow procedures such as post-coital testing, hCG administration, intercourse, donor and husband insemination and egg collection to be timed optimally. Patients shown not to be ovulating may be treated with ovulation induction agents.

A baseline scan early in the menstrual cycle should always be done to identify and record cystic structures which could later be misinterpreted as developing follicles. A luteal cyst (from the previous cycle) is commonly seen and may decrease in size during the follicular phase. A coiled hydrosalpinx may be mistaken as a group of follicles if care is not taken to identify continuity of the tubal lumen (Fig. 8).

Natural cycles In the natural unstimulated ovarian cycle precursor follicles (2 to 4 mm) grow in each ovary in response to the intercycle FSH rise. There are usually about 20 of such follicles, their number decreasing with age.[25] Under optimal conditions they may be identified on ultrasound. At a mean diameter of 10 mm (range 7 to 14) 7 days (range 9 to 6) before the LH surge a dominant follicle takes over and there is very little further growth of other follicles. Non-dominant follicles within the ovary that contains the dominant follicle, tend to decrease in size during the late follicular and luteal phases of the cycle.[26]

Occasionally (5% of cycles) two dominant follicles develop.[27,28]

Stimulated and superovulation cycles Anovulation is treated by artificially raising the woman's serum follicle stimulating hormone level to initiate the growth of follicles. This may be done with oral anti-oestrogens (e.g. clomiphene or cyclofenil) which bind to cytoplasmic oestrogen receptors in the pituitary causing a secondary rise in endogenous follicle stimulating hormone (FSH), or parenterally with human menopausal gonadotrophin (hMG) or pure FSH. Preferably this therapy should stimulate the development and ovulation of one, but no more than three follicles. If more follicles are allowed to develop and ovulate, a high multiple pregnancy can result and there is a risk of the ovarian hyperstimulation syndrome (see below). Clomiphene (25 to 200 mg given for 5 days early in the follicular phase) rarely causes such problems; 10% of pregnancies are twin while triplets are very unusual (Fig. 9). Parenteral ovulation induction was previously monitored by measuring serum or urinary levels of oestrogen. When the levels rose excessively, the treatment had to be abandoned and a lower dose of gonadotrophin used in subsequent cycles. This technique does not differentiate one follicle from many follicles producing the same total amount of oestrogen. Ultrasound allows accurate monitoring of the numbers of follicles developing, but it may still be difficult to predict how many will ovulate (Fig. 8) because of the wide range of size at which follicles rupture. Patients with polycystic ovaries are particularly difficult to manage.

Superovulation therapy is used prior to assisted conception techniques such as gamete intra-fallopian transfer (GIFT) or in vitro fertilisation (IVF). HMG or pure FSH,

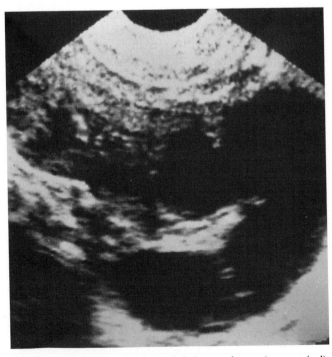

Fig. 8 A hydrosalpinx showing coiled shape and septa (trans-vaginal).

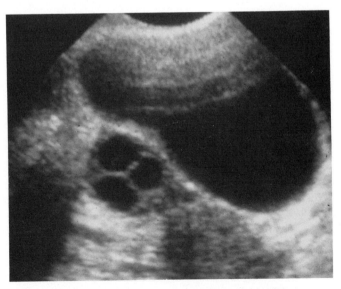

Fig. 9 Stimulated ovary. An ovary stimulated with clomiphene citrate (transabdominal).

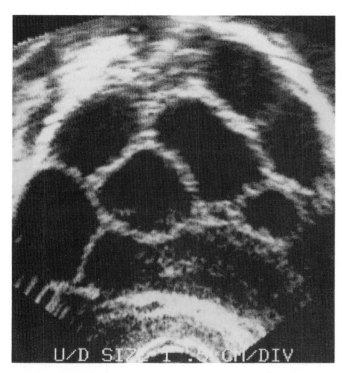

Fig. 10 **Stimulated ovary.** A trans-vaginal ultrasound scan of an ovary stimulated with hMG.

or a combination of both, with or without an anti-oestrogen are used. The objective is to stimulate the synchronous development of many follicles from which eggs are collected prior to ovulation (Fig. 10). Follicles which would have become suppressed by the dominant follicle are 'rescued' by the higher than physiological levels of FSH.[29] In some patients this strategy fails and one follicle remains dominant. Aspiration of this leading follicle may prevent it from triggering an endogenous luteinising hormone (LH) surge[30,31] and allow the treatment cycle to continue. Patients concerned that their increased production of eggs will mean an early menopause will usually be reassured when a simple explanation of the mechanism of superovulation is given. The risk of high multiple pregnancies is obviated by limiting the number of eggs or embryos replaced, but the risks of the ovarian hyperstimulation syndrome remain.

Ovarian blood supply before ovulation Taylor in 1985[32] originally obtained Doppler signals from the ovarian arteries scanning transabdominally through a full bladder. However, due to technical limitations and patient obesity, it was not possible to obtain signals in 27% of the women studied. They found that the impedance of the ovarian artery decreased throughout the menstrual cycle, possibly before the dominant follicle could be recognised by its size or increased hormone production. This effect was noted to be more marked in clomiphene stimulated cycles. Obtaining satisfactory ovarian artery Doppler signals trans-vaginally

is difficult because from this direction the artery traverses the infundibulopelvic ligament at approximately 90° to the insonating ultrasound beam. A recent study using a trans-vaginal colour flow system has raised doubts as to whether intra-ovarian vessels can be identified during the follicular phase of the menstrual cycle.[33]

During gonadotrophin-stimulated cycles for IVF, the ovarian artery impedance reduces during the follicular phase, in parallel to the increasing production of oestradiol. Furthermore, in an hMG stimulated cycle, the ovarian impedance is inversely proportional to the number of follicles greater than 15 mm which are present in the ovary, and to the number of oocytes subsequently harvested from the ovary.[34]

Follicle measurement In the unstimulated ovary follicles are approximately spherical. They may, however, be flattened in one plane or have their shape altered by pressure from the ultrasound transducer or the bladder so a mean of the maximum diameter in three planes is a better estimate of follicular size than measurements in only two planes (Figs 11 and 12).

Errors in measurement may arise as a result of difficulty in defining the follicle margin; this is more likely to occur when using transabdominal ultrasound.[35]

A blind comparison between the two ultrasound approaches has shown that although the mean readings by a single observer of follicle size are likely to be similar, whichever route is used, there is more scatter in the transabdominal readings and therefore more potential for inaccuracy.[36] The inter-observer variation of measurement is

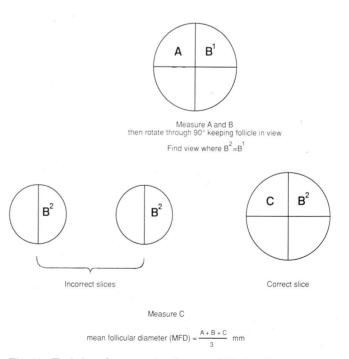

Fig. 11 **Technique for measuring the mean follicular diameter.**

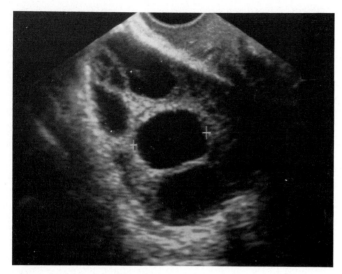

Fig. 12 Follicle measurement: the widest diameters should be selected.

larger than the intra-observer measurement by either route, the least inter-observer variation being ± 1.6 mm (95% confidence limit) for the trans-vaginal route. This suggests that serial follicular measurement is best done by the same observer using the trans-vaginal route.[37]

There is a significant correlation (r = 0.64) between the mean follicular diameter measured trans-vaginally and the follicular fluid volume aspirated laparoscopically.[38]

Follicular measurement is more difficult in stimulated and superovulation cycles as pressure from abutting follicles distorts the follicles so that measurements often have to be a 'best estimate'. When there are many follicles, assessment may have to be limited to measurement of the two or three largest and a count of the total number. The count is performed by sweeping through the ovary from one edge to the other, in any plane.

Rate of follicular growth During the 5 days prior to ovulation the dominant follicle in the natural cycle grows in a linear fashion at an average rate of 2 to 3 mm per day.[6,39] In clomiphene stimulated cycles the growth rate during the 3 days preceding ovulation has been found to be greater than in the natural cycle.[40]

Subtle changes in the rate of follicular growth in patients with endometriosis have been detected.[41]

Prediction of ovulation Follicular rupture occurs at a wide range of follicular sizes (13 to 30 mm) with a mean of 21 mm and is unaffected by prior ovulation induction therapy.[28] There is a linear correlation between the mean level of serum oestradiol and the mean follicular diameter.[42] In stimulated cycles, where there are several follicles, this relationship holds good for total follicular volume.[43] The peak serum oestradiol (1500 to 1650 pmol/l per follicle) and the peak luteinising hormone levels occur in the majority of cases 2 and 1 day respectively before ovulation.[39,44]

Because follicular size is no indication of imminent ovulation, other morphological parameters have been assessed in the hope that they will be a better guide. A poorly reflective halo around the follicle, thought to represent oedema in the theca cell layer, and a crenated lining to the follicle, thought to indicate separation of the granulosa cell layer from the basement membrane, have been described as occurring within 24 and 6 to 10 hours respectively prior to ovulation.[45] A number of authors have identified echoes within the follicle which they ascribe to the presence of an expanded cumulus oophorus, either attached to the follicular wall or free floating (Fig. 13).[46] Unfortunately none of these ultrasound signs has proved to be of practical value in the investigation or management of infertility.

Preceding ovulation, associated with the LH rise, perifollicular ovarian blood flow can be identified using trans-vaginal colour Doppler. In the few hours preceding ovulation there is a rapid increase both in the number of blood vessels that can be identified supplying the follicle and in the blood velocity within them.[33]

Ovulation pain (mittelschmerz) occurs in a minority of menstrual cycles;[28,47] it may occur either before or after ovulation,[48] though usually before,[49] and does not necessarily correspond to the side on which ovulation occurs.[47]

Timing of investigations and procedures

Because of the wide range of follicular size prior to ovulation, follicular monitoring can only give a guide to when ovulation might occur. During the 1980s, follicle monitoring was used extensively but it has now been largely superseded by urinary LH dipsticks which give 12 to 36 hours warning of ovulation; they may be purchased by the patient and used at home, which is convenient. Follicle

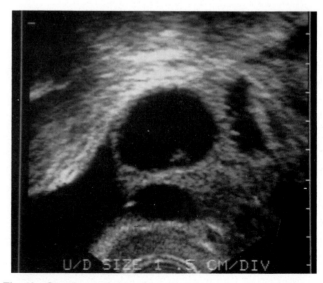

Fig. 13 Cumulus oophorus. Cone shaped cumulus mass clearly visible within pre-ovulatory follicle.

monitoring may identify a growing follicle to enable the most appropriate moment to begin testing the urine for LH to be chosen. This is particularly useful when the menstrual cycles are irregular or long.

Post-coital testing (PCT) Cervical mucus varies in consistency during the menstrual cycle in response to the changes in ovarian oestrogen production. Sperm can only swim well in the clear viscid mucus that is produced during the peri-ovulatory period. A positive post-coital test (many sperm swimming progressively through copious clear mucus) confirms that ejaculation of motile sperm has occurred into the vagina of an ovulatory woman and carries a good prognosis.

A poor or negative PCT (no sperm or few immotile or non-progressively motile sperm in low volume cellular mucus) may indicate either a significant problem (apareunia, poor sperm quality, an immunological disorder, anovulation) or a mistimed test. Assessment with ovarian ultrasound, with or without urinary LH testing, improves the likelihood that post-coital tests are timed appropriately, sparing couples the unnecessary anxiety caused by a false negative test.

Sexual intercourse and artificial insemination Serial ovarian ultrasonography may help women with irregular cycles identify their peri-ovulatory period and thus increase their chance of conception. Accurate identification of the fertile period is particularly important when artificial insemination of the partner's or donor semen is being used, as such treatment is demanding both of staff and patient time.

Donor semen is in short supply and it is therefore important to ensure that it is used efficiently. Insemination timed using ultrasound has been shown to be more successful than insemination timed using only knowledge of previous menstrual cycle lengths and basal body temperature recording.[28]

Administration of human chorionic gonadotrophin Oocyte maturation and ovulation may be induced with human chorionic gonadotrophin (hCG) when the follicle has reached a size at which it is likely to contain a suitably responsive egg. This approach is used during ovulation induction or superovulation with gonadotrophins as therapy with these drugs may reduce or completely suppress the endogenous LH surge. Ovulation occurs 32 to 40 hours after the administration of hCG. If hCG is administered late at night procedures, such as insemination and egg collection, may be performed at convenient times during the working day.

The actual follicular size at which hCG should be administered varies. Premature administration will damage the developing oocytes. When using clomiphene or hMG and sexual intercourse, good results may be achieved when hCG is administered at 17 mm. When using these drugs for superovulation prior to an egg collection, the hCG must be given before the endogenous LH surge to maintain con-

trol of the cycle. If serum or urinary LH measurements detect a premature surge or there is a fall in the serum oestradiol level, there is a risk that the oocytes will be aged when collected 36 hours later and the treatment cycle should therefore be abandoned. When the endogenous gonadotrophins have been suppressed with a luteinising hormone releasing hormone (LHRH) analogue (such as Buserelin®) there is no danger of being pre-empted by the endogenous LH surge and the hCG may then be delayed until the follicles are very much larger, without detrimental effect.[50] Delaying hCG administration allows smaller follicles to grow thereby increasing the subsequent yield of oocytes and makes the timing of the egg collection more flexible.

Ovulation

Usually the follicle simply disappears at ovulation.[28] However, an increase or decrease in size of the follicle, a change in shape or the development of irregular margins or internal echoes (Fig. 14) may all indicate that ovulation has occurred. During the peri-ovulatory period it is always possible to detect fluid in the pouch of Douglas. Only a relatively small percentage of women have a detectable increase in volume of this fluid at ovulation.[28]

Contrary to popular belief ovulation need not alternate between the two ovaries: there is a 75% chance of ovulation from the same ovary as the preceding cycle and this may continue for several consecutive cycles.[51]

Ovarian blood flow after ovulation The impedance in the artery supplying the ovary containing the corpus luteum falls significantly in comparison to the contralateral

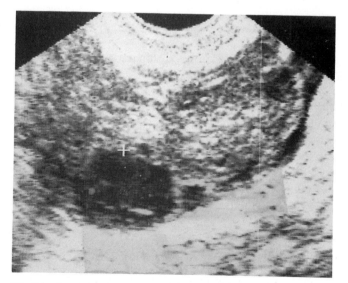

Fig. 14 Corpus luteum. A scan on the preceding day showed a 21 mm follicle. This has now developed an irregular outline and internal echoes following ovulation.

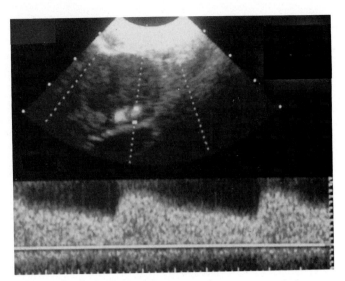

Fig. 15   Corpus luteum Doppler. Low impedance vessels near a corpus luteum (trans-vaginal Doppler).

ovary.[52] Presumably this signifies an increased blood supply and the vessels within the ovarian substance may be seen relatively easily with colour flow imaging during the luteal phase. Immediately following ovulation there is a dramatic increase in blood velocity within the vessels supplying the newly formed corpus luteum. This is due to the rapid formation of new blood vessels (neovascularisation). In the adult these blood vessels only develop in the corpus luteum, wound healing and malignancy. They are unique in that they produce very low impedance Doppler waveforms because the resistance vessels (arterioles) lack muscle lining in the media (Fig. 15).

In a group of women having IVF treatment, intra-ovarian flow velocity waveforms analysed 3 days following embryo transfer showed that those who became pregnant had a lower impedance in comparison to those who did not conceive.[53]

Corpus luteum   The corpus luteum may have a variety of ultrasound appearances. After ovulation the collapsed 'follicle' may fill in almost completely and be difficult to differentiate from the surrounding ovarian stroma. There is, however, usually a cystic component which aids identification. It often increases in size and fills with echoes of varying amplitude. A haemorrhagic corpus luteum or luteal cyst (Fig. 14) may exceed 40 mm in diameter. Since the ultrasound appearance of the corpus luteum is so varied, serial examinations may be required to document its resolution at the end of the secretory phase of the cycle.

Ultrasound assessment of non-conception cycles

Serial ovarian ultrasound can detect anovulation in both natural or stimulated cycles. Lower conception rates than expected after ovulation have led to attempts to define the characteristics of unsuccessful ovulations. Asynchrony between oestrogen and luteinising hormone levels and follicular rupture has been documented[54] and some patients appear to undergo premature rupture of follicles.[55] Failure to detect follicular collapse but with infilling of the follicle suggests luteinisation without ovulation. The luteinised unruptured follicle (LUF) syndrome, occurs more often in infertile than fertile patients and could possibly be a cause of unexplained infertility.[56] The absence of an ovulatory stigma in such patients has been confirmed laparoscopically[57] but the ultrasonic diagnosis was found to have a 15% false positive rate. The LUF syndrome may be more common with endometriosis.

Great care should be taken in diagnosing this syndrome as ovulation may be associated with an increase in the size of apparent 'follicles' and these cystic corpora lutea may even indicate a conception cycle.[58]

Ovarian hyperstimulation syndrome

The ovarian hyperstimulation syndrome (OHSS) is potentially the most serious complication of ovulation induction with gonadotrophins. The syndrome occurs after hCG administration to patients with a large number of follicles and high serum oestradiol levels and is particularly likely to occur in patients with a polycystic ovarian morphology. HCG administration is less likely to be followed by clinically significant hyperstimulation syndrome if the follicles are subsequently aspirated at egg collection. This is probably because a substantial proportion of the oestrogen secreting granulosa cells are removed with the follicular fluid. In principle, if the ovarian response is monitored with oestrogens or ultrasound, and cycles causing concern abandoned before hCG administration, hyperstimulation is avoidable. In practice, however, even in the most careful hands, cases occur, particularly following superovulation therapy prior to assisted conception techniques. The syndrome may be divided into mild, moderate and severe depending on the degree of ovarian enlargement, symptoms and signs.

Mild OHSS (lower abdominal discomfort, ovaries enlarged up to 5 × 5 cm) occurs in most patients who successfully superovulate prior to egg collection. Such patients may be observed and managed symptomatically. They do not require admission to hospital.

Patients with more serious OHSS may be divided on ultrasound criteria into moderate (ovaries measuring more than 5 × 5 cm) (Fig. 16) and severe (ovaries measuring more than 12 × 12 cm).[59] The clinical features which cause concern are nausea, vomiting, ascites, pleural and pericardial effusions. These features all compound to worsen the haemoconcentration, causing hyperviscosity and hypercoaguability, which predispose to thrombosis, embolism and renal failure. Gross ascites may aggravate the discomfort, nausea and vomiting. Previously paracentesis

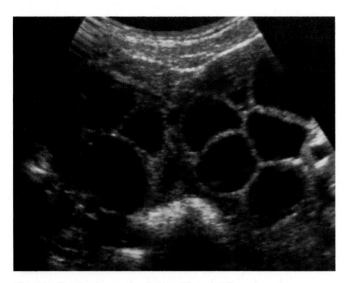

Fig. 16 Ovarian hyperstimulation. There is bilateral ovarian enlargement with multiple follicles.

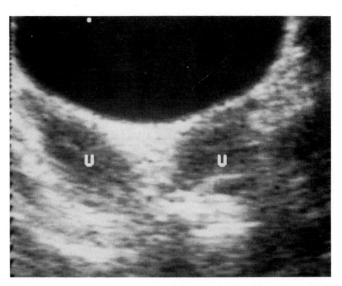

Fig. 17 Transabdominal scan of uterus didelphys; the separate uteri (U) may be seen.

was proscribed[59] because of the risk of damage to the fragile luteal cysts but, when performed under ultrasound control,[60] it has been found to be a safe and useful procedure.

Uterine ultrasound

Identification

The uterus is usually easily identifiable in the midline, its uniformly reflective myometrium contrasting with the varying reflectivity of the adjacent bowel. The opposing surfaces of the endometrium produce a characteristic midline echo usually of high reflectivity. In patients with the pelvic anatomy distorted by an adnexal mass or fibroids it may be helpful to identify the external os and follow the endometrial cavity to the fundus. There is no relationship between uterine position (anteversion or retroversion) and infertility.

Congenital abnormalities

Trans-vaginal ultrasonography can be used to identify congenital uterine malformations,[61] the most common of which is the partially septate uterus, which is a leading cause of repeated first trimester miscarriage.[62] However, major malformations such as uterus didelphys (Fig. 17) are not usually associated with infertility.[63]

Visualisation of uterine malformations can be improved by filling the uterine cavity with saline.[64]

Cervix

Mucus retention cysts are commonly seen within the substance of the cervix (Fig. 18) (see Ch. 3). During the

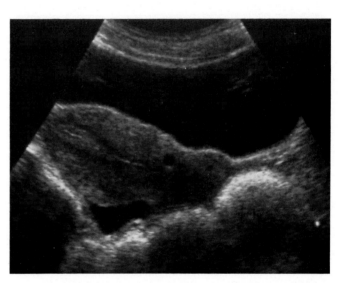

Fig. 18 Nabothian cyst. Endocervical mucus retention cyst. Note a little fluid in the pouch of Douglas.

periovulatory period a column of mucus may be seen extending from the external os to the uterine cavity.

Myometrium

Changes during the menstrual cycle The uterine cross-sectioned area increases in response to the rising oestradiol levels during the follicular phase of the cycle.[65]

Rhythmic contractions of the sub-endometrial myometrium causing fluid within the uterine cavity to move may be observed with the trans-vaginal probe (Fig. 19). The amplitude and frequency of these contractions peak during the peri-ovulatory period.[66]

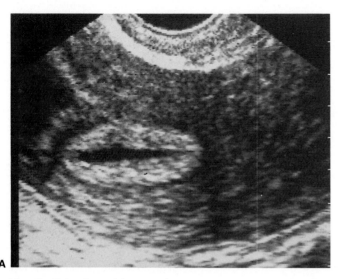

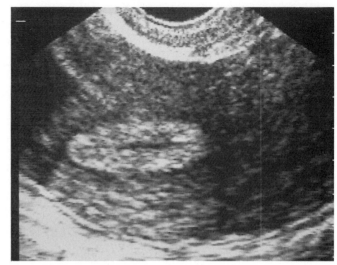

Fig. 19 Subendometrial contractions (every 18 seconds) moving fluid in endometrial cavity; 1 day post-ovulation in conception cycle.

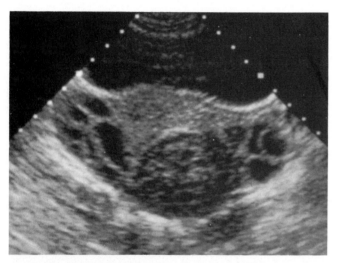

Fig. 20 Posterior wall fibroid seen with transabdominal ultrasound. The ovaries have been superovulated. (Figure courtesy of Ms V Sharma, St James' Hospital, Leeds.)

Leiomyoma Fibroids may be identified by their disruption of either the uniform myometrial reflectivity or the smooth uterine outline (Fig. 20). They often contain highly reflective areas which may cast an acoustic shadow. Large fibroids are best seen with transabdominal ultrasound as they often extend beyond the effective range of the trans-vaginal probe. The relationship of fibroids to the uterine cavity may be examined closely with trans-vaginal ultrasound. The effect of fibroids on fertility probably depends on their site: large fibroids may anatomically disturb oocyte pick-up by the fimbrial end of the tube while those near the cornua may obstruct the fallopian tube. Submucous fibroids may interfere with implantation, particularly if they are pedunculated.

Endometrium

Changes during the menstrual cycle During the menses the endometrium may be identified as a narrow strip of variable reflectivity on either side of the midline echo (Fig. 21).

The endometrium thickens as the serum oestrogen level rises. It is initially seen as a poorly reflective zone on either side of the midline echo (Fig. 22). Its outer margin, where it meets the myometrium, is defined by a band of increased reflectivity. Immediately outside this band is a 'halo' of reduced reflectivity thought to represent the inner layers of compact and vascular myometrium.[67] The reflectivity of the endometrium increases so that by mid-cycle it is

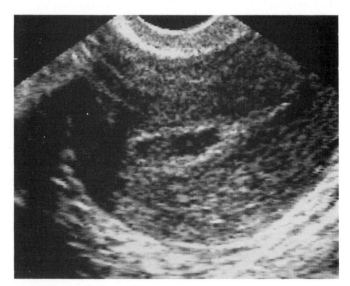

Fig. 21 Day 2 of menses; blood in endometrial cavity, thin endometrium.

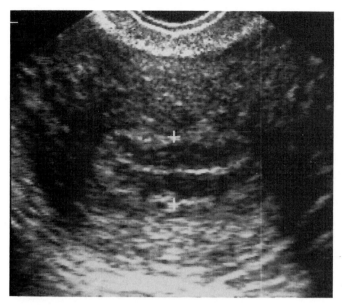

Fig. 22 Poorly reflective mid-follicular endometrium.

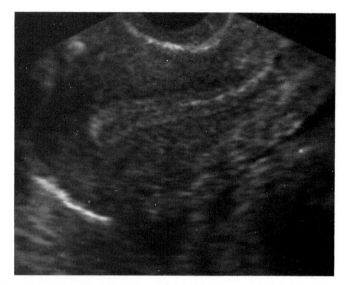

Fig. 24 Moderately reflective mid-luteal endometrium.

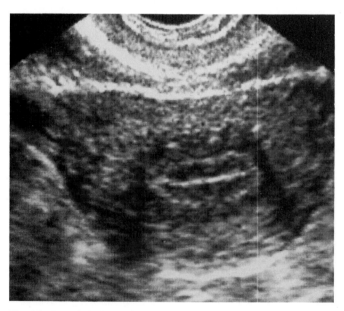

Fig. 23 Isoechoic late follicular endometrium.

isoechoic with the myometrium (Fig. 23) but by the mid-luteal phase it is more reflective (Fig. 24).[68] Enlargement and tortuosity of the glands along with an increase in glycogen and mucus content are presumed to cause the increasing reflectivity.

The endometrial thickness increases through to the mid-luteal phase then plateaus before falling, prior to the next menses.[69] If conception occurs the thickness increases further.

Endometrial indices and fertility Endometrial growth in a stimulated cycle is very similar to the normal cycle in spite of much higher oestrogen levels. This suggests that the uterine response in the natural cycle is virtually maximal. There is a tendency for the endometrium to be thinner when clomiphene citrate is used.[69,70] A positive correlation between endometrial thickness in the follicular phase and subsequent conception has been reported[71,72] but the majority of authors have failed to confirm such a relationship.[67,69,73,74]

Endometrial reflectivity may be used as a guide to variations in the end organ response to oestrogen, thus allowing earlier administration of hCG than adherence to a fixed minimum mean follicular diameter would allow.[75]

Both in the late follicular phase and after egg collection in superovulated IVF cycles an endometrium of low reflectivity is associated with higher pregnancy rates than when the endometrium is more reflective.[74,76] This ultrasonic 'advancement' may be indicative of premature luteinisation which would be expected to have an adverse effect on the cycle outcome.

Suboptimal levels of mid-luteal serum progesterone correlated with an endometrial thickness below 10 mm.[77] An attempt has been made to use endometrial thickness in the luteal phase to predict conception. A minimum thickness 11 days after hCG has been defined but increased growth does not occur early enough to be useful.[73] In practice assessment of the endometrium is of little use in the management of the infertile couple.

Adhesions Intra-uterine adhesions may form following surgical trauma or infection. If these adhesions occur in the cervical canal or lower uterine segment, amenorrhoea will ensue (Asherman's syndrome) and a haematometra may be demonstrable. It may be possible, under ultrasound guidance, to relieve the obstruction with a uterine sound.[78]

Benign polyps Endometrial polyps may be identified

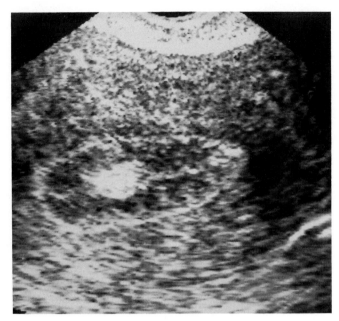

Fig. 25   Polyp. Small, clearly defined highly reflective ellipsoid polyp within the upper endometrial cavity.

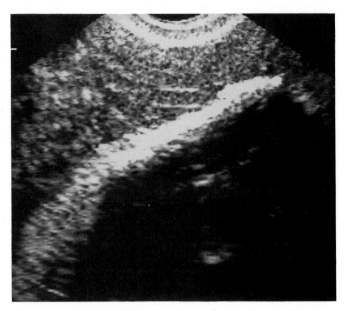

Fig. 26   Endometrial ossification – intensely reflective endometrium with acoustic shadow.

by ultrasound. Their relevance to fertility is unknown. The ultrasound appearances are variable and range from apparent endometrial thickening to clearly defined lesions which may be either poorly or highly reflective (Fig. 25).

Endometrial ossification   The aetiology of this rare condition is unknown. Pieces of cartilage or bone are found at hysteroscopy or dilatation and curettage. They may act like an intra-uterine contraceptive device and inhibit implantation.[79] The highly reflective bone has a striking appearance (Fig. 26).

Intra-uterine contraceptive device   Very occasionally examination of the uterine cavity reveals an intra-uterine contraceptive device, the removal of which should rapidly resolve the patient's infertility problem!

Uterine artery blood flow

Trans-vaginal colour Doppler allows the ascending branch of the uterine artery to be identified and insonated at an optimal angle to obtain a spectral tracing. Changes in the uterine blood supply during the menstrual cycle of normal women,[80] subfertile women and in stimulated cycles have been investigated using this technique. Normally the rise in oestrogens in the follicular phase is associated with decreasing uterine artery impedance (Figs 27 and 28). At mid-cycle there is a transitory rise in resistance, followed by a further fall to the lowest value at 7 days after ovulation. Prior to menstruation the impedance rises as the ovarian hormone levels fall.

Patients with a high uterine artery impedance immediately prior to embryo transfer during treatment with in vitro fertilisation, fail to conceive.[81] Attempts to improve

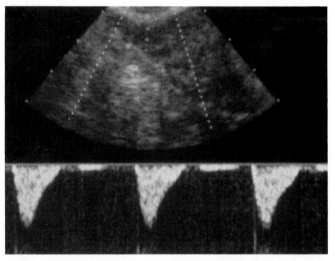

Fig. 27   Uterine blood flow – early follicular phase. No end diastolic flow.

results with oestrogen therapy and by cryopreserving the embryos for replacement in an artificial cycle have met with some success.[82,83]

Tubal ultrasound

The normal tube

The fallopian tube is not usually visible with ultrasound though it is sometimes possible to visualise the reflective fimbrial end within fluid in the pouch of Douglas.[84] Fimbrial cysts are common and may be seen as echo-free structures separate from the ovary.

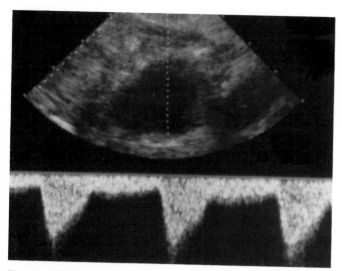

Fig. 28 Uterine blood flow – mid-luteal phase. Continuous flow through systole and diastole. (Figure courtesy of R Schlief, Clinical Research Diagnostics, Schering AG, PO Box 65 03 11, Berlin.)

The abnormal tube and pelvic inflammatory disease

Blockage of the fallopian tube with accumulation of fluid (hydrosalpinx) may be demonstrated with ultrasound. Typically the distended tube is coiled around the ovary and the folds produce septa which do not completely cross the lumen (Fig. 8). Conception rates following salpingostomy are less than 25% if the hydrosalpinx has a thick wall or a diameter greater than 15 mm.[85] Other damage from pelvic infection may be detectable with ultrasound. A tubo-ovarian abscess may be differentiated from an ovarian cyst by its thick wall and reflective contents. Pelvic adhesions may be seen as loculated fluid collections.

Tubal patency testing

Tubal patency is usually assessed either by hystero-salpingography or at laparoscopy. Following injection of saline through the cervix ultrasound may be used to detect fluid in the pouch of Douglas for assessment of tubal patency.[64] It is as sensitive as hysterosalpingography at demonstrating the patency of at least one tube but is less good at establishing the side that is patent. An ultrasound contrast medium (Echovist: Schering, Berlin) consisting of a suspension of galactose monosaccharide microparticles in an aqueous (20%) solution, has been used to assess tubal patency. Unfortunately this technique overestimates the incidence of tubal blockage.[86] Ultrasound is unlikely to replace conventional techniques for the assessment of tubal patency.

Ultrasound directed procedures

Introduction

Transabdominal ultrasound directed oocyte harvesting was the first ultrasound directed procedure used in the treatment of infertility.[87] Since that time ultrasound has played an increasingly important role in the treatment of infertility.

Follicle aspiration

Historical review In the first successful in vitro fertilisation attempts, oocytes were collected during laparoscopy. This is an expensive procedure, requiring in-patient care and general anaesthesia; it fails when there are peri-ovarian adhesions and it has a significant serious complication rate,[88] including haemorrhage and infection. Demand for in vitro fertilisation and other assisted conception techniques requiring egg collection has increased as

Table 1 Ultrasound directed follicle aspiration. King's College Hospital, London. 1983–1990

Year	TA/TV	PU/TV	Direct TA	TV (abd. probe)	TV (vag. probe)	Mixed routes	Total
1983	45						45
1984	145	6		6			157
1985	48	188	1	1		55	293
1986	2	291	2	0	60	30	385
1987	0	57	0	0	338	23	418
1988	1	14	0	0	515	9	539
1989	4	4	0	0	648	3	659
1990	0	0	0	0	813	5	818
Total	245	560	3	7	2374	125	3314

TA/TV – transabdominal trans-vesical
TA – transabdominal
PU/TV – perurethral trans-vesical
TV – trans-vaginal

results have improved. Cost considerations have provided pressure to simplify the procedures. Ultrasound directed follicle aspiration (UDFA) has reduced costs considerably because egg collection becomes an outpatient technique that requires minimal analgesia.

UDFA was initially guided by transabdominal ultrasound developed from experience with ultrasound directed amniocentesis.[89] The ovary was either approached through the full bladder (transabdominal, through the bladder),[90] or directly, through the anterior abdominal wall (direct transabdominal). Subsequently trans-vaginal,[91] trans-vaginal/trans-vesical[92] and perurethral approaches were developed.[93] However, these techniques, though as effective as laparoscopy,[94] were not easy to learn and were not widely adapted. Oocyte collection using a trans-vaginal ultrasound transducer was first described by Wikland in 1985.[95] This approach has become the technique of choice. Table 1 shows how the preferred route for egg collection at King's College Hospital has moved from transabdominal trans-vesical in 1983/84 to perurethral in 1985/86 and finally to trans- vaginal with the trans-vaginal probe since 1987.

Patient preparation and analgesia   Most patients require some form of analgesia such as pethidine and a tranquilliser, such as diazepam; the risk of vomiting necessitates starving for 6 hours and careful titration of the drugs against the patient's level of consciousness and an oxygen supply should respiratory support become necessary. A benzodiazepine tranquilliser may be used as premedication pre-operatively to reduce anxiety. UDFA may be performed with no analgesia if there are few follicles or if the patient is particularly stoical and some patients may find hypnotherapy adequate. Good rapport between patient and operator is crucial: excessive intravenous sedation may make the patient confused and uncooperative.

A paracervical block with lignocaine may be used prior to trans-vaginal egg collection and, though this local anaesthetic is a known parthenogenetic activator and appears in the follicular fluid, it has not been found to have an adverse effect on oocyte quality.[96] Epidural anaesthesia renders the patient pain-free but the subsequent recovery time precludes its routine use.

Vaginal route   The patient is placed in the lithotomy position; preparation varies from simply cleansing the vagina with saline and culture medium[96] to preparation with povidone iodine on the day before and of the procedure.[97] Antibiotics, both oral and intravenous, have been used.[98]

The trans-vaginal transducer is covered with a sterile spermicide-free condom. A biopsy guide is attached and the assembly is inserted into the vagina. The end of the transducer rests in the lateral fornix of the vagina on the side of the ovary to be punctured (Fig. 29). The follicles are identified and the electronic biopsy guides lined up with a follicle in the middle of the ovary. The distance from the end of the probe to the centre of the follicle is

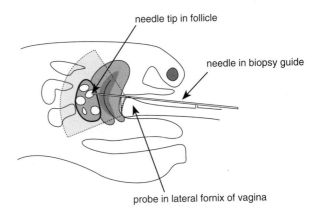

needle tip in follicle

needle in biopsy guide

probe in lateral fornix of vagina

Fig. 29   Diagram of trans-vaginal ultrasound directed follicle aspiration.

measured and, after warning the patient to expect a sharp stabbing sensation, the needle is passed rapidly into the ovary (Fig. 30). A single channel needle is preferred[99] though a double channel needle that allows aspiration and flushing through separate channels has been used,[100] but this is slower and no more productive.

The follicular fluid is aspirated by applying suction from a pump at approximately 100 mmHg. It is important to ensure that the follicle is entirely empty before re-aligning the needle or moving on to the next follicle. It is usually possible to empty all the follicles in each ovary with one puncture on each side.

Alternative routes   Occasionally some or all the follicles are not accessible by the trans-vaginal approach. If an ovary is fixed on the posterior aspect of the uterus the operator has a choice between needling the follicles through the myometrium (Fig. 31) (avoiding the endometrium[101]) or filling the bladder and reaching them over the fundus of the uterus (Fig. 32; needle A). If an ovary is out of the range of the trans-vaginal transducer and does not descend with pressure on the lower abdominal wall, it may be approached using the direct transabdominal route (Fig. 32; needle B) or the perurethral route (Fig. 32; needle C).

i) Transabdominal trans-vesical follicle aspiration
The patient is placed in the lithotomy position and catheterised with a Foley catheter (12 French gauge). Throughout the procedure the bladder volume is adjusted with Hartmann's solution to optimise viewing of the follicles to be aspirated with as little discomfort to the patient as possible.

After anaesthetising a small area of the skin on the anterior abdominal wall with 10 ml of 1% lignocaine, a needle is passed under freehand ultrasound guidance into the bladder. The needle is then manipulated within the bladder to a suitable angle (Fig. 33) before passing it through the posterior bladder wall into the ovary. It is often possible to aspirate all the follicles in each ovary

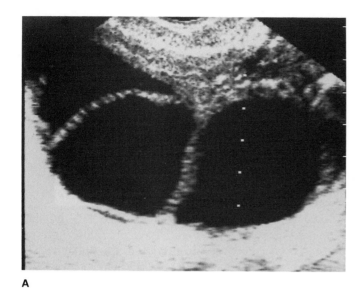

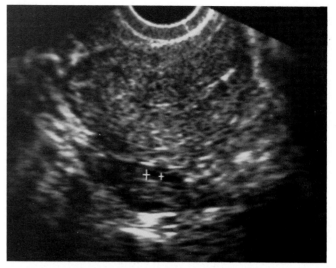

Fig. 31 Posteriorly sited ovary. Oocyte recovery from an ovary in this position is not practicable via the trans-vaginal route.

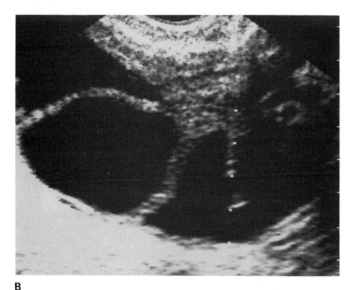

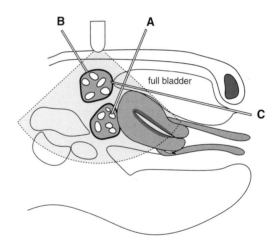

Fig. 32 Alternative routes for ultrasound directed follicle aspiration.

Fig. 30 Ultrasound guided oocyte recovery. A: Ovary before and **B:** after needle passed into follicle under trans-vaginal ultrasound guidance.

through a single posterior bladder wall puncture, but withdrawal into the bladder and realignment may be necessary. The contralateral ovary is approached through a second anterior abdominal wall puncture.

ii) Direct transabdominal follicle aspiration The patient is placed supine, a full bladder may help by steadying the ovary but it is not always necessary. An ultrasound transducer with a short focal length and high frequency, such as a trans-vaginal probe, gives good images of the ovaries (Fig. 3).

After anaesthetising the skin and abdominal wall, a needle is passed directly into a target follicle either freehand or using a biopsy guide.

Withdrawal of the needle to the ovarian surface enables the operator to realign the needle for subsequent follicles. This procedure is more difficult than either of the other techniques, particularly if the anterior abdominal wall is thick.

iii) Perurethral route The patient is placed in the lithotomy position. A needle is introduced into the bladder with the tip sheathed in the side hole of a Foley catheter (14 French gauge). Under transabdominal ultrasound control the bladder is filled with Hartmann's solution until the follicles are seen clearly. The needle is disengaged from the catheter and the follicles aspirated in a similar manner to that described under the transabdominal trans-vesical technique. As the needle is nearly at right angles to the transducer, its entire length should be seen (Fig. 34).

Results In 1990 in our unit (King's College Hospital, London) a total of 818 cases of UDFA were performed with a mean of 17 follicles aspirated (range 1 to 54). Each

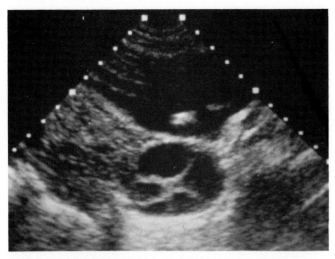

Fig. 33 Transabdominal trans-vesical UDFA; highly reflective needle tip seen immediately prior to posterior bladder wall and follicle puncture.

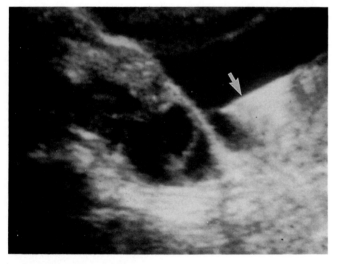

Fig. 34 Perurethral UDFA; needle (arrow) poised to puncture posterior bladder wall and enter follicle. The entire length of the needle is visible.

procedure took 35 minutes on average and 10 eggs were collected (range 1 to 37). During 1990 the follicles were aspirated and then routinely flushed. At the beginning of 1991 a policy of aspiration only was adopted unless there were less than five follicles available, in which case we flushed as often as was necessary.

From 1 March to 28 May 1991 a total of 160 aspirations were performed with a mean of 18 follicles (range 3 to 55). The time for each procedure was shortened to 22 minutes (range 5 to 60), while on average 12 eggs were collected (range 1 to 36). The very significant reduction in procedure time with no reduction in the number of eggs collected per follicle is striking.

In 1990 it was necessary to resort to an alternative route in five cases. In one case an ovary was inaccessible on the posterior aspect of the uterus. In four cases an ovary was too high to be approached trans-vaginally.

Complications All patients feel some pain as the needle is initially placed in the ovary. The amount of discomfort felt as the needle is moved within the ovary is variable and much depends on the patient's personality and the theatre staff's ability to promote a relaxed atmosphere. The commonest complaint is of occasional sharp pain. Some patients feel virtually no pain whilst a few find it very uncomfortable indeed.

Removal of the needle at the end of a trans-vaginal ultrasound directed follicle aspiration procedure may be followed by haemorrhage. Inspection of the puncture site will reveal a spurting blood vessel which invariably responds to direct pressure.

One patient collapsed 18 hours after follicle harvest: laparotomy revealed significant bleeding from a large number of ruptured follicles without specific vascular damage.

It is common for the patients to complain of lower abdominal pain for a few days after the procedure. It may be difficult to determine whether this is due to a small intra-peritoneal bleed, to infection or to the hyperstimulation syndrome. Six cases of severe pelvic infection following trans-vaginal UDFA occurred in our series but there were none when the transabdominal or perurethral routes were used. In several of these cases large abscesses developed insidiously over a number of weeks.

Pelvic infections have occurred even after the administration of prophylactic antibiotics.[98] During UDFA using the transabdominal or perurethral technique, if the bladder pressure becomes too high urine may extravasate into the tissues (Fig. 35). Post-operative clot retention (Fig. 36) or urinary tract infection may occur.

It is important that patients are warned of these complications before the procedure to ensure that significant symptoms are reported immediately.

Ultrasound directed embryo transfer

Cervical embryo transfer Routine blind trans-cervical transfer of embryos to the uterine cavity is followed by implantation in approximately 10% of procedures.[102] There are many factors which may explain this poor implantation rate but mechanical failure may be contributory.

Ultrasound may be used to measure the distance from the external os to the fundus before blind transfer to ensure that the embryos are placed in the uterine cavity rather than the cervical canal. This is particularly useful when the uterus is enlarged with fibroids. The most appropriate place to deposit embryos within the uterine cavity is not known. Embryo transfer may be observed ultrasonically but in practice the catheters are not seen easily without

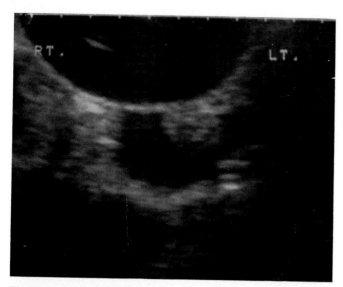

Fig. 35 **Urinary extravasation** into paravesical tissues during transabdominal trans-vesical UDFA.

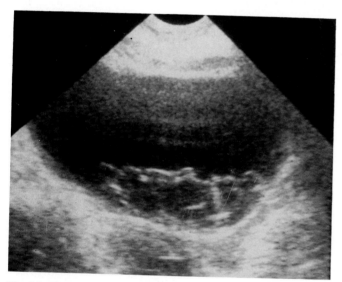

Fig. 36 **Blood clot within the bladder.** Clot causing retention after transabdominal trans-vesical UDFA.

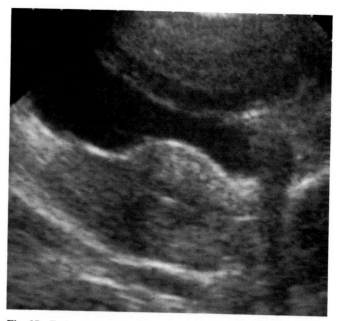

Fig. 37 **Embryo transfer catheter.** Longitudinal view of uterus pushed into an axial position by a full bladder. The embryo transfer catheter in the endometrial cavity is seen only with difficulty.

Surgical embryo transfer Very occasionally, when the cervix is severely stenosed or tortuous and both fallopian tubes are blocked, the only way to transfer embryos is surgically[104] through the myometrium.

The patient is placed in the lithotomy position, the vagina cleansed and a vaginal probe, mounted with a biopsy guide, inserted. The electronic guide line on the monitor is carefully lined up with the endometrial cavity just below the fundus. A 25 cm 19 gauge needle primed with culture medium is passed through the biopsy guide then, with a quick thrust, into the uterus. When the needle is correctly sited, injected culture medium will be seen transiently separating the reflective anterior and posterior surfaces of the endometrial cavity (Fig. 38). A long embryo transfer catheter with the embryos at its tip is then passed down the needle into the endometrial cavity. The embryos are injected and the catheter and needle withdrawn. Surgical embryo transfer may lead to pregnancy in up to 70% of cases in animals but the success rate is very low in the human.

Direct intraperitoneal insemination (DIPI)

When this relatively simple assisted conception technique was introduced in 1986[105] it was hoped that it would prove to be an effective low cost treatment for patients with patent fallopian tubes. It has been used to treat couples with unexplained infertility, cervical mucus hostility, oligospermia, failed donor insemination and women who have ovulated prior to egg collection.[106] The patient is gently superovulated with clomiphene and hMG or LHRH

moving them back and forth which risks damage to the endometrium (Fig. 37). The only randomised controlled study comparing blind with ultrasound guided embryo transfer failed to show a significant difference in pregnancy rate between the two groups.[103]

Some patients have a tortuous cervical canal which can only be negotiated under ultrasound control. Patients with a history of a difficult embryo transfer may benefit from a trial transfer between treatment cycles, during which ultrasound is used to assess the best way to manipulate the transfer catheter. The bladder volume may have a significant effect on the ease with which the catheter passes by altering the degree of uterine flexion.

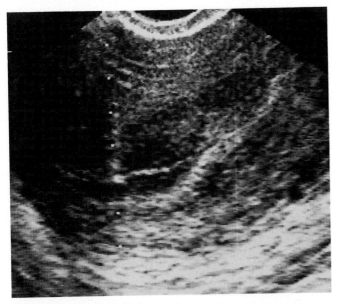

Fig. 38 Surgical embryo transfer; the needle may be seen passing through the myometrium, its tip in the endometrial cavity the anterior and posterior surfaces of which are separated by injected fluid.

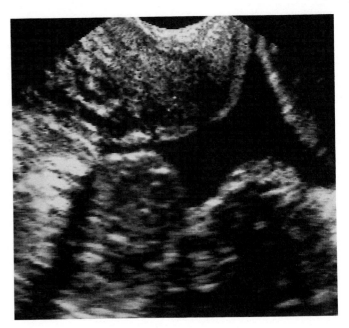

Fig. 39   Pool of fluid in pouch of Douglas.

analogue and hMG. Care is taken to avoid stimulating the development of more than three follicles greater than 14 mm. If more do develop the cycle may either be abandoned or the follicles aspirated and the patient treated with either GIFT, peritoneal oocyte sperm transfer or IVF and embryo transfer.

The procedure is performed 36 hours after administration of hCG. The patient is placed in the lithotomy position with a head up tilt so that the peritoneal fluid gravitates to the pouch of Douglas. The vagina is cleaned with an antiseptic solution and a vaginal probe with a biopsy guide attached inserted. A pool of peritoneal fluid is identified (Fig. 39). After warning the patient that she will feel a sharp pain, a 19 gauge needle is passed along the guide and into the pool with a single rapid movement. Aspiration of peritoneal fluid confirms that the needle tip is correctly sited before the injection of a prepared sperm sample. The pregnancy rate after DIPI is 10%[107] or less.[108] This is better than after superovulation alone but not better than after controlled superovulation and the intra-uterine insemination (IUI) of prepared sperm.[108] IUI probably achieves intraperitoneal insemination without the need for a surgical procedure. DIPI is unlikely to find a role in the routine treatment of infertility.

Peritoneal oocyte sperm transfer (POST)

The establishment of ultrasound directed follicle aspiration for oocyte collection removed the need for laparoscopy during treatment with IVF and embryo transfer. To units promoting the use of ultrasound techniques the introduction of GIFT in 1984 seemed like a retrograde step as it requires tubal catheterisation under laparoscopic control.

Reasoning that most patients with unexplained infertility will have gamete abnormalities rather than a problem with ovum pick up by the fallopian tube, Mason and colleagues[109] placed both sperm and oocytes in the pouch of Douglas in the hope that they would achieve results comparable to GIFT.

The patients are first superovulated as if for in vitro fertilisation, with a view to collecting a minimum of three oocytes. Initially the follicles were aspirated by the trans-abdominal trans-vaginal route, but more recently the trans-vaginal approach has been used.[110] When all the follicles have been emptied, the needle is introduced, under ultrasound guidance into the pouch of Douglas which is repeatedly rinsed with culture medium until the aspirated fluid is clear. A long embryo transfer catheter, loaded with three eggs and 4 000 000 prepared sperm, is then passed down the needle and its contents injected into the pouch of Douglas.

Sharma et al[110] have reported a pregnancy rate of 24% per POST procedure. This technique is simpler to perform than either GIFT or IVF and embryo transfer. It has two advantages over DIPI; firstly egg release from the follicle is guaranteed, secondly spare eggs not transferred may be inseminated to confirm the fertilising capability of the gametes.

This is an under-rated procedure and its role has yet to be fully evaluated.

Transuterine intrafallopian transfer (TIFT)

Fertilisation and early embryo development to the morula stage normally occur in the fallopian tube. In vitro fertilisation is performed in culture medium, designed for rodents, in the artificial environment of the laboratory. The resultant embryos are transferred to the uterus at the two to six cell stage. The culture conditions may not be optimal and the uterine environment may not suit the embryo at this early stage of development. There are therefore good reasons to believe that results will be improved by the transfer of either gametes or embryos to the fallopian tube.

This hypothesis is supported by the higher implantation rates achieved after zygote intrafallopian transfer (ZIFT) and tubal embryo stage transfer as compared to IVF and ET[111] and the good results achieved with zygote transfer.[112]

No prospective randomised trial to compare intrafallopian transfer techniques with conventional methods has been performed so the relative success rates are not known. Intrafallopian tube methods require general anaesthesia and laparoscopy with their associated risks. TIFT has been, and still is being, developed to overcome these major disadvantages.

The technique was first used to transfer sperm[113] but has since been used to transfer egg and sperm together,[114] zygotes[115] and cleavage stage embryos.[116]

The transfer device most commonly used for TIFT has been developed in Australia (William Cook; Jansen Anderson Intratubal Transfer Set). It consists of a flexible Teflon® 5.5 French gauge outer cannula with a lateral curve designed to fit into the uterine angles, a metal obturator and a soft 3 French gauge Teflon® inner cannula which tapers to 2 French at its distal 5 cm.

The patient is placed in the lithotomy position and the cervix cleaned with antiseptic solution. The metal obturator is bent to the shape of the uterine cavity and placed inside the 5.5 French gauge cannula overriding its lateral curve. The two are then inserted into the uterus. A recent design change has been the addition of an olive tip to the end of the outer cannula which allows it to be slid more smoothly into position.

The obturator is then removed allowing the outer cannulas memory to carry the cannula tip into one or other of the uterine angles. The inner 3 French cannula, containing the sperm, eggs or embryos is then passed through the outer cannula. The position of the cannulae may be confirmed with either trans-vaginal[113] or abdominal ultrasound.[115] Using a combination of operator 'feel' and ultrasound the cornual orifice is found and the tube catheterised. When this is successful the patient typically complains of lateralised discomfort. The flow of fluid as the contents of the inner cannula are injected may be seen on ultrasound.

Seven of 28 having eggs and sperm transferred and 18 of 76 having zygotes transferred conceived using this technique in Sydney, Australia between 1989 to 1990.[116] TIFT certainly has the potential to replace laparoscopic techniques but ultrasonic screening may prove unnecessary as operator skills and confidence improve.[117]

Conclusion

The modern investigation of infertility would be incomplete without pelvic ultrasound. A very significant proportion of patients requiring treatment for infertility will need monitoring with ultrasound or an ultrasound guided procedure or both.

Colour flow Doppler equipment is generating more information on reproductive events during health and disease from which we can expect the development of improved methods of treatment for infertile women.

REFERENCES

1 von Micsky L I. Ultrasonic tomography in obstetrics and gynaecology. In: Grossman C C, Holmer J H, Joyner C, Purnell E. eds. Diagnostic ultrasound. New York: Plenum Press. 1966: p 348–368

2 Kratochwil A, Urban G, Friedrich F. Ultrasonic tomography of the ovaries. Ann Chirur Gynae Fenniae 1972; 61: 211–214

3 Hackelöer B J, Hansmann M. Ultraschalldiagnostik in der fruhschwangerschaft. Gynakologe 1976; 9: 108–122

4 Hackelöer B J, Nitschte S, Daume E, Sturm G, Buchholz R. Ultraschalldarstellung von ovarveranderungen bei gonadotropinstimulierung. Geburtsh u Frauenhheilk 1977; 37: 185–190

5 Sample W F, Lippe B M, Gyepes M T. Grey-scale ultrasonography of the normal female pelvis. Radiology 1977; 125: 477–483

6 Hackelöer B J, Robinson H P. Ultraschalldarstellung des wachsenden follikels und corpus luteum in normalen physiologisschen zyklus. Geburtsh u Frauenhheilk 1978; 38: 163–168

7 Macler J, Jacquetin B, Ehret C, Dervain I, Plas-Roger S, Aron R, Renaud C. La surveillance echographique de l'induction de l'ovulation. J Gynecol Obstet Biol Reprod 1978; 7: 746–748

8 Robertson R D, Picker R H, Wilson P C, Saunders D M. Assessment of ovulation by ultrasound and plasma estrodiol determinations. Obstet Gynecol 1979; 54: 686–691

9 Hackelöer B J, Fleming R, Robinson H P, Adam D H, Coutts J R T. Correlation of ultrasonic and endocrinologic assessment of human follicular development. Am J Obstet Gynecol 1979; 135: 122–128.

10 Queenan J T, O'Brien G D, Bains L M, Simpson J, Collins W P, Campbell S. Ultrasound scanning of ovaries to detect ovulation in women. Fertil Steril 1980; 34: 99–105

11 Morimoto N, Noda Y, Takai I, Yamada I, Tojo S. Ultrasonographic observation of ovarian follicular development via vaginal route. Acta Obstet Gynaecol Jpn 1983; 35: 151–158

12 Williams S R, Rothchild I, Wesolowski D, Austin C, Speroff L. Does exposure of preovulatory oocytes to ultrasonic radiation affect reproductive performance. In Vitro Fertil Embryo Transfer 1988; 5(1): 18–21

13 Polson D W, Wadsworth J, Adams J, Franks S. Polycystic ovaries – a common finding in normal women. Lancet 1988; i: 870–872

14 Adams J, Polson D W, Franks S. Prevalence of polycystic ovaries in women with anovulation and idiopathic ligutism. BMJ 1986; 293: 355–359

15 Homburg R, Armar N A, Eshel A, Adams J, Jacobs H S. Influence of serum luteinizing hormone concentrations on ovulation, conception and early pregnancy loss in polycystic ovary syndrome. BMJ 1988; 297: 1024–1026

16 Eshel A, Abdulwahid N A, Armar N A, Adams J M, Jacobs H S.

Pusatile luteinizing hormone – releasing hormone therapy in women with polycystic ovary syndrome. Fertil Steril 1988; 49: 956–960

17 Adams J, Polson D W, Abdulwahid N, et al. Multifollicular ovaries: clinical and endocrine features and response to pulsatile gonadotrophin releasing hormone. Lancet 1985; ii: 1375–1379

18 Editorial. Follicular multiplicity. Lancet 1985; ii: 1404

19 Granberg S, Wikland M. Ultrasound in the diagnosis and treatment of ovarian cystic tumours. Hum Reprod 1991; 6: 177–185

20 Hornstein M D, Barbieri R L, Ravnikar V A, McShane P M. The effects of baseline ovarian cysts on the clinical response to controlled ovarian hyperstimulation in an in vitro fertilization program. Fertil Steril 1989; 52: 437–440

21 Thatcher S S, Jones E, Decherney A H. Ovarian cysts decrease the success of controlled ovarian stimulation and in vitro fertilization. Fertil Steril 1989; 52: 812–816

22 Rizk B, Tan S L, Kingsland C, Steer C, Mason B A, Campbell S. Ovarian cyst aspiration and the outcome of in vitro fertilisation. Fertil Steril 1990; 54: 661–664

23 Bourne T, Campbell S, Steer C, Whitehead M, Collins W. Transvaginal colour flow imaging: a possible new screening technique for ovarian cancer. BMJ 1989; 299: 1367–1370

24 Dlugi A M, Coy R A, Dieterle S, Bayer S R, Seibel M M. The effect of endometriomas on in vitro fertilisation outcome. In Vitro Fertil and Embryo Transfer 1989; 6: 338–341

25 Glasier A F, Baird D T, Hillier S G. FSH and the control of follicular growth. J Steroid Biochem 1989; 32: 167–170

26 Packe T D, Wladimiroff J W, DeJon F H, Hop W C, Fauser B C. Growth patterns of non-dominant ovarian follicles during the normal menstrual cycle. Fertil Steril 1990; 54: 638–642

27 O'Herlihy C, DeCrespigny L, Lopata A, Johnston I, Hoult I, Robinson H. Preovulatory follicular size: a comparison of ultrasound and laparoscopic measurements. Fertil Steril 1990; 34: 24–26

28 Marinho A O, Sallam H N, Goessens L K V, Collins W P, Rodeck C H, Campbell S. Real time pelvic ultrasonography during the periovulatory period of patients attending an artificial insemination clinic. Fertil Sertil 1982; 37: 633–638

29 Hillier S G, Afrian A M M, Margara R A, Winston R M L. Superovulation strategy before in vitro fertilisation. Clin Obstet Gynaecol 1985; 12: 687–723

30 Barash A, Shoham Z, Lunenfeld B, Segal I, Insler V, Borenstein R. Can premature luteinization in superovulation protocols be prevented by aspiration of an ill-timed leading follicle? Fertil Steril 1990; 53: 865–869

31 Pampiglione J S, Tan S L, Steer C V, Wren M, Parsons J H, Campbell S. Drainage of the dominant follicle in in-vitro fertilisation. Assisted Reproduction, Technology and Andrology 1991; 1: 76–80

32 Taylor K J W, Burns P N, Woodcock J P, Wells P N T. Blood flow in deep abdominal and pelvic vessels: ultrasonic pulsed Doppler analysis. Radiology 1985; 54: 487–493

33 Bourne T, Jurkovic D, Waterstone J, Campbell S, Collins W. Intrafollicular blood flow during human ovulation. Ultrasound Obstet Gynecol 1991; 1: 53–59

34 Dentinger J, Reinthaller A, Bernaschek G. Transvaginal pulsed Doppler measurement of blood flow velocity in the ovarian arteries during cycle stimulation and after follicle puncture. Fertil Steril 1989; 51: 466–470

35 Andreotti R F, Thompson G H, Janowitz W, Shapiro A, Zusmer N R. Endovaginal and transabdominal sonography of ovarian follicles. J Ultrasound Med 1989; 8: 555–560

36 Gonzalez C J, Curson R, Parsons J. Transabdominal versus transvaginal ultrasound scanning of ovarian follicles: are they comparable? Fertil Steril 1988; 50: 657–659

37 Eissa M K, Hudson K, Docker M F, Sawers R S, Newton J R. Ultrasound follicle diameter measurement: an assessment of inter observer and intra observer variation. Fertil Steril 1985; 44: 751–754

38 Yee B, Barnes R B, Vargyas J M, Marrs R P. Correlation of transabdominal and transvaginal ultrasound measurements of follicle size and number with laparoscopic findings for in vitro fertilisation. Fertil Steril 1987; 47: 828–832

39 Renaud R L, Macler J, Dervain I, et al. Echographic study of follicular maturation and ovulation during the normal menstrual cycle. Fertil Steril 1980; 33: 272–276

40 Leerentveld R A, Gent I, Stoep M, Wladimiroff J W. Ultrasonographic assessment of follicle growth under monofollicular and multifollicular conditions in clomiphene citrate – stimulated cycles. Fertil Steril 1985; 43: 565–569

41 Doody M C, Gibbons W E, Zamah N M. Linear regression analysis of ultrasound follicular growth series: statistical relationship of growth rate and calculated date of growth onset to total growth period. Fertil Steril 1987; 47: 436–440

42 Hackelöer B J, Sallam H N. Ultrasound scanning of ovarian follicles. Clin Obstet Gynaecol 1983; 10: 603–620

43 Hillier S G, Parsons J H, Morgara R A, Winston R M L, Crofton M E. Serum oestradiol and preovulatory follicular development before in-vitro fertilisation. Endoc 1984; 101: 113–118

44 Smith D H, Picker R H, Sinosich M, Saunders D M. Assessment of ovulation by ultrasound and oestradiol levels during spontaneous and induced cycles. Fertil Steril 1980; 33: 387–390

45 Picker R H, Smith D H, Tucker M H, Saunders D M. Ultrasonic signs of imminent ovulation. JCU 1983; 11: 1–2

46 Kerin J F, Edmonds D K, Warners G M, et al. Morphological and functional relations of Graafian follicle growth to ovulation in women using ultrasonic, laparoscopic and biochemical measurements. Br J Obstet Gynaecol 1981; 88: 81–90

47 Marinho A O, Sallam H N, Goessens L, Collins W P, Campbell S. Ovulation side and occurrence of mittleschmerz in spontaneous and induced ovarian cycles. BMJ 1982; 284: 632

48 Depares J, Ryder R E J, Walker S M, Scanlon M F, Norman C M. Ovarian ultrasonography highlights precision of symptoms of ovulation as markers of ovulation. BMJ 1986; 292: 1562

49 O'Herlihy C, Robinson H P, Crespigny L J. Mittleschmerz is a preovulatory symptom. BMJ 1980; 986

50 Rutherford A J, Subak-Sharpe R J, Dawson K J, Margara R A, Frank S, Winston. Improvement of in vitro fertilisation after treatment with buserelin an agonist of lutenising hormone releasing hormone. BMJ 1988; 296: 1765–1768

51 Werlin L B, Weckstein L, Weathersbee P S, Parenicta K, White D, Stone S C. Ultrasound: a technique useful in determining the side of ovulation. Fertil Steril 1986; 46: 814–817

52 Scholtes M C W, Wladimiroff J W, Van Rijen H J M, Hop W C J. Uterine and ovarian flow velocity waveforms in the normal menstrual cycle: a transvaginal Doppler study. Fertil Steril 1989; 52: 981–985

53 Baber R J, McSweeney M B, Gill R W, et al. Transvaginal pulsed Doppler ultrasound assessment of blood flow to the corpus luteum in IVF patients following embryo transfer. Br J Obstet Gynaecol 1988; 95: 1226–1230

54 Polan M L, Totora M, Caldwell B V, Decherney A H, Haseltine F P, Kase N. Abnormal ovarian cycles as diagnosed by ultrasound and serum estodiol levels. Fertil Steril 1982; 37: 342–347

55 Ying Y K, Daly D C, Randolph J F, et al. Ultrasonographic monitoring of follicular growth for luteal phase defects. Fertil Steril 1987; 48: 433–436

56 Bateman B G, Kolp L A, Nunley W C, Thomas T S, Mills S E. Oocyte retention after follicle luteinization. Fertil Steril 1990; 54: 793–798

57 Liukkonen S, Koskimies A I, Tenhunen A, Ylostalo P. Diagnosis of luteinized unruptured follicle (LUF) syndrome by ultrasound. Fertil Steril 1984; 41: 26–30

58 Hackelöer B J. Ultrasound scanning of the ovarian cycle. In Vitro Fertil Embryo Transfer 1984; 1: 217–220

59 Schenker J G, Weinstein D. Ovarian hyperstimulation syndrome: a current survey. Fertil Steril 1978; 30: 255–268

60 Borenstein R, Elhalah U, Lunenfeld B, Schwartz Z S. Severe ovarian hyperstimulation syndrome: a reevaluated therapeutic approach. Fertil Steril 1989; 51: 791–795

61 Nasri M N, Setchell M E, Chard T. Transvaginal ultrasound for diagnosis of uterine malformations. Br J Obstet Gynaecol 1990; 97: 1043–1045

62 Rrock J A, Schlaff W D. The obstetric consequences of uterovaginal anomalies. Fertil Steril 1985; 43: 681–692

63 Jones H W. Reproductive impairment and the malformed uterus. Fertil Steril 1981; 36: 137–148

64 Randolph J R, Ying Y K, Maier D B, Schmidt C L, Riddick D H. Comparison of real-time ultrasonography, hysterosalpingography and laparoscopy/hysteroscopy in the evaluation of uterine abnormalities and tubal patency. Fertil Steril 1986; 46: 828–832

65 Adams J M, Tan S L, Wheeler M J, Morris D V, Jacobs H S, Franks S. Uterine growth in the follicular phase of spontaneous ovulatory cycles and during luteinizing hormone-releasing hormone induced cycles in women with normal or polycystic ovaries. Fertil Steril 1988; 49: 52–55

66 Lyons E A, Taylor P J, Zheng X H, Ballard G, Levi C S, Kredenster J V. Characterisation of subendometrial myometrial contractions throughout the menstrual cycle in normal fertile women. Fertil Steril 1991; 55: 771–774

67 Fleischer A C, Herbert C M, Sacks G A, Wentz A C, Entiman S S, James A E. Sonography of the endometrium during conception and non-conception cycles of in vitro fertilisation and embryo transfer. Fertil Steril 1986; 46: 442–447

68 Randall J M, Fisk N M, McTavish A, Templeton A A. Transvaginal ultrasonic assessment of endometrial growth in spontaneous and hyperstimulated menstrual cycles. Br J Obstet Gynaecol 1989; 96: 954–959

69 Imoedemke D A G, Shaw R W, Kirkland A, Chan R. Ultrasound measurement of endometrial thickness on different ovarian stimulation regimens during in vitro fertilisation. Hum Reprod 1987; 2: 545–547

70 Leng S, Lindenberg S. Ultrasonic evaluation of endometrial growth in women with normal cycles during spontaneous and stimulated cycles. Hum Reprod 1990; 5: 377–381

71 Glissant A, Mouzon J, Frydman R. Ultrasound study of the endometrium during in vitro fertilisation cycles. Fertil Steril 1985; 44: 786–790

72 Gonen Y, Casper R, Jacobsen W, Blankier J. Endometrial thickness and growth during ovarian stimulation: a possible predictor of implantation in in vitro fertilisation. Fertil Steril 1989; 52: 446–450

73 Rabinowitz R, Laufer N, Lewin A, et al. The value of ultrasonographic endometrial measurement in the prediction of pregnancy following in vitro fertilisation. Fertil Steril 1986; 45: 824–828

74 Walker B G, Gembruch U, Diedrich K, Al-Hasani S, Krebs D. Transvaginal sonography of the endometrium during ovum pick-up in stimulated cycles for in vitro fertilisation. J Ultrasound Med 1989; 8: 549–553

75 Smith B, Porter R, Ahuja K, Craft I. Ultrasonic assessment of endometrial changes in stimulated cycles in an in vitro fertilisation and embryo transfer program. In Vitro Fertil Embryo Transfer 1984; 1: 233–238

76 Sher G, Herbert C, Maassarani G, Jacobs M H. Assessment of the late proliferative phase endometrium by ultrasonography in patients undergoing in-vitro fertilisation and embryo transfer (IVF/ET). Hum Reprod 1991; 6: 232–237

77 Deichert I, Hackelöer B J, Dawne E. The sonographic and endocrinologic evaluation of the endometrium in the luteal phase. Hum Reprod 1986; 1: 219–222

78 Spitznagel E, Daly D. Sector ultrasound in the diagnosis and treatment of hematometria secondary to Asherman's syndrome. Fertil Steril 1988; 49: 370–372

79 Ombelet W. Endometrial ossification, an unusual finding in an infertility clinic. A case report. J Reprod Med 1989; 34: 303–306

80 Steer C, Campbell S, Pampiglione J, Kingsland C, Masson B, Collins W. Transvaginal colour flow imaging of the uterine arteries during the ovarian and menstrual cycles. Hum Reprod 1990; 5: 391–395

81 Steer C, Tan S L, Mills C, Rizk B, Mason B, Campbell S. Vaginal colour Doppler assessment of uterine artery impedance on the day of embryo transfer: a new screening technique for unsuccessful in vitro fertilisation. Lancet 1991; submitted

82 Goswany R K, Williams G, Steptoe P C. Decreased uterine perfusion – a cause of infertility. Hum Reprod 1988; 3: 955–959

83 Steer C, Mason B, Sathanandan M, et al. Pituitary ovarian axis down regulation with LHRH agonist therapy increases frozen embryo pregnancy rates abstract. In: Serono Symposia – Neuro Endocrinology of Reproduction California, 4–9 Nov 1989

84 Rattern S, Thaler I, Goldstein S R, Timor-Tritsch I E, Brandes J M. Transvaginal sonographic technique: targeted organ scanning without resorting to 'planes'. JCU 1990; 18: 243–247

85 Donnez J, Casanas-Roux F. Prognostic factors of fimbrial microsurgery. Fertil Steril 1986; 46: 200–204

86 Schlief R, Deichert U. Hysterosalpingo – contrast sonography of the uterus and fallopian tubes: results of a clinical trial of a new contrast medium in 120 patients. Radiology 1991; 178: 213–215

87 Lenz S, Lauritsen J G, Kjellow M. Collection of human oocytes for in vitro fertilisation by ultrasonically guided follicular puncture. Lancet 1981; i: 1163–1164

88 Chamberlain G, Carron Brown J. eds. Gynaecological laparoscopy. In: Report on the confidential enquiry into gynaecological laparoscopy. Royal College of Obstetricians and Gynaecologists. London: 1978

89 Lenz S, Lauritsen J G. Ultrasonically guided perentaneous aspiration of human follicles under local anaesthesia: a new method of collecting oocytes for in vitro fertilisation. Fertil Steril 1982; 38: 673–677

90 Wickland M, Nilsson L, Hansson R, Hamberger L, Janson P O. Collection of human oocytes by the use of sonography. Fertil Steril 1983; 39: 603–608

91 Gleicher N, Friberg J, Fullan N, et al. Egg retrieval for in vitro fertilisation by sonographically controlled vaginal culdocentesis. Lancet 1983; i: 508–509

92 Dellenbach P, Nisand I, Moreau L, Feger B, Plumere C, Gerlinger P. Transvaginal sonographically controlled follicle puncture for oocyte retrieval. Fertil Steril 1985; 44: 656–662

93 Parsons J, Riddle A, Booker M, et al. Oocyte retrieval for in vitro fertilisation by ultrasonically guided needle aspiration via the urethra. Lancet 1985; 1: 1076–1077

94 Lewin A, Laufer N, Rabinowitz R, Margalioth E J, Bar I, Schenker J G. Ultrasonically guided oocyte collection under local anaesthesia: the first choice method for in vitro fertilisation – a comparative study with laparoscopy. Fertil Steril 1986; 46: 257–261

95 Wikland M, Lennart E, Hamberger L. Transvesical and transvaginal approaches for the aspiration of follicles by the use of ultrasound. NY Sci 1985; 442: 182

96 Wikland M, Hamberger L, Enk L, Nilsson L. Sonographic techniques in human in vitro fertilisation programmes. Hum Reprod 1988; 3: 65–68

97 Itskovity J, Boldes R, Levron J, Thaler I. Transvaginal ultrasonography in the diagnosis and treatment of infertility. JCU 1990; 18: 248–256

98 Meldrum D R. Editorial. Antibiotics for vaginal oocyte aspiration. J In Vitro Fertil Embryo Transfer 1989; 6: 1–2

99 Scott R T, Hofmann G E, Muasher S J, Aeosta A A, Kreiner D K, Rosenwaks Z. A prospective randomized comparison of single- and double-lumen needles for transvaginal follicular aspiration. J In Vitro Fertil Embryo Transfer 1989; 6: 98–100

100 Parsons J, Pampiglione J S, Sadler A P, Booker M W, Campbell S. Ultrasound directed follicle aspiration for oocyte collection using the perurethral technique. Fertil Steril 1990; 53: 97–102

101 Wisanto A, Bollen N, Camus M, DeGrauwe E, Devroey P, Van Steirteghern A C. Effect of transuterine puncture during transvaginal oocyte retrieval on the results of human in vitro fertilisation. Hum Reprod 1989; 4: 790–793

102 Waterstone J, Parsons J H, Bolton V. Elective transfer of two embryos. Lancet 1991; 337: 975–976

103 Hurley V A, Osborn J C, Leoni M A, Leeton J. Ultrasound-guided embryo transfer: a controlled trial. Fertil Steril 1991; 55: 559–562

104 Parsons J H, Bolton V N, Wilson L, Campbell S. Pregnancies following in vitro fertilisation and ultrasound-directed surgical embryo transfer by perurethral and transvaginal techniques. Fertil Steril 1987; 48: 691–693

105 Forrler A, Dellenback P, Nisand I, et al. Direct intraperitoneal insemination in unexplained and cervical infertility. Lancet 1986; 1: 916–917

106 Pampiglione J S, Davies M C, Steer C, Kingsland C, Mason B A, Campbell S. Factors affecting direct intraperitoneal insemination. Lancet 1988; 1: 1336

107 Curson R, Parsons J H. Disappointing results with direct intraperitoneal insemination. Lancet 1987; i: 112

108 Hovatta O, Kurunmaki H, Tutinen A, Lahteenmaki P, Kaskimies A I. Direct intraperitoneal or intrauterine insemination and superovulation in infertility treatment: a randomised study. Fertil Steril 1990; 54: 339–341

109 Mason B, Sharma V, Riddle A, Campbell S. Ultrasound-guided peritoneal oocyte and sperm transfer (POST). Lancet 1987; 1: 386

110 Sharma V, Pampiglione J S, Mason B A, Campbell S, Riddle A. Experience with peritoneal oocyte and sperm transfer as an out-patient based treatment for infertility. Fertil Steril 1991; 55: 579–582

111 Yovich J L, Yovich J M, Edirisinghe W R. The relative chance of pregnancy following tubal or uterine transfer procedures. Fertil Steril 1988; 49: 858–864

112 Devroey P, Staessen C, Camus M, DeGrauwe E, Wisanto A, Van Steirteghem A C. Zygote intrafallopian transfer as a successful treatment for unexplained infertility. Fertil Steril 1989; 52: 246–249

113 Jansen R P S, Anderson J C, Radonic I, Smit J, Sutherland P. Pregnancies after ultrasound-guided fallopian insemination with cryostored donor semen. Fertil Steril 1988; 49: 920–922

114 Lucena E, Ruiz J A, Mendoza J C, et al. Vaginal intratubal insemination (VITI) and vaginal GIFT, endosonographic technique: early experience. Hum Reprod 1989; 4: 658–662

115 Scholtes M C W, Roozenburg B J, Alberda A, Zeilmaker G H. Transcervical intrafallopian transfer of zygotes. Fertil Steril 1990; 54: 283–286

116 Bauer O, Van der Ven H, Diedrich K, al Hasani S, Krebs D, Gembruch U. Preliminary results on transvaginal tubal embryo stage transfer (TV-TEST) without ultrasound guidance. Hum Reprod 1990; 5: 553–556

117 Jansen R P S. Personal Communication 1991

Embryology

Ian G. Parkin

INTRODUCTION

This chapter summarises the development of the major organ systems. All timings are based on the time of fertilisation, about 2 weeks after the last menstrual period. Although the fetal period is not considered to start until the ninth week (and most obstetric ultrasonic scanning is not done until about 16 weeks) the events of the previous 6 weeks (i.e. weeks 2 to 8) are crucial to the developing embryo and also to the understanding of organogenesis.

By the beginning of the third week (i.e. at the time of the first missed menstrual period) implantation has taken place, chorion is forming and the embryo forms the bilaminar germ disc with the prochordal plate (fused entoderm and ectoderm with no intervening mesoderm) visible at the cephalic end, and the primitive streak at the caudal end.

The primitive streak becomes a groove, cells turn inwards and multiply in between the ectoderm and entoderm to form intra-embryonic mesoderm, which spreads in all directions to reach the extra-embryonic mesoderm and create the trilaminar disc.

The cephalic end of the streak forms the primitive pit which sinks inwards to create the notochord in the midline, pushing towards the prochordal plate. The neural plate, which then becomes the neural tube, forms from the ectoderm overlying the notochord.

The mesoderm forms somites (paired cubes) in the paraxial region, with intermediate mesoderm just adjacent, and lateral mesoderm outside that. The intra-embryonic coelom forms as a horseshoe-shaped cavity in the lateral mesoderm, its posterior wall being somatic and its ventral wall (lining the entoderm) being splanchnic and forming the muscular wall of the developing gastrointestinal tract. Within the remainder of the mesoderm angiogenetic clusters coalesce to form the primordia of blood vessels, and the urogenital system will develop in the intermediate mesoderm.

During the fourth week these primordia fold in both cephalo-caudal and lateral directions and the majority of organ systems commence their development. The prochordal plate becomes buccopharyngeal membrane, while structures initially anterior to it rotate downwards to become the thorax, closed by lateral folding. Behind and above bulges the developing neural tube. The entoderm is pinched off to become the intestinal tract (epithelium). The intra-embryonic coelom becomes pericardial, pleural and peritoneal cavities. The mesoderm, which was originally at the anterior end of the horseshoe, swings inferiorly to become the septum transversum, and later the central tendon of the diaphragm.

The two-directional folds (cephalo-caudal and lateral) ensure a purse-string closure of the anterior abdominal wall around the umbilicus, with ectoderm forming the epithelium. Failure of fusion of the lateral folds causes a defect in the body wall allowing the intestine to lie in the extra-embryonic coelom. Such a defect may also cause failure of thoracic closure, resulting in ectopia cordis.

Central nervous system

The rapidly growing central nervous system is thought to control and induce much of the cephalo-caudal embryonic folding, and consequently is the logical system to consider first. During the third week of embryonic life, the cephalic end of the primitive streak forms the primitive knot (Hensens Node). From here cells move towards the prochordal plate and form the rod-like notochordal process between the entoderm and ectoderm (Fig. 1). The knot becomes pitted and the pit burrows along the notochordal process converting it into a canal which fuses with the underlying entoderm and opens up to communicate with the yolk sac. (At this stage, through the original primitive pit, the yolk sac and amnion communicate via this neurenteric canal. As the surrounding ectoderm is induced to form the neural tube, and the entoderm the intestine, if this neurenteric canal remains open a connection between the intestine and the spinal cord central canal will exist.)

The notochordal canal effectively becomes a plate in the roof of the yolk sac, the plate folds inwards ventrally to again separate from the yolk sac and become the notochord (Fig. 2). The overlying ectoderm thickens to become the neural plate (motor cells) and the immediately lateral cells become neural crest (sensory and autonomic cells).

Axially the plate grooves and cranially becomes broader, appearing almost bilobed. Caudally the plate envelops the primitive pit. As the embryonic disc grows so does the neural plate, and its groove. By the seven somite stage the edges of the groove meet dorsally in the midline and fuse, opposite the fourth to sixth somites. Cranial to this fusion the plate will become brain and caudally will be the upper cervical part of the cord. Continued caudal growth of the plate will form the remainder of the spinal cord (Fig. 3).

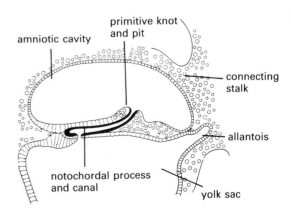

Fig. 1 Formation of notochordal process and its canal.

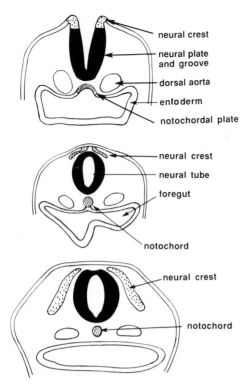

Fig. 2   Neural plate, groove and tube, with notochordal plate becoming notochord.

bone and cartilage of the vertebral column is growing more quickly, outstripping the spinal cord. Consequently by birth the cord is 15 to 17 cm long and ends opposite L3.

Failure of closure of the neuropores causes neural tube defects as well as abnormalities in the overlying meningeal and skeletal elements. The various degrees of spina bifida are due to lack of closure of the posterior neuropore. Defects at the anterior neuropore are responsible for abnormalities of brain and cranium, including exencephaly and anencephaly.

Brain development

The somewhat bilobed cranial end of the neural tube becomes the familiar brain shape as a result of ventral cervical and mesencephalic flexures, dorsal pontine and telencephalic flexures and three primary dilatations, forebrain, midbrain and hindbrain (Fig. 4). Other secondary dilatations or vesicles are developed from the forebrain (prosencephalon) and hindbrain (rhombencephalon). The forebrain buds laterally on each side, to become the lateral ventricles and overlying cerebral hemispheres, leaving the original dilatation as the third ventricle and its wall the diencephalon (thalamus). The pineal primordium separates forebrain and midbrain dilatations.

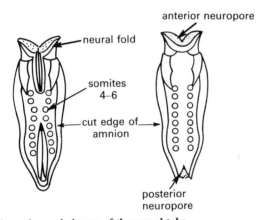

Fig. 3   Elongation and closure of the neural tube.

As fusion occurs anterior and posterior neuropores remain at either end. But the 'zip up' extends in both directions, so that the anterior neuropore closes to become the lamina terminalis by the 20 somite stage (3.5 weeks) and the posterior neuropore closes by the 25 somite stage (4 weeks). Consequently, by late somite stage the neural tube is present, with cranial swellings and a caudal part still forming to extend the full length of the embryo. As the disc folds the tube follows the concavity and the swollen cranial end is thrown forwards over the stomodeum, creating the cervical flexure at the junction of the cord and rhombencephalon. By 3 months the developing

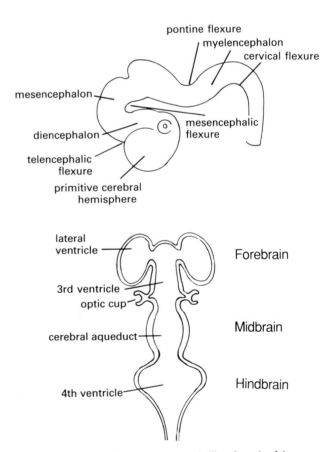

Fig. 4   Neural tube (brain) flexures and dilatations (early).

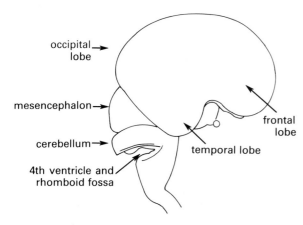

Fig. 5 Brain flexures (late).

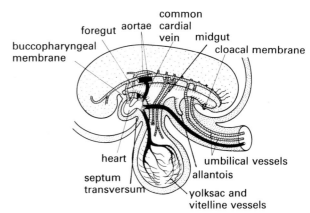

Fig. 6 Gastrointestinal tube and relations.

The midbrain shows the flexure but is largely unchanged as the cerebral aqueduct with tectum posteriorly, tegmentum and cerebral peduncles anteriorly.

The hindbrain thickens in its upper part, anteriorly to form the pons and posteriorly to form the cerebellum. The lower part remains as medulla oblongata. Between the two the dorsal concavity of the pontine flexure draws out the dorsal wall of the tube to create the thin roof of the fourth ventricle and the floor of the rhomboid fossa.

The telencephalic flexure throws the developing cerebral hemispheres dorsally over the diencephalon, which is consequently buried and the hemispheres grow to overlap the midbrain and extend backwards to contact the cerebellum, as well as growing ventrally and rostrally to form the temporal lobes (Fig. 5).

As the lateral ventricles and fourth ventricle are formed the neural thinning allows ependyma and pia mater to come together, forming tela choroidea, and eventually the cerebrospinal-fluid-producing choroid plexus. Defective circulation (aqueduct stenosis) or absorption of cerebrospinal fluid causes hydrocephaly.

Gastrointestinal tract

Following the cephalo-caudal and lateral folding of the trilaminar disc the entoderm becomes converted into a tube which will form the epithelium of the alimentary canal. This stretches from the buccopharyngeal to the cloacal membranes where entoderm and ectoderm stick to each other. Elsewhere the tube has a covering of splanchnic mesoderm which will differentiate to become the musculature and mesothelium (or surrounding fascia) of the tract. Mesoderm which remains and tethers the tract to either the dorsal or ventral body walls will become the corresponding mesentery. The entoderm maintains continuity with the yolk sac via the vitelline duct at what will become the umbilicus (Fig. 6).

Posterior to the tract lie the developing vertebral bodies and central nervous system. Anteriorly, throughout the length of the embryo, lie a number of structures: the septum transversum forms a division with the intra-embryonic coelom (peritoneal cavity) inferiorly while the heart tube, pericardial and pleural cavities lie superiorly. The cephalic end of the heart tube (aortic sac) gives rise to the two dorsal aortae which curve backwards to lie postero-lateral to the canal. Further growth of the embryo and descent of the heart stretches the tube creating a series of regions; oropharynx, oesophagus, foregut, midgut, hindgut and cloaca.

Oropharynx

Starting at the buccopharyngeal membrane this entodermal tube lies surrounded by mesoderm and ectoderm which will become the body wall. At the start of the fourth week, sequentially with embryonic growth, and not all clearly defined, a series of five pouches bulge outwards from the pharynx towards four ectodermal, surface, clefts and create six intervening arches of mesoderm.

Each arch receives; migrating neural crest cells which surround the mesenchymal core and later become specific skeletal structures, an artery which runs from the aortic sac through the mesoderm to the dorsal aorta, and a nerve direct from the brain stem which lies posteriorly.

Between the fourth and eighth weeks the facial structure develops from five primordia. Cranial to the buccopharyngeal membrane (now broken down) a mesodermal thickening, the frontonasal process, grows towards first arch thickenings (maxillary processes) at each side (upper cheek). Inferiorly lie the mandibular thickenings of first arch mesoderm, overlying Meckel's cartilages (derived from neural crest cells). Ectodermal thickenings, the nasal placodes, appear in the frontonasal process and the surrounding mesoderm thickens to form medial and lateral nasal swellings around the placodes so that they become sunken and lie at the base of nasal pits (Fig. 7).

Each lateral swelling is initially separated from the maxillary arch by the naso-lacrimal groove, but fusion occurs along these lines by the end of week 5. The medial prom-

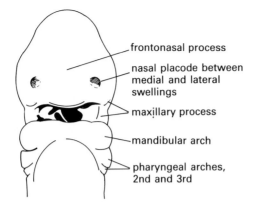

Fig. 7 Upper face development.

frontonasal process

nasal placode between medial and lateral swellings

maxillary process

mandibular arch

pharyngeal arches, 2nd and 3rd

inences fuse with each other a week later to create the inter-maxillary segment which will form the philtrum of lip, the premaxilla and associated gum, the primary palate and the nasal septum. At the same time maxillary prominences move medially, inferior to the lateral nasal swellings, to fuse with the medial swellings (inter-maxillary segment). All the underlying mesenchyme is continuous, therefore there are no actual divisions underlying the grooves created externally by these prominences (Fig. 8).

The central part of the frontonasal process remains as the forehead, dorsum and apex of nose. The alae curve from the lateral nasal swellings, which are now continuous with the cheeks. These early lips and cheeks, although structured originally from the first and second arch prominences are invaded by second arch mesoderm which differentiates to become the muscles of facial expression carrying the VII cranial nerve with it. The residual first arch mesoderm becomes the muscles of mastication, supplied by the mandibular nerve.

As the prominences above grow and develop around the nasal placode, the latter sinks more deeply so that the nasal pit becomes a nasal sac which grows backwards, in front of the overlying brain. The floor of this sac is the oronasal membrane, separating the nasal and oral cavities, but this soon disappears leaving a single chamber. In the upper,

nasal part, superior, middle and inferior conchae develop from the lateral wall.

While these developments have been continuing, the secondary palate has started its growth during the fifth week, to be completed by 12 weeks, with weeks 6 to 8 as the most critical. The primary palate, from the inter-maxillary segment, is already in situ but forms only the most anterior (incisive) part of the adult structure. Behind this two shelves (lateral palatine processes) push out horizontally from the internal aspect of the maxillary prominences and hang on each side of the tongue (Fig. 9).

By the seventh week further growth makes the tongue relatively smaller, and lie more inferiorly, allowing these palatal processes to elongate, swing upwards into a horizontal position and fuse with each other, the primary palate, and the nasal septum (a downgrowth from the internal aspect of the inter-maxillary segment). The fusion starts anteriorly during the eighth week and extends posteriorly until complete fusion, at the uvula, occurs by the twelfth week.

Clefts occur anteriorly following deficiencies in the inter-maxillary segment (medial nasal prominences) and/or the maxillary prominences, so that they fail to fuse. Posterior clefts are due to faults in formation of the secondary palate, usually the lateral palatal processes.

Once into the fetal period (week 9) facial development is slow and depends on a reproportioning of the rather flat, underdeveloped, but completed, face as described above. The growing brain forces a prominent forehead, the eyes move medially and the external ears grow from buds which

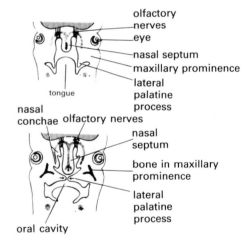

olfactory nerves

eye

nasal septum

maxillary prominence

lateral palatine process

tongue

nasal conchae

olfactory nerves

nasal septum

bone in maxillary prominence

lateral palatine process

oral cavity

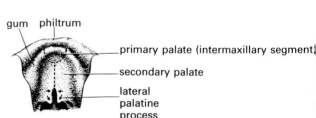

gum philtrum

primary palate (intermaxillary segment)

secondary palate

lateral palatine process

Fig. 9 Palate formation.

Line of fusion of maxillary and lateral nasal prominences

Maxillary prominence

Lateral nasal prominence (alae)

Fused medial nasal prominences (intermaxillary segment)

Fusions of maxillary prominence and the fused medial nasal prominences

Fig. 8 Facial lines of fusion.

appeared during week 5, from first and second arch components. By birth the lower face is still small and grows after birth as dictated by the developing oronasal apparatus.

The primitive pharynx is wide behind the stomodeum and narrow towards the oesophagus. The laterally situated pouches give rise to many non-pharyngeal structures. The first pouch becomes the Eustachian tube and middle ear while the second pouch forms the epithelium and crypts of the palatine tonsil (lymphoid tissue being derived from the underlying mesoderm). During weeks 6 and 7 buds of oral epithelium grow into the underlying mesoderm to become the salivary glands.

The floor of the pharynx, by the end of the fourth week, produces the midline tuberculum impar (median tongue bud) from first arch mesoderm. Beside this, also from first arch mesoderm, develop the lateral lingual swellings which soon grow over, completely envelop, and bury the tuberculum impar to form the connective tissue, lymphatic and blood vessels of the oral tongue while overlying entoderm becomes the epithelium (Fig. 10).

A similar story exists for the pharyngeal tongue, which starts with a midline second arch swelling, the copula, which is soon overgrown and buried by the hypobranchial eminence of third, and far posteriorly, fourth arch origin.

This accounts for the sensory innervation of the tongue being anteriorly trigeminal (lingual) and posteriorly glossopharyngeal and vagus nerves. The second arch is represented only by taste buds, supplied by the chorda tympani branch of the facial nerve.

Tongue musculature is derived from occipital somites which bring the hypoglossal nerve with them.

Slightly further caudally, at the fourth/sixth arch level as the pharynx narrows to become the oesophagus, the laryngotracheal groove develops, during week 4, in the pharyngeal floor. The groove enlarges to become the laryngotracheal diverticulum, and its entodermal lining will become the epithelium and glands of the larynx, trachea and lungs. The diverticulum is separated from the pharynx and oesophagus by the tracheo-oesophageal septum which leaves at its cranial end an opening (the laryngeal inlet) into the laryngotracheal tube. Consequently the developing larynx, trachea and lung bud now lie anterior to the oesophagus (Fig. 11).

Should the tracheo-oesophageal septum deviate posteriorly the oesophagus narrows (atresia) and will not completely separate from the laryngotracheal tube (tracheo-oesophageal fistula).

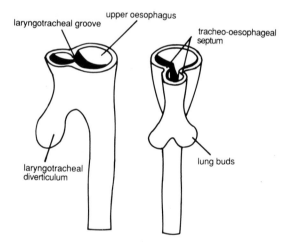

Fig. 11 Laryngotracheal diverticulum.

Oesophagus

At the early stage (fourth week) the oesophagus is short, but heart descent and lung growth force it to elongate and reach its relative adult proportion by 7 weeks. During this time the epithelium (entoderm) proliferates to occlude the lumen. However by the end of the eighth week the oesophagus usually reopens. Failure of this recanalisation causes oesophageal atresia and stenosis.

Epithelium and glands are derived from entoderm while the surrounding musculature has two origins: cephalic, skeletal muscle comes from surrounding fourth and sixth

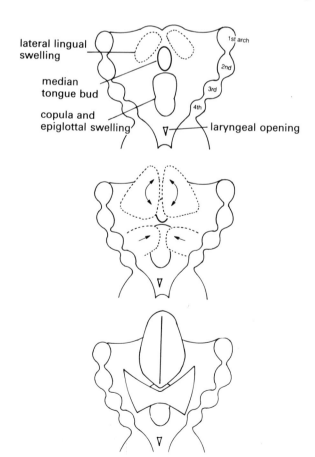

Fig. 10 Tongue development.

arch mesoderm; caudal, smooth muscle from splanchnic mesoderm. (Both are supplied by branches of the vagus nerve). At this stage the oesophagus also has a flange of mesoderm behind it forming a dorsal mesentery.

In front of the oesophagus, and fused with its ventral mesoderm, is the septum transversum which now separates the pericardial cavity from the abdominal cavity and will become the central tendon of the diaphragm. Laterally the growing lungs and pleural cavities burrow into the body wall creating medial pleuro-peritoneal membranes which fuse with the septum transversum and the dorsal mesentery of the oesophagus to form a complete diaphragm separating the thoracic and abdominal cavities. Further body wall excavation forms costo-diaphragmatic recesses while myoblasts invade this thoraco-abdominal septum to eventually create the recognised musculotendinous sheet of the adult diaphragm.

Fusion of the various diaphragmatic elements (septum transversum, pleuro-peritoneal membranes and dorsal mesentery of the oesophagus) occurs by 6 weeks and the sheet then 'descends' due to relative body growth. Should this fusion fail, or the pleuro-peritoneal membranes be defective, the abdominal contents will herniate into the thorax when they return from the physiological hernia at 10 weeks.

Foregut

The foregut is the entodermal tube from the distal end of the oesophagus to the mid-duodenum supplied by the coeliac axis. It also gives the epithelial primordia of liver, gall bladder, pancreas and associated ducts. Surrounding mesoderm forms the musculature and connective tissue of these structures, as well as the peritoneum and mesenteries. During the fifth week the stomach makes its first appearance as a dilatation of the tube. This portion then undergoes rotation around longitudinal and anteroposterior axes (the adult position of the left and right vagus nerves providing good landmarks for following the former). The clockwise rotation in the longitudinal axis moves the left vagus to the anterior wall, the right vagus to the posterior wall and swings the dorsal mesentery in a curve out to the left (Fig. 12).

The left (previously posterior) aspect grows more quickly than the right and forces the stomach to bend. Rotation of this curved tube around an anteroposterior axis throws the left side (greater curvature) to face inferiorly and slightly left while the right side (lesser curvature) faces superiorly and slightly right.

The mesenteries are taken with these rotations so that the dorsal mesentery, which grows considerably, appears to hang off the greater curvature (originally the posterior aspect of the dilatation) as the greater omentum which maintains its connection to the posterior abdominal wall. The ventral mesentery connects the lesser curvature (orig-

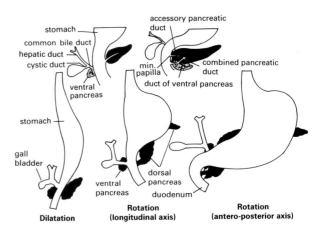

Fig. 12 Foregut development.

inally anterior aspect) to the liver, developing in the septum transversum superiorly and to the right, then past the liver to the ventral wall as falciform ligament (the umbilical vein lies in its free border). The repositioning pinches off a part of the peritoneal cavity to create the lesser sac posterior to the stomach and lesser omentum.

The caudal, pyloric, end of the stomach is also pushed to the right and takes the duodenum with it so that the latter forms a C-shaped curve which rotates back onto the posterior abdominal wall where its mesentery resorbs and it becomes mainly retroperitoneal.

As in the oesophagus epithelial proliferation causes duodenal obliteration (sixth week) which recanalises after the eighth week. Failure to recanalise, which may have a number of causes (including Down's Syndrome and vascular abnormalities) leads to duodenal atresia and stenosis.

During the fourth week the hepatic diverticulum arises, from the lower end of the foregut ventrally. This bud of entoderm grows into the septum transversum (ventral mesentery) to become the cords of hepatocytes surrounded by mesodermally derived sinusoids, connective tissue, Kupffer cells and haemopoietic tissue. The embryonic liver is relatively large. Haemopoiesis commences by 6 weeks and bile production by 12 weeks.

The connection of the hepatic diverticulum to the duodenum sends another bud to become cystic duct with gall bladder, while the diverticulum itself remains as the bile duct (following obliteration and recanalisation).

In a similar way the pancreas springs from the entodermal tube, but as two buds. The ventral pancreas arises near the bile duct and the dorsal pancreas a little further cranially. The clockwise duodenal rotation forces the ventral bud to sweep all the way around to lie behind the dorsal bud. Both buds fuse and straddle the midline to nestle in the left aspect of the duodenal C-curve (Fig. 12). While rotating around the duodenum the pancreatic buds may form a ring around it (annular pancreas) which may, at birth, cause duodenal obstruction.

The main pancreatic duct is derived from the ventral pancreatic duct and the distal portion of the dorsal duct, opening with the bile duct into the duodenum. The proximal portion of the dorsal duct may remain as the accessory duct, opening into the minor papilla, cranial to the ampulla of Vater (major papilla).

Midgut and hindgut

Caudal to the bile duct opening, the duodenum, jejunum, ileum, caecum, ascending colon and proximal two thirds of the transverse colon are formed, as the midgut, from the entoderm of the yolk sac. This part of the tube communicates with the yolk sac via the vitelline duct (until 10 weeks), is supplied by the superior mesenteric artery and is suspended on a dorsal mesentery. Similarly, the hindgut continues to the rectum supplied by the inferior mesenteric artery.

The midgut grows and outpaces the abdomen. Consequently, it forms the primary intestinal loop, pushing into the physiological umbilical hernia (6 weeks) with a much folded cranial limb and a straighter caudal limb containing the caecal diverticulum. The loop rotates, in an anti-clockwise direction, around the superior mesenteric axis (viewed from the front) so that the cephalic limb (small intestine) moves downwards and to the right while the caudal limb (large intestine) moves up and left (Fig. 13).

As the hernia reduces (10 weeks) the small intestine returns first to lie centrally in the abdomen, posterior to the artery. (The vitello-intestinal duct should regress but may remain as Meckel's ileal diverticulum.)

Failure of the lateral folds to fuse causes defects in the anterior abdominal wall omphalocele allowing the abdominal contents to lie externally, covered by the amnion. This problem often extends inferiorly to affect the cloaca, causing bladder extrophy. Failure of the physiological hernia to reduce leaves loops of intestine in the umbilical cord. As this reduction should occur during the tenth week neither of these types of omphalocele can be diagnosed before that time.

As the large intestine returns to the abdomen it rotates further in the anti-clockwise direction, so that the descending colon (part of the hindgut) falls into the left flank, transverse colon across upper abdomen and ascending colon to the right flank. The liver still takes up so much space that the caecum (last to return) has to lie tucked up close to its right lobe. Relative growth of body and decrease in liver size then causes apparent descent of the caecum to the right iliac fossa.

The appendix is formed from the caecum due to a slower rate of growth than that of the rest of the caecal diverticulum.

The dorsal mesentery for the full length of midgut and hindgut is forced into different positions, away from its initial midline. Where it is forced against the posterior abdominal wall it resorbs, and that part of the intestine becomes retroperitoneal and fixed. The small intestine, transverse and sigmoid colon keep their mesentery.

Cloaca

The distal end of the developing intestinal tract is sealed by the cloacal membrane, an apposition of ectoderm and entoderm with no intervening mesoderm. The allantois develops (second week) as a diverticulum of the yolk sac entoderm but cephalo-caudal folding moves its position so that it becomes a ventral bud of the entodermal tube lying between the cloacal membrane and the vitelline duct/umbilicus.

The mesoderm between the duct and the allantois proliferates and pushes into the developing intestinal tube, behind the allantois, all the way to the cloacal membrane (Fig. 14). The mesoderm becomes the urorectal septum which has the intestinal tube (lower end) posterior to it and the allantois in front. As the septum fuses with the cloacal membrane (7 weeks) it divides it into a dorsal anal membrane and a ventral urogenital membrane. Slight posterior deviation of the urorectal septum causes stenosis of the anorectal region.

Mesodermal proliferation around the anal membrane raises ectodermal swellings on either side and it comes to lie in the anal pit (proctodeum). Consequently, when at 8 weeks the anal membrane disappears, the lower one third of the anal canal is formed from ectoderm and the upper two thirds, joining the rectum, is entodermal hindgut (Fig. 15).

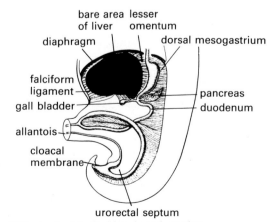

Fig. 13 Midgut, physiological hernia and rotation.

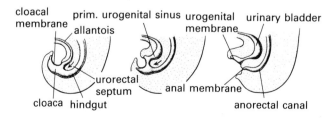

Fig. 14 Division of cloaca.

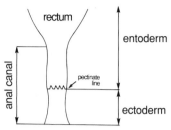

Fig. 15 Anal canal.

Failure of anal membrane breakdown causes imperforate anus, while (similar to the duodenum) failure of rectal recanalisation is another cause of stenosis.

Cardiovascular system

During week 3 (prior to folding) angiogenetic clusters form from proliferation in the intra-embryonic and extra-embryonic mesodermal cells. Clefts develop within the clusters and become confluent to form a lumen. The central cells detach into the lumen as primitive blood cells while the peripheral ones flatten and form the endothelium of what are now called blood islands. These coalesce to form a vascular network, with circulation by the end of week 3. In this way a horseshoe forms in the mesoderm around the cephalic end of the notochord and prochordal plate (Fig. 16). This horseshoe will become the heart tube, and has vascular extensions: dorsal aortae and cardinal veins in the intra-embryonic mesoderm on each side of the notochord; vitelline vessels in the mesoderm around the yolk sac; and umbilical vessels in the mesoderm of the chorion and connecting stalk (Fig. 6).

Cephalo-caudal folding throws the horseshoe, and the tube of the intra-embryonic coelom initially anterior to it, forwards and downwards to lie ventral to the developing pharynx (cervical region). Lateral folding ensures that the two limbs of the horseshoe move together and combine into a single tube which lies dorsal to the single pericardial tube formed from similar fusion of the coelomic limbs. Growth

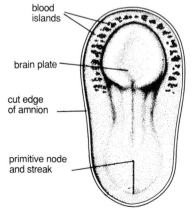

Fig. 16 Blood islands forming a cephalic horsehoe.

of the heart and lungs later pushes both systems inferiorly into the definitive thoracic cavity. The heart tube invaginates into the pericardial cavity. Its superior end is arterial, receiving the two dorsal aortae into the aortic sac or truncus arteriosus. The inferior end is venous, receiving the cardinal, vitelline and umbilical veins into the sinus venosus.

Again as a result of folding, the dorsal aortae, which were continuations of the original horseshoe heart tube, curve bilaterally from the aortic sac past the pharynx to lie behind and parallel to the developing alimentary canal. This curve becomes incorporated into the first pharyngeal arch as the first aortic arch. As each pharyngeal arch develops an aortic arch grows into it, from the aortic sac dorsally to join the dorsal aorta (Fig. 6).

These events occur sequentially between weeks 3 and 7. Heart descent and evolution of the pharyngeal derivatives forces the aortic arches to become (Fig. 17):

1: maxillary artery
2: hyoid, stapedal arteries
3: left common carotid, innominate arteries (the external carotid is a branch of the third arch)
4: left becomes arch of aorta, right becomes right subclavian artery
5: disappears
6: pulmonary arteries.

The aortic sac (truncus arteriosus) divides as the ascending aorta and pulmonary trunk. The initially paired dorsal aortae fuse to become a single aorta which is continuous with the arch of the aorta, derived from the left fourth aortic arch. The vitelline arteries become the coeliac axis, superior and inferior mesenteric arteries. The umbilical arteries originally carry deoxygenated blood to the placenta, but remain only as the internal iliac and superior vesical arteries.

The venous end of the heart remains for longer as a right and left horn of the sinus venosus. Each horn receives vitelline (yolk sac), umbilical (connecting stalk, oxygenated blood to embryo), and common cardinal veins. The latter are formed by the fusion of the anterior (head end) and posterior (rest of body) cardinal veins. Following left sided venous obliteration the left sinus horn regresses to remain as part of the coronary sinus and the right horn becomes incorporated into the atria.

The vitelline veins, on their way through the septum transversum to the sinus venosus, form a plexus around the duodenum and also link with the hepatic sinusoids of the developing liver. Consequently they become portal and hepatic veins as well as contributing to the proximal inferior vena cava.

The umbilical veins run alongside the liver. The right degenerates and the left develops a large channel, the ductus venosus, sunk into the liver, to shunt deoxygenated blood directly to the inferior vena cava without circulating

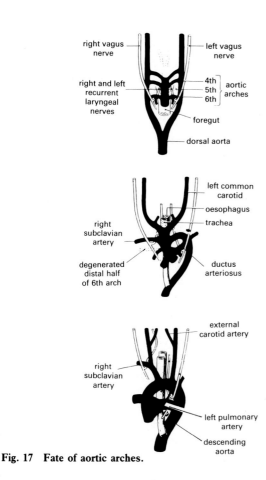

Fig. 17 Fate of aortic arches.

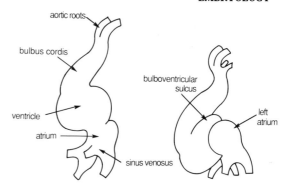

Fig. 18 Heart tube flexion and rotation to create septa.

through the liver. After birth the left umbilical vein and ductus venosus become the ligamentum teres and ligamentum venosum.

The paired anterior and posterior cardinal veins develop further cardinal systems stimulated by the appearance of, in particular, the urogenital organs. These systems create anastomoses either in, or crossing, the midline. These anastomotic channels, along with the proximal portions of the right cardinal systems, tend to remain and contribute to the larger, central veins (inferior vena cava, common iliacs, azygos root, brachiocephalic, renal). The distal portions, and left veins either obliterate or remain as specific organ or body wall veins (left gonadal, hemi-azygos, left superior intercostal).

Heart

The endothelium of the heart tube becomes surrounded by cardiac jelly and the mesodermal myo-epicardial mantle. These form the myocardium and epicardium as the tube invaginates into the ventrally situated pericardial cavity. Each end of the tube is anchored so that growth causes kinking and rotation of the tube to push it into the pericardium and place the atrium and sinus venosus dorsal to the truncus arteriosus and bulbus cordis end of the ventricle (Fig. 18). The partitions of the heart (concurrent, weeks 4 to 5) are created by: the constrictions formed at the sites of these flexures; dilatations on either side of these constrictions; and by the active growth of endocardial cushions (invaded by mesoderm) which push into the lumen and cause either narrowing or septum formation.

Flexural constriction narrows the junction between the bulbus cordis and the ventricle. The atrioventricular canal is divided into right and left openings by the growth and fusion of dorsal and ventral atrioventricular cushions. At the apex of the ventricle, opposite the bulbo-ventricular constriction, a further endomyocardial ridge develops and pushes towards the fused atrioventricular cushions to become the inter-ventricular septum (Fig. 19). Initially, the apparent growth of this septum is by the ventricles dilating and enlarging on either side of it and, consequently, there is free communication between the ventricles over the upper edge of this ridge (the inter-ventricular foramen).

In the meantime the fused atrioventricular cushions produce a thin extension which pushes into the

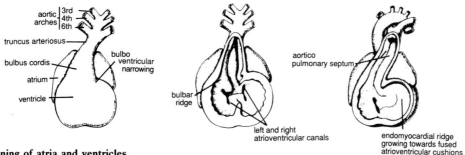

Fig. 19 Early positioning of atria and ventricles.

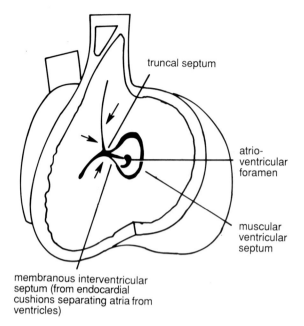

Fig. 20   Complete partitioning of heart chambers.

inter-ventricular foramen towards the upper edge of the muscular ridge. This will soon form the membranous part of the inter-ventricular septum and should it fail to develop there will be a resultant membranous ventricular septal defect.

Simultaneously truncal and bulbar ridges, continuous with each other, form in the truncus arteriosus and bulbus cordis. These ridges take a spiral course as they grow and fuse to form a spiral aorticopulmonary septum which divides the truncus arteriosus into aorta and pulmonary trunk which wind around each other. (Failure to spiral causes transposition of the great vessels.)

The bulbus cordis becomes incorporated into the ventricles to form the right ventricular infundibulum and the left ventricular aortic vestibule. This incorporation, together with active growth of the septa, ensure that the bulbar ridges, the membranous extension of the atrioventricular cushions and the muscular inter-ventricular septum fuse to obliterate the inter-ventricular foramen (end of seventh week), producing separate right and left ventricles and outflows (Fig. 20). These divisions form the 'crux' seen on fetal cardiac ultrasonic scans.

Cavitation of the ventricular wall undercuts the tissue to produce the trabeculae carneae, papillary muscles, chordae tendineae and atrioventricular valve cusps. The aortic and pulmonary valves are developed by the hollowing out and reshaping of three subendocardial valve swellings.

During weeks 4 and 5, as the ventricles and major arteries have been growing and partitioning, so has the primitive atrium. It divides by the active growth of septa which meet and fuse with the endocardial cushion that divides the atrioventricular canal into right and left halves (the atrioventricular septum). But the septa develop in a

way which ensures communication from left to right atrium.

The septum primum grows downwards from the atrial roof and creates the foramen primum between its advancing inferior edge and the atrioventricular septum. As the septum primum fuses with the atrioventricular septum to obliterate the foramen primum, its upper aspect develops a series of perforations which coalesce and form the foramen secundum (Fig. 21).

Just to the right of the septum primum the thicker, stiffer septum secundum begins to grow inferiorly from the atrial roof. It advances to overlap the foramen secundum and form an incomplete partition with the foramen ovale in its inferior aspect. The lower part of the septum primum forms a flap valve allowing the passage of blood from right to left atrium via the foramen ovale.

As mentioned above, many left sided veins obliterate early, shunting blood to the right. Consequently the right sinus horn increases in size and the sinu-atrial orifice moves to the right. As the right atrium grows it incorporates the sinus venosus and right sinus horn, which now receives from the superior and inferior vena cavae. In the adult, the original fetal atrium is represented by the auricle and that part of the atrial wall with musculi pectinati. Posteriorly, demarcated by the crista terminalis, the atrium is smooth and developed from the sinus venosus.

On the left, initially, a single pulmonary vein develops by budding from the atrium and branching to the lungs. Atrial growth incorporates the vein so that only the left auricle is original atrium, the rest is vein derived and four pulmonary veins enter the chamber.

The ultimate division of the early heart tube into atrial and ventricular portions, each divided into separate left and right chambers, and each chamber connected to a specific vessel or vessels, is dependent upon the growth and fusion of many septa. Therefore septal defects may have isolated consequences (probe patency of foramen ovale, atrial septal defect, ventricular septal defect) or may lead to multiple abnormalities such as Fallot's tetralogy.

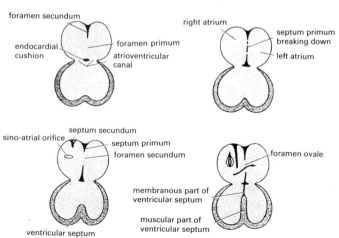

Fig. 21   Formation of atrial septa.

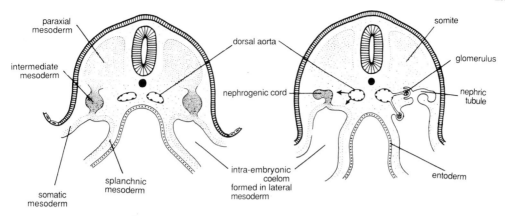

Fig. 22 Folding to position the mesodermal regions and kidney development in the intermediate mesoderm.

Urogenital system

The excretory and reproductive systems must be considered together as they develop adjacent to each other and utilise structures common to both. Growth tends to be sequential, as cranial sections regress, caudal sections proliferate. The primordia develop from intermediate mesoderm with its overlying coelomic epithelium and form the allantois and cloaca lying anterior to the urorectal septum.

The embryo grows and creates new somites, with segments of intermediate mesoderm just laterally. These segments fuse and create a nephrogenic cord which runs to the cloaca. As the lateral mesoderm splits to form somatic and splanchnic layers around the coelomic (peritoneal) cavity, folding then ensures that the intermediate mesoderm comes to lie on the posterior abdominal wall with a covering of coelomic epithelium (Fig. 22).

The first, and therefore most cranial, 'kidney' to develop in the nephrogenic cord is the non-functional pronephros. The remainder of the cord, caudal to the pronephros, forms the nephric duct to connect pronephros and cloaca.

As the pronephros regresses the mesonephros develops caudal to it (4 to 5 weeks), in the nephrogenic cord, and opens into the nephric duct. Consequently the nephric duct is renamed the mesonephric or Wolffian duct. The mesonephros creates a ridge on the posterior abdominal wall. The coelomic epithelium on the medial aspect of the ridge proliferates to form the genital ridge which grows inwards into the underlying mesoderm to form the gonadal primordium. Germ cells migrate into this primordium so that the gonad is created from three tissue types (mesoderm, mesothelium, yolk sac) (Fig. 23).

At this stage, on the posterior wall, there is a definite, joint, urogenital ridge with the gonadal blastema medially and the mesonephros (nephrogenic cord) laterally. There is then an invagination of coelomic epithelium on the lateral aspect of the ridge (i.e. lateral to the mesonephros and its duct) to form the paramesonephric duct (Mullerian) which maintains an opening into the coelom. Caudally the urogenital ridges swing medially to fuse in the midline, i.e. in the urorectal septum which divides the cloaca. As each ridge runs over the pelvic brim it gains a mesodermal connection, the inguinal fold, to the anterior abdominal wall. The fate of structures within the urogenital ridge may be considered under the separate areas of urinary and reproductive development.

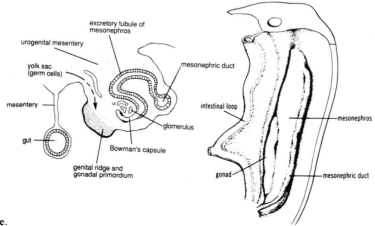

Fig. 23 Urogenital ridge.

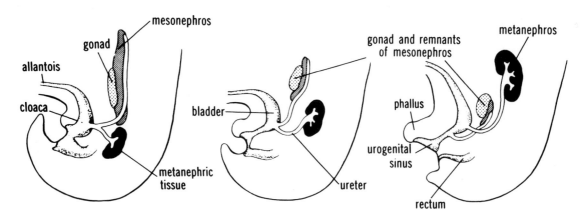

Fig. 24 Ureter and metanephric development.

Kidney and ureter

As the mesonephros begins to regress cranially the meta-nephros forms in the nephrogenic cord (5 to 6 weeks) in the sacral region, caudal to the mesonephros. Just above its point of entry into the cloaca the mesonephric duct gives off the ureteric bud on its posteromedial aspect. The bud grows dorsally and migrates around the mesonephric duct to enter its posterolateral aspect. During its dorsal growth the ureteric bud expands and meets the metanephric blastema which appears to ascend due to embryo growth, reaching the adult position by week 9 (Fig. 24).

The ureteric bud may duplicate or divide abnormally to create double ureters. The developing kidneys may fail to ascend and remain in the pelvis or fusion may occur at their lower poles resulting in horseshoe kidney.

The ureteric bud develops into major, then minor calyces, followed by further subdivision and decrease in size to form collecting tubules (fifth month). Where the metanephros contacts a collecting tubule it forms a double-cell mass, the renal vesicle. Each vesicle becomes a nephron and differentiates to form a glomerulus, then proximal and distal convoluted tubules with the loop of Henle between. The nephrons cluster around the collecting tubules as lobules and the lobules cluster around the major divisions of the ureteric bud as lobes. (The lobar nature of the kidney is visible into infancy but usually is lost by adulthood.) The metanephros begins to function at about 11 weeks. Abnormal development of the collecting tubules allows the formation of blind renal vesicles which become the cysts of congenital polycystic kidney.

The ureter enters the mesonephric duct, the caudal part of which is now termed the common excretory duct. The latter duct joins the cloaca which is divided by the urorectal septum so that the rectum lies posteriorly, with the allantois, urogenital ducts and primitive urogenital sinus anteriorly (6 weeks). The lower end of this urinary part of the cloaca is sealed by the urogenital membrane around which mesoderm flows to create lateral genital swellings

and an anterior midline genital tubercle (4 weeks) so that the membrane comes to lie in a depression, the external cloaca, which is forced to face inferiorly due to formation of the anterior abdominal wall. The primitive urogenital sinus is considered in two parts. Cranial to the entry of the common excretory ducts is the vesico-urethral canal, continuous with the allantois, and caudal to their entry is the definitive urogenital sinus.

Bladder and urethra

The vesico-urethral canal will form the lining mucosa of the bladder, while muscle comes from the surrounding mesoderm. Most of the bladder remains an abdominal organ and does not enter the true pelvis until after puberty.

The canal grows and incorporates the common excretory ducts so that the mesonephric ducts and ureters now enter separately. (Failure to do so causes ectopic ureteric orifices.) The ureteric openings migrate cranially and laterally leaving the trigone at what will be the base of the bladder (Fig. 25).

The vesico-urethral canal develops a dilated upper part, becoming the bladder, and remains narrow inferiorly to form the bladder neck and upper urethra which, in the male, receive the mesonephric ducts. The allantois degenerates with eventual obliteration of its lumen to leave the urachus (which later forms the median umbilical ligament) between bladder and umbilicus.

Below the entry of the mesonephric ducts, which obliterate in the female or become the male ejaculatory ducts/vas deferens, the definitive urogenital sinus forms the mucosa of the upper pelvic portion of the urethra above the urogenital membrane. This pelvic portion in the female becomes the whole urethra while in the male it will form the prostatic and membranous parts. (The prostate gland being formed by buds from the urogenital sinus with surrounding mesoderm forming the stroma) (Fig. 26).

Below the urogenital membrane the external cloaca is

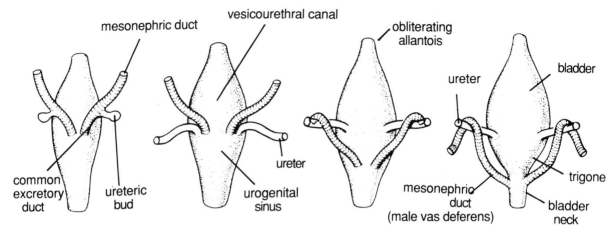

Fig. 25 Bladder, ureter and genital ducts.

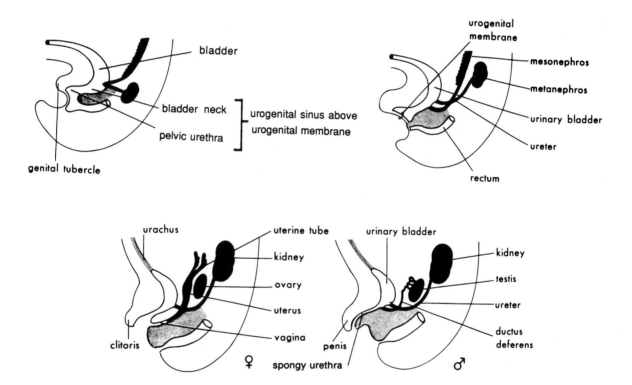

Fig. 26 Urethral development with breakdown of urogenital membrane and sex differentiation.

formed from the surface ectoderm in a depression between the genital tubercle (which will form penis or clitoris) anteriorly, and the genital swellings (scrotal wall or labia majora) laterally. Sandwiched just medial to each genital swelling, immediately below the urogenital membrane, are the bilateral, ectodermal urogenital folds. At about 7 weeks the urogenital membrane ruptures and sex differentiation, phallic development, starts at about 9 weeks.

In the male the genital tubercle grows and lengthens to form the penis, drawing the urogenital folds with it to form the lateral walls of the urethral groove on the ventral aspect of the penis. Meanwhile entoderm from the membranous urethra (lower urogenital sinus) proliferates downwards as the urethral plate to line the walls of the urethral groove (Fig. 27).

The urethral folds begin to fuse in the ventral midline to form the penile raphe and enclose the entodermally lined spongy urethra. This zipping-up, which can be abnormally halted at any stage to produce hypospadias, ensures that the spongy urethra progresses down the length of the penis

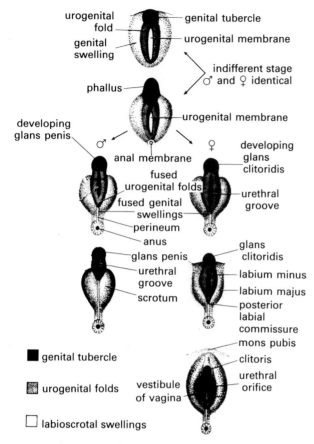

urogenital fold

genital tubercle

urogenital membrane

genital swelling

indifferent stage ♂ and ♀ identical

phallus

urogenital membrane

developing glans penis

♂

♀

developing glans clitoridis

anal membrane

fused urogenital folds

urethral groove

fused genital swellings

perineum

anus

glans penis

glans clitoridis

urethral groove

labium minus

scrotum

labium majus

posterior labial commissure

mons pubis

clitoris

urethral orifice

vestibule of vagina

■ genital tubercle

▨ urogenital folds

☐ labioscrotal swellings

Fig. 27 Development of cloaca, below urogenital membrane.

and meets the urethral canal of the glans, formed by ectodermal ingrowth.

In the female the genital tubercle, not stimulated by androgens, remains as the clitoris. The urogenital folds become the labia minora and the external cloaca the vestibule of the vagina which receives the vagina and urethra between the labia majora (genital swellings).

Gonads and reproductive ducts

The gonadal ridge, described earlier, forms as an 'indifferent' stage at about 5 weeks, from mesodermal proliferation and the ingrowth of primary sex cords from the overlying coelomic epithelium (mesothelium). The primordial germ cells, from the yolk sac, are incorporated into the cords by week 6.

In the male, during week 7, and influenced by the Y-chromosome, the primary sex cords form the seminiferous tubules (also the sustentacular cells) and the blastema becomes surrounded by the characteristic, tough, fibrous tunica albuginea. The yolk sac germ cells give rise to spermatogonia while the mesoderm provides the interstitial cells (Fig. 28).

In the female, development occurs slightly later as the primary sex cords degenerate and (at 10 weeks) are replaced by secondary sex cords which break into primordial follicles, each containing an oogonium (16 weeks). The developing ovary is surrounded by a tunica albuginea but it is rather thin (Fig. 29).

Within the ovary, during the fetal period only, the oogonia (from yolk sac germ cells) undergo active mitosis to form thousands of these primitive germ cells. Many of these regress but by birth about two million are left as primordial follicles which remain quiescent until puberty.

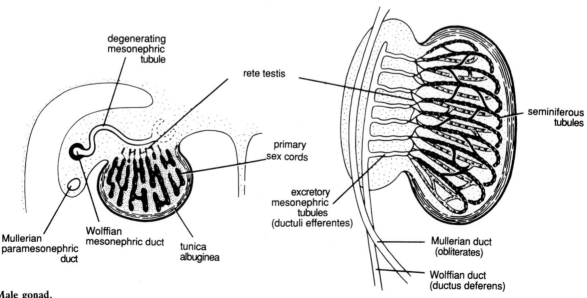

degenerating mesonephric tubule

rete testis

seminiferous tubules

primary sex cords

excretory mesonephric tubules (ductuli efferentes)

Mullerian paramesonephric duct

Wolffian mesonephric duct

tunica albuginea

Mullerian duct (obliterates)

Wolffian duct (ductus deferens)

Fig. 28 Male gonad.

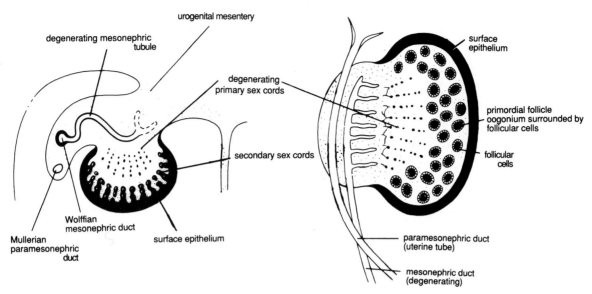

Fig. 29 Female gonad.

Both male and female gonads become tethered to the anterior abdominal wall and genital swellings by a gubernaculum of mesonephric duct origin. Pelvic enlargement and abdominal elongation causes the apparent decent of the gonads, guided by the gubernaculum. The testis descends, through the inguinal canal, into the scrotum (formed from the genital swelling) while the ovary goes only as far as the pelvic brim.

The development of the reproductive duct system is controlled by the presence, or absence of testicular androgens. Consequently, in the male, the paramesonephric ducts degenerate while the mesonephric duct joins to the testis to form epididymis, then vas deferens and ejaculatory duct entering the pelvic urethra.

However, in the female, the mesonephric ducts regress while the paramesonephric ducts form the genital duct system. Cranially, fimbriae form where the ducts enter the coelomic (peritoneal) cavity and this part becomes the uterine tube (Fig. 30). Further caudally the paramesonephric ducts fuse, behind the bladder, to form the uterovaginal canal. The cranial point of fusion forms the uterine fundus, and the uterovaginal canal then grows caudally down the urorectal septum to meet, and fuse with a pair of sinovaginal bulbs which grow upwards from the entoderm of the urogenital sinus. These bulbs also fuse to create a solid plate of entoderm, the vaginal plate, which eventually canalises to receive the uterus (Fig. 31). The common sources of origin of the urinary and reproductive duct systems, the dependence of development upon local hormone production, duct fusions, regressions and canalisations create many opportunities for congenital malformations to occur in this region.

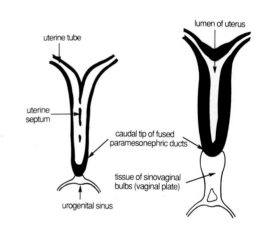

Fig. 30 Paramesonephric ducts fusing to form uterus.

Fetal period

As described above, the major organ systems have largely developed by the start of the ninth week. Between that time and birth (38 weeks post-fertilisation) there is rapid growth and reproportioning of these systems, but the fetus is less susceptible to teratogenic agents.

At the start of the fetal period the head is half the fetal length, male and female external genitalia are indistinguishable, coils of intestine protrude into the physiological hernia in the umbilical cord, the liver is the major site of erythropoiesis and the pronephros is non-functional.

By the twelfth week the head is still relatively large but its growth has slowed in relation to the rest of the body, external genitalia show obvious sex differentiation, the intestine has returned to the abdomen, the spleen also

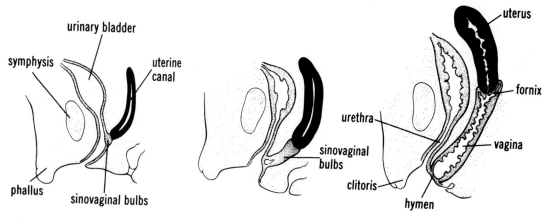

Fig. 31 Vaginal development.

SOMITES	POST–FERTILISATION TIME	CROWN–RUMP LENGTH (APPROX.)	EVENTS				
			EMBRYOLOGICAL TIMING				
			C.V.S.		G.I.T.	C.N.S.	G.U.T.
	6 days		Early implantation				
	8 days		Bi-laminar disc				
	15 days		Tri-laminar disc (Mesoderm from primitive streak)				
Early pre-somite	16/17 days		Angiogenetic clusters (Intra and extra embryonic) Development of allantois			Notochord	
Late pre-somite	18/19 days	1.4 mm				Neural plate Neural groove	
1–4	20		Folding of tri-laminar disc		Formation of gut tube and pharyngeal system	Neural tube starts to form. Neural crest lies dorsolaterally	Pronephros – cells visible in intermed. mesoderm
10–12	23	2.2 cm	Formation of single heart tube Beating Folding of heart tube			'Zips up'. Ant., then Post. Neuropores close / Brain dilatations	Mesonephros developing/degenerating cranio-caudally
26–29	28 days	4 mm					
42–44	5 weeks	5–8 cm	Oblitn. of umb. and vit. vs. Formation of cardiac septae	Development and reformation of aortic arches / S.A. Node	Liver forming Gut rotating Physiological hernia	Ant. spinal roots / Brain flexures / Cerebral vesicles	Sex gland primordia / Ureteric bud / MN duct and ureter open separately into the V.U. canal
	6 wks	10–14 mm			Cloaca faces caudally / Uro-rectal septum fuses		Paramesonephric ducts appear / Renal vesicles in metanephros
	7 wks	17–22 cm	Complete ventricular septum		U.G. membrane disappears		Male gonadal blastema obvious
	9 wks	5 cm	Oblitn. L Cardinal V	Formation of main veins	Sex of ext. genit. Anal canal opens		Testicular tunica albuginea Prostatic buds appear.
	12 wks	8 cm			Gut returns to abdomen	Cord same length as whole embryo / Obvious adult brain architecture	
		9 cm					Rete canalises, joins to mesonephric tubules
	16 wks	10 cm					
	20 wks	15 cm					Distinction between uterus and vagina
	24 wks	20 cm					Processes vaginalis

commences erythropoiesis and urine is produced by the metanephros (kidney). Primary ossification centres appear, particularly in the skull and long bones and the fetus will move in response to stimuli.

Over the following 4 weeks (to the sixteenth week) a more 'human' form is seen as the eyes face forwards, ears are close to their final position and there is rapid growth. Skeletal ossification continues so that bones are visible on X-ray and both upper and lower limbs have almost reached normal relative proportions, although the lower ones are still rather small. Soon after this, limb movements may be felt by the mother.

By 20 weeks scalp hair, eyebrows, lanugo and vernix caseosa are well-established. The ovary has had primordial follicles with oogonia for about 4 weeks, but now the uterus is formed and vagina begins to canalise. The testis has begun its descent but is still on the posterior abdominal wall.

The next 4 weeks see substantial weight gain. But weeks 26 to 29 are important as the lungs, pulmonary circulation and nervous system have matured enough to sustain life. The eyes re-open, subcutaneous fat develops and bone marrow takes over erythropoiesis.

The last 9 weeks are for final maturation so that the pupillary light reflex and the grasp reflex have developed and the head circumference approaches that of the abdomen. Fetuses reach an average crown-rump length of 360 mm and a weight of 3400 gm. In the male, by full term the testes have moved into the scrotum.

FURTHER READING

1 Moore K L. The Developing Human. 4th Edition. Philadelphia: W B Saunders. 1988
2 Langman J. Medical Embryology. 3rd Edition. Baltimore: Williams and Wilkins. 1975
3 Hamilton W J, Boyd J D, Mossman H W. Human Embryology. 3rd Edition. Cambridge: W Heffer. 1962
4 Snell R S. Clinical Embryology for Medical Students. 2nd Edition. Boston: Little and Brown. 1975
5 Williams P L, Warwick R, Dyson M, Bannister L M. Gray's Anatomy. 37th Edition. Edinburgh: Churchill Livingstone. 1989
6 Beck F, Moffat D B, Davies D P. Human Embryology. 2nd Edition. Oxford: Blackwell Scientific Publication. 1985

The illustrations, as indicated above, have been reproduced by the kind permission of the publishers:

Fig. 6 Beck F, Moffat D B, Davies D P. Human Embryology 2nd Edition. Blackwell Scientific Publications.
Figs 9, 26 and 27 Moore K L. The Developing Human. 4th Edition. W B Saunders. 1988.
Fig. 21 Snell R S. Clinical Embryology for Medical Students. 2nd Edition. Little and Brown.
Figs 13, 14, 16, 22, 23, 24, 25, 28, 29 and 31. Langman J. Medical Embryology 3rd Edition. Williams and Wilkins.

All other illustrations have been redrawn and labelled by Mr. S J Gover.

8

The first trimester Transabdominal ultrasound

Paul A. Dubbins

Ultrasound imaging of the first trimester of pregnancy produces an anatomical record of the embryological development of the human. Recent advances in transducer technology have led to the introduction of trans-vaginal ultrasound probes which are particularly useful for the evaluation of early pregnancy and its problems (see Ch. 9).[1] However, transabdominal scanning will probably remain the 'routine' approach in the evaluation of early pregnancy for some time.

Technique

A full bladder is required for ultrasound evaluation of the pelvic organs by the transabdominal approach.[2] This requires a considerable fluid load: up to a pint and a half of liquid in the hour prior to the examination. The full bladder displaces gas filled bowel out of the pelvis, providing an acoustic window to the pelvic organs, and usually places the axis of the uterus parallel to the anterior abdominal wall (Fig. 1). The uterus and adnexal structures can then be demonstrated by a series of sweeps of the transducer, first in longitudinal planes to right and left of midline, then in transverse planes angling both cephalad and caudad to make maximal use of the bladder as an acoustic window. It is also useful in both longitudinal and transverse planes to place the transducer on the right side of the pelvis and angle to the left, and vice versa, to achieve optimum visualisation of the adnexal structures; turning the patient into an oblique position may further improve visualisation. Modified scan planes may be necessary, particularly to demonstrate the long axis of the uterus and its contiguity with the cervical canal. This is particularly so when the uterus is deviated to one or other side of the midline.

Although the full bladder technique is the starting point for most transabdominal evaluations of the pelvis, it is not without its problems and a flexible approach should be used. Not only is an overdistended urinary bladder[2] uncomfortable for the patient but it may also prevent visualisation of a normal gestation sac, distort the appearance of twin sacs and prevent the visualisation of a normal embryo. This is partly as a result of distortion of the gestation sac, but also because the uterus is moved into the far field of the ultrasound beam where resolution is degraded. These problems can usually be resolved by partial emptying of the bladder.

It is not always necessary to prepare patients for ultrasound examination in early pregnancy. In the slim patient with an anteverted uterus or a uterus in neutral position, simple compression on the anterior abdominal wall sometimes allows visualisation of the fundus, body and contents of the uterus in great detail (Fig. 2).

The retroverted uterus remains difficult to assess whether the bladder is filled or empty. The axis of the retroverted uterus is not along the ultrasound beam and the uterus and its contents are further from the transducer

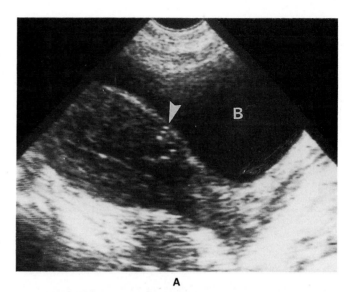

A

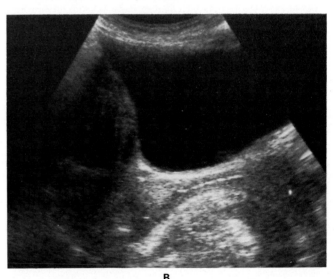

B

Fig. 1 Normal pelvis. A: Long axis scan through the mid-pelvis. The filled urinary bladder is identified (B). The normal pear shape of the uterus is seen. The large arrowhead indicates the site of a caesarean section scar. **B:** A scan showing the vaginal 'stripe'.

(Fig. 3). Trans-vaginal scanning provides a better approach to the retroverted uterus.

Ultrasound signs of early pregnancy

Although the blastocyst forms in the first week following fertilisation, it only embeds in the endometrium during the second week.[3] The earliest sonographic sign of pregnancy, at 25 days menstrual age, is a focus of high reflectivity with thickening of the adjacent decidua. The focus probably corresponds to the implantation site, the decidual thickening being the endometrial response (Fig. 4A).[4] This decidual thickening is echo-poor and allows significant

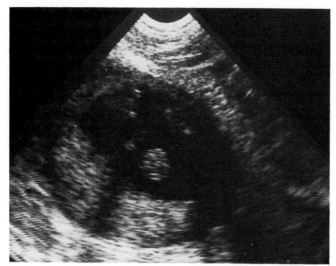

Fig. 2 Pregnant uterus. Scan through the lower abdomen in a pregnant patient. There has been no preparation but with pressure of the transducer on the anterior wall of the pelvis, the fundus of the pregnant uterus can be demonstrated.

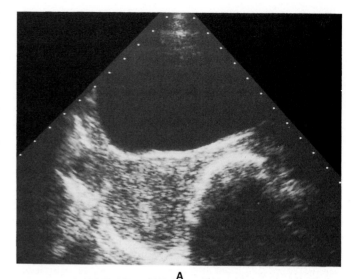

A

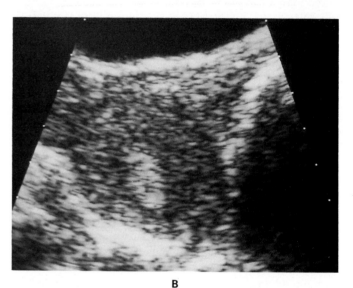

B

Fig. 4 Early pregnancy. A: 4 week intra-uterine gestation with a focus of increased reflectivity in the fundus of this retroverted uterus. **B:** Magnified view of the same early gestation demonstrates the area of increased reflectivity surrounded by a narrow echo-poor area with the whole demonstrating some increased through transmission. This is termed the intradecidual sign.

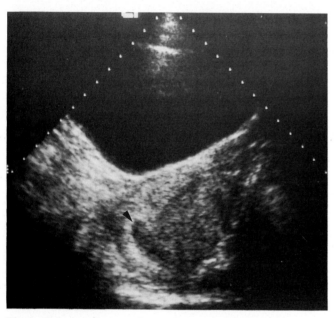

Fig. 3 Retroverted uterus. Long axis scan through the pelvis in a patient with a retroverted uterus. The gestation sac (arrowhead) is only poorly seen and the contents of the sac are not identified.

sound through transmission giving posterior acoustic enhancement. Known as the intradecidual sign, this is said to be specific for early pregnancy and to allow the differentiation from other causes of increased endometrial reflectivity such as endometrial carcinoma and endometrial polyps (Figs 4B and 5). However, the sign may be difficult to demonstrate, particularly in patients of larger build or when bladder filling is suboptimal. In the retroverted uterus demonstration may also be difficult and

these appearances may be mimicked occasionally by the secretory endometrium.

As early as 5 weeks menstrual age an intra-uterine gestation can be demonstrated as a fluid space. This gestation sac correlates with decidua and the extra-embryonic coelom which will become the chorionic cavity (Fig. 5). Differentiation of the normal early gestation sac from other causes of fluid within the cavity of the uterus such as the 'pseudogestation sac' of ectopic pregnancy has been the subject of much discussion.

The 'double decidual sac' sign, 'crescent' sign or 'decidua chorionic sac' sign are all terms used to describe

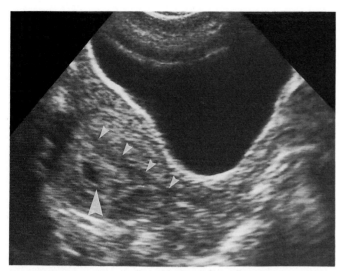

Fig. 5 Pregnancy of 5 weeks and 3 days. Long axis scan. The linear uterine canal is indicated by the small arrows. The appearances of the endometrium are not altered by the intradecidual gestation sac (arrowheads).

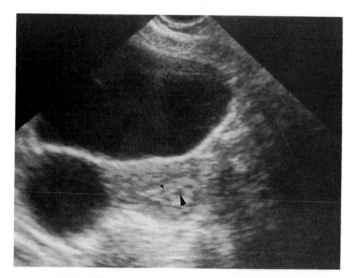

Fig. 6 'Double decidual sac' sign. 5 week gestation with the gestation sac (large arrowhead). The sac projects into the uterine cavity producing a double decidual appearance (small arrowhead). The reliability of this appearance and the explanation for its cause are challenged.

which becomes wrapped around it. Some authors claim this to be developmentally inexact, and moreover can be demonstrated to be false by the demonstration of a normal linear uterine cavity with no evidence of 'wrap around' (Fig. 5).[4] Notwithstanding the dispute of the cause of the decidua chorionic sac (DCS) sign, its reliability has been demonstrated in the differentiation of intra-uterine pregnancy from ectopic pregnancy where the DCS sign does not occur.[5–7] However, the DCS sign is not seen in all normal pregnancies, being reported in as few as two thirds of cases in some series. Furthermore it may also occur in abnormal intra-uterine pregnancies such as blighted ova.[4] Thus when present it may be of value, when absent it is of less diagnostic significance.

The embryonic disc is formed early during the fourth week of menstrual age (Fig. 7).[3,4] It is divided from the trophoblast on the one side by the developing amniotic cavity and on the other by the yolk sac and the extra-embryonic coelom (chorionic cavity). The yolk sac and the amniotic sac increase in size and become visible as two small bubbles or blebs, sometimes as early as 5½ weeks gestation. Recognition of these two blebs allows identification of the embryonic disc. Subsequently both sacs enlarge, the amniotic cavity enveloping the embryo and obliterating the chorionic sac, while the yolk sac becomes a more obvious spherical cyst-like structure adjacent to the developing embryo (Figs 8 and 9). Occasionally the stalk attaching the yolk sac to the embryonic gut can be identified. The yolk sac may reach 5 mm in diameter and may be demonstrated between weeks 7 and 11 but is gradually resorbed and so is not seen after week 12 (see Ch. 11) (Fig. 9).[8]

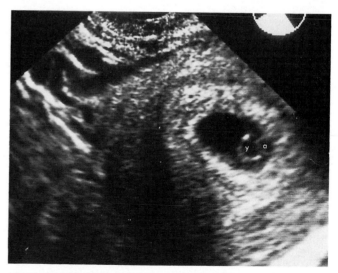

Fig. 7 'Double bleb' sign. Trans-vaginal scan demonstrating 'double bleb' appearance. The gestation sac is clearly seen. Within the gestation sac the embryonic plate is separated from the trophoblast by the developing amniotic cavity (a). The yolk sac (y) lies on the other side of the embryonic plate. The 'double bleb' sign is seen only occasionally on transabdominal ultrasound.

the appearance of a normal gestation sac in which the decidua parietalis appears to diverge and surround a portion of the chorionic sac (Fig. 6).[5] The appearance of double concentric rings or a crescent is therefore presumed to be due to the adjacent structures of the chorionic ring and decidua parietalis separated by uterine cavity fluid. Other workers suggest that the appearances are due to the adjacent location of decidua capsularis and decidua parietalis.[6] These explanations however, require that the gestation sac projects significantly into the uterine cavity

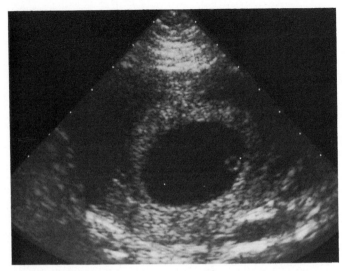

Fig. 8   Yolk sac. Normal yolk sac within the gestation sac. This examination was performed by lower abdominal compression with an empty bladder.

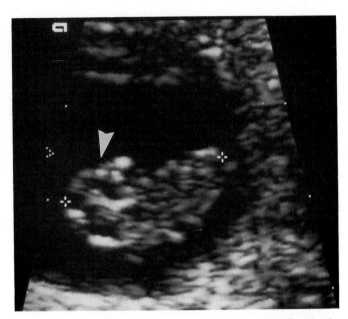

Fig. 10   10 week gestation, showing a clearly recognisable fetal head (arrowhead), in which the developing hemispheres and ventricles are seen.

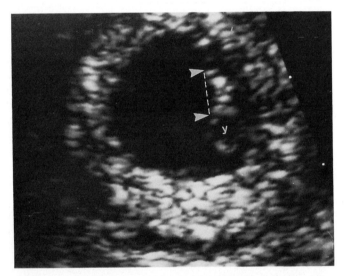

Fig. 9   Crown-rump length measurement indicated by arrowheads in a 6 week gestation. Care must be taken not to include the yolk sac (y) in this measurement if overestimation of gestational age is not to be made.

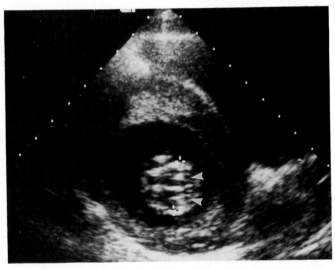

Fig. 11   Biparietal diameter at 12 weeks. The relatively large size of the lateral ventricles is demonstrated on this scan together with two small posteriorly located choroid plexus cysts (arrowheads).

The heart begins to beat on day 22 post-ovulation i.e. at the beginning of the sixth post-menstrual week,[3] and at this stage viability of the embryo can be confirmed. Between 41 and 43 days of gestation the heart rate averages 90 beats per minute, increasing to approximately 125 beats per minute by the seventh week.[9] The heart rate increases to a maximum of between 170 and 180 beats per minute in the ninth week, slowing to about 150 by the thirteenth week.[10]

Detailed embryological development of the human cannot be documented by transabdominal ultrasound.[11] The head appears as a recognisable structure between the ninth and tenth weeks (Fig. 10). Axial scans at this stage demonstrate the intracerebral structures dominated by the large lateral ventricles (Fig. 11). These are more regularly visualised between the tenth and twelfth weeks and during this time the reflective choroid plexuses may be identified. Indeed choroid plexus cysts have been reported as early as 12 weeks (Fig. 11), presumably indicating that, in most cases, these form part of normal development. Facial structures can be appreciated between the tenth and twelfth weeks (Fig. 12).

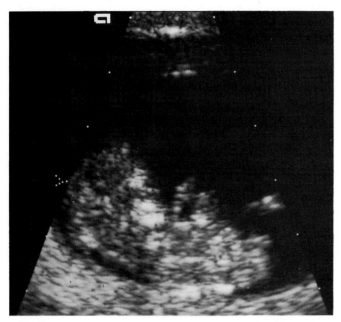

Fig. 12 Fetal face. 11 week gestation showing identifiable facial structures.

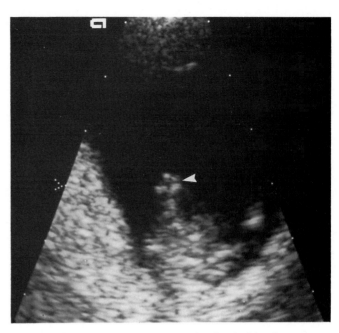

Fig. 14 Fetal hand. 11 week gestation showing fetal hand (arrowhead), the thumb and forefinger are seen.

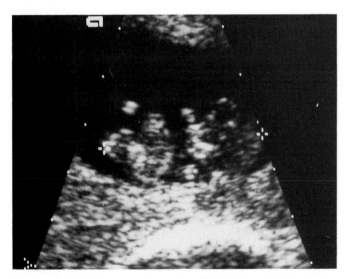

Fig. 13 Fetal limbs. 11 week gestation showing arms and legs.

In the abdomen the fetal stomach may be seen as early as 10 weeks and the fetal bladder at 12 weeks; some claims that the kidneys can also be recognised in the first trimester have been made[11,12] but this is only possible under ideal imaging conditions.

Limb buds may be seen by 9 weeks, individual bones and joints between 11 and 12 weeks (Fig. 13) and individual digits at 12 weeks (Fig. 14).

At 12 weeks a full fetal structural survey is possible including assessment of the heart, the neural axis and the limbs, but is rarely achieved with current transabdominal probes. The renal and gastrointestinal tracts require later assessment because abnormalities here are manifested later.

The improved resolution of ultrasound equipment allows confirmation of structural integrity of a first trimester pregnancy and is a considerable incentive to attempt to diagnose fetal abnormalities earlier than the mid-second trimester. It is important .however, to recognise that approximately 40% of embryos in Carnegie Stage 21 (gestational age 9½ weeks) have nuchal blebs, which, although they may be associated with a meningomyelocele, usually disappear later in gestation. Similarly, at Carnegie Stage 23 (gestational age 10 weeks), the small and large bowel are extra-abdominal.[3,13] The diagnosis, therefore, of neural tube defects (other than anencephaly) and of abdominal wall defects should probably be avoided before the end of the first trimester. Trans-vaginal ultrasound may allow a better understanding of embryology and better early diagnosis (see Ch. 9).

Cardiac motion is the first detectable embryonic activity, seen from as early as 5½ weeks.[14] From between 6 and 7 weeks smooth vermiform body movements of the embryo can be detected; they become more rapid by the eighth week, at which stage some flexion and extension of the trunk may be observed. During the ninth week sudden spasmodic trunk extensions and trunk curling occur. By the tenth week the vermiform movements have ceased and are replaced by more co-ordinated movement with, for example, head and lower limb extension. The movement of the limbs increases in the eleventh week and there are frequent 'jumps' involving sudden, violent movements particularly of the trunk and lower limbs, the fetus propelling itself through the amniotic fluid and then subsequently sinking down again.

Measurements in the first trimester[15]

Obstetric measurement has an important role in the evaluation of gestational age, of embryonic growth and well-being and in the assessment of structural abnormality. In the first trimester three measurements have been used to assess gestational age and to document normal embryonic growth. The first, the uterine size or uterine length, has been superseded by measurement of the gestation sac and of the crown-rump length (see Ch. 11).

Gestation sac

The size of the gestation sac can be measured as a diameter or as a volume. The volume can be calculated either by planimetry, taking parallel scans at 5 mm intervals, or by assuming an ellipsoid shape and halving the product of the three diameters. The accuracy of sac volume in the assessment of the gestational age is said to be as good as ± 1 week (see Appendix).

Crown-rump length

Since its first description by Robinson in 1975, the measurement of crown-rump length of the embryo has become the most widely accepted method of assessment of gestational age in the first trimester. With real time ultrasound it is not difficult to establish and measure the longest length of the embryo. By about 9 weeks the head can be routinely distinguished from the body, making the measurement of crown-rump simpler since embryonic structure is more clearly recognised and doubts about measurement end points less likely. Earlier in the gestation, a yolk sac lying at one or other end of the embryo might inadvertently be included in the measurement (Fig. 9). As the pregnancy advances however, progressive curling of the fetal trunk and flexion of the fetal neck may result in a 5% to 10% underestimation of crown-rump length measurement. This fetal flexion becomes more marked after the first trimester so the crown-rump length is not used after 14 weeks.

The placenta

Initially chorionic villi are present across the entire surface of the implanted embryo.[16] Subsequently however, there appears to be a nutritional disparity favouring the development of the trophoblast that lies adjacent to the endometrium. This is the site of the development of the placenta with further stimulus to the development of the chorionic villi (chorion frondosum) and their loss elsewhere (chorion laeve). This polarisation or placental development

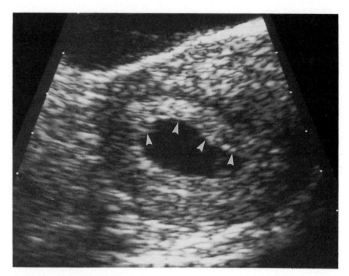

Fig. 15   Early placental polarisation with the arrowheads indicating thickening in the region of the chorion frondosum.

can be observed as early as 7 weeks and is fully established by 12 weeks (Fig. 15).

Multiple pregnancy

It is possible to identify more than one gestation sac as early as 5 weeks of gestation (Figs 16 and 17). Similar criteria as in singleton pregnancies must be applied to document the viability of each gestation. It is more difficult to demonstrate the intradecidual sign and the decidua chorionic sac sign in multiple pregnancies to evaluate viability. The identification of two or more gestation sacs and two or more embryos in the first trimester does not, however, guarantee continued survival of the embryos, even to the end of the first trimester; the 'vanishing twin' (see below) appears to be a common phenomenon with a resultant surviving singleton pregnancy (see *Abdominal and General Ultrasound*, Vol. 1, Ch. 4).[17]

Assessment of abnormalities

The assessment of abnormalities in the first trimester may be divided into two broad groups. The first is the evaluation of the symptomatic patient, the second the evaluation of the pregnancy for structural abnormalities. However, it is only recently that the resolution of ultrasound equipment has allowed the recognition of anatomical detail during the first trimester. An increasing amount of information is available about the embryo, but there are currently only a few reports of the detection of structural abnormalities before 12 weeks. However, there is significant potential for earlier assessment of structural integrity of the developing embryo, provided dose levels of ultrasound during the critical period of organogenesis can be minimised (see Ch. 7).[11]

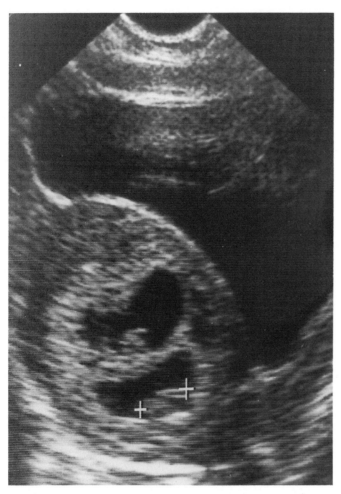

Fig. 16   8 week twin pregnancy. Two gestation sacs are seen, both containing live embryos.

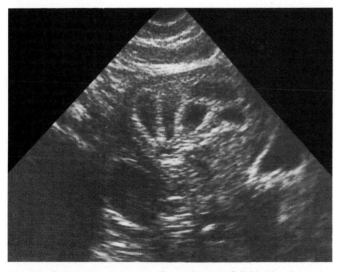

Fig. 17   Quintuplet pregnancy. Even without a full bladder the enlarged uterus can be seen with five separate gestation sacs. Embryos were identified within all five at 6½ weeks gestation.

Symptoms and signs of problems in early pregnancy

Most patients present for first trimester ultrasound with one or more symptoms or signs. The commonest is vaginal bleeding which is the cardinal symptom of threatened abortion, although it may be present in other conditions.[18,19] Pelvic and lower abdominal pain may be present, with or without bleeding.[20] The normal symptoms of pregnancy such as nausea, vomiting, breast tenderness etc. may be accentuated in hyperemesis gravidarum, suggesting high levels of human gonadotrophin. Pregnancy symptoms may be diminished, implying that HCG levels are low and suggesting that the pregnancy is not viable. Physical signs may include a uterus of inappropriate size for gestational age, either large or small; focal or generalised abdominal tenderness with guarding and cervical excitation. Although clinical features may point to a specific diagnosis, there is often a wide differential diagnosis. Ultrasound examination is directed to establish the site of the pregnancy, confirm morphological normality of the uterus and gestation and to demonstrate embryonic viability.

Ultrasound findings

The most reliable sign of viability is the demonstration of an embryonic heart beat. However, this may be difficult or impossible to demonstrate in pregnancies of less than 6 weeks, especially when the patient is obese, the uterus is retroverted or there are abdominal scars etc. Other sonographic signs may be used to predict the outcome in pregnancies complicated by threatened abortion.

The gestation sac

The initial appearance of a highly reflective focus followed by the development of a fluid containing intra-uterine sac are the earliest signs of pregnancy. Features to refine the prediction of pregnancy outcome have been described. These include an assessment of gestation sac size and growth, the characteristics of the rim or rind of the gestation sac and the appearances of the gestation sac contents, including the embryo.

Gestation sac size and growth   The growth of the gestation sac, as measured by linear dimensions or volumetrically, is linear in the first trimester. Charts correlating gestation sac size with gestational age are well-established (Fig. 18) (see Ch. 11 and Appendix). It is therefore possible to use discrepancies between size and the history of pregnancy, or between size and other sonographic features of pregnancy, as prognostic indicators. A gestation sac too small for the menstrual age implies pregnancy failure. However, this interpretation depends upon certain knowledge of the date of conception (which is only possible when there is a regular menstrual cycle with predictable ovulation each month). In practice

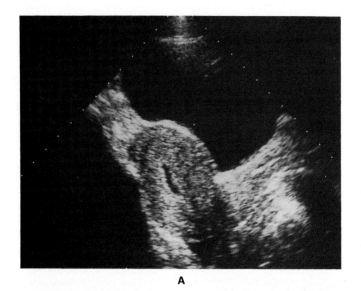

A

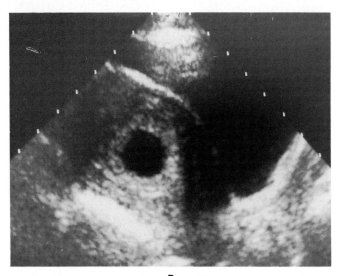

B

Fig. 18 Growth of the gestation sac. A: Long axis scan through the pelvis, a gestation sac is shown in the uterus at 5 weeks and 2 days of amenorrhoea. **B:** Gestation sac 10 days after the first scan showing growth of the sac.

therefore, it is only completely specific and sensitive in cases where ovulation is being monitored or induced, or following in vitro fertilisation. It is only in these patients that 'menstrual dates' are accurate enough to compare with ultrasound criteria of gestational age. Robinson suggests that a gestation sac whose volume is greater than 2.5 ml and which does not contain a visible embryo is not viable.[21] This gestation sac volume/embryo relationship has been variously reported between 2.5 and 5 ml.[22,23] The assessment of gestation sac growth in normal pregnancies reveals a mean diameter growth rate of 1.2 mm per day. This compares with 0.25 mm per day in cases of blighted ovum. In cases of threatened abortion, a follow up examination can be performed in 10 to 14 days to assess gestation sac

growth rate: a sac that fails to double in volume each week between weeks five and eight is suggestive of gestational failure.[24] However, while the assessment of gestation sac growth is an interesting ancillary finding, it is of limited diagnostic value. Follow up examination in doubtful cases is certainly important but rather to establish the appearance of a viable embryo with cardiac activity than to assess growth of a gestation sac. This is particularly important with embryonic demise (missed abortion) since, in these cases, a gestation sac may continue to grow at a normal rate (Fig. 19). It might be expected that, since gestation

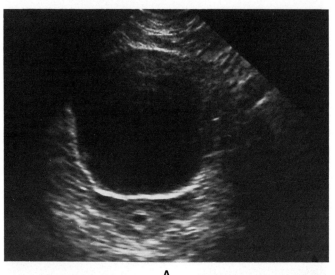

A

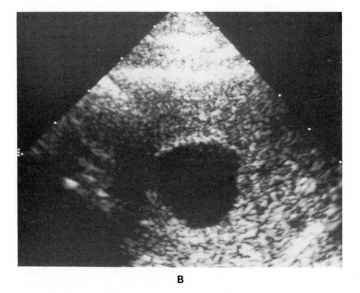

B

Fig. 19 Blighted ovum. A: Transverse scan of the pelvis with an overfull urinary bladder. There is, however, no distortion of the gestation sac which remains rounded. The sac diameter is 7 mm indicating a gestational age of 5 weeks. **B:** 15 days later the gestation sac has grown to a mean diameter of 2 cm which would indicate a gestational age of 7½ weeks. However the margins of the sac are irregular and there is no reflective rind. This is a blighted ovum with no evidence of an embryo in spite of gestation sac growth.

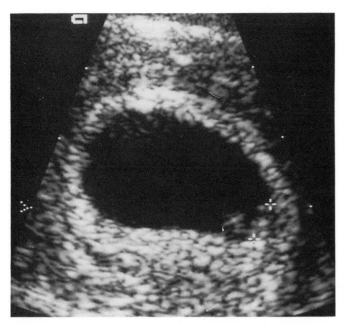

Fig. 20   Large gestation sac with inappropriately small embryo. The crown-rump length of the embryo at 5 mm is equivalent to a gestational age of 6 weeks but the gestation sac volume was measured at 3.8 ml which is that of a 7½ week pregnancy. This pregnancy developed normally to term. There was no evidence of polyhydramnios.

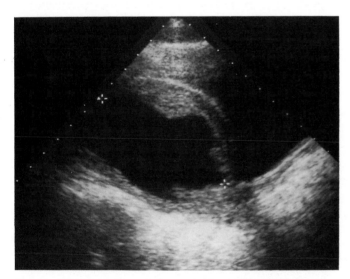

Fig. 21   Large irregular gestation sac without evidence of an embryo. The sac size is consistent with a gestation of approximately 11 weeks.

cursor of polyhydramnios but our experience does not support this.

Gestation sac characteristics

Gestation sac shape   The normal sac has a uniform round or oval shape; in missed abortion it is often distorted, angulated and irregular (Fig. 21). These features are useful as supportive diagnostic criteria of pregnancy failure but may be absent in many cases.[23] Similarly they may be mimicked by a number of different pathological and normal conditions.[19] An overfilled urinary bladder may distort the gestation sac producing flattening and angulation (Fig. 22). Similar appearances may be produced by Brax-

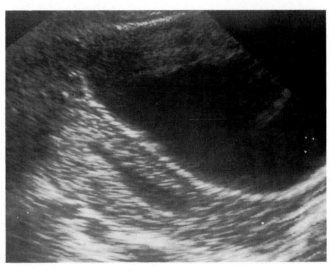

Fig. 22   Flattened gestation sac. Flattened and pointed gestation sac in this long axis scan. The compression of the gestation sac is caused by an overfilled urinary bladder.

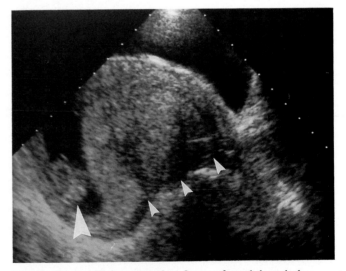

Fig. 23   Braxton Hicks contraction. Scan performed through the pelvis with an empty bladder of a 10 week gestation. The gestation sac is distorted by a prominent Braxton Hicks contraction (small arrowheads). A transverse section of the embryonic abdomen is indicated by the large arrowhead.

sac size and crown-rump length may be used to assess gestational age, there would be a correlation between these two. This implies, however, that standard deviations of gestation sac size are small throughout early development and in all pregnancies.[25] There are cases where large sac volumes are present in the first trimester with an apparently inappropriately small crown-rump length measurement of the embryo (Fig. 20). This appearance may be the pre-

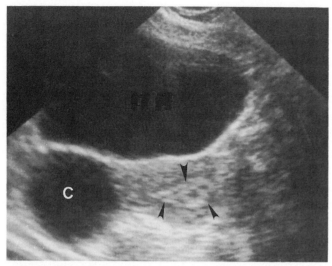

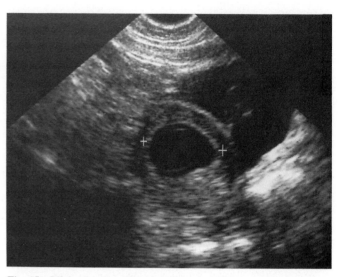

Fig. 24 Double decidual sac sign. Transverse scan of a normal 5 week gestation. The gestation sac demonstrates a double decidual sac sign (arrowheads) with the reflective rim of the gestation apparently projecting into the uterine cavity with its decidual reaction. There is a corpus luteum cyst in the right ovary (C).

Fig. 25 Blighted ovum. The gestation sac shows no features of sac morphology commensurate with viability. There is no reflective rind.

ton Hicks contractions (Fig. 23) and the sac is frequently distorted by coexistent uterine pathology such as fibroids.[26] Irregular gestation sacs may also be seen in uterine anomalies such as bicornuate uterus.

Features of gestation sac morphology   Various signs have been described as indicating a good prognosis for pregnancy outcome.[5–7] Of these the intradecidual sign and the double decidual sac sign or chorionic decidual reaction are best known (Fig. 24). The implication is that the absence of these signs indicates a poor prognosis for pregnancy outcome (Fig. 25). However, these characteristics of early gestation sacs are an inconstant feature even in normal pregnancies. The double decidual sacs sign is reported as being observed in some three quarters of pregnancies.[27] Moreover, the double decidual sign may also be seen in pregnancies which subsequently fail (Fig. 26). The intradecidual sign (Fig. 27) has been reported in 92%

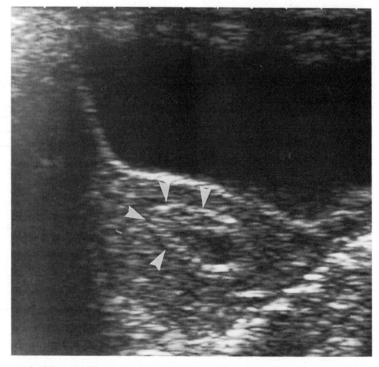

Fig. 26 Missed abortion. Apparent double decidual sac sign (arrowheads) in a missed abortion.

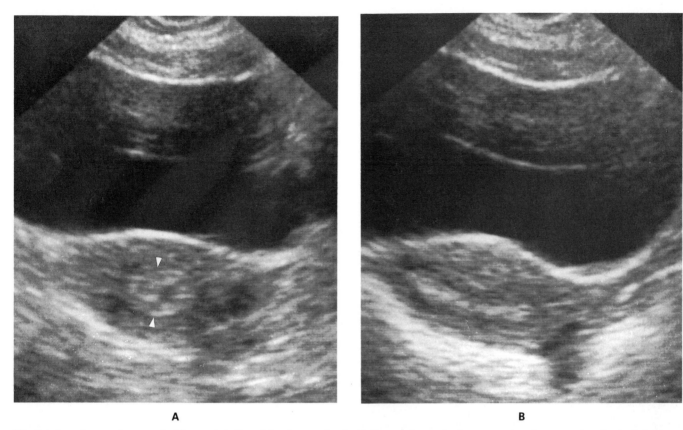

Fig. 27 5 week gestation sac. A: The sac is indicated by the arrowheads. **B:** Long axis scan in the same patient demonstrating clearly defined endometrial line without projection of the sac into the 'cavity'. This has been described as the intradecidual sign.

of pregnancies, but this has not been independently confirmed.[4]

The yolk sac sign The appearance of the yolk sac as a normal feature in the first trimester has been taken to be an indicator of the viability of the pregnancy (Fig. 28).[8,28–30] A gestation sac of diameter greater than 2 cm should contain a demonstrable yolk sac. A gestation without a yolk sac would therefore be expected to be non-viable. These criteria are however, a little confusing in practice. A gestation sac diameter of 2 cm is at approximately the 'double bleb' stage of embryonic development at which the embryo itself should be visualised along with the yolk sac (Figs 29 and 30).[4] While the yolk sac later separates from the embryo (remaining attached by the vitelline stalk) by this stage the live embryo should be clearly visible without the need to rely upon demonstration of the yolk sac (Fig. 31). Furthermore, the yolk sac is reported to be visible in only two thirds of normal intra-uterine pregnancies even when the embryo is visible. In addition the yolk sac can persist even after embryonic demise and is reported to be present in as many as 16% of non-viable pregnancies. Indeed a gestation sac of 25 mm or more and empty except for the yolk sac is abnormal (Fig. 32). It appears that the location and size of the yolk sac are important in making the dis-

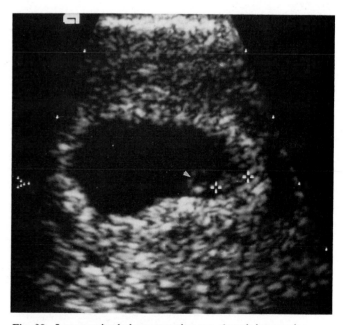

Fig. 28 Inappropriately large gestation sac. 6 week intrauterine pregnancy of crown-rump length 5 mm. This is equivalent to a gestational age of approximately 6 weeks. The 'cystic' yolk sac is noted immediately adjacent to the embryo (arrowhead). Incidentally the gestation sac is inappropriately large for dates but the course of the pregnancy was normal.

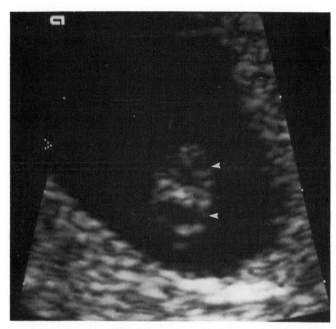

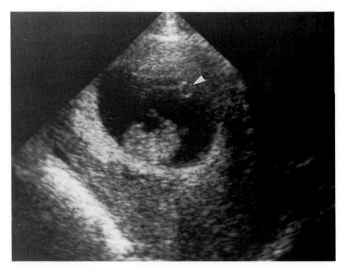

Fig. 31   Yolk sac. 8 week gestation. The yolk sac (arrowhead) is now clearly separated, via the vitelline stalk, from the embryo.

Fig. 29   'Double bleb' sign. Magnified transabdominal scan of a 5½ week pregnancy demonstrating the 'double bleb' sign (two arrowheads) with the embryonic plate interposed.

of the gestation sac with an echo-poor or echo-free space interposed (presumably representing blood) (Figs 34 and 35). This may be subchorionic and be related to the surface of the placenta, or chorio-amniotic and related to the non-placental portion of the gestation sac. There is some dispute about the importance of this finding. While some have suggested that there is no correlation between the presence and size of a separation and the eventual outcome of the pregnancy,[31] others indicate that fetal loss rate is increased to approximately 20%, even without other abnormal findings.[19,32] However, the statistical significance is difficult to evaluate when considering expected fetal loss rates in the presence of vaginal bleeding. It seems likely that small intra-uterine haematomas do not prejudice the continuation of the pregnancy although the possibility of late growth retardation has not been fully evaluated.[33]

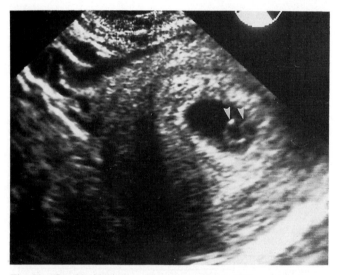

Fig. 30   'Double bleb' sign. Trans-vaginal scan of 5½ week pregnancy demonstrating the 'double bleb' sign (arrowheads).

tinction between viable and non-viable pregnancy. A peripherally placed yolk sac measuring 3 mm or less is likely to be normal and associated with the 'double bleb' sign. A yolk sac measuring 4 mm and free floating within the centre of an otherwise empty amniotic sac implies pregnancy failure (Figs 32 and 33).

Chorio-amniotic separation or subchorionic haematoma

This feature may be seen in early pregnancy as a separation of the linear echo of the chorionic membrane from the wall

Embryonic viability

The most important indicator of the viability of a pregnancy is demonstration of the embryonic heart beat.[34,35] This can be detected from the end of the sixth week at the 'double bleb' stage of development.[4] Obviously this sign is more use as a positive indicator of viability than in the accurate diagnosis of pregnancy failure. In pregnancies after 7 weeks, when the embryo can be clearly seen, the absence of a heart beat is diagnostic of a missed abortion. Passive motion of the embryo in response to percussion of the maternal abdominal wall with the ultrasound probe has been described. This is an interesting if somewhat macabre feature but, in fact, adds nothing to the diagnosis because cardiac activity can always be assessed in an embryo large enough to demonstrate this sort of abnormal movement. The demonstration of an embryonic heart beat not only confirms a live intra-uterine pregnancy but, irrespective of

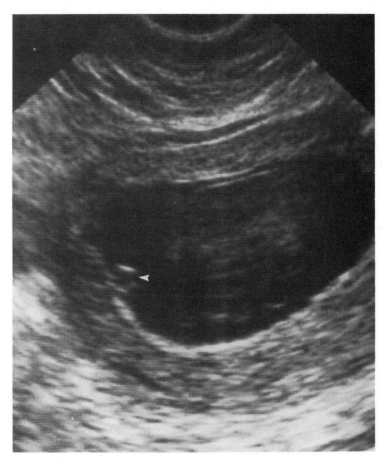

Fig. 32 Blighted ovum. Transabdominal scan (empty bladder) in a non-viable 10 week gestation. Although the yolk sac (arrowhead) was identified peripherally the embryo was too small to visualise. The features confirm the diagnosis of a blighted ovum.

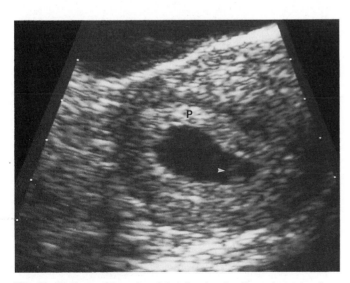

Fig. 33 Yolk sac. Normal peripherally placed yolk sac (arrowhead). Although the embryo is not identified on this scan the features of the gestation sac show polarisation of the placenta (P) and the embryo was demonstrated on other scan planes.

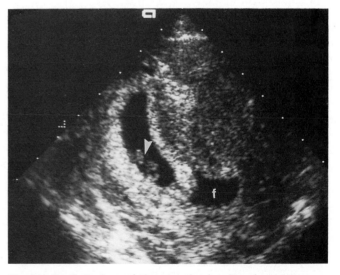

Fig. 34 Small chorio-amniotic separation in a 7 week pregnancy. Scan performed with an empty bladder. The gestation sac is clearly seen with an embryo (arrowhead). There is a small amount of fluid (f) adjacent to the gestation sac, this presumably represents an intra-uterine haematoma. At 7 weeks of gestation this is unlikely to be a so-called implantation bleed.

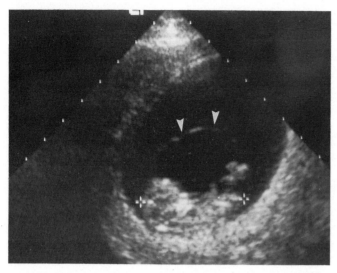

Fig. 35 Chorio-amniotic separation with the membrane indicated by the arrowheads.

other ancillary signs, is of prognostic significance, with a low likelihood of spontaneous abortion (2% to 4%) after confirmation of a viable embryo.

Hormone pregnancy tests and beta HCG

Although much more sensitive than earlier pregnancy tests, these can be positive in other conditions and may remain positive for some time after pregnancy failure.[36] Quantification of the beta subunit of human gonadotrophin in maternal serum may be correlated with the ultrasound findings in the pelvis.[37,38] Thus an intra-uterine gestation sac should be visible with serum HCG levels of greater than 1800 mIu/ml. Although this may be useful in the demonstration or diagnosis of ectopic pregnancy (see below) its value in the differentiation of normal from abnormal intra-uterine pregnancies is less well-defined. The demonstration of a live intra-uterine embryo remains the most reliable prognostic indicator for the viability of a pregnancy. Knowledge of a previous pregnancy test may be useful in the interpretation of the ultrasound findings. The finding of an inappropriately small gestation sac in a patient with good menstrual history and an early positive pregnancy test may allow the firm diagnosis of blighted ovum/missed abortion without the need for follow up examination.

Low implantation

The site of implantation of the gestation sac in the uterus is of doubtful importance in determining fetal outcome. A low implantation has been reported to have a poor prognosis,[19] others indicate that it may only be a minor risk factor for placenta praevia rather than a predictor of early fetal loss.[4]

Summary of ultrasound signs

The 'gold standard' for the diagnosis of a normal viable first trimester pregnancy remains the demonstration of an embryonic heart beat. While other findings may be useful when counselling the mother for an unfavourable outcome, none is reliable enough to state unequivocally that the outcome will be poor. There are many instances of a poor prognosis being confounded by clear demonstration of an embryonic heartbeat on a follow up scan. Unless therefore, there is a combination of clinical history, findings of hormonal pregnancy tests and ultrasound features, it is prudent to arrange to re-examine the patient after an interval. A flexible approach should be adopted, re-examining as early as possible. Thus if on the first examination the gestation sac is of 6 week size or more, re-examination in 1 week will allow the confident assessment of embryonic cardiac motion. If the gestation is less than 6 weeks in size then a delay of 7 to 10 days is more appropriate. The use of trans-vaginal ultrasound often makes such delays unnecessary because cardiac activity can be detected earlier. If trans-vaginal ultrasound is unavailable and if the uterus is anteverted, scanning with an empty urinary bladder will often allow the use of a higher frequency transducer with improved resolution and improved detection of embryonic cardiac motion (Fig. 36).

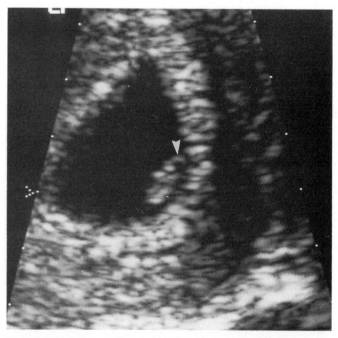

Fig. 36 Normal 6 week gestation. Transabdominal ultrasound with an empty bladder demonstrating an intra-uterine gestation sac. The embryo is seen within the sac. The yolk sac (arrowhead) lies at one end of the embryo. This is a 7 mm embryo of approximately 6 weeks gestation. Cardiac motion was not detectable using a 3 MHz transducer with a full urinary bladder but at 5 MHz following bladder emptying fetal viability was confirmed.

Pregnancy failure

Inevitable abortion

Inevitable abortion is a clinical diagnosis in which uterine bleeding in the first trimester is accompanied by dilatation of the cervical canal.[20] It is rarely necessary to perform ultrasound in these cases but occasionally the ultrasound features of inevitable abortion are demonstrated. The gestation sac has separated from the endometrium and, together with the embryo and intraluminal blood, is found low in the uterus with a dilated cervical canal. Even if the embryonic heart beat continues, this is a sign of inevitable and indeed impending embryonic loss (Fig. 37).

Blighted ovum and missed abortion

The term 'blighted ovum' is applied to a gestation sac without an embryo.[22,23] While it is known that approximately half of all spontaneous abortions contain no embryo, the differentiation of this condition from a missed abortion on ultrasound criteria alone is not always possible, since a tiny non-viable embryo may be too small to resolve. Furthermore, an empty gestation sac may be seen in a normal, very early pregnancy for the same reasons of lack of resolution, particularly when the uterus is retroverted or retroflexed. Abnormal morphological features of the gestation sac may be useful as ancillary findings in these conditions (see above).

The vanishing or blighted twin

The incidence of liveborn twins is reported as 2% of pregnancies (Fig. 38).[39,40] Ultrasound studies, however, suggest

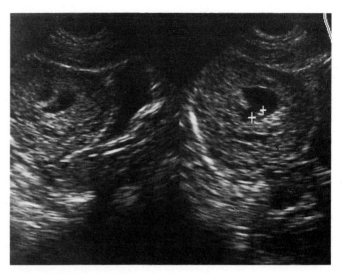

Fig. 38   Twin gestation sacs. Longitudinal and transverse scans through the uterus. There are twin gestation sacs. One of these contains a live embryo, the other is empty.

that twin conception is more common than this with reports of twin gestation sacs varying between 3% and 6% of all pregnancies.[41] Documented evidence of a live embryo that is subsequently lost is only available for a small proportion of these cases, but the presence of a second gestation sac with characteristics typical of a blighted ovum or a missed abortion is well-documented. This may be associated with uterine bleeding and the gestation sac is subsequently resorbed. The vanishing twin appears to have few prognostic sequelae for its sibling, most proceeding to normal delivery. It is important therefore, to temper the early diagnosis of twin pregnancy with a caveat to take account of the possibility of loss of one of the twins in the first trimester. Overall the loss rate of one of the twins is probably of the order of 50%, although it is possible that overdiagnosis of blighted twin may be made as a result of confusion of the diagnosis of a distorted second gestation sac with subchorionic haemorrhage, implantation bleeds or pseudo-second sac (see *Abdominal and General Ultrasound, Vol. 1, Ch. 4*).[42]

Incomplete abortion

The appearances on ultrasound of an incomplete abortion are relatively non-specific (Fig. 39). The sonographic appearances of blood are so variable, ranging from echo-free to highly reflective, that the differentiation between simple residual retained clot and retained products of conception (including trophoblast and/or embryonic parts), is difficult. Unless there is reflective material within the uterine cavity, a cautious approach to interpretation of the ultrasound findings, and therefore to management is advisable. Patients should be managed on a combination of ultrasound findings and clinical grounds. A patient whose vaginal bleeding is settling and in whom ultrasound

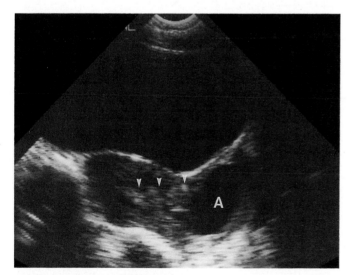

Fig. 37   Inevitable abortion. Long axis scan through the pelvis in a patient in the process of aborting. The amniotic fluid and/or blood (A) is within a distended cervical canal. Some products of conception (arrowheads) remain within the uterus.

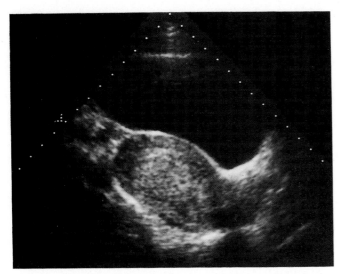

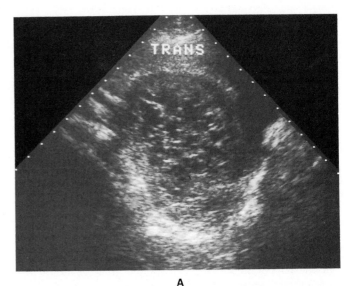

A

Fig. 39 Incomplete abortion. Long axis scan through the pelvis. The uterus contains considerable reflective material. This represents a combination of retained products of conception and blood clot. It is difficult in this situation to differentiate between incomplete abortion and an early molar pregnancy.

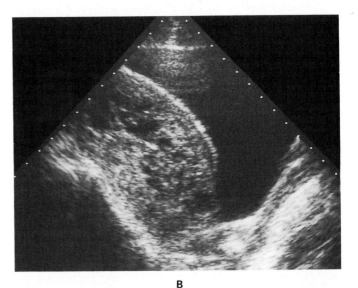

B

Fig. 40 Hydatidiform mole. A: Transverse and **B:** longitudinal scan through the pelvis. The uterus is enlarged and contains multiple cystic spaces of varying sizes. The cysts allow increased through transmission of sound.

demonstrates either fluid only, or in association with little reflective material, is managed expectantly with follow up ultrasound being performed as clinically indicated.

Hydatidiform mole

Hydatidiform moles are thought to be due to failure of development of an embryo, i.e. a blighted ovum, or to arise from a defective embryo (see Ch. 23).[4,18–20] The transformation of intact apparently viable gestations at 8 weeks into molar pregnancies has been documented with ultrasound. The reported reduction of incidence of molar pregnancies over recent years can be accounted for by earlier uterine evacuation consequent upon earlier diagnosis of blighted ovum and missed abortion by ultrasound. Hydatidiform mole is the proliferation of trophoblast at the expense of embryonic tissue.

The proliferative trophoblast forms numerous vesicles which produce a typical ultrasonic appearance: the uterus is filled with tiny cystic spaces. These may be interposed with more normal appearing trophoblastic or placental tissue and there may be varying amounts of fluid within the uterine cavity. The multiple vesicles accounted for the so-called 'snowstorm' appearance originally described using early bistable static equipment. However, it is no longer appropriate to use this descriptive term with modern equipment and the description should therefore be abandoned. Because of the fluid content of the cysts or vesicles there is marked increase in transmission through the uterus which makes correct adjustment of the TGC important if the more deeply placed vesicles are to be well-seen. Although the appearance of multiple 'cysts' is frequently

encountered, the appearances of trophoblastic disease are variable (Figs 40 and 41). There may be several larger vesicles or cysts within the uterine cavity or heterogeneous solid tissue, reflecting hydropic change within less atypical trophoblast. In addition, intra-uterine blood may be seen as echo-free fluid or blood clot of varying reflectivity. Molar pregnancy is frequently, but not invariably, associated with multiple theca lutein ovarian cysts (Fig. 42). These are large luteal cysts stimulated by the high HCG levels; they produce either a 'soap bubble' or 'spoke wheel' appearance of the ovaries which are remarkably enlarged. Because tumour invasion cannot be assessed, the distinction between hydatidiform mole, invasive mole or chorion

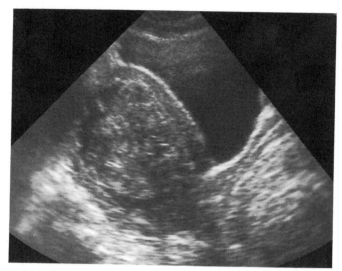

Fig. 41 **Hydatidiform mole**, long axis scan through the pelvis. The uterus is filled with heterogeneous material. Postero-superiorly this would appear to extend outside the uterus. At hysterectomy an invasive mole was demonstrated.

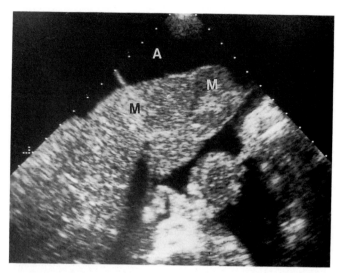

Fig. 43 **Malignant trophoblastic disease.** Right upper quadrant scan showing ascites (A) and a liver containing multiple metastases of differing reflectivity (M).

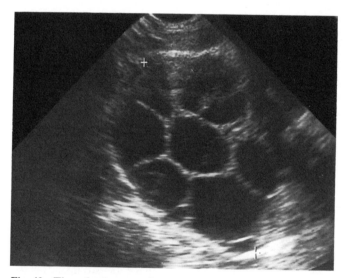

Fig. 42 **Theca lutein cysts.** Scan in the left iliac fossa in a patient with an hydatidiform mole shows a markedly enlarged ovary containing multiple theca lutein cysts.

carcinoma cannot be made with transabdominal scanning unless ancillary signs such as the presence of ascites or metastatic lesions, for example in the liver (Fig. 43) are demonstrated. The foregoing description of hydatidiform mole applies to gestations of between 9 and 12 weeks of amenorrhoea. Prior to this, the demonstration of abnormal trophoblast is more difficult, though the pathological processes are the same but on a small scale. It may be possible to demonstrate tiny cystic structures similar to those seen in the late first and early second trimester but, more frequently, irregular thickening of the endometrium is seen. This may be difficult to differentiate from an in-complete abortion and it is therefore important that all curettings are sent for histological examination. Doppler flow characteristics to a uterus containing molar tissue are abnormal with decreased resistance to flow (decreased PI); this may be of value in the early diagnosis of hydatidiform mole, detection of persistent molar tissue following uterine evacuation, and in the early detection of recurrence.[43]

Partial mole This is a relatively uncommon compli-cation of pregnancy characterised by restricted involvement of trophoblastic tissue in the molar degeneration (see Ch. 23).[44,45] It is associated exclusively with chromosomal triploidy (69 chromosomes). Sonographic features have been reported in the second and third trimesters. There may be a large placenta which contains numerous irregular cystic spaces in association with an embryo or fetus show-ing various degrees of growth abnormality. This may manifest itself as an empty gestation sac, a gestation sac with a dead fetus or, later in the pregnancy, a growth retarded fetus. The diagnosis is however, rarely made by ultrasound and is often only discovered by pathological examination of the placenta after fetal loss.

Ectopic pregnancy

Ectopic pregnancy remains a diagnostic problem.[4,6,46–50] Lower abdominal pain and tenderness in any woman of child bearing age should raise the suspicion of an ectopic pregnancy. Typically there is a history of amenorrhoea, perhaps with other symptoms of early pregnancy, followed by a brown vaginal loss in association with the pain. Physi-cal examination is often non-contributory although uterine enlargement, adnexal tenderness with or without a mass and lower abdominal and pelvic peritonism may be found.

However, these features may be present in patients without ectopic pregnancy and may be absent in patients with ectopic pregnancy. It might be advocated that all patients presenting with these symptoms undergo a diagnostic laparoscopy but in one series of such patients over 50% were found to have normal intra-uterine pregnancies, only 11% subsequently being proved to be ectopic in location.

Much was expected of ultrasound in the differentiation of ectopic pregnancy from other causes of lower pelvic pain. However, the pathognomonic sign of ectopic pregnancy on ultrasound, i.e. an intact gestation sac outside the

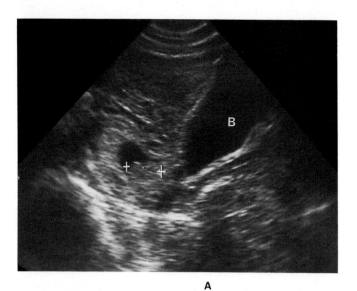

A

B

Fig. 44   Ectopic pregnancy. A: Long axis scan to the left of the midline. A gestation sac containing a live embryo (between the crosses) is shown outside the uterus. B – bladder. **B:** Transverse scan through the pelvis. There is a live ectopic pregnancy in the right adnexa. The crown–rump length is indicated by the calipers. There is free fluid in the pouch of Douglas and to the left of the uterus (f). An IUCD (arrowhead) is noted within the uterine cavity, this predisposes to ectopic pregnancy.

uterus containing a viable embryo, is only seen in 1% to 5% of all cases and even in these it is usually impossible to localise the site of the pregnancy as tubal, ovarian or abdominal except on statistical grounds (Figs 44 and 45). The most common additional feature on ultrasound is the demonstration of an adnexal mass which may be complex or completely cystic. A complex mass is seen in just under half of all extra-uterine pregnancies, and presumably represents blood within the tube or within the peritoneal cavity. There is usually free fluid in the pouch of Douglas, and occasionally intraperitoneal fluid elsewhere, for example in Morrison's pouch, following rupture of the ectopic pregnancy (Figs 46 and 47). However, in approximately 20% of cases there is no peritoneal fluid and indeed in normal subjects, particularly in the post-ovulatory phase, there may be a small amount of free fluid in the pouch of Douglas. Furthermore, the demonstration of complex, cystic or solid masses in the adnexa is not specific of an ectopic pregnancy (Fig. 48).[51]

Similar findings will be seen in ovarian cysts, which may have complex appearances as well as give rise to pelvic pain if there is intracystic haemorrhage. Ovarian tumours, tubovarian abscesses, endometriosis, para-ovarian cysts and torsion of a pedunculated fibroid can also mimic these findings. The sonographer may be further confused by the presence of intracystic haemorrhage when blood clot may mimic a dead embryo. Finally the adnexae appear normal in 20% of patients with ectopic pregnancies.

From the foregoing it may be supposed that ultrasound has no value in the diagnosis of ectopic pregnancy. However, of all the patients presenting with symptoms suggestive of this diagnosis over half will have normal intra-uterine pregnancies. The demonstration of a normal intra-uterine gestation sac with a live embryo is reassuring and, for the most part, can be used to avoid the necessity for diagnostic laparoscopy. However, there is a caveat. With the increasing use of ovarian stimulation with GIFT techniques and IVF the coexistence of an intra-uterine pregnancy with an extra-uterine pregnancy, originally considered to be exceptionally rare, is now increasing. When ovulation induction or ovum implantation has been performed, the sonographer needs to be somewhat circumspect about excluding an ectopic pregnancy purely on the basis of a live uterine pregnancy.

The most accurate assessment of ectopic pregnancy is made by a combination of hormonal assessment and ultrasound. Quantification of serum beta HCG levels allows correlation with expected size of intra-uterine gestation. Using the second international unit standard, an HCG level of 1800 mIu/ml should be associated with the presence of an intra-uterine gestation sac of greater than 5 mm in diameter. The diagnosis of abnormal pregnancy then relies on lack of correlation between the sonographic findings and the level of beta HCG.[37,38,47] With beta HCG levels of less than 1800 mIu/ml the presence of a gestation sac may be

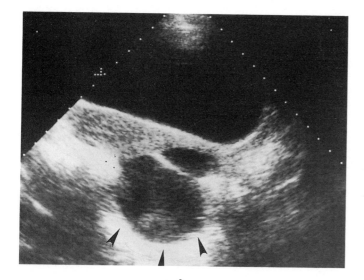

A

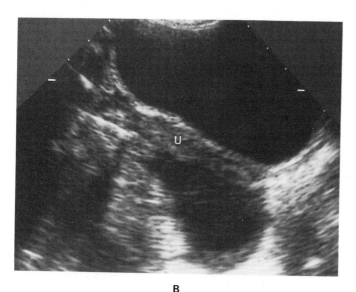

B

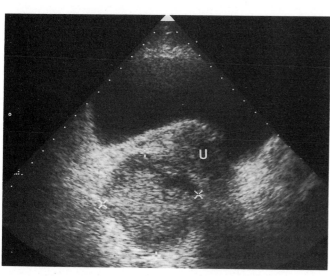

C

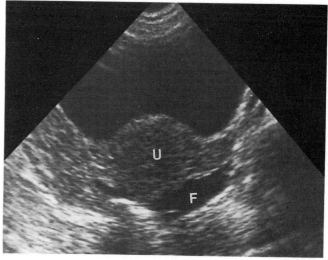

Fig. 46 Ectopic pregnancy, transverse scan through the pelvis. The uterus is identified (U). There is free fluid in the pouch of Douglas (F). This is occasionally the only finding in ectopic pregnancy.

taken to indicate an abnormal pregnancy. This may be a blighted ovum or a missed abortion, or may instead represent the pseudogestation sac of ectopic pregnancy. This has been termed a decidual cast or decidual reaction and may be confusing to the sonographer trying to exclude an ectopic pregnancy purely on the basis of the demonstration of an intra-uterine gestation sac. A number of authors have suggested methods of morphological differentiation of this decidual cast from a true gestation sac, e.g. by the use of the deciduo-chorionic sac sign (double decidual sac sign). This has been reported to be visualised in 90% of cases although other reports indicate a much lower sensitivity and specificity. The intradecidual sign (see above), is also proposed as a discriminator of the true from pseudo-gestation sac but experience indicates that this also is of limited value.

In patients with beta HCG of greater than 1800 mIu/ml, the absence of an intra-uterine gestation sac is virtually pathognomonic of an ectopic pregnancy. Elevated levels of HCG may also be recorded in early molar pregnancy. In this situation an intra-uterine gestation sac is not seen but usually irregular uterine contents may be identified suggesting pregnancy failure either as a result of molar degeneration or an incomplete abortion. Accurate evalu-

Fig. 45 Ectopic pregnancy. A: Long axis scan through the pelvis. The uterus is not enlarged but there is a complex mass containing a septum and both cystic and solid elements posterior to this (arrowheads) in the pouch of Douglas. **B:** Long axis scan through the pelvis demonstrating a normal sized uterus (U). There is a large complex mass in the pouch of Douglas which represents an ectopic pregnancy. **C:** Transverse scan through the pelvis. The uterus is identified (U). There is a large reflective mass posterior and to the right of this which represented a haemorrhagic ectopic pregnancy.

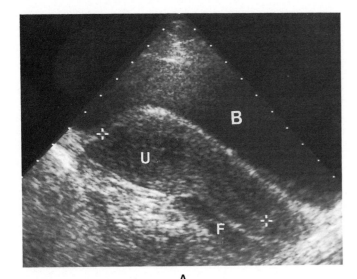

A

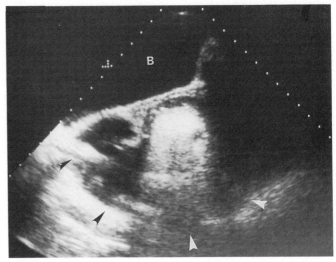

Fig. 48 **Dermoid cyst.** Complex mass in the left adnexa on this transverse scan (arrowheads). This was a large dermoid cyst in association with very early pregnancy. B – bladder.

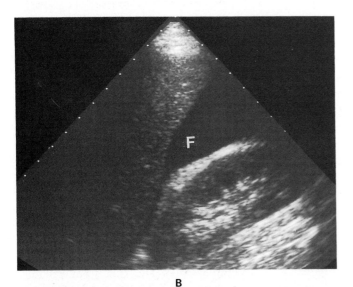

B

ation of a suspected ectopic pregnancy requires a quantitative beta HCG combined with careful ultrasound, perhaps with the addition of Doppler. Trans-vaginal ultrasound seems likely to be the best ultrasound method (see Ch. 9).

In chronic ectopic pregnancy, a condition marked by an insidious onset with ill-defined symptomatology, the ultrasound findings are even less constant. There is usually an adnexal mass which is most often complex, representing an inflammatory haematoma,[52] but this may be totally obscured by adherent bowel consequent upon adhesions. The beta HCG is frequently negative in these cases. If a chronic ectopic pregnancy is suspected on clinical grounds, even a negative ultrasound should not preclude recourse to laparoscopy.

Tumours in early pregnancy

Although gynaecological tumours of all types may occur in early pregnancy, the commonest are physiological corpus luteum cysts.[18,51] These may be demonstrated in as many as 20% of normal pregnancies, and may reach a size of 6 to 8 cm. Although usually asymptomatic, they may be associated with pain or discomfort, particularly if haemorrhage occurs into the cyst. They are usually echo-free and regular in outline, although, if haemorrhagic, they

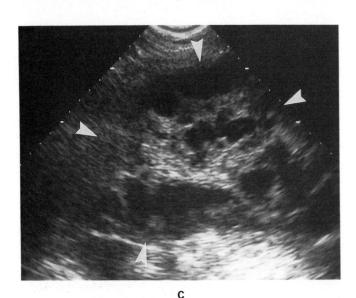

C

Fig. 47 **Ruptured ectopic pregnancy. A:** The uterus is slightly enlarged (U) with a small amount of fluid in the pouch of Douglas (F). B – bladder. **B:** There is free fluid (F) in Morrison's pouch representing intra-abdominal haemorrhage. **C:** There is a large complex mass (arrowheads) extending from the pelvis into the abdomen. This was a large pelvi-abdominal haematoma consequent upon rupture of an ectopic pregnancy.

may contain echoes. With the increasing use of assisted conception, luteal stimulation is more common and corpus luteum cysts are more frequently seen, are larger and frequently multiple. The ovarian hyperstimulation syndrome of multiple theca lutein cysts with ascites may be seen in association with an early intra-uterine gestation sac (or sacs). Other ovarian tumours may occur but are extremely rare. These include ovarian dermoids and cystic or solid benign and malignant tumours. Similar diagnostic criteria must be used as in the absence of a pregnancy. However, the diagnosis is complicated because of the possibility of confusion with ectopic pregnancy.

Uterine tumours are uncommon. Uterine fibroids are a contributory cause to relative infertility, presumably because of the distortion of the endometrial canal and the poor placentation that may result.[19] However, fibroids, particularly when small, may be demonstrated in association with early pregnancy (Fig. 49). The appearances are the same as fibroids in the absence of a pregnancy but they may cause distortion of a gestation sac, thereby suggesting the possibility (at least in very early pregnancy) of an abnormal or non-viable gestation (Fig. 50). Fibroids may grow rapidly in early pregnancy and may subsequently undergo necrosis, producing pain. They are rarely confused with other causes of pelvic pain, such as an ectopic pregnancy.

Uterine anomalies

Pregnancy may occur in any of the uterine anomalies. In septate or sub-septate uteri it is possible to demonstrate the uterine septum as well as the gestation sac. In a bicornuate uterus the gestation sac may be seen in one horn while in the other horn a decidual cast may be demonstrated

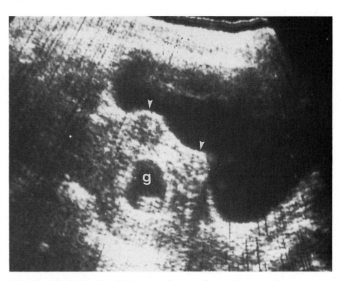

Fig. 50 **Multiple fibroids** in association with an intra-uterine pregnancy. At least two fibroids are present (arrowheads) in this long axis scan of the uterus. There is no evidence of distortion of the gestation sac (g).

(Figs 51 to 53). Care must be taken to avoid confusing this with an ectopic pregnancy. Longitudinal scans oblique to either side of the midline will usually allow the demonstration of the continuity of both horns with the cervix.

Doppler in early pregnancy

Doppler studies of the uterine artery and of the region of the trophoblast in the uterus have been performed in an attempt to assess normal and abnormal gestations (see Ch. 15). Although the uterine artery has high impedance flow, there are complex low impedance flow signals from the region of the developing placenta. In trophoblastic disease the low impedance signals from the uterine artery are said to be easily distinguishable from those of normal early pregnancy and missed abortion.[53] In ectopic pregnancy Doppler examination of an adnexal mass may demonstrate characteristic flow patterns of a corpus luteum which are of low impedance. This finding serves only to confirm a viable or recently viable normotopic or ectopic pregnancy but it may be possible to combine Doppler waveform characteristics with morphological data to refine the diagnosis. In addition, some ectopic pregnancies are reported to demonstrate what has been termed peritrophoblastic flow: high velocity, somewhat disordered low impedance signals similar to those seen in a normal intra-uterine pregnancy. Although early reports indicate a potential use for Doppler in the assessment of pregnancy failure and ectopic pregnancy, it is known that pulsed Doppler ultrasound produces high dose levels to the developing embryo. The use of Doppler ultrasound in the first trimester of pregnancy should be restricted to research institutions working to a strict protocol and with ethical approval. There should

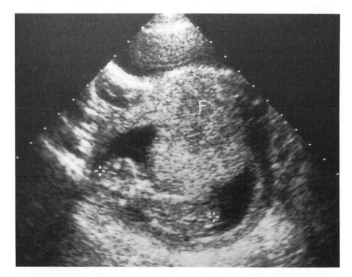

Fig. 49 **Uterine fibroid** in association with pregnancy. Transverse scan of the pelvis. There is a large fibroid (F) distorting the uterine cavity and impinging upon the fetus whose crown-rump length is indicated by crosses.

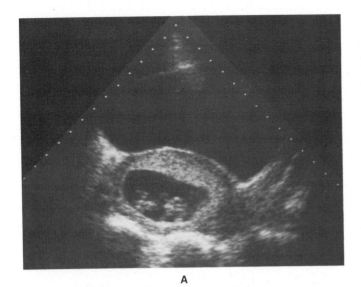

A

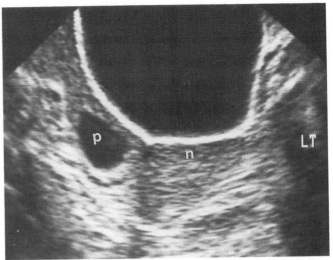

Fig. 52 Pregnancy in bicornuate uterus. Transverse scan of the pelvis showing pregnant (p) and non-pregnant (n) horns.

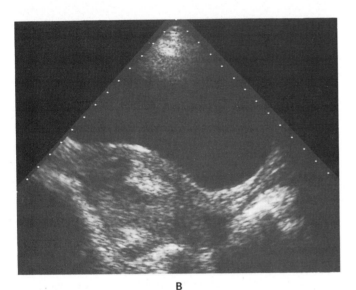

B

Fig. 51 Pregnancy in a bicornuate uterus. A: Long axis scan through the pregnant horn shows a clearly defined gestation sac and a contained embryo. **B:** The non-pregnant horn is enlarged and there is a decidual reaction. This is presumably due to hormonal effects of the pregnancy in the other horn rather than pregnancy loss in one horn.

be a careful and formal assessment of bio-effects within the protocol. Normal pregnancies should not be included in such studies unless termination is planned. The power output levels of the equipment in use should be known and kept as low as possible.

Diagnosis of structural anomalies in the first trimester

The potential for ultrasound diagnosis of abnormalities earlier than the second trimester is extremely attractive. Organogenesis is complete by 12 weeks of gestation. Theoretically therefore, some of the structural abnormalities now diagnosed at 18 weeks scan might be

demonstrable earlier. Skull ossification begins before 12 weeks and therefore the diagnosis of anencephaly is possible at this stage. However, a reappraisal of embryological development is required if errors are to be avoided. The diagnosis of anencephaly has been missed on an ultrasound scan performed at 10 weeks.[13] The reliability of ultrasound for evaluation of the remainder of the neural axis for fetal anomaly detection remains to be proven. Although it is possible to examine the fetal spine in axial and sagittal views in the late first trimester, there is as yet no report of the diagnosis of spina bifida.[11] Visualisation of the cerebellum in the first trimester might allow the earlier detection of the Chiari II malformation associated with spina bifida. However, as yet the chronology of migration of the fetal cerebellum in this condition is not known.

There have been a few reports of the diagnosis of abdominal abnormalities in first trimester fetuses. The demonstration of omphalocele has, for example, been made in a 12 week gestation, with a soft tissue mass noted anterior to the abdomen. The association of this with an abdominal diameter significantly smaller than the biparietal diameter allowed the diagnosis to be made.[54] As previously mentioned, diagnosis of abdominal wall defects in the first trimester should be made with caution because of the normal extra-abdominal position of the embryonic gut. Indeed in one study gut was apparently documented outwith the anterior abdominal wall as late as 12 weeks of gestation in 20% of cases (Fig. 54).[11]

The appearance of embryonic kidneys has been reported as early as 9 weeks of gestation. While this observation is not yet routine, it offers the potential for diagnosis of severe abnormalities of the renal tract by the demonstration of abnormally dilated collecting systems. One such case reported as early as 10 weeks of gestational age was associated with a distended bladder.[12]

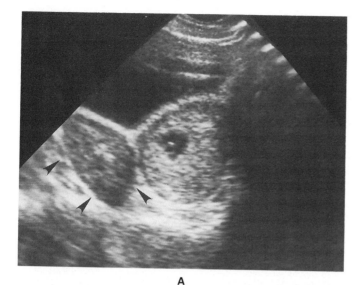

A

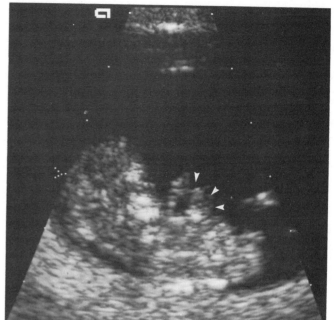

Fig. 54 Pseudo-omphalocele. In this 11 week gestation gut (arrowheads) remains outside the anterior abdominal wall reflecting its normal rotation. This normal pregnancy proceeded to term.

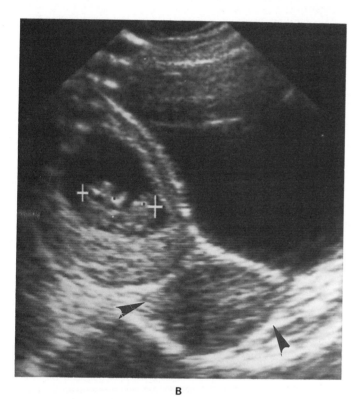

B

Fig. 53 Pregnancy in association with a pelvic kidney.
A: Transverse scan of the pelvis showing an early pregnancy with a yolk sac. To the right of the uterus there is a mass (arrowheads). This might be confused for a non-pregnant horn but was in fact a pelvic kidney. **B:** The uterus later in the pregnancy (10 weeks) now lies above the kidney (arrowheads).

The limbs can be measured by the end of the twelfth week raising the possibility that the more severe forms of dwarfism might be detectable at a time when pregnancy termination is less traumatic both physically, psychologically and morally. However, many forms of short limbed dwarfism are associated with normal limb bone lengths in the first trimester, the reduced growth of the limbs only being manifest later.

Other structural abnormalities seem unlikely to be diagnosable in the first trimester, at least for the foreseeable future. The lateral ventricles, for example, occupy most of the intracranial hemidiameter, making the early diagnosis of hydrocephalus difficult if not impossible. It is interesting however, that choroid plexus cysts have been demonstrated at 12 weeks and, although none of these have been shown to be associated with chromosomal abnormalities, this remains a potential source of information.

Evaluation of the heart in the first trimester, except for demonstration of the variation in heart rate, awaits greater sonographic resolution and the subsequent documentation of embryological development. This remains true for the majority of structural abnormalities.

REFERENCES

1 Timor-Tritsch I E, Farine D, Rosen M G. A close look at early embryonic development with the high-frequency transvaginal transducer. Am J Obstet Gynecol 1988; 159: 676
2 Baker M E, Mahony B S, Bowie J D. Adverse effect of an overdistended bladder on first trimester sonography. AJR 1985; 145: 597
3 Moore K L. Before we are born: basic embryology and birth defects. 3rd edition. Philadelphia: WB Saunders. 1989

4 Yeh H-C. Sonographic signs of early pregnancy. Crit Rev Diagn Imaging. 1988; 28: 181

5 Cadkin A V, McAlpin J. The decidua–chorionic sac: a reliable sonographic indicator of intrauterine pregnancy prior to detection of a fetal pole. J Ultrasound Med 1984; 3: 539

6 Nyberg D A, Laing F C, Filly R A, Uri-Simmons M, Brooke Jeffrey R. Ultrasonographic differentiation of the gestational sac of early intrauterine pregnancy from the pseudogestational sac of ectopic pregnancy. Radiology 1983; 146: 755

7 Nelson P, Bowie J D, Rosenburg E R. Early intrauterine pregnancy or decidual cast: an anatomic–sonographic approach. J Ultrasound Med 1983; 2: 543

8 Crooij M J, Westhuis J, Schoemaker J, Exalto N. Ultrasonographic measurement of the yolk sac. Br J Obstet Gynaecol 1982; 89: 931

9 Cadkin A V, McAlpin J. Detection of fetal cardiac activity between 41 and 43 days of gestation. J Ultrasound Med 1984; 3: 499

10 Shenker L, Astle C, Reed K, Anderson C. Embryonic heart rates before the seventh week of pregnancy. J Reprod Med 1986; 31: 333

11 Green J J, Hobbins J C. Abdominal ultrasound examination of the first trimester fetus. Am J Obstet Gynecol 1988; 159: 165

12 Bulic M, Podobnik M, Korenic B, Bistricki J. First-trimester diagnosis of low obstructive uropathy: an indicator of initial renal function in the fetus. JCU 1987; 15: 537

13 Hill L M, Thomas M L, Kislak S, Runco C. Sonographic assessment of the first trimester fetus: a cautionay note. Am J Perinatol 1988; 5: 13

14 Bowerman R A. Atlas of normal fetal ultrasonographic anatomy. Chicago: Year Book Medical Publishers. 1986

15 Kurtz A B, Goldberg B B. Obstetrical measurements in ultrasound. Chicago: Year Book Medical Publishers. 1988

16 Terinde R. The placenta. In: Hansmann M, Hackelöer B-J, Staudach A, Wittman BK. eds. Ultrasound diagnosis in obstetrics and gynaecology. Berlin: Springer-Verlag. 1985: p 325–341

17 Landy H J, Weiner S, Corson S, Batzer F R, Bolognese R J. The 'vanishing twin': ultrasonographic assessment of fetal disappearance in the first trimester. Am J Obstet Gynecol 1986; 155: 1

18 Jirous J, Kaswari R, Dejmek M, Hanousek L. Differential diagnosis of the early pregnancy failure by ultrasound. SB VED Lek Fak Univ Karlovy 1984; 27: 569

19 Mantoni M. Ultrasound studies of patients with bleeding in early pregnancy. Danish Medical Bulletin 1987; 34: 250

20 Clinical ultrasonographic correlations of metrorrhagias of the first trimester of pregnancy. Panminerva Medica 1987; 29: 123

21 Robinson H P. Gestation sac volumes as determined by sonar in the first trimester of pregnancy. Hum Reprod 1975; 2: 739

22 Bernard K G, Cooperberg P L. Sonographic differentiation between blighted ovum and early viable pregnancy. AJR 1985; 144: 596

23 Nyberg D A, Laing F C, Filly R A. Threatened abortion: sonographic distinction of normal and abnormal gestation sacs. Radiology 1986; 158: 397

24 Nyberg D A, Mack L A, Laing F C, Patten R M. Distinguishing normal from abnormal gestational sac growth in early pregnancy. J Ultrasound Med 1987; 6: 23

25 Goldstein S R, Subramanyam B R, Snyder J R. Ratio of gestational sac volume to crown-rump length in early pregnancy. J Reprod Med 1986; 31: 320

26 Schaffer R M, Gottesman R, Tortora B M, Fox F, Borland M M, Noyes M B. The eccentric gestational sac: sonographic appearance and differential diagnosis. Medical Ultrasound 1983; 7: 157

27 Nyberg D A, Filly R A, Mahony B S, Monroe S, Laing F C, Brooke Jeffrey R. Early gestation: correlation of HCG levels and sonographic identification. AJR 1984; 144: 951

28 Mantoni M. Pederson J F. Ultrasound visualisation of the human yolk sac. JCU 1979; 7: 459

29 Hurwitz S R. Yolk sac sign: sonographic appearance of the fetal yolk sac in missed abortion. J Ultrasound Med 1986; 5: 435

30 Nyberg D A, Mack L A, Harvey D, Wang K. Value of the yolk sac in evaluating early pregnancies. J Ultrasound Med 1988; 7: 129

31 Vitse M, Boulanger J C, Ballot J J, Seron G, Camier B. Pronostic des hematomes deciduaux ou decollements ovulaires de decouverte echographique au premier trimestre de la grossesse. Rev Fr Gynecol Obstet 1984; 79: 775

32 Goldstein S R, Subramanyam B R, Raghavendra B N, Horii S C, Hilton S. Subchorionic bleeding in threatened abortion: sonographic findings and significance. AJR 1983; 141: 975

33 Stabile I, Campbell S, Grudzinskas J G. Threatened miscarriage and intrauterine hematomas: sonographic and biochemical studies. J Ultrasound Med 1989; 8: 289

34 Simpson J L, Mills J L, Holmes L B, et al. Low fetal loss rates after ultrasound proved viability in early pregnancy. JAMA 1987; 258: 2555

35 McFadyen I R. Missed abortion and later spontaneous abortion in pregnancies clinically normal at 7–12 weeks. Eur J Obstet Gynecol Reprod Biol 1985; 20: 381

36 Melis G B, Strigini F, Fruzzetti F, Paoletti A M, Battistelli P, Boldrini A. Ultrasound and estriadol plasma levels in threatened abortion. Acta Europaea Fertilitatis 1984; 15: 287

37 Batzer F R, Weiner S, Corson S L, Schlaff S, Otis C. Landmarks during the first 42 days of gestation demonstrated by the B-subunit of human chorionic gonadotropin and ultrasound. Am J Obstet Gynecol 1983; 146: 973

38 Nyberg D A, Filly R A, Filho D L, Laing F C, Mahony B S. Abnormal pregnancy: early diagnosis by US and serum chorionic gonadotropin levels. Radiology 1986; 158: 393

39 Brown B.St.J. Disappearance of one gestational sac in the first trimester of multiple pregnancies – ultrasonographic findings. Can Assoc Radiol J 1982; 33: 273

40 Gindoff P R, Yeh M N, Jewelewicz R. The vanishing sac syndrome. Ultrasound evidence of pregnancy failure in multiple gestations, induced and spontaneous. J Reprod Med 1986; 31: 323

41 Jeanty P, Rodesch F, Verhoogen C, et al. The vanishing twin. Ultrasonics 1981; 2: 25

42 Lloyd S A. The double sac – pitfalls to avoid in diagnosis. Medical Ultrasound 1983; 7: 49

43 Taylor K J, Schwartz P E, Kohorn E I. Gestational trophoblastic neoplasia: diagnosis with Doppler US. Radiology 1987; 165: 445

44 Callen P W. Ultrasonography in evaluation of gestational trophoblastic disease. In: Callen P W, ed. Ultrasonography in obstetrics and gynecology. Philadelphia: WB Saunders. 1983: p 259

45 Hertzberg B S, Kurtz A B, Wapner R J, et al. Gestational trophoblastic disease with coexistent normal fetus: evaluation by ultrasound-guided chorionic villus sampling. J Ultrasound Med 1986; 5: 467

46 Spirt B A, O'Hara R, Gordon L. Pseudogestational sac in ectopic pregnancy: sonographic and pathologic correlation. JCU 1981; 9: 338

47 Kadar N, Taylor K J, Rosenfield A T, Romero R. Combined use of serum HCG and sonography in the diagnosis of ectopic pregnancy. AJR 1983; 141: 609

48 Coleman B G, Baron R L, Arger P H, et al. Ectopic embryo detection using real time sonography. JCU 1985; 545

49 Zwiebel W J, Haning R V. A rational approach to diagnosis and management in ectopic pregnancy. Semin Ultrasound 1983; 3: 235

50 Nyberg D A, Filly R A, Laing F C, Mack L A, Zarutskie P. Ectopic pregnancy: diagnosis by sonography correlated with quantitative HCG levels. J Ultrasound Med 1987; 6: 145

51 Pennes D R, Bowerman R A, Silver T M. Echogenic adnexal masses associated with first-trimester pregnancy: sonographic appearance and clinical significance. JCU 1985; 13: 391

52 Bedi D G, Fagan C J, Nocera R M. Chronic ectopic pregnancy. J Ultrasound Med 1984; 3: 347

53 Dillon E H, Taylor K J. Doppler ultrasound in the female pelvis and first trimester pregnancy. In: Taylor K J, Strandness D E, eds. Duplex Doppler ultrasound. Clinics in diagnostic ultrasound. New York: Churchill Livingstone. 1990: p 93

54 Curtis J A, Watson L. Sonographic diagnosis of omphalocele in the first trimester of fetal gestation. J Ultrasound Med 1988; 7: 97

9

The first trimester
Trans-vaginal ultrasound

Introduction
Selection of ultrasound equipment
The technique of trans-vaginal ultrasound
examination
The viable intra-uterine pregnancy
Threatened abortion and the non-viable
pregnancy
Extra-uterine pregnancy
Early diagnosis
Hormone assays
Trans-vaginal ultrasound examination
The management of ectopic pregnancy
The future of ectopic pregnancy management

Rajat K. Goswamy

INTRODUCTION

Trans-vaginal ultrasonography is gradually replacing trans-abdominal ultrasonography for most early pregnancy problems because of improved image quality and its ability to detect ectopic pregnancies as early as 1 week after a missed period. The convenience of being able to perform ultrasound examinations without the need for a full bladder makes it preferred by patients, eases scheduling and is especially important in urgent cases. Frequency of micturition, a well-established symptom of early pregnancy, may make bladder filling difficult or impossible.

Selection of ultrasound equipment

The selection of the right ultrasound equipment is probably the most difficult decision that one has to make when starting with new imaging techniques.

Mechanical and electronic (phased array) sector transducers are available in a range of frequencies, some being end-firing and others off-set to allow imaging of lateral structures. The mechanical systems at present appear to have superior resolution to electronic probes, though the former are less reliable. Orientation is easier with end-fire than with off-set probes though lateral structures in the pelvis may be seen more easily with the latter. Probes where the sector, which is normally on-line, can be steered to either side have the benefits of easy orientation as well as superior imaging of laterally displaced organs and are the most flexible and satisfactory.

The choice of probe frequency is dependent on the fact that higher frequencies give greater resolution in the near field, but their depth range is limited. For example, a 7.5 MHz probe gives high resolution images within a range up to 5 cm, whereas a 5 MHz transducer images structures between 3 cm and 10 cm but with reduced resolution. With a 5 MHz probe, if a structure to be imaged lies within 3 cm, one can still obtain good images by withdrawing the transducer slightly to increase the distance between the probe and the imaged structure. In general 5 MHz is preferable, especially in early pregnancy scanning where deep insertion of the probe is better avoided. Multi-frequency probes are now becoming available; these can be switched between 5, 6.5 and 7.5 MHz.

The technique of trans-vaginal examination

Prior to performing a thorough examination it is of utmost importance to obtain an adequate clinical history. The date and nature of the last menstrual period allow a decision, for example, as to whether the presence of an 18 mm cystic area in the ovary is a Graafian follicle or a cystic corpus luteum. An abnormal bleed, which was lighter than usual could be associated with a threatened abortion or an ectopic pregnancy. A heavier than normal bleed could be associated with an incomplete abortion or with pelvic inflammatory disease.

Previous pelvic surgery is important because this may indicate a higher risk of ectopic pregnancy, especially if the fallopian tubes have been affected.[1] A history of an ovariectomy can save time spent looking for an ovary that is not present and even diagnostic error when a structure is mistaken for an ovary.

Use of contraception and drug therapy can alert the sonographer to search for ectopic pregnancies, in the case of the intra-uterine contraceptive device, while heterotopic pregnancies are more likely to occur when ovulation induction agents or assisted reproduction techniques, such as in vitro fertilisation (IVF) or gamete intra-Fallopian transfer (GIFT) have been used.[2]

In history taking it is therefore important to ask the following questions before embarking on a trans-vaginal examination:

a) When was your last menstrual period?
b) Was the bleeding normal in duration and amount?
c) What contraceptive method, if any, do you use?
d) Have you been on any sort of fertility treatment?
e) Have you had any pelvic surgery?

In positioning the patient for trans-vaginal ultrasound examination every effort should be made to ensure that there is enough room to manoeuvre the probe. This can be achieved either by placing the patient's feet in lithotomy stirrups or by placing a ledge just at the end of the couch (Fig. 1) so that the patient can lie on her back with the buttocks close to the end of the couch, her legs flexed and her heels resting on the ledge placed approximately 6

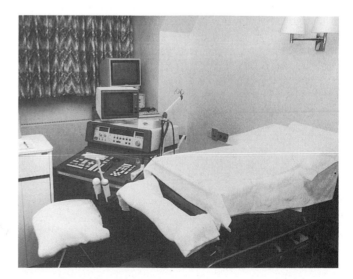

Fig. 1 Examination couch. Note that stirrups are not required for adequate trans-vaginal examination and the patient's buttocks are positioned at the edge of the couch with her feet resting on the lower ledge.

inches below the height of the couch. A wedge or pillow may be placed below the patient's buttocks but this does not always provide adequate room to angle the probe sufficiently, especially where the uterus is acutely anteverted.

Prior to insertion, ultrasound transmission gel is placed on the active surface of the probe and the probe is then covered by a condom. In early pregnancy the vagina has enough natural secretion to provide adequate contact for imaging so that the tip of the covered transducer does not need further gel. The labia should be parted gently to avoid unnecessary discomfort to the patient.

The urethra is visualised as it exits from the bladder neck (Fig. 2) and the probe is then passed within the vagina so that it points towards the anterior vaginal wall which appears as an echo-poor linear structure immediately

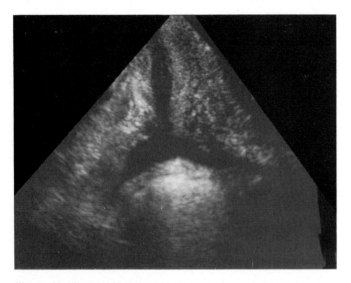

Fig. 2 Urethra and bladder neck. In the transverse plane the urethra can be seen leaving the bladder.

adjacent to the transducer head (Fig. 3). Following the vagina superiorly leads to the anteverted uterus. Once the uterus has been located, its cavity should be identified and any contents imaged. Even when an intra-uterine pregnancy has been identified a systematic examination of the other pelvic organs should be carried out.

Trans-vaginal ultrasound examination is target orientated rather than governed by ultrasound planes, in contrast to abdominal ultrasonography.[3] A scan transverse to the uterine axis may not necessarily be the transverse plane of the patient because the uterus may be deviated from the midline. Scans should be performed in the transverse, oblique and longitudinal planes of the organ being imaged to understand the orientation of the pelvic organs and their relationship to each other.

After imaging the uterus the probe is directed towards the pelvic side walls to search for the ovaries.[4] These contain small primordial follicles and one usually contains a corpus luteum. If the ovaries are not detected immediately lateral to the uterus, the probe should be directed further laterally to image the internal iliac vessels (Fig. 4) which appear as long echo-free structures as they pass down the pelvic side wall. The ovaries can often be visualised just anterior to these vessels. If the ovaries are still not demonstrated the probe should be angled towards the rectum. The pouch of Douglas often contains some free fluid and ovaries may be located here. If one has still not imaged the ovaries, the probe should be angled to point towards the anterior abdominal wall to look for the ovaries lying above the uterus. This is the most difficult ovarian position for trans-vaginal imaging and the gain or output of the machine needs to be increased considerably before satisfactory images are obtained. If there is still difficulty in visualising one or other ovary, pressure placed with a

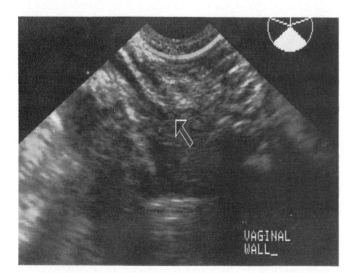

Fig. 3 Anterior vaginal wall. The anterior vaginal wall is seen as a zone of low reflectivity close to the transducer.

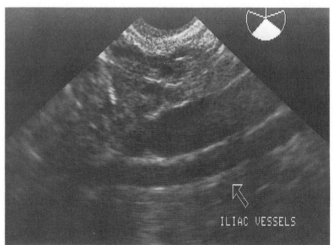

Fig. 4 Internal iliac vessels. These are seen as two longitudinal echo-free structures in the lateral aspect of the sector. They are extremely useful landmarks to help in location of ovaries.

second hand on the abdomen may bring a high ovary into the pelvis and within range of the imaging transducer. Sometimes it may be useful to place the patient in reverse Trendelenburg position. If these manoeuvres fail, a trans-abdominal scan should be performed.

While looking for the ovaries, any fluid spaces in the adnexal region should be noted. Cystic structures that are separate from the ovaries include tubal swellings and loculated ascites associated with adhesions (i.e. pelvic pseudocysts) which are common after major or repeated pelvic surgery. A hydrosalpinx is usually tubular or retort-shaped and contains incomplete septa. Loculated adhesions do not usually have septa and exclude bowel loops from within them. The presence of bowel loops within the fluid mass is usually indicative of free fluid within the pelvis.

Before removing the probe, the pouch of Douglas should be examined for signs of fluid, blood clots or an ectopic sac (Fig. 5).

Finally a scan in the longitudinal axis of the uterus should be performed and the endometrial canal should be followed into the cervical canal. It is not necessary to measure the canal, but any free fluid or blood clot in the canal can be seen easily and the internal os can be visualised to check for dilatation (Fig. 6).

The viable intra-uterine pregnancy

Ever since Kratochwil[5] first described that pregnancy could be diagnosed as early as the first week after missed menses (that is 5 weeks after the last period or 3 weeks after ovulation) early diagnosis of pregnancy by ultrasound has been important. Pregnancies are conventionally dated from the first day of the last menstrual period (LMP), as-suming a 4 week menstrual cycle. Patients do not always

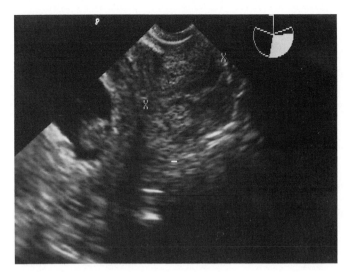

Fig. 6 The cervical canal. The cervix is seen as a poorly reflective area inferior to the uterus with the canal seen as a thin reflective line between the crosses. Note the embryo in the uterus.

remember the date of the LMP accurately, though women trying to conceive are usually reliable.

With the use of trans-vaginal ultrasound it is possible to image a gestation in the uterus within a day of a missed period. Thus by 4 weeks and 1 day the uterine cavity shows a thickened endometrium with the gestation sac seen as a 2 to 3 mm echo-free structure surrounded by a reflective trophoblastic ring (Fig. 7). The gestation sac is invariably located eccentrically within the uterine cavity; an echo-free space in a central position is more likely to be a pseudosac that raises the possibility of an ectopic pregnancy, requiring a careful search of the adnexal areas. If there is a past history of ectopic pregnancy, a scan per-

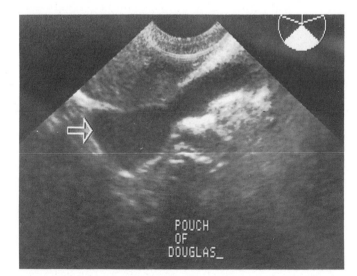

Fig. 5 Fluid in the pouch of Douglas is seen as an echo-free space (arrow) posterior to the uterus. Loops of bowel are often visualised here.

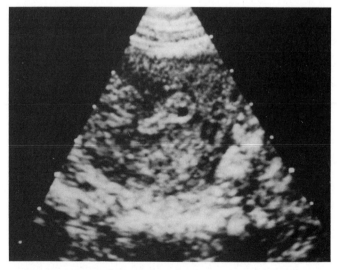

Fig. 7 Intra-uterine pregnancy. 4 weeks gestational age. A gestation sac measuring 3 mm is seen at the time of the missed period. Typically the sac is eccentric.

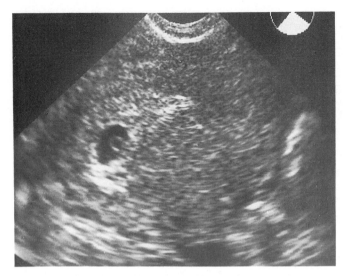

Fig. 8 5 week intra-uterine pregnancy. The yolk sac occupies most of the gestation sac and is surrounded by a moderately reflective decidua.

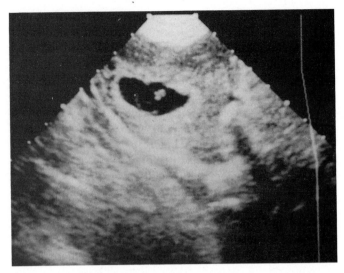

Fig. 9 5½ week intra-uterine pregnancy. The embryo is seen as a highly reflective structure lying next to the yolk sac and measures approximately 3 mm.

formed at the first suspicion of pregnancy is reassuring. In the case of IVF or GIFT pregnancies it is possible to diagnose multiple pregnancy at this very early stage. However it is important to realise that the diagnosis of pregnancy at this stage does not indicate that it is viable; this can only be assessed reliably when heart motion is demonstrated. The demonstration that the sequence of developmental events is taking place at a normal rate is a more reliable prognostic indicator than a single ultrasound finding on one occasion.

By 5 weeks the yolk sac is demonstrable and this now measures between 3 and 4 mm. The gestation sac is double the size of the yolk sac (Fig. 8). The need to measure these structures is discussed later in this section although the presence of normal shaped structures and their relationship to each other in size is enough to estimate gestational age to within a few days.

By 5½ weeks heart motion is seen at the edge of the yolk sac and the embryo appears as three thin lines located between the yolk sac and the chorionic plate (Fig. 9). The gestation sac has a mean diameter of approximately 1 cm at this stage.

By six weeks lacunar structures become visible on one side of the gestation sac. This is the region where the placenta will develop. In real time it is sometimes possible to see blood flow in these spaces. Locating the placenta is important where chorion villus sampling is being considered (hardly ever performed at 6 weeks of pregnancy) or when there is evidence of intra-uterine bleeding (see next section). The embryo is now the same size as the yolk sac, which has a diameter of 4 to 5 mm (Fig. 10). By this stage heart motion can almost always be demonstrated with a trans-vaginal probe, though this may be more difficult when the embryo is very closely applied to the side wall of

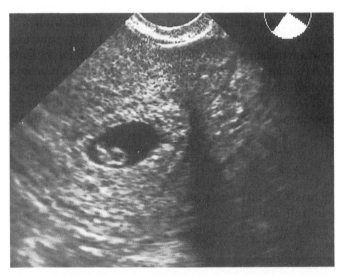

Fig. 10 6 week intra-uterine pregnancy. The embryo is approximately the same size as the yolk sac (5 mm). Cardiac pulsation is always seen in live embryos at this stage. Note the lacunar areas in the lateral wall of the gestation sac.

the gestation sac. Careful examination of the region between the yolk sac and the side wall of the chorionic cavity helps in detecting heart motion. Using transabdominal ultrasound heart motion can be detected in 17% to 60% of patients at 6 weeks.[5-7]

At 7 weeks, the embryo measures 7 mm in length and the yolk sac 5 mm in diameter. The head of the embryo is just distinguishable from the body (Fig. 11). The head appears to be larger than the body which can be recognised by the presence of heart motion within it. The heart rate is below 120 beats per minute[8] and Doppler signals can be detected.

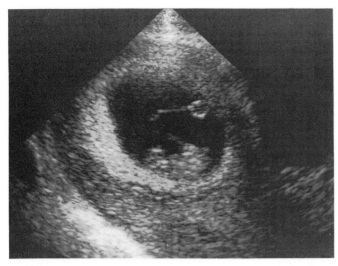

Fig. 11   7 week embryo. The head and body are distinguishable and a yolk sac is visible close to the embryo.

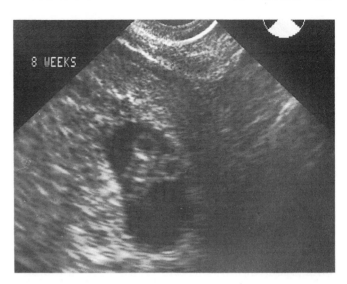

Fig. 13   8 week embryo. Note that the yolk sac and embryonic head appear identical in size and appearance. (Can be mistaken for a twin pregnancy or double headed monster.)

At 8 weeks gestational age the ultrasound findings are most dramatic. Embryonic movements, the recognition of limb buds and the development of the central nervous system are all obvious landmarks of development (Fig. 12). The embryo measures 1 cm, twice the diameter of the yolk sac which remains at 5 mm for the rest of the first trimester of pregnancy. The head contains a single cerebral ventricle which may simulate a second yolk sac, and must not be mistaken for a double-headed monster. The finding of equal sized yolk sac and head is typical of this gestational age (Fig. 13).

The placental site is easily distinguishable at this stage and the umbilical cord insertion can be traced to both placental and embryonic ends (Fig. 14). The gestation sac diameter is twice the size of the embryo and the amniotic sac is seen wrapped closely around it (Fig. 15).

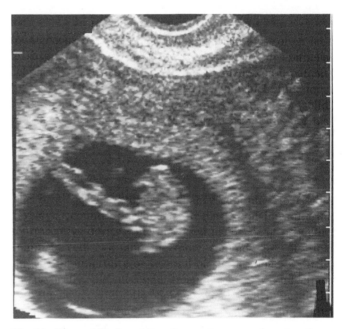

Fig. 14   The umbilical cord insertion can be seen at the point of entry in the abdomen.

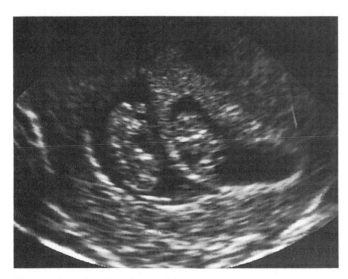

Fig. 12   8 week twin embryos with a limb bud visible.

By the ninth week, knees and elbows become obvious and the lower limbs are seen with legs crossed (Fig. 16). The coccygeal region is prominent at this stage and umbilical cord pulsations are marked. At the site of the cord insertion in the abdomen, the physiological umbilical herniation of the gut may be seen to peristalse: this appearance must not be diagnosed as an exomphalos. The choroid plexus becomes distinguishable with the formation of the falx cerebrum (Fig. 17) and the spinal column is seen along the dorsal aspect. The crown-rump length is greater than 2 cm.

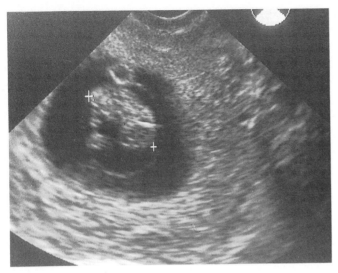

Fig. 15   **9 week embryo** with amniotic sac in close apposition to it. Crown-rump length is approximately 2 cm at this stage.

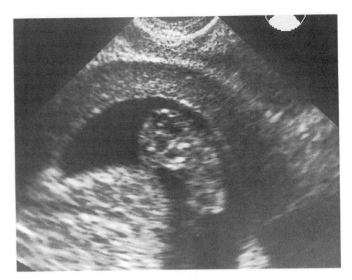

Fig. 17   **A 9½ week intra-uterine pregnancy.** There is early differentiation of intracranial anatomy.

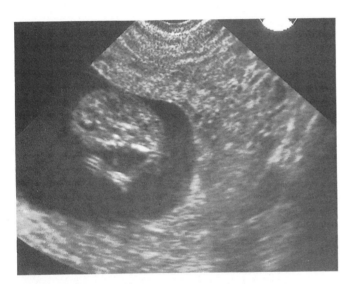

Fig. 16   **A 9½ week intra-uterine pregnancy** showing an arm.

At 10 weeks, the yolk sac gradually disappears and the fetal heart, stomach, urinary bladder and kidneys may be seen. Organogenesis is complete well before this, but organs are difficult to distinguish until they have grown to be larger than 2 to 3 mm in size. The limbs flex and extend with kicking and punching actions which, along with jerky movements of the trunk, help in visualisation of most of these structures. The physiological umbilical hernia starts to reduce and disappears by 12 weeks.

After 10 weeks gestational age, the uterus enlarges out of the true pelvis and many fetal and uterine structures are out of range for a trans-vaginal probe. The main use of trans-vaginal scanning at this stage is in combination with abdominal ultrasound in an attempt at early diagnosis of congenital malformations. By using a 5 MHz transducer trans-vaginally, all structures within 8 cm are easily distin-

guishable. The same transducer can then be used per abdomen to image structures in the upper part of the uterine cavity, with the patient's bladder half full.

A simple scheme of anatomical landmarks and their correlation with gestational age is shown in Table 1. This table can be used in everyday practice when performing trans-vaginal ultrasound in amenorrhoeic patients with an accuracy greater than any table presently used to estimate gestational age. If a gestation sac is seen alone without a yolk sac, the pregnancy must be less than 5 weeks if it is viable. The presence of the yolk sac dates the pregnancy as being at least 5 weeks and the detection of cardiac pulsation along with this indicates a 6 week gestation. Embryonic movements are not seen before 7 weeks and limb buds appear at 8 weeks. The head and yolk sac are equal in size at 8 weeks and the falx indicates a gestational age of at least 9 weeks. The physiological umbilical hernia is only seen in gestations beyond 9 weeks and limb flexion and extension do not occur before this age. Crown-rump length or biparietal diameter measurements do not improve on this accuracy. After 10 weeks measurements of the biparietal diameter can be accurately recorded and current obstetric charts help date pregnancies with an error of less than 1 week as previously described.

Table 1   Chronological assessment of structures in early pregnancy

Ultrasound findings	Gestational age
Gestation sac	4 weeks
Yolk sac	5 weeks
Cardiac pulsation	6 weeks
Embryonic movements	7 weeks
Head and limb buds	8 weeks
Yolk sac and head equal in size	8 weeks
Falx cerebri	9 weeks
Cord insertion	9 weeks

Threatened abortion and the non-viable pregnancy

The incidence of spontaneous abortions varies between 20% and 30% in spontaneous or assisted conception pregnancies.[9] Where ovulation induction agents or procedures such as in vitro fertilisation have been carried out, the loss rate may appear to be higher than with spontaneous conception because the diagnosis of pregnancy is made definitively by blood testing in almost all instances. Many who conceive spontaneously without realising it, have a so-called late period which is actually an early miscarriage which goes undiagnosed.

The ultrasound findings in incomplete and inevitable abortion have been described in the preceding chapter. These same features are more clearly demonstrated with trans-vaginal ultrasound and the diagnosis of an open internal cervical os is definitive because the whole length of the cervix can be visualised by withdrawing the probe from the fornices.

The shape and size of the gestation sac may help predict the outcome of the pregnancy, though hard data are difficult to acquire because of the variation in sac size after 7 weeks gestational age (Fig. 18). Though gestation sac size does seem to have some prognostic value in the diagnosis of abnormal early gestation, it is particularly important in multiple pregnancies.[10] A small sac (mean diameter < 50% of the coexisting sac(s)) is more likely to undergo spontaneous resorption (Figs 19 and 20). In more than 90% of IVF multiple gestations, unequal gestation sacs are followed by spontaneous resorption of one embryo. This condition, described as the 'vanishing twin', occurs in at least 10% of twin pregnancies and 25% of triplet or quadruplet pregnancies, improving pregnancy outcome in the long run.

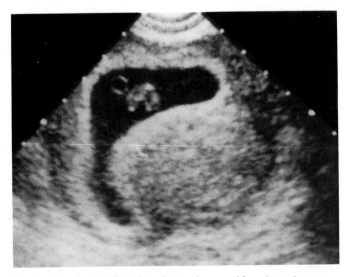

Fig. 18 An abnormally enlarged gestation sac. Note the embryo that is rather curled up in position and the sac measures more than six times the size of the embryo. Trisomy 18 was detected on chromosome examination of the embryo.

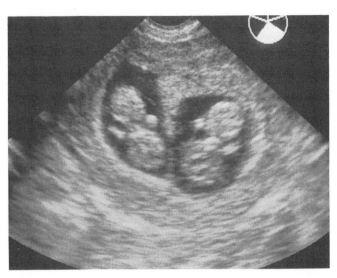

Fig. 19 Normal 9 week twin pregnancy. Both embryos and sacs are of equal size.

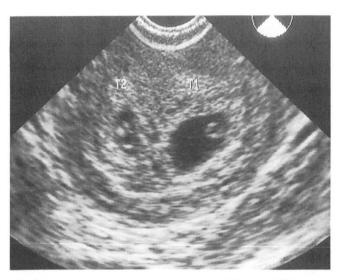

Fig. 20 Abnormal twin pregnancy at 6 weeks. Twin one (T1) gestation sac is much larger than twin two (T2). Spontaneous absorption of T2 occurred 3 weeks later.

It is in missed abortions and threatened abortions that trans-vaginal ultrasound has its greatest impact. The greater detail obtained with high frequency probes facilitates detection of heart motion and increases confidence when no activity can be demonstrated. With abdominal ultrasound, cardiac pulsations are difficult to detect before 7 weeks gestational age. In obese women, or those with abdominal scarring, it may be necessary to wait a further week before one can be sure that failure to detect cardiac activity is significant. With trans-vaginal ultrasound, heart motion can often be detected as early as $5\frac{1}{2}$ weeks gestational age (when the embryo measures only 2 to 3 mm) and always after 6 weeks. This gives trans-vaginal ultrasound an edge over abdominal imaging such

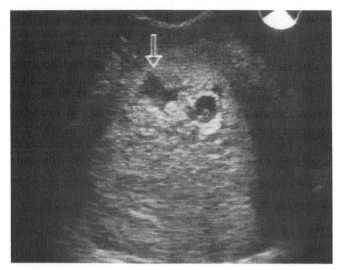

Fig. 21   Retro-implantation bleed. Detected in a 6 week pregnancy with low HCG levels.

that patients can be reassured immediately that all is still well with their pregnancy.

Trans-vaginal ultrasound is superior for imaging the implantation site. The small lacunae that become visible at the implantation site as early as the sixth week have been mentioned. Blood flow is seen in real-time examinations with high frame rates. Early detection of the implantation site is an advantage when a patient is seen with vaginal bleeding in early pregnancy. It should direct the search for intra-uterine fluid collections (Fig. 21). These fluid collections may be seen to track from the implantation site to the internal cervical os.[11] Small bleeds near or behind the implantation site are less well-visualised by transabdominal ultrasound because they are compressed by the full urinary bladder.

Retro-implantation bleeds can be demonstrated in patients undergoing early pregnancy monitoring after IVF treatment when low levels and low rates of rise in β-HCG are found (Table 2). This retro-implantation bleed, or sub-chorionic haemorrhage, corresponds with partial placental detachment in later pregnancy. Whether these occur because of defective implantation in the first instance or whether they are the result of injury to the sac or are due to decreased uterine perfusion is as yet undetermined. What is even more striking in these cases is that the outcome of the pregnancy is not related to the size of the bleed. In some cases cardiac activity continues despite large

Table 2   Outcome after diagnosis of retro-implantation bleeds

Missed abortion	18 (48.6%)
Delivered	19 (51.4%)
Total	37

All patients were monitored with serum hCG levels every 5 days and ultrasound weekly until resolution.

retro-implantation bleeds (Fig. 22), and in others very small bleeds are associated with early embryonic death (Fig. 23). The HCG levels of the first recorded case in the author's experience are shown in Figure 24, where these levels are compared to those seen with ongoing intra-uterine pregnancies. When these cases are scanned every 5 days, it is possible to visualise organising blood clot (Fig. 25) and the gradual resorption followed by repair at the implantation site.

The outcome of these pregnancies is rather unpredictable, approximately 50% resulting in missed abortions or blighted ova. Perhaps, comparing this condition to placental abruption, the outcome depends on the relation

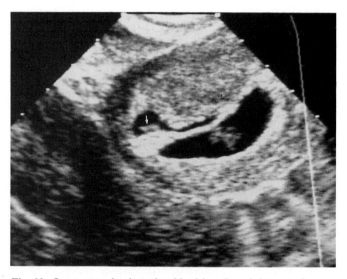

Fig. 22   Large retro-implantation bleed in a 7 week intra-uterine pregnancy. The reflective area in the fluid (arrow) is probably a blood clot.

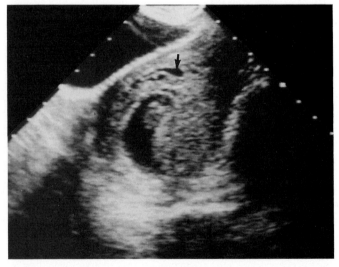

Fig. 23   A small retro-implantation bleed (arrow) is seen adjacent to the gestation sac in the uterus. This embryo died.

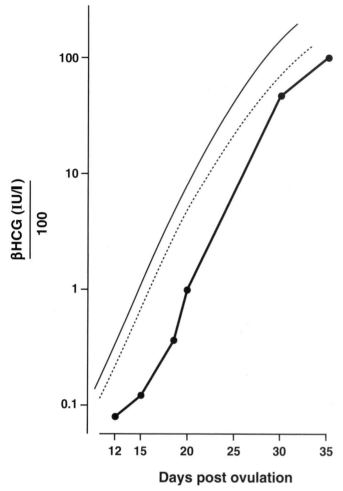

Fig. 24 β-HCG levels. Plasma levels of β-HCG in normal single intra-uterine pregnancies (mean and – 1SD) and in a patient with a retro-implantation bleed.

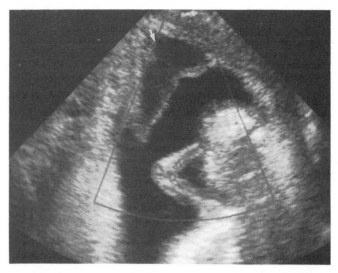

Fig. 25 Subchorionic haematoma in a 12 week gestation (arrow).

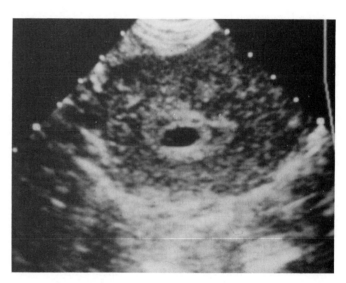

Fig. 26 7 week intra-uterine pregnancy with a small retro-implantation bleed and no clear evidence of an embryo.

between the area of placental haemorrhage and the site of cord insertion, which can be located by 9 weeks.

In some cases of retro-implantation haemorrhage the embryo may die and be rapidly resorbed. If the patient is not scanned within 1 week, a diagnosis of blighted ovum will be made, rather than a missed abortion (Fig. 26).

Another predictor of poor outcome that is seen with trans-vaginal, but not with abdominal ultrasound, is the presence of large vascular spaces surrounding the whole gestation sac. This is common when there is no evidence of a retro-implantation bleed and no live embryo. It may be a late consequence of retro-implantation bleeding.

At present the only documented clinical use of trans-vaginal Doppler in predicting the outcome of early pregnancy is in studying flow in the corpus luteum. A viable corpus luteum has a low resistance bed with relatively high diastolic flow, whereas diastolic flow is reduced or absent with failure of the corpus luteum.

In summary the principal uses of trans-vaginal ultrasound in the abnormal first trimester are in providing a rapid assessment of fetal heart activity, accurate localis-ation of the implantation site, the detection of implantation defects and prognostic indicators such as intramural blood flow which can avoid prenatal tests being blamed for spon-taneous abortions. The superior imaging of blood clot and debris in and around the gestation sac improves the con-fidence in the diagnosis of embryonic death. The limited use of Doppler should be stressed.

Some major congenital abnormalities can be detected in the first trimester with trans-vaginal probes. Anencephaly is easily demonstrated by the ninth week. Also obvious are cystic hygromas, which are an indication for chromosome testing even when transient, since most of these are as-sociated with trisomy 21 or 18; chorionic villus sampling avoids the trauma of second trimester terminations of pregnancy in these patients. Though the detection of other deformities and anomalies has been reported[12] these are difficult situations where an anatomical confirmation may not be possible if the pregnancy is terminated by curettage in the first trimester. This raises difficult ethical issues with the risk of normal pregnancies being terminated because of misdiagnosis.

Extra-uterine pregnancy

Ectopic or extra-uterine gestation is the leading cause of maternal mortality in the United Kingdom and was one of the most difficult diagnoses in gynaecological practice until recently. With the development of sensitive bio-assay methods and new imaging techniques, such as trans-vaginal ultrasound and colour flow mapping, we may be entering a new era in the management of ectopic pregnancies.

Nearly 78 400 cases of ectopic pregnancies were reported to the Centres of Disease Control in USA in 1985,[13] giving a prevalence of 1 in 66 pregnancies. Factors contributing to this high incidence include the use of intra-uterine contraceptive devices, tubal surgery, pelvic inflammatory disease due to use of non-barrier methods of contraception and ovulation induction methods, including multiple embryo or gamete transfer in in vitro fertilisation (IVF) and gamete intra-fallopian transfer (GIFT). The fallopian tubes are the commonest site for ectopic gestations, the ovaries being affected in only 1%. Other sites, such as intra-abdominal and cervical are even rarer.

The use of laparoscopy in the diagnosis and treatment of ectopic pregnancy has resulted in earlier diagnosis in the last decade, with tubal rupture being encountered in only 10% of cases in some centres.[14]

Early detection of ectopic pregnancy is crucial to reducing mortality and morbidity and this is even more important if future fertility is to be maintained. A combination of hormone assays and ultrasound examination form the corner-stones for diagnosis.

Early diagnosis

Hormone assays
Ascheim and Zondek[15] developed a biological urine assay in 1928, to diagnose pregnancy but more recently rapid in vitro quantitative testing kits have become available which give much greater sensitivity than older methods, so that the diagnosis of implantation is possible within 2 days.

Several studies have reported that blood levels of HCG are lower in ectopic pregnancies than in viable intra-uterine pregnancies.[16–18] The use of different reference standards in different studies have lead to different thresholds being recommended but the levels of HCG are consistently lower with ectopic pregnancies than with intra-uterine pregnancies. However, HCG levels are also lower with abnormal intra-uterine pregnancies, for example when there is evidence of bleeding behind the implantation site as seen by trans-vaginal ultrasonography.

A useful additional distinguishing feature is the mean doubling time of HCG; in a normal gestation this is 2 days, in an abnormal intra-uterine gestation it is 3 days or more.[19] If these criteria alone are used, the diagnosis would be delayed by at least 48 hours in 13% of ectopic gestations.

In assisted fertilisation progesterone is an additional useful marker. The serum progesterone level is significantly lower on day 15 after oocyte recovery in ectopic gestation than with an intra-uterine gestation (a mean of 20 ng/ml as compared to 60 ng/ml).[20] Thus a low progesterone level is an indication for a trans-vaginal ultrasound examination.

Trans-vaginal ultrasound examination

It is most important that trans-vaginal ultrasonography is performed by an operator with a good knowledge of pelvic anatomy and with a high level of suspicion for an ectopic gestation. In cases of IVF or GIFT therapy the timing of the examination is also important.

The fallopian tubes lie lateral to the fundus of the uterus, usually between the uterus and the pelvic side wall. However, they are often tortuous so that parts of the length of the tube may lie behind, above or even anterior to the uterus. Previous pelvic surgery or inflammatory disease, predisposing factors for ectopic pregnancy, may add to the anatomical variability so that it must be remembered that an ectopic gestation can be found anywhere in the pelvis. Ectopic pregnancies outside the true pelvis cannot be detected by trans-vaginal ultrasound examination; fortunately, they are extremely rare.

The timing of the ultrasound examination is important. In general the scan should be performed as soon as there is a suspicion of pregnancy. An intra-uterine gestation sac is identifiable within 2 days of a missed period and a yolk sac is identifiable within 5 days. The demonstration of structures within the gestation sac helps in the distinction from a pseudogestation sac, seen in ectopic pregnancies (Fig. 27).

In women who have had ovulation therapy (IVF or GIFT), low β-HCG and progesterone levels warn of the possibility of an ectopic pregnancy; trans-vaginal ultrasound examination should be carried out on day 25 post-ovulation, or post-oocyte recovery. By this stage one can expect to see cardiac pulsation which forms the basis for further management (see below).

A definitive diagnosis of ectopic gestation depends on the identification of a gestation sac outside the uterine cavity. It appears as a highly reflective ring with an echo-free area within it. Though ovarian ectopic pregnancies are extremely rare, it is important that this is differentiated

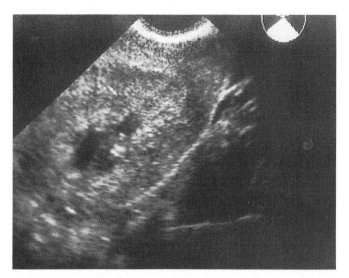

Fig. 27 A pseudogestation sac. There is fluid in the centre of the uterus with irregular echoes within it. These echoes may be mistaken for an embryo.

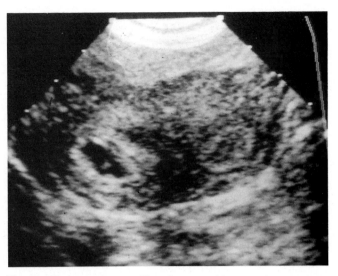

Fig. 29 Bicornuate uterus. There is a normal intra-uterine gestation sac seen in one horn whereas only decidual echoes are seen in the other. Note the myometrium surrounding both areas.

from a corpus luteum cyst, especially in superovulation, when rings are seen within the ovary (Fig. 28). Once a gestation sac has been located, the contents must be scrutinised for the presence of a yolk sac, the embryo and heart motion.

Only when embryonic structures are seen is the diagnosis of ectopic pregnancy certain. Otherwise assays of β-HCG and the absence of an intra-uterine pregnancy form the basis for a presumptive diagnosis of anembryonic ectopic pregnancy. The importance of making this diagnosis and its application in clinical practice are elaborated when discussing conservative management in the section below.

A difficulty when making the diagnosis of a cornual or interstitial ectopic pregnancy is the possibility of a bicor-

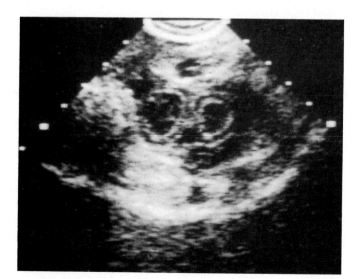

Fig. 28 Multiple corpora lutea after IVF treatment. An intra-uterine pregnancy was also present.

nuate uterus containing an intra-uterine pregnancy in one horn with a decidual reaction in the other (Fig. 29). A pregnancy in the uterus is surrounded by an echo-poor band of myometrium, whereas an interstitial ectopic pregnancy (Fig. 30) lacks such echoes lateral to the gestation sac.

Despite all the points discussed, it is possible to miss an ectopic pregnancy even with trans-vaginal ultrasonography. This is most likely to occur when the uterus contains a gestation sac-like structure with so-called 'yolk sac remnants'. The appearance of blood clot within a pseudo-gestation sac is very similar to that seen with an incomplete or inevitable spontaneous abortion. In these cases, curettage of the uterus will confirm the presence of chorionic villi and refute the diagnosis of ectopic gestation. The absence of chorionic villi necessitates checking β-HCG levels a few days after curettage. If these are rising then laparoscopy is needed to make a definitive diagnosis.

Fluid in the cul de sac is generally an unhelpful sign since it is not always seen with ectopic pregnancies and its presence does not indicate an ectopic pregnancy unless there are also blood clots within it.

Colour flow mapping and spectral Doppler to diagnose ectopic pregnancy have been proposed as useful additional studies but probably do not improve sensitivity. Their place in monitoring ectopic pregnancies after conservative therapy is yet to be determined.

The management of ectopic pregnancy

The management of ectopic pregnancy has changed dramatically in the last decade with the development of laparoscopic surgery. Lawson Tait first described the treatment of ectopic pregnancy with salpingectomy in 1884.[21]

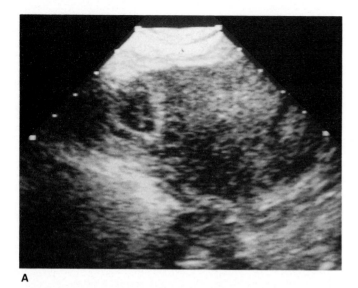

A

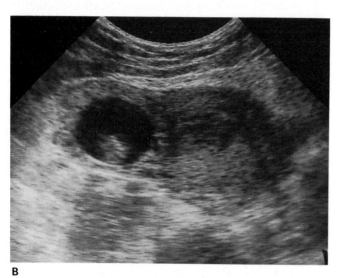

B

Fig. 30 Ectopic pregnancies. A: An ectopic pregnancy in the interstitial part of the right fallopian tube. Note that there is no myometrium lateral to the ectopic pregnancy thus differentiating this from a cornual pregnancy. **B:** Cornual pregnancy, surrounded by myometrium. (Transabdominal scan, empty bladder technique.)

All five cases he reported had ruptured. Up to then ectopic pregnancies were managed expectantly with a mortality rate of 69%.[22] In 1953 Stromme reported the use of salpingotomy,[23] the first report of conservative surgery in ectopic pregnancy. Several other conservative operations to conserve the tube have been attempted, such as fimbrial expression, segmental resection and salpingostomy.

Laparoscopic surgery for both intact and ruptured sacs has revolutionised the conservative management of ectopic gestation.[24–26] However, it is an invasive procedure and it can be argued that in many cases surgery may not have been necessary if β-HCG monitoring along with trans-vaginal ultrasonography had been available.

Non-surgical management of ectopic pregnancies has been practised for many years. Managed expectantly with monitoring of HCG levels and pelvic examination,[27] over half of ectopic pregnancies resorb spontaneously. A difficulty with this study is that the ectopic pregnancies that underwent tubal abortion never had the diagnosis confirmed by any other means though our experience with monitoring by trans-vaginal ultrasonography and β-HCG levels confirms these findings.

Several recent papers report the use of laparoscopic guided injection of drugs directly into the fallopian tube or gestation sac, including prostaglandin,[28] methotrexate[29,30] and hyperosmolar glucose.[31] However, all the surgical treatments required laparoscopy until Feichtinger and Kemeter[32] injected methotrexate directly into the ectopic sac guided by trans-vaginal ultrasound. They proposed this technique for the treatment of unruptured ectopic pregnancies and postulated that the same technique may be used for the treatment of intra-uterine blighted ova or missed abortions.

In our series of 46 IVF cases with ectopic gestations monitored by trans-vaginal ultrasound and β-HCG assays, more than half resolved spontaneously: in this group no cardiac activity could be detected by ultrasound. Laparoscopy or laparotomy were required in the 30% in whom cardiac activity was detected and the β-HCG levels rose. Patients where there was no cardiac activity but rising hormone levels were candidates for ultrasonically guided injections into the sac – six of the eight were heterotopic pregnancies. Methotrexate, used in one case, led to severe side effects so potassium chloride was chosen for the remainder and in six of these the intra-uterine pregnancy continued to term.

Some important interim conclusions can be derived from this study. The data of Lund published 35 years ago,[27] showing that more than 50% of ectopic pregnancies resolve spontaneously, are confirmed. The use of ultrasound to direct injection for the treatment of ectopic pregnancies seems feasible, though the numbers are as yet too small to draw firm conclusions. With these developments laparotomy may become outdated as a treatment for ectopic pregnancy, except in rare cases.

All patients who received ultrasound guided injection developed colicky lower abdominal pain approximately 1 week later. Trans-vaginal ultrasonography revealed evidence of intraperitoneal bleeding in only one case but bleeding within the tubal lumen and the gestation sac was noted to be in the centre of the tubal lumen (Fig. 31). The pathogenesis of tubal abortion is demonstrated in these cases. After injection, fetal demise results in trophoblastic detachment from the tubal wall, with consequent intra-tubal bleeding. The resulting pain is probably caused by tubal distension and contractions. Gradual resorption of the tubal contents then occurs over a period of 3 to 6 weeks. This was demonstrated in all cases of tubal pregnancy which resolved following ultrasound directed injection.

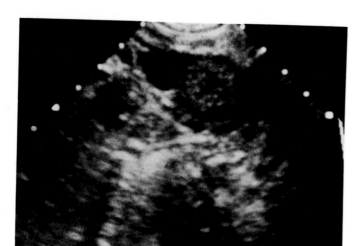

Fig. 31 Infected ectopic pregnancy. An ectopic pregnancy 1 week after injection of potassium chloride. Fluid is seen around the conceptus. There was no fluid in the peritoneal cavity.

The future of ectopic pregnancy management

It seems likely that less invasive techniques may replace conventional laparoscopy or laparotomy, at least in some patients.

Doppler ultrasound is already being used to detect ectopic trophoblastic tissue. However, colour flow mapping is not always able to detect the typical blood flow in trophoblastic tissue (2 out of 9 cases of confirmed ectopic pregnancies).[33] It may be that the trophoblast was no longer viable in the Doppler negative cases. Colour flow mapping may be useful as an alternative to β-HCG levels to monitor trophoblastic activity.

Laparoscopic injection of ectopic pregnancies may be replaced by ultrasound directed injection. Difficulties in seeing the sac mean that the injection is not as precisely directed as with ultrasound.

The best agent for injection is yet to be established, results thus far being similar whether hyperosmolar glucose, saline, potassium chloride, methotrexate or prostaglandins are chosen. With the development of thermal needles it may be possible to dispense with all drug injections. It may even be possible to direct a microwave or powerful ultrasound beam accurately at the ectopic sac alongside an imaging transducer, thus obviating the need for any injection.

Overall it seems probable that trans-vaginal ultrasound will eventually replace abdominal ultrasound in early pregnancy. Its potential as a diagnostic aid in threatened abortion and the speed with which a diagnosis of non-viability can be made, make it a necessity for all emergency gynaecological admissions when bleeding has occurred in the first trimester.

Its superiority in imaging the cervix and intra-uterine contents needs little elaboration. Finally, advances in early diagnosis and treatment of ectopic pregnancy may be expected to decrease morbidity and increase future fertility potential in these patients, as well as decrease maternal mortality.

REFERENCES

1 Langer R, Bukovsky I, Herman A, Ron-el R, Lifsjitz Y, Caspi E. Fertility following conservative surgery for tubal pregnancy. Acta Obstet Gynecol Scand 1987; 66: 649
2 Robertson D E, Smith W, Craft I. Reduction of ectopic pregnancy by ultrasound methods. Lancet 1987; 2: 1524
3 Timor-Tritsch I, Peisner D, Raju S. Sonoembryology: an organ orientated approach using a high frequency vaginal probe. JCU 1990; 18: 286
4 Goswamy R, Campbell S, Whitehead M I. Screening for ovarian cancer. Clin Obstet Gynecol 1983; 10: 621
5 Kratochwil A, Eisenhut L. Der fruheste nachweis der fetalen herzaktion durch ultraschall. Geburtshilfe Frauenheilkd 1967; 27: 176
6 Robinson H P. Early detection of fetal heart movement by sonar. Ultrasonics 1973; 11: 52
7 Schillinger H. Detection of heart action and active movements of the human embryo by ultrasonic time motion techniques. Eur J Obstet Gynecol Reprod Biol 1976; 6: 333
8 Rempen A. Diagnosis of viability in early pregnancy with vaginosonography. J Ultrasound Med 1990; 9: 711
9 Hertz J B. Diagnostic procedure in threatened abortion. Obstet Gynecol 1984; 66: 223
10 Schatts R, Brandsma G, Cleveringa L M, Lankhorst P H, Vroegrop I S, Jansen C A M. Evidence of asynchronous implantation in IVF multiple pregnancies. Human Reproduction 1988; 3: Supl 1, 17
11 Goldstein S R. Early detection of pathologic pregnancy by transvaginal sonography. JCU 1990; 18: 262
12 Rottem S, Bronshtein M. Transvaginal sonographic diagnosis of congenital anomalies between 9 weeks and 16 weeks, menstrual age. JCU 1990; 18: 307
13 MMWMR. Ectopic Pregnancy – United States, 1984 and 1985. MMWMR 1988; 7: 637
14 DeCherney A, Kase N. The conservative surgical management of unruptured ectopic pregnancy. Obstet Gynecol 1979; 54: 451
15 Ascheim Zondek, Manual of pregnancy testing. In: Hoe E H. ed. Pregnancy testing. Boston: Little Brown. 1928: p 1961
16 Pittaway D. Diagnosis of ectopic pregnancy. Obstet Gynecol 1986; 68: 440
17 Kadar N, Romero R. HCG determinations in early pregnancy. Fertil Steril 1987; 47: 722
18 Kadar N, Romero R. Serial human chorionic gonadotrophin measurements in ectopic pregnancy. Am J Obstet Gynecol 1988; 158: 1239
19 Kadar N, Romero R. A method for screening for ectopic pregnancy and its indications. Obstet Gynecol 1982; 58: 156
20 Milwidsky A, Adoni A, Segal S. Chorionic gonadotrophin and progesterone levels in ectopic pregnancy. Obstet Gynecol 1977; 50: 1945
21 Lawson Tait R. Five cases of extrauterine pregnancy operated upon at the time of rupture. BMJ 1884; 1: 1250
22 Parry J S. On extrauterine pregnancy: its causes, species, pathologic anatomy, clinical history, diagnosis, prognosis and treatment. Lea and Febiger. 1876: p 1
23 Stromme W B. Salpingotomy for tubal pregnancy: report of a successful case. Obstet Gynecol 1953; 1: 472
24 Reich H, Freifeld M L, McGlynn F, Reich E. Laparoscopic treatment of ectopic pregnancy. Obstet Gynecol 1987; 69: 275–279

25 Bruhat M A, Manhes H, Mage G, et al. Traitement par coelioscopique de la grossesse extrauterine. Acta Med Rom 1982; 20: 398

26 Semm K. New methods of pelviscopy for myomectomy, ovariectomy, tubectomy and adnexectomy. Endoscopy 1979; 2: 85

27 Lund J. Early ectopic pregnancy: comments on conservative management. J Obstet Gynaecol Br Emp 1955; 62: 70

28 Husslein P, Fitz R, Pateisky N, Egarter C. Prostaglandin injection for termination of tubal pregnancy: preliminary results. Am J Perinatol 1989; 6: 117

29 Li M C, Hertz R, Spencer D B. Effect of Methotrexate therapy on choriocarcinoma and chorioadenoma. Proceedings Soc Exp Biol Med 1956; 93: 361

30 Ichinoe K, Wake N, Shinkai N, Shiina Y, Miyazaki Y, Tanaka T. Nonsurgical therapy to preserve oviduct function in patients with tubal pregnancies. Am J Obstet Gynecol 1987; 156: 484

31 Lang P F, Weiss P A M, Mayer H O, Haas J G, Honigl W. Conservative treatment of ectopic pregnancy with local injection of hyperosmolar glucose solution or prostaglandin-F2: a prospective study. Lancet 1990; 1: 78–80

32 Feichtinger W, Kemeter P. Conservative treatment of ectopic pregnancy by transvaginal aspiration under sonographic control and Methotrexate injection. Lancet 1987; 1: 381

33 Kurjak A, Zalud I, Alfirevic Z, Jurkovic D. The assessment of abnormal pelvic blood flow by transvaginal color and pulsed Doppler. Ultrasound Med Biol 1990; 16: 437

The normal fetus

David R. Griffin

INTRODUCTION

In this chapter the normal fetal anatomical appearances are described from the time of a routine examination at approximately 18 post-menstrual weeks to term. The detailed embryology and developmental anatomy is described in Chapter 7. Recognition of abnormal fetal anatomy is founded upon a sound knowledge of normal appearances, which can only be attained through 'hands on' experience.

A systematic approach to the examination of the fetus ensures that all regions are covered. Starting with the number of fetuses, the presentation, fetal activity, liquor volume, placental site and morphology and the number of cord vessels are assessed systematically. The fetal examination can conveniently begin with the head so that gestational age can be confirmed by measurement of the biparietal diameter. The skull, brain and face are examined before progressing caudally to scan the thorax, heart, abdominal cavity and urogenital tract. Finally the spine and limbs complete the picture. Fetal lie may make this order of examination impossible, but if deviated from, a check list will serve as a reminder so that no parts are missed. This approach is particularly important when the ultrasonologist's attention is directed toward a particular fetal part or system because of suspected abnormality. It is all too easy to become so involved in abnormal features that other parts are forgotten. It is good practice to examine the whole fetus first and to return to a detailed examination of abnormal features afterwards.

A three-dimensional image of the fetus is built up by scanning in three orthogonal planes (Fig. 1). Unfortunately there is no agreed terminology for these planes and terms used in the head may differ from those in the trunk. The axial plane may also be known as horizontal or transverse plane, the coronal plane as the frontal plane and the sagittal plane as the median plane. In this chapter the terminology in Figure 1 is used. An experienced operator frequently deviates from these standard views to obtain optimal imaging of a particular organ.

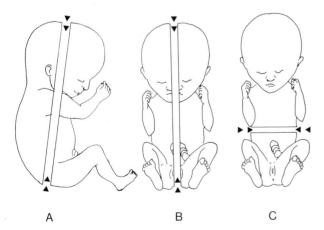

Fig. 1 Basic planes of ultrasound examination. A: The coronal plane. **B:** The sagittal plane. **C:** The axial plane.

Head

Cranium and cranial contents

In examining the fetal head attention needs to be directed to:

a) the cranial vault;
b) the intracranial contents;
c) the soft tissue features of the face.

Examination of these structures is performed in the three planes described above. Most routine measurements of the head and intracranial structures are performed in the axial plane which should be orientated parallel to the fronto-occipital diameter (Fig. 2).

The skull The skull is best examined in the axial plane.[1] Throughout pregnancy it should have an ovoid shape, the biparietal diameter (BPD) being 80% to 90% of the occipitofrontal diameter (OFD), and narrower in the frontal than in the occipital region (Fig. 3). If the fetus is

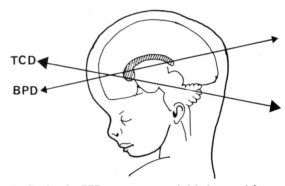

Fig. 2 Section for BPD measurement. Axial plane used for examination of the fetal head at the level used for measurement of the BPD, head circumference and ventricle-hemisphere ratios.

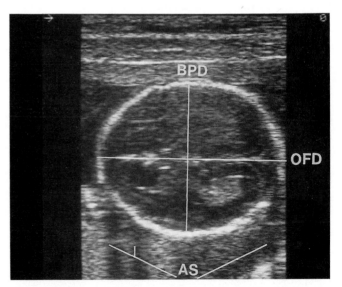

Fig. 3 Axial scan – 18 weeks. Axial scan of the fetal head at 18 weeks at approximately the level in Figure 2 to show BPD and OFD measurements. Note acoustic shadows (AS).

presenting by the breech, the head may be <u>dolichocephalic</u> with an unusually low BPD/OFD ratio. Echoes from the vault should be very strong and an acoustic shadow should be evident across more distal structures in the ultrasound beam. These are more noticeable beyond the lateral extremities of the skull image where the ultrasound beam is attenuated by a greater thickness of skull. This acoustic shadowing becomes more pronounced with increasing maturity so that it becomes more difficult to examine intracranial structures at later stages without using the acoustic windows afforded by the sutures and fontanelles. Conversely defective skull mineralisation may be suspected when there is enhanced imaging of intracranial detail. Breaks in the integrity of the skull outline will be evident at the sutures but, except in the mid-sagittal plane where the anterior and posterior fontanelles are best seen, these gaps should be small.

Difficulty in obtaining a good axial view may occur in a cephalic presentation when the head is deep in the pelvis, when there is asynclitism or when the spine lies perpendicular to the scanning plane, with the vertex immediately beneath the abdominal wall. This may be overcome by displacing the uterus upwards out of the pelvis and applying pressure to the anterior fetal shoulder. If this manoeuvre fails then tilting either the couch or the patient into a head down position may be effective. Occasionally the patient may need to return for a further examination after an interval in the hope that the adverse position has changed.

The sagittal plane is mainly used in examining the fetal facial profile. Parasagittal sections clearly outline the full extent of the lateral ventricles but they can be difficult to obtain except when the fetus lies in a direct occipito-anterior or occipitoposterior position.

In the coronal plane the skull should have a semicircular outline. This view is used to examine soft tissue features of the face.

Abnormalities may occur in skull size (microcephaly, neural tube defects, macrocephaly), skull shape (brachycephaly, the 'lemon sign', scaphocephaly, clover leaf skull, microcephaly), skull integrity (anencephaly, encephalocele, exencephaly) or skull mineralisation (some skeletal dysplasias).

Intracranial structures From the sixteenth week to term there is considerable growth of brain structures both in size and in complexity (Fig. 4). The lateral cerebral ventricles are a prominent feature of the brain in the early second trimester but they shrink as the cerebral hemispheres grow. At 16 weeks the lateral ventricles consist of little more than an anterior horn, body and small inferior horn. The inferior and posterior horns become elongated

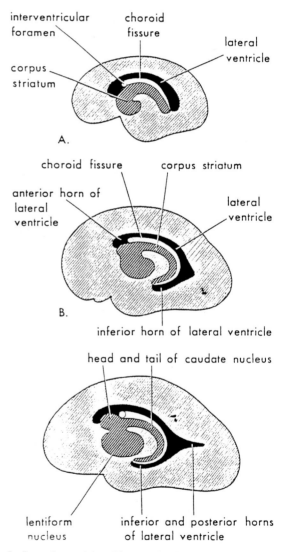

Fig. 5 **Lateral ventricles.** Diagram showing development of the lateral ventricular system. (From: Moore K L. The developing human. Philadelphia: WB Saunders. 1982: p 400.)

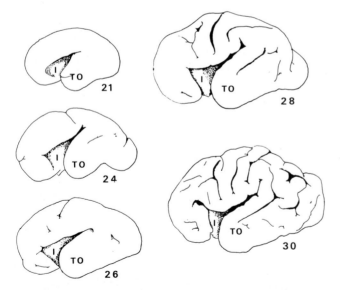

Fig. 4 **Opercularisation of the brain.** Diagrammatic representations of the fetal brain from 21 to 30 weeks showing opercularisation of the insula (I) and formation of gyri. TO – temporal operculum. (Drawn from Gray's Anatomy.)

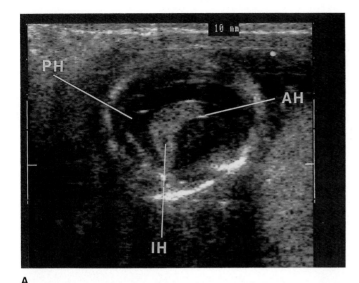

A

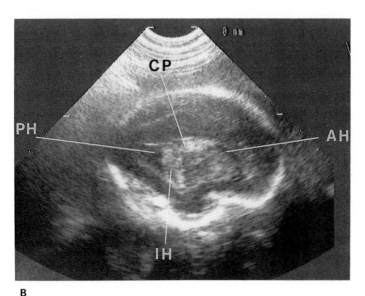

B

Fig. 6 Developing ventricle. A: 18 week and **B:** 23 week parasagittal scans to demonstrate developing anterior (AH), posterior (PH) and inferior horns (IH) and the choroid plexus (CP) with the ventricular outlines highlighted.

with growth of the temporal and occipital lobes of the cerebrum (Figs 5 and 6). Until the twentieth post-menstrual week, the choroid plexus is a prominent highly reflective feature on the inferolateral wall of the body of the lateral ventricle (almost filling it) and the roof of the inferior horn. The choroid plexus becomes progressively less prominent thereafter until in the third trimester it is barely visible.

Most of the essential structures of the fetal brain may be demonstrated in the axial plane at two positions (Figs 2 and 7). The first transects the anterior horns of the lateral ventricles, the cavity of the septum pellucidum, the thalamic nuclei and third ventricle, the body and posterior horns of the lateral ventricles and the insula and Sylvian fissure (lateral cerebral sulcus). The second is more caudal and angled to include the brain stem, cerebellum and cisterna magna.

As a consequence of disturbance of the ultrasound beam as it passes through the convex proximal skull table, detail of intracranial structures in the proximal hemisphere is frequently poor. The distal hemisphere therefore is chosen for measurements. This phenomenon should be borne in mind when intracranial pathology such as a choroid plexus cyst is detected unilaterally. Every effort should be made to view the brain from the other side so that obscured contralateral pathology is not missed.

In the normal fetal brain the lateral wall of the body of the lateral ventricle runs parallel to the midline in the second trimester so that measurement of the anterior horn is representative of the body. As the medial wall of the anterior horn is rarely seen, measurement is taken from the midline echo. This measurement rarely exceeds 9 mm in the normal second trimester brain. The body of the lateral ventricle has a measurable width posteriorly between its medial and lateral walls. The lateral wall is frequently obscured by the choroid plexus and the lateral wall should then be taken to be the lateral border of the choroid plexus (Fig. 8). Later in the second trimester the posterior horns converge in the occipital poles so that measurement of their maximum width will no longer be perpendicular to the midline but angled posteriorly (Fig. 9). Until about 20 weeks the width of the body of the lateral ventricle is similar to the anterior horn measurement but as the medial wall of the body and posterior horn become indented by the calcar avis the width of the lateral ventricle decreases. Traditionally the anterior and posterior ventricle measurements have been compared as a ratio with the maximum width of the cerebral hemisphere. This ratio should be less than 0.5 from the sixteenth week onwards. Nomograms are available (see Appendix).[2]

Until the twentieth week the brain has a smooth surface with few sulci or gyri (Fig. 4). The gyri and sulci extend and become more convoluted as the brain grows. Of particular clinical significance is the development of the lateral sulcus (Sylvian fissure) between the insula medially and the anteriorly migrating temporal operculum. From about the twenty-second week this process, known as opercularisation, produces a linear echo in the same scanning plane as, but lateral to, the lateral ventricles. This may be mistaken for the lateral wall of the lateral ventricle and can lead to an erroneous diagnosis of ventriculomegaly (Fig. 10). If in doubt the identification of the pulsations of the middle cerebral artery running in the lateral sulcus confirm the origin of the echo.

The medial walls of the lateral ventricle are formed anteriorly by the septum pellucidum, a double membrane enclosing a narrow cavity (cavum septum pellucidum). This structure may be seen throughout gestation as a pair

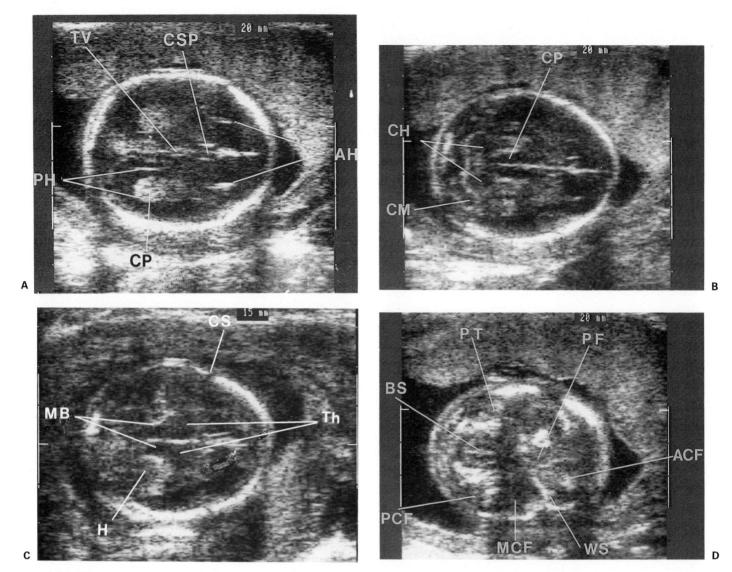

Fig. 7 Normal sections – 18 weeks. Axial sections of the fetal head at 18 weeks, each section slightly more caudal than the last. **A:** To show the lateral and third ventricles. AH – lateral wall of anterior horn of lateral ventricle, PH – posterior horn, CP – choroid plexus, CPS – cavity of the septum pellucidum, TV – third ventricle. **B:** Plane angulated about 15° to show the cerebellar hemispheres (CH), cisterna magna (CM), CP – cerebral peduncles. **C:** Section at the level of the thalamus (Th). H – hypocampus, MB – midbrain, CS – coronal suture. **D:** Section at the level of the base of the skull showing cranial fossae. ACF – anterior cranial fossa, MCF – middle cranial fossa, PCF – posterior cranial fossa, PF – pituitary fossa, WS – wing of the sphenoid bone, PT – petrous part of the temporal bone, BS – brain stem in the foramen magnum.

of parallel echoes close to the midline and just posterior to the echoes from the lateral walls of the anterior horns. The cavum septum pellucidum interrupts the midline (interhemispheric) echo about one third of the distance from the frontal to the occipital calvarium. It should not be confused with the third ventricle which lies postero-inferior to it between the thalamic nuclei (Fig. 7A) and is rarely visualised in the normal fetus. The bodies or antra of the lateral ventricles diverge and the medial wall can be identified. The choroid plexus is a highly reflective structure arising from the floor of the lateral ventricle (Figs 7A, 11 and 12). It usually either fills the lateral ventricle from its medial to lateral wall or a small anechoic rim may be seen on its

medial border. The lateral border of the choroid plexus may generally be taken to be that of the ventricle also.

The cerebellar hemispheres are seen at 18 weeks as bilaterally symmetrical, almost circular structures of low reflectivity but with a more reflective rim (Fig. 13). As pregnancy progresses the cerebellar hemispheres become more triangular in axial section and the highly reflective vermis becomes more prominent between the cerebellar hemispheres (Fig. 14). Anterior to the cerebellum the poorly reflective cerebral peduncles are evident. Posteriorly the cisterna magna is seen as an anechoic space between the posterior aspect of the cerebellum and the inner aspect of the occipital bone. The cerebellar hemispheres may also

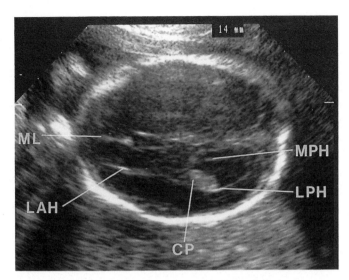

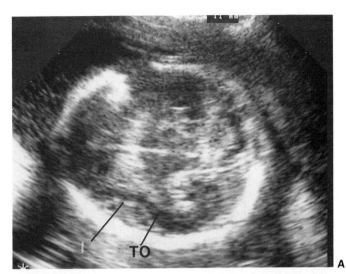

Fig. 8 Fetal head – 19 weeks. The anterior horn of the lateral ventricle is measured from the midline (ML) to the lateral wall (LAH). The posterior horn is measured from the medial wall (MPH) to the lateral wall (LPH) at its maximal width. The lateral wall of the posterior horn is frequently outlined by the choroid plexus (CP).

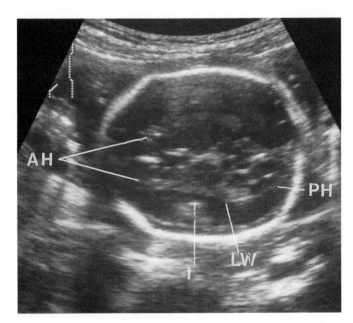

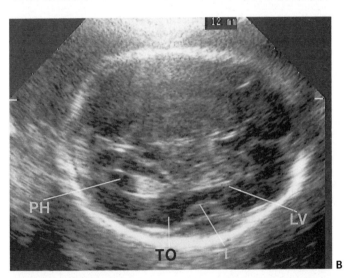

Fig. 9 Posterior horn – 25 weeks. Axial scan of the fetal head at 25 weeks to show narrowing and convergence of the posterior horn (PH). The lateral wall (LW) of the lateral ventricle can be followed to the anterior horn (AH) and should not be confused with the insula (I).

be well-demonstrated in a posterior coronal plane (Fig. 15).

The face

An examination of the fetal face should be an essential part of any routine examination for fetal normality. It is not difficult or particularly time consuming and may be

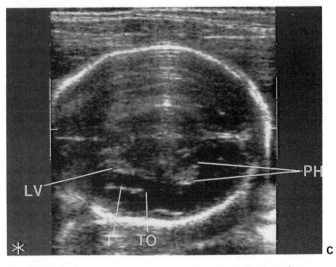

Fig. 10 Development of the insula. Axial scans at **A:** 18 weeks, **B:** 22 weeks and **C:** 25 weeks to demonstrate the insula. PH – posterior horn, LV – lateral wall of lateral ventricle, TO – temporal operculum, I – insula.

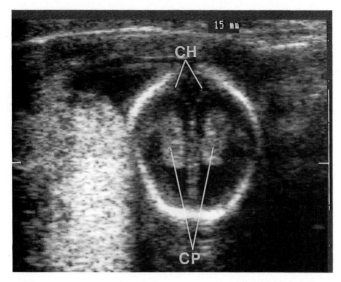

Fig. 11 Choroid plexus. Axial scan (17 weeks) from the occipital aspect showing the choroid plexus (CP) in each lateral ventricle. The occipital poles of the cerebral hemispheres (CH) are demonstrated.

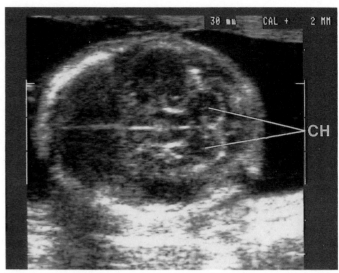

Fig. 13 Cerebellum – 21 weeks. Axial scan to show cerebellar hemispheres (CH) at 21 weeks.

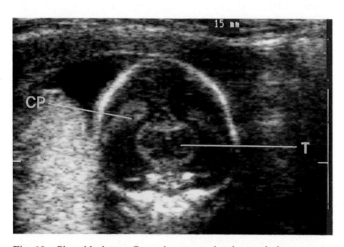

Fig. 12 Choroid plexus. Coronal scan angulated posteriorly to demonstrate the choroid plexus (CP) following the lateral ventricle into the inferior horn as it curves round the thalamus (T).

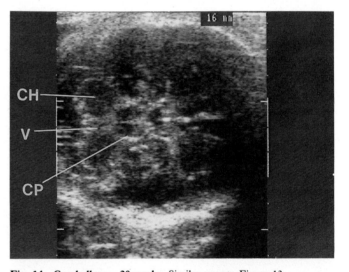

Fig. 14 Cerebellum – 30 weeks. Similar scan to Figure 13 showing cerebellar hemispheres (CH) and vermis (V) at 30 weeks. CP – cerebral peduncles.

rewarded by the discovery of a facial cleft, one of the more common congenital defects and a marker for a lethal or severely disabling genetic syndrome.

Coarse facial features start to be recognisable on ultrasound examination in the late first trimester. By the fourteenth post-menstrual week the nose, lips, ears etc. are evident and by the time of a routine 18 week scan a detailed three-dimensional image of the face may be constructed (Fig. 16). The added resolution of a 5 MHz transducer will often help in examining the finer details of the lips and ears.

Three views are employed: axial, coronal and sagittal (Fig. 17). In the coronal plane the chin, lips, external nares

(Fig. 18), eyelids, lenses, cheeks and forehead may be demonstrated as if in a direct frontal portrait. Slight adjustments of the plane are necessary to demonstrate all these features but the technique can be mastered with a little perseverance. The axial plane demonstrates the orbits, lenses * (Fig. 19), nasal bones (Fig. 20), palate, oral cavity, upper and lower lips and mandible (Fig. 21). The sagittal plane reveals the fetal profile (Fig. 22) and is useful when

---

* Editor's note: Although to date these structures have been considered to be the lenses, their size suggests that they are in fact the complete globe of the eye.

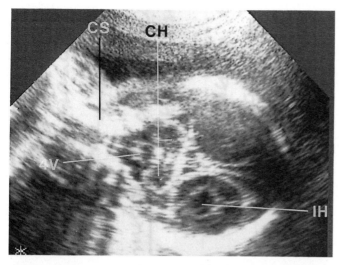

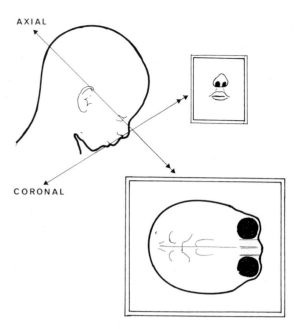

Fig. 15 Cerebellum – 19 weeks. Coronal scan to show cerebellar hemispheres (CH), fourth ventricle (4V) and inferior horn of the lateral ventricle (IH). CS – cervical spine.

Fig. 17 Scan planes for the fetal face. Diagram of scanning planes for examination of the fetal face.

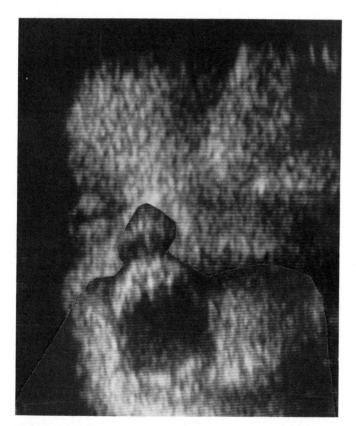

Fig. 16 Fetal face. Composite picture from two scans of the same fetal face at slightly different angles to give an indication of the three-dimensional mental image that can be built up during real time scanning.

demonstrating the chin, tongue (with the mouth open), forehead, nasal bridge etc.

The lips, nose and ears (Fig. 23) become increasingly clear as pregnancy advances although they are more likely

to be obscured by the upper limbs. It is unusual to be able to demonstrate both ears on a single occasion. The palate is most easily demonstrated in the axial plane at about 16 to 18 weeks whereafter it becomes increasingly obscured by the maxilla.

The neck

The fetal neck may be examined for its external contours and its internal structure.

In axial section the neck should be circular with the cervical vertebrae centrally. Soft tissue or fluid filled irregularities or swellings should suggest the possibility of neoplasms or cystic hygroma. Nuchal oedema posteriorly may be a marker for trisomy 21.[3]

The larynx is best demonstrated in the coronal plane. The epiglottis and the vestibular folds can usually be demonstrated (Fig. 24) and can be seen to move with fetal breathing and swallowing. Swallowing dysfunction from bulbar palsy may be a rare cause of polyhydramnios. The carotid vessels can be identified laterally for pulsed Doppler studies of carotid blood flow velocities.

Trunk

The fetal trunk is comprised of the axial skeleton (spine, shoulder and pelvic girdles and ribs) and the thorax and its contents divided from the abdominal cavity by the diaphragm.

Before attending to the detailed examination of the thoracic and abdominal contents an overall view of the whole trunk should be obtained to ensure that the relative

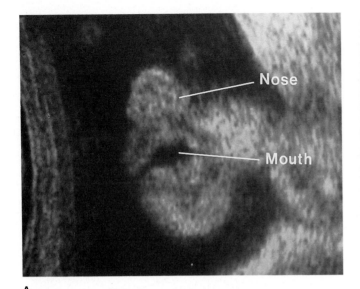

A

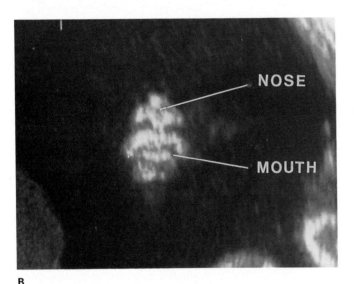

B

Fig. 18 Fetal mouth and nose. Coronal views of the fetal face, **A:** with the mouth open and **B:** mouth closed. The contours of the nostrils and lips are clearly demonstrated.

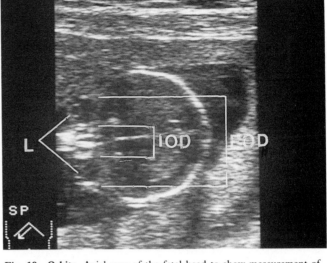

Fig. 19 Orbits. Axial scan of the fetal head to show measurement of the internal (IOD) and external orbital diameters (EOD) and the lenses.

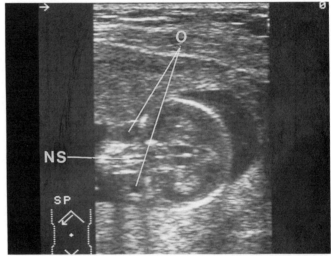

Fig. 20 Orbits and nasal bones. Axial scan to show the orbits (O) and nasal bones. Note that the nasal septum (NS) and turbinate bones normally give a double echo.

proportions are correct. In sagittal and coronal planes the transition from the thoracic to abdominal wall should be a smooth curve (Fig. 25). Angulation between the base of the thorax and the abdominal wall (particularly in the sagittal plane) should suggest the possibility of a reduced thorax (short ribs) or an abdominal mass (e.g. multicystic or polycystic kidneys). Similarly, in transverse section the thoracic circumference at the level of the heart should be roughly similar to the abdominal circumference at the umbilical vein. In the same views the integrity of the skin coverings should be checked to exclude omphalocele, gastroschisis, bladder extrophy, spina bifida, sacral teratoma or other surface tumours. Ensure that the umbilical cord contains one vein and two arteries and that it has

a normal insertion into the anterior abdominal wall (Fig. 26).

The spine

The vertebrae have three centres of ossification in fetal life; the vertebral body and each lamina of the neural arch (Fig. 27). The spinous process does not start to ossify until after birth. Thus, ultrasonically in transverse section there are three reflective foci surrounding the echo-free neural canal which represent these ossification centres. In the cervical, thoracic and upper lumbar vertebrae they have an equilateral triangular orientation with its base posterior.

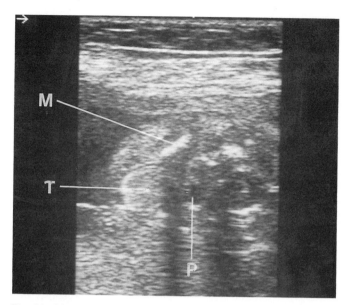

Fig. 21   **Mouth.** Axial scan demonstrating the tongue (T), ramus of the mandible (M) and pharynx (P).

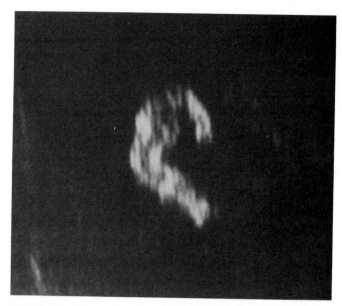

Fig. 23   **Ear.** Scan of the fetal ear in the mid-second trimester.

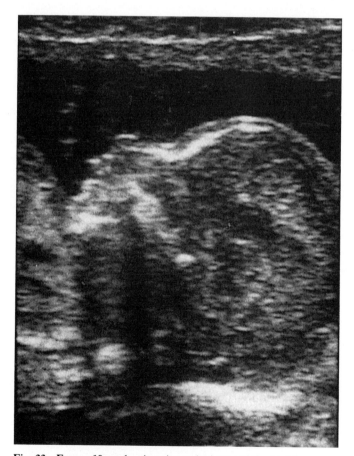

Fig. 22   **Face – 19 weeks.** Anterior sagittal scan of the fetal face demonstrating the profile.

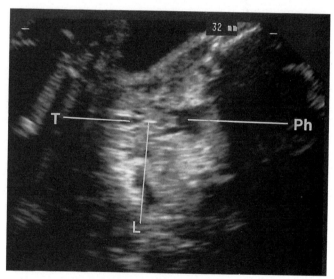

Fig. 24   **Larynx.** Sagittal scan of the fetal larynx (28 weeks). T – trachea, L – larynx, Ph – pharynx.

Owing to the lumbar expansion of the neural canal the laminar echoes are more widely spaced in the lower lumbar vertebrae and may give a U-shaped appearance. The arms of the U should be parallel or convergent. Divergent arms should raise suspicions of spina bifida and initiate a search for signs of a meningocele and Arnold-Chiari malformation in the fetal head (see Ch. 16). The normal lumbar and cervical expansions of the neural canal are best appreciated in the coronal plane. As part of a spinal examination the integrity of the overlying skin should be noted.

The spinal curvatures are best examined in the sagittal plane (Fig. 28) where the posterior and anterior elements of vertebral bodies are recognised as a double row of strong

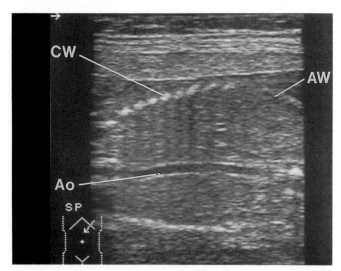

Fig. 25 Trunk – coronal. Longitudinal coronal section of the fetal trunk to show the smooth transition from the chest wall (CW) to the abdominal wall (AW). Ao – aorta.

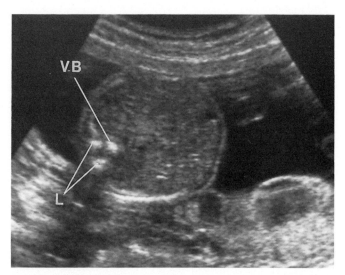

Fig. 27 Lumbar spine. Transverse section of the fetal lumbar spine (20 weeks) to show the three major ossification centres. Note the integrity of the skin overlying the spine. L – laminae, VB – vertebral body.

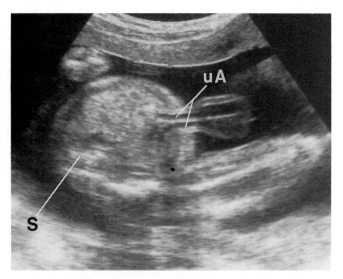

Fig. 26 Abdomen – transverse. Transverse scan of the fetal lower abdomen to show the insertion of the umbilical cord. uA – umbilical arteries, S – spine. Figure courtesy of the Portland Hospital.

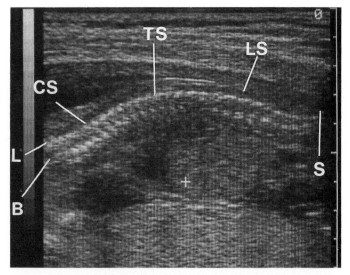

Fig. 28 Spine – sagittal. Sagittal section of the spine (18 weeks). The vertebrae are seen as paired reflective dots, the posterior representing the laminae (L) and the anterior representing the vertebral bodies (B). The spinal curvatures can be identified, convex in the thoracic (TS) and upper lumbar spine (LS) and concave in the cervical (CS) and lumbo-sacral (S). The skin can be seen overlying the cervical and thoracic spine.

echoes (the laminae posteriorly and the vertebral bodies anteriorly). The usual posture of the fetal spine is convex posteriorly (kyphotic). There may be a slight lordosis of the cervical spine when the head is extended but the lumbar lordosis is variably evident depending upon fetal attitude. The spine approaches the skin surface in the sacral region. Spinal flexion may be very marked if there is limited amniotic fluid. The spine should be examined throughout its length for symmetry of both its curvature and vertebral sequence. In low-risk cases this is first accomplished by a sagittal view including the complete length of the spine if possible. The transducer is then rotated through 90° and the spine studied in transverse

section, maintaining an orthogonal orientation to the vertebrae by following the curvatures. A quick sweep along the spine will reveal gross defects. When an abnormality is suspected, such as spina bifida or Charcot-Levine syndrome (see Ch. 16), more care is needed to examine each vertebra in succession. With good equipment and scanning conditions detail of the vertebrae, spinal canal and spinal cord may be seen with increasing clarity as pregnancy advances (Fig. 29).

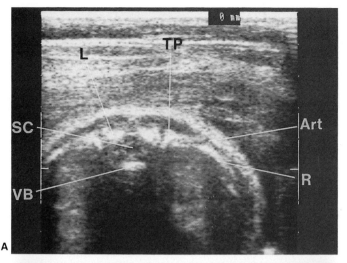

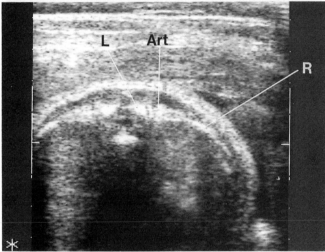

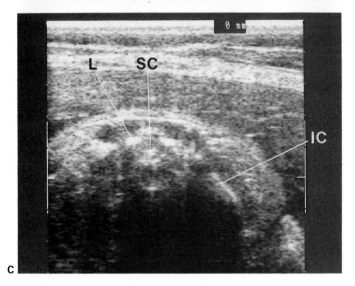

Ribs

The ribs are difficult to image in their full length. They should enclose about two thirds of the thorax which should be almost circular in transverse section. They should be evenly spaced and follow a smooth curve round the thorax. Where it is necessary to examine the ribs in detail the best views have been found to be:

a) tangential to the lateral thoracic wall to examine spacing and contour;
b) longitudinal paramedian for counting;
c) transverse for length and thoracic circumference.
Detailed examination of the rib cage tends to be time consuming, frustrating and hampered by fetal movement and shadowing by the shoulder girdle.

The shoulder and pelvic girdles

The clavicles are S-shaped and easily identified and measured on a transverse scan in the upper thorax (Fig. 30). The triangular outline of the scapula and the spine of the scapula are seen in coronal section tangential to the rib cage (Fig. 31).

The iliac crest may be clearly seen in transverse and tangential scans (Figs 29C and 32). The pubis is usually obscured by the femora. It may show separation in cloacal extrophy.

Thoracic contents

The major thoracic contents are the heart and great vessels and the lungs. The heart occupies about one third of the chest and is situated with the apex towards the left side. The left ventricle lies posterolaterally and the right ventricle lies anteromedially. Detailed normal anatomy of

Fig. 29 Spine – third trimester. Transverse scans of the spine in the third trimester (33 weeks) to show detail. **A:** Mid-thoracic vertebra. The three major ossification centres in the vertebral body (VB) and the laminae (L) surround the spinal canal (SC). Detail of the transverse process (TP) and its articulations (Art) with the neck and head of the rib (R) are clear. **B:** The twelfth rib (R) articulates with the lamina (L). **C:** Lumbar vertebra with lamina (L) spinal canal (SC) and iliac crest (IC).

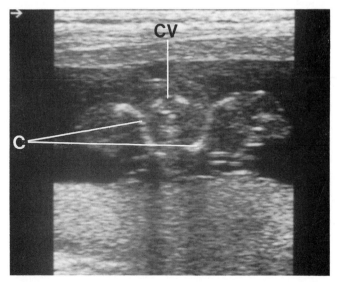

Fig. 30 Clavicles. Transverse scan to show the clavicles (18 weeks). CV – cervical vertebra, C – clavicles.

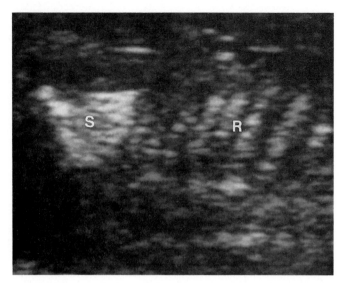

Fig. 31 Scapula. Scan tangential to the chest wall to demonstrate the scapula (S). R – ribs.

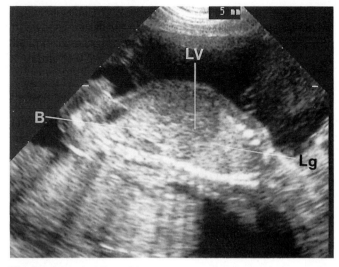

Fig. 33 Lung and liver. Right anterior parasagittal scan (19 weeks) to show relative intensity of lung (Lg), liver (LV) and bowel (B).

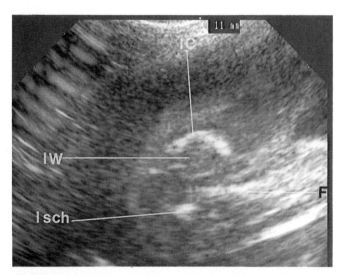

Fig. 32 Pelvis. Scan at 22 weeks to show the pelvic bones. IC – iliac crest, IW – wing of ilium, Isch – ischium, F – femur.

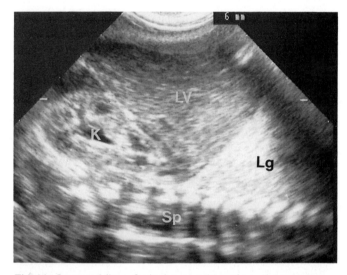

Fig. 34 Lung and liver. Sagittal scan at 34 weeks to demonstrate contrast between lung (Lg) and liver (LV) reflectivity (compare with Fig. 33). K – kidney, Sp – spine.

the heart is described in Chapter 19. The left lung lies behind the heart and is smaller than the right. The lobar divisions are not normally evident. The heart is normally in contact with the chest wall through most of its anterior border and at the apex. This relationship may be lost with a left sided diaphragmatic hernia or in cystic adenomatoid malformation type III of the lung. The reflectivity of the lung at most gestational ages is greater than the liver and often similar to the bowel (Fig. 33). As the bronchioles proliferate and the alveoli develop, lung reflectivity increases compared to the liver (Fig. 34).[4] Normally the pleural and pericardial cavities are not evident.

Breathing movements of the chest wall are evident from early in the second trimester. They can be recognised in either longitudinal or transverse section as rhythmic changes in thoracic diameter or excursions of the diaphragm or kidneys. Fetal breathing is a useful indicator of fetal well-being.[5]

The diaphragm

The diaphragm is a thin fibromuscular membrane that separates the thorax from the abdomen. Under good scanning conditions it is seen in sagittal and coronal views as a thin, upwardly convex, echo-poor line separating liver from lung and heart from stomach. In any routine examination it is important to confirm the normal relationships of these organs (Fig. 35). The chest should

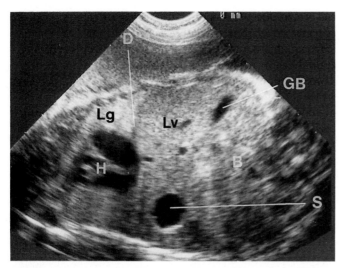

Fig. 35 Trunk. Coronal scan of the trunk. The heart (H) and lungs (Lg) are separated from the liver (Lv) by the diaphragm (D). The stomach (S) and gallbladder (GB) are seen at the lower border of the liver. Between them a faint line separates liver from bowel (B).

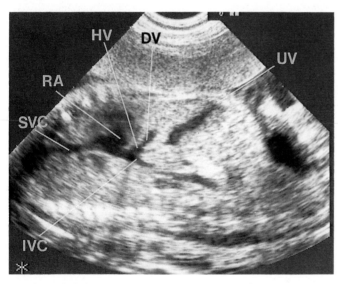

Fig. 36 Umbilical venous circulation. Longitudinal anteroposterior view of the fetal trunk to demonstrate the course of the umbilical venous circulation. The umbilical vein runs an oblique course through the liver from the cord insertion to the ductus venous (DV) and then into the right atrium (RA) via the hepatic vein (HV) and inferior vena cava (IVC). SVC – superior vena cava.

contain no echo-free structures apart from the heart and great vessels. The stomach should be beneath the left ventricle of the heart and separated from it by the diaphragm.

The abdomen

On general examination the abdominal portion of the trunk contains the liver, intestines, renal tract and great vessels.

It should routinely contain two cystic structures, the stomach and the bladder, both of which must be identified.

The liver

The liver occupies the upper third of the abdominal cavity. Its right lobe is larger than the left so that its outline in coronal sections approximates to a right-angled triangle, the hypotenuse being the base of the liver that faces caudally and to the left. It is of uniformly low reflectivity, lower than the lung or bowel which form its upper and lower borders and similar to renal parenchyma. The umbilical vein enters the liver anteriorly and runs a 45° oblique course cephalad and posteriorly to join the portal veins and enter the inferior vena cava via the ductus venosus (Fig. 36). Just prior to its junction with the portal veins it takes a J-shaped turn which is the level at which an abdominal circumference should be measured. At the right inferior border of the liver a further oblique, anechoic structure, the gallbladder is usually seen. This can be distinguished from the umbilical vein by its lateral position and lack of continuity with the umbilical insertion (Fig. 37).

The spleen

The left upper quadrant of the abdominal cavity is occupied by the spleen. Although its ultrasonic visualisation has been described and biometric tables have been published[6] (see Appendix) it may be difficult to identify routinely. It lies above the left kidney and behind the stomach. It has a uniform reflectivity, similar to the liver.

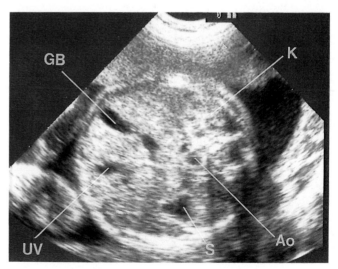

Fig. 37 Trunk. Transverse scan of the fetal abdomen showing stomach (S), umbilical vein (UV), gallbladder (GB) and kidney (K). The aorta (Ao) is anterior to the spine.

The stomach

The stomach should be identified in all routine scans and if it is not the patient should be re-examined later the same day or on another occasion. The stomach may be evident from the ninth to tenth week onwards. In most cases it will be seen from the fourteenth week and always by the time of a routine 18 to 20 week examination (Fig. 38). Its shape will vary with fullness and gestation, the greater and lesser curvatures becoming more recognisable with increasing age. After the sixteenth week peristalsis may be seen on prolonged observation. Considering its dynamic state, the

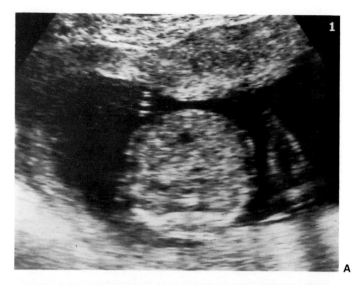

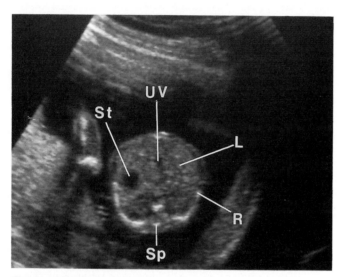

Fig. 38 Abdominal circumference. Typical transverse scan (17 weeks) at the level of the umbilical vein (UV) and stomach (St) suitable for abdominal circumference measurement. Sp – spine, L – liver, R – rib.

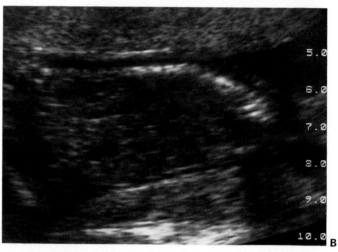

Fig. 40 Kidneys at 16 weeks. A: Transverse scan to show kidneys on either side of the lumbar spine. They have little architectural detail at this stage apart from the echo-free renal pelvis. **B:** Longitudinal scan of the same kidney.

volume of the stomach has been found to be remarkably constant and biometric nomograms are available (see Appendix).[7] The stomach contents are echo-free.

The small intestine

In the second and early third trimesters the lumen of the small bowel is not usually obvious but nearer term it can be identified with occasional peristalsis. Widespread visualisation of the lumen and peristalsis should alert the sonographer to the possibility of bowel obstruction.

The colon

Like the small intestine the lumen of the colon is not normally evident in the second trimester. However in the third

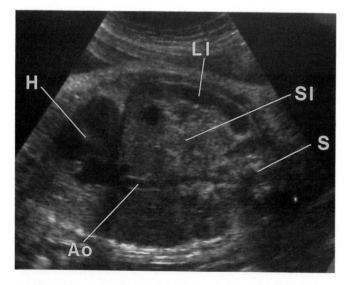

Fig. 39 Colon. Scan showing large intestine (LI) at 32 weeks containing meconium and enclosing the more reflective small intestine (SI). Heart – H, Ao – aorta, S – spine.

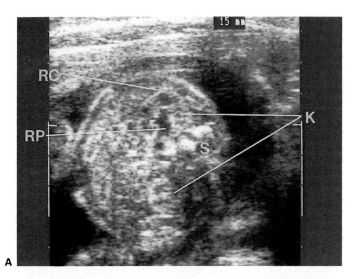

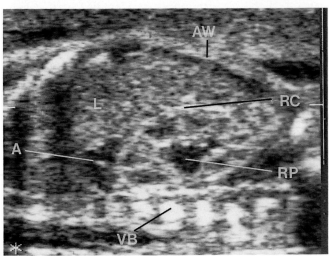

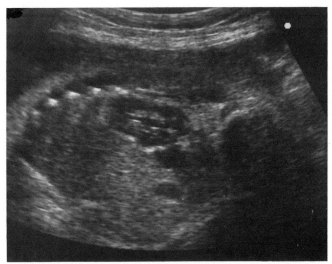

Fig. 42 Longitudinal scan of kidney at 36 weeks. The lobation is apparent and the renal capsule is highly reflective. Note shadowing of the adrenal by the 11th rib.

Fig. 41 Kidneys and adrenal at 24 weeks. A: The perimeter of the kidney (K) is more easily identified from the reflective renal capsule (RC). Renal architecture and the renal pelvis (RP) are evident. S – spine. **B:** Longitudinal scan clearly showing echo-poor pyramids and lobation of the kidney, the renal capsule (RC) and the intrarenal pelvis (RP). The adrenal gland is seen as a triangular structure above the upper pole of the kidney. VB – vertebral body, L – liver, AW – abdominal wall.

trimester colonic contents can be identified in the ascending colon at first and progressively filling the transverse, descending and sigmoid colons by term. Haustrations are seen. Cellular debris produces low level echoes in colonic contents which distinguish them from the echo-free fluid in the stomach or urinary tract or other cystic abdominal or pelvic masses (Fig. 39).

The urinary tract

The urinary tract is comprised of the kidneys, renal pelves, ureters, bladder and urethra. The ureters and urethra are not seen under normal circumstances although the urethra may be evident in males during micturition.

The kidneys

The kidneys are situated on either side of the lumbar spine and may be consistently visualised from about the fourteenth week. At this stage they have an homogeneous appearance with slightly lower reflectivity than the surrounding bowel and similar to the liver. At this early stage they are most readily demonstrated in a posterior transverse scan below the level of the liver. The renal pelvis may be seen as an echo-free, slit-like space in the centre of the kidney (Fig. 40).

As pregnancy progresses further details of the renal architecture appear. A thin reflective rim, representing the renal capsule, appears at about the nineteenth week. From about the twenty-fourth week fetal lobation becomes increasingly apparent, particularly in coronal and parasagittal sections. The medullary pyramids are arranged round the renal pelvis as a rosette of echo-poor foci with poorly defined margins (Figs 41 and 42). They should not be confused with cysts which are echo-free and have well-defined margins.

At all gestational ages the circumference of the kidney should be about one third of the abdominal circumference.[8] The renal volume is calculated by measuring longitudinal, transverse and anteroposterior dimensions and dividing by two. Growth in all dimensions is roughly linear throughout pregnancy (see Appendix).[9]

Comparison of size and structure between the kidneys is best accomplished when they are simultaneously imaged in the prevertebral coronal plane. As in the adult, the left kidney lies slightly higher than the right and both should have an ovoid structure, the longitudinal axis is virtually parallel to the spine. In this view the renal pelves drain medially. In later pregnancy the renal vasculature may be seen at the hilum.

In the early stages of pregnancy the kidneys may be quite difficult to image in obese patients or if the fetus is lying with its spine either posteriorly or vertically in the scanning plane. Identification may be facilitated during fetal breathing which causes longitudinal excursions of the kidneys against the spine. Visualisation is also often difficult in oligohydramnios when kidneys must be identified to exclude renal agenesis. A vaginal transducer may be helpful in these cases as the fetus is often a breech presentation deep in the pelvis.

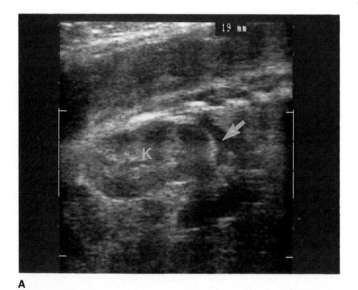

A

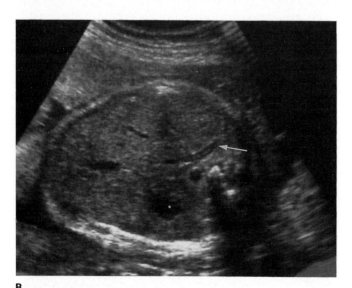

B

Fig. 43 Adrenal glands. A: Parasagittal and **B:** transverse scans at 36 weeks to show adrenal glands (arrow). K – kidney.

The renal pelvis The prominence of the intrarenal pelvis is the subject of much debate. Studies are in hand to ascertain the limits of normal size. For the present an arbitrary figure of 5 mm for the mean transverse and anteroposterior diameters has been chosen as the accepted upper limit.

Normally the extrarenal pelvis cannot be seen but slight prominence may be a normal variant.

The bladder

The bladder is seen as an echo-free structure of variable size arising from the pelvis. Prior to the fourteenth week urine production is limited so that the bladder may not be identified easily. Thereafter urine production progressively increases to a rate of approximately 50 ml per hour at term.[10] If the bladder cannot be identified or if it seems excessively full a repeat examination after about half an hour should show filling in the former and emptying in the latter. Bladder volume is assessed by measuring the bladder outline in three dimensions and halving their product. The bladder should have no internal echoes.

The adrenal glands

The adrenal glands are situated between the upper pole of each kidney and the liver on the right and the spleen on the left (Figs 41B and 43). They may be difficult to identify owing to shadowing from the ribs. Nevertheless normal ranges for adrenal dimensions have been constructed (see Appendix).[11,12] Of importance in diagnostic ultrasonography is that the adrenal glands may take on an enlarged ovoid shape in cases of renal agenesis and be mistaken for kidneys.

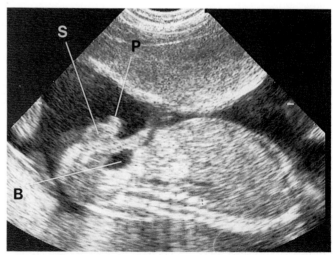

B

Fig. 44 Male genitalia. Sagittal scan of a 20 week fetus to show male genitalia. B – bladder, P – penis, S – scrotum.

Fetal genitalia

The male phallus may be demonstrated from quite early in the second trimester if the fetus is in a favourable supine position with its hips abducted (Fig. 44). However, sex assignation at this stage is imprudent as the clitoris may also be prominent. Later in pregnancy the scrotum is more evident and contains the testes (Fig. 45). These are best seen in a scan tangential to the upper thigh with the fetal legs flexed. In this plane the vulva may also be seen as fine lines (labia minora) between the mounds of the labia majora (Fig. 46).

Musculoskeletal system

Long bones (see Appendix)

It is important to measure femur length and to examine limb morphology in any routine 18 to 20 week scan. Firstly because femur length has been shown to be as accurate an indicator of fetal gestational age as biparietal diameter[13-15] and serves as a useful alternative in dating a pregnancy when the head is in a difficult position for measurement. Furthermore, when checked against other fetal measurements, pathologies such as limb reductions or microcephaly should be detected. Fetal limb reductions or deformities are a feature of many lethal or crippling congenital disorders (trisomy 18, the chondrodysplasias, arthrogryposis multiplex congenita, TAR syndrome, etc.) most of which should be detected in the second trimester by careful ultrasound examination.

The femur is best located initially by scanning the fetus across the trunk in the axial plane and running down the fetal axis until the pelvic bones are identified. The proximal ends of one or both femora will then be seen. Keeping the femur in the image, the transducer is then rotated about the axis of the scanning plane until the whole of the ossified diaphysis (shaft) of the bone is in view (Fig. 47A). It is common practice to align the femur parallel to the transducer. However, this may give rise to an overestimate of the femoral length owing to beam spread effects. Alignment of the femur at about 45° to the transducer minimises this artefact, which can be reduced further by lowering the transmit power. Slight lateral shift of the scanning plane should cause the whole bone to disappear from view. If this manoeuvre causes apparent shortening or lateral shift of the bone in the image then the full length of the bone is not within the scanning plane and further rotational adjustment of the transducer is necessary. Inclusion of the limb extremities (knee and buttock, elbow and shoulder etc.) in the image will help in correct alignment. Finally ensure that the diaphysis to be measured is not overshadowed by other bony structures and that adjacent bones are not included in the measurement. Accuracy may be improved if several measurements of the bone are taken until they are consistent.

The technique for humerus measurement is similar to that for the femur (Fig. 47B). With older machines it is sometimes difficult to differentiate the humeral extremities from their adjacent articulations (scapula/clavicle and olecranon process of ulna) but with modern high resolution equipment this should not be a problem. Humerus length is a useful alternative measure of fetal age if the femur is obscured, as may occur in a breech presentation.

The distal long bones are identified by following on from the proximal. One forearm is often obscured behind the fetal head or body but will eventually move into view. Because radial hypoplasia or aplasia is a feature of many important syndromes the radius and ulna (Figs 47D and 48) should be visualised independently in all cases and measured separately in high-risk examinations. The tibia

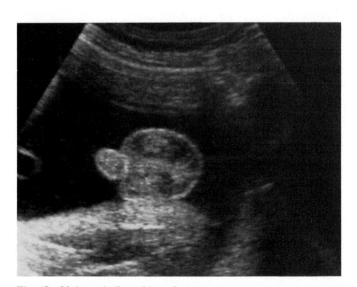

Fig. 45 Male genitalia at 36 weeks.

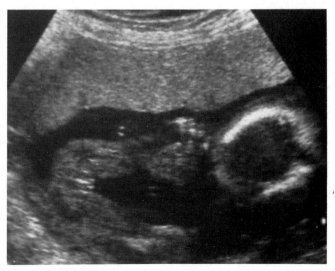

Fig. 46 Female genitalia. Scan of a female fetus at 22 weeks gestation.

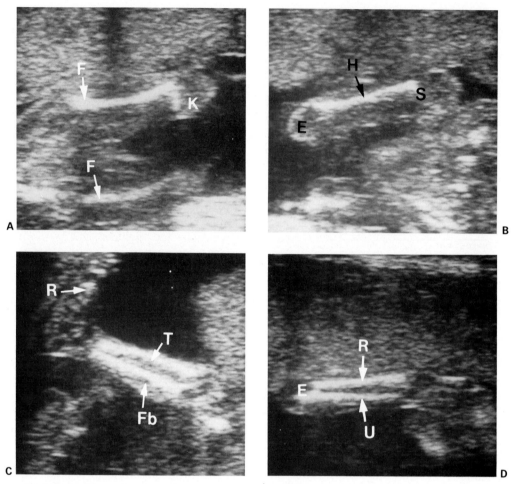

Fig. 47 Measurements of the long bones in a fetus of 18 weeks. Note the soft tissue extremities beyond the diaphysis at each articulation.
A: Femur (F). Only the proximal femur is fully visualised. Note the expansion of the diaphysis at the femoral condyles and the knee (K) beyond.
B: Humerus (H). S – shoulder, E – elbow. **C:** Tibia (T) and fibula (Fb). The heel and toes can be seen on the foot. **D:** Radius (R) and ulna (U).
The ulna is longer owing to the olecranon. E – elbow.

and fibula (Fig. 47C) are of such similar lengths that they need not be measured independently but should be individually identified.

The upper tibial and lower femoral epiphyses will appear in the third trimester (Fig. 49). The exact timing of their appearance is variable and may be affected by growth impairment. The value of using them to date pregnancies in the third trimester is limited.

The feet may be viewed in three major planes (Figs 50 to 52) to identify deformities such as talipes, rocker bottom feet, poly/syndactyly etc. Recently interest has been aroused in the ultrasonic recognition of the 'sandal gap'[16] between the big and second toes and its application to the diagnosis of Down's syndrome. Its application to clinical practice has yet to be evaluated. Foot length (heel to big toe) and femur length should be approximately equal in the second trimester, the foot usually being slightly larger. Hands should be examined so as to reveal four fingers and

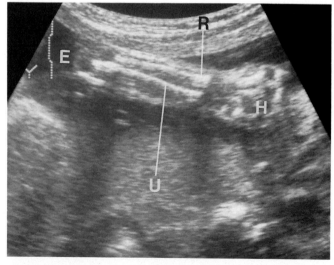

Fig. 48 Forearm. Radius (R) and ulna (U) at 28 weeks showing greater anatomical detail than in Figure 47D. E – elbow, H – hand.

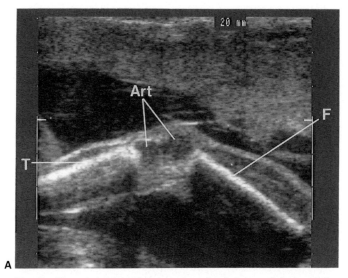

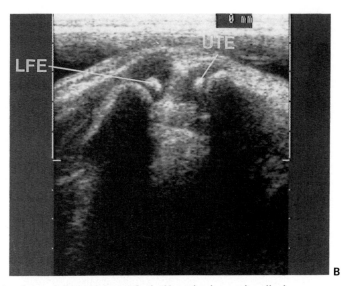

Fig. 49 Knee epiphyses. Scans to show development of the lower femoral and upper tibial epiphyses. **A:** At 29 weeks the unmineralised epiphyseal cartilages of the knee (Art). T – tibia, F – femur. **B:** At 38 weeks the lower femoral (LFE) and the upper tibial epiphyses (UTE) have begun to ossify.

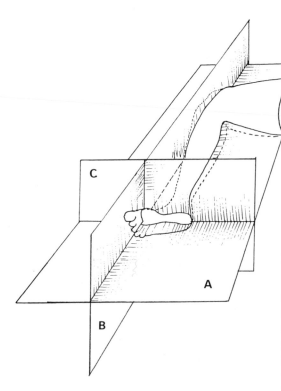

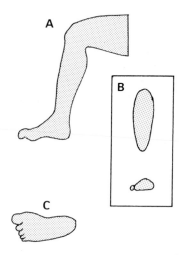

Fig. 50 Diagram of planes for measurement of the foot.

a normal thumb (Fig. 53). It may take a little time before the fetus opens the hand to reveal all digits.

Hip, knee, ankle, elbow, wrist and finger joints should be studied for normal position and movement.

Amniotic fluid

Prior to the fourteenth week of pregnancy the amniotic fluid is chiefly a transudate across the fetal skin and membranes. Thereafter fetal urine production increasingly contributes to amniotic fluid so that by the twentieth week urine accounts for the majority. Amniotic fluid volume rises progressively from about 250 ml at 16 weeks to a fairly constant mean of 800 ml in the third trimester with a slight reduction post-term.[16] Production is most rapid between 24 and 28 weeks. The constant volume is obtained by a balance of fetal swallowing and micturition. Any disturbance in this balance such as reduced urine outflow (urinary tract obstruction, renal pathology or disturbed physiology), impaired intestinal absorption of fluid (duodenal atresia) or possibly excessive contribution of transudate from disrupted skin coverings (omphalocele, meningocele, teratoma) will cause the volume to rise or fall.

Accurate measurement of amniotic fluid is time consuming. A simple estimate may be obtained by measuring

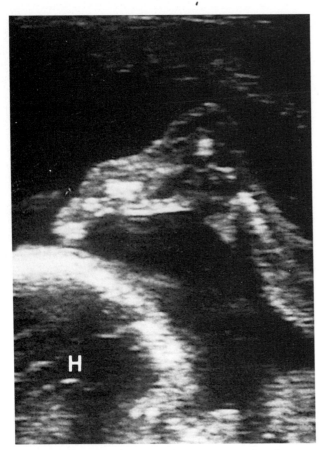

Fig. 51   Foot. Sagittal scan of the foot (22 weeks) – plane A. H – head.

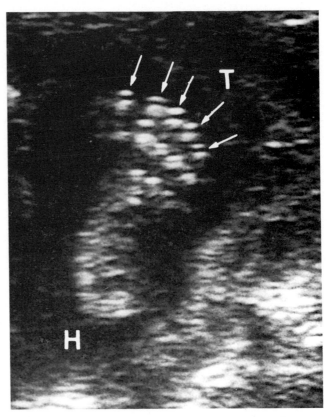

Fig. 52   Foot. Axial scan of the foot – plane C. H – heel, T – toes.

the largest pool of amniotic fluid in two dimensions at right angles. In the third trimester measurements between 2 and 8 cm are considered to be normal. Measurements below or above this range indicate oligohydramnios or polyhydramnios respectively (see Ch. 14).

Multiple pregnancy

The accepted incidence of twin pregnancies is one in 80. There are more dizygotic twins than monozygotic. The incidence of triplets is about one in 6000 pregnancies. These incidences are increasing with the more widespread use of ovulation stimulation and extracorporeal fertilisation.

Multiple pregnancies are at increased risk of fetal malformation, spontaneous abortion, growth retardation, placenta praevia, polyhydramnios and preterm labour. Routine ultrasound examination enables early detection of multiple pregnancy and timely institution of management regimes designed to reduce morbidity from these complications. All mothers of multiple pregnancy should be offered a full anomaly scan and serial scans for fetal growth. It is prudent to scan at 4 weekly intervals with extra examinations according to clinical need.

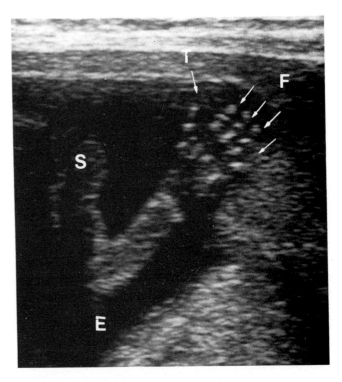

Fig. 53   Scan of the forearm and fanned hand (17 weeks). Contours of the shoulder (S), elbow (E), thumb (T) and fingers (F) can be seen. The fifth finger is partly obscured.

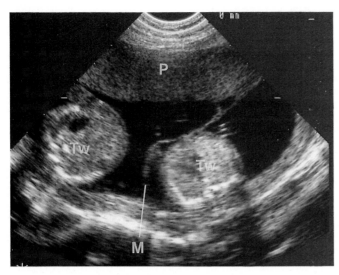

Fig. 54 Twin pregnancy showing the trunk of each twin (Tw) in transverse section and the membrane (M) dividing the two sacs. The attachment of the membrane to the placenta (P) can be seen on the left.

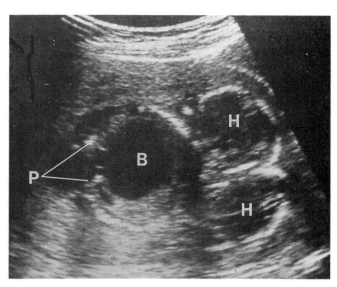

Fig. 55 Conjoint twins. Two heads (H) can be seen above a common trunk with fused pelvis (P) and common, distended bladder (B). There were two complete spines, two legs and four arms.

The only certain way to distinguish binovular from monovular twins is to identify different sexes. The thickness of the dividing membrane between the sacs (Fig. 54) or apparent placental unity are unreliable indications. When no dividing membrane can be seen the differential diagnosis is between severe oligohydramnios in one sac and a mono-amniotic pregnancy. Both situations carry a high risk and require skilled examination as fetal abnormality or a shared circulation are distinct possibilities.

In examining a multiple pregnancy a highly systematic approach should be adopted, starting with examination of the head and carefully following the continuity of the body through the trunk and onto the limbs. With mobile fetuses, and particularly with triplets, this is the only way to ensure full examination of each fetus. Ensuring that each fetus moves independently from the other excludes conjoint twins (Fig. 55). Shadowing of one fetus by the other is a frequent impediment to full examination but patience will eventually be rewarded!

REFERENCES

1 Shepard M, Filly R A. A standard plane for biparietal diameter measurement. J Ultrasound Med 1982; 1: 145–147
2 Chudleigh P, Pearce J M. Obstetric ultrasound: how, why and when. Edinburgh: Churchill Livingstone. 1986: p 65
3 Benaceraff B R, Chann A, Gelman R, Laboda L A, Frigoletto F D Jnr. Can sonography reliably identify anatomic features associated with Down's syndrome in fetuses? Radiology 1989; 173: 377
4 Fried A M, Loh F K, Umer M A, Dillon K P, Kryscio R. Echogenicity of fetal lung: relation to fetal age and maturity. AJR 1985; 145: 591–594
5 Griffin D. Fetal activity. In: Studd J. ed. Progress in obstetrics and gynaecology, volume 4. Edinburgh: Churchill Livingstone. 1984: p 92–117
6 Schmidt W, Yarconi S, Jeanty P, Grannum P, Hobbins J C. Sonographic measurements of the fetal spleen: clinical implications. J Ultrasound Med 1985; 4: 667–672
7 Goldstein I, Reece E A, Yarkoni S, Wan M, Green J C, Hobbins J C. Growth of the fetal stomach in normal pregnancies. Obstet Gynecol 1987; 70: 641–644
8 Grannum P, Bracken M, Silverman R, Hobbins J C. Assessment of fetal kidney size in normal gestation by comparison of ratio of kidney circumference to abdominal circumference. Am J Obstet Gynecol 1980; 136: 249–254
9 Jeanty P, Dramaix-Wilmet M, Elkhazen N, Hubinont C, van Regemorter N. Measurements of fetal kidney growth on ultrasound. Radiology 1982; 144: 159–162
10 Nicolaides K H, Peters M T, Vyas S, Rabinowitz R, Rosen D J, Campbell S. Relation of rate of urine production to oxygen tension in small-for-gestational-age fetuses. Am J Obstet Gynecol 1990; 162: 387–391
11 Jeanty P, Chervenak F, Grannum P, Hobbins J C. Normal ultrasonic size and characteristics of the fetal adrenal glands. Prenat Diagn 1984; 4: 21–28
12 Lewis E, Kurtz A B, Dubbins P A, Wapner R J, Goldberg B B. Real time ultrasonographic evaluation of normal fetal adrenal glands. J Ultrasound Med 1982; 1: 265–270
13 O'Brien G D, Queenan J T, Campbell S. Assessment of gestational age in the second trimester by real time ultrasound measurement of the femur length. Am J Obstet Gynecol 1981; 139: 540–545
14 Hadlock F P, Harrist R B, Deter R L, Park S K. Fetal femur length as a predictor of menstrual age: sonographically measured. AJR 1982; 138: 875–878
15 Quinlan R W, Brumfield C, Martin M, Cruz A C. Ultrasonic measurement of femur length as a predictor of fetal gestational age. J Reprod Med 1982; 27: 392–394
16 Nicolaides K H. Personal communication. 1990

Establishing gestational age

J. Malcolm Pearce and Richard De Chazal

Introduction

Ultrasound measurements in the first half of pregnancy are now widely used to confirm or establish gestational age despite the paucity of objective evidence of benefit in the low-risk population. In the high-risk patient it appears to be logical to establish gestational age by means of ultrasonic measurements as changes in such parameters will be used subsequently to determine intra-uterine growth (see Ch. 13). This section details the methods of obtaining the measurements used to determine gestational age, reviews the currently available charts and examines the evidence for routinely establishing gestational age in all pregnancies.

Clinical methods of establishing gestational age

The gestational age of a pregnancy can only be reliably estimated if the date of conception is known. This is rarely known in spontaneous conceptions but is accurately known in assisted conception cycles. In most cases the gestational age is estimated by assuming that the date of conception occurs 2 weeks after the date of the last period, but this only holds if the following conditions apply:

a) the date of the last period is accurately known;
b) the menstrual cycle is a regular 28 days;
c) there is no history of bleeding in early pregnancy;
d) the woman has not been taking the oral contraceptive pill for 2 months prior to the last period.

In these circumstances the expected date of delivery (EDD) can be determined from Naegele's formula and the current gestational age can be determined by the use of a gestational calculator.

Unfortunately some 25% to 40% of patients[1,2] will not have fulfilled the above criteria and therefore the length of pregnancy based upon the date of the last period is usually known as the post-menstrual age. Additional clinical evidence of the gestational age may be gained from:

a) the date of the onset of pregnancy symptoms – these may be completely absent in a multigravid and in any pregnancy may vary in presentation from 3 to 8 weeks post-menstrual age;
b) the date of the first positive pregnancy test. Modern tests are based upon monoclonal antibodies to human chorionic gonadotrophin (HCG) and are positive from about 10 days after conception. Traditional urinary pregnancy tests become positive at 6 weeks gestation but become negative again at 16 to 18 weeks gestation as the urinary HCG levels decline;
c) the date of onset of fetal movements. This is widely quoted as 22 weeks in primigravidae and 16 weeks in multigravidae. In all patients, however, there is approximately a 7 week range in maternal perception of first fetal movements;[3]
d) clinical examination by an experienced obstetrician in

the first 12 weeks of pregnancy is accurate to within ± 2 weeks gestation but ultrasonic measurement of crown-rump length is more reliable;[4]

e) X-rays of the fetus to determine gestational age were often used in the last 6 weeks of pregnancy prior to planned elective delivery. Ultrasonic determination of gestational age in early pregnancy has been shown to be superior to X-rays in late pregnancy.[4]

Evaluation of ultrasound charts used to determine gestational age

Introduction Any variable that changes with increasing gestational age may be used to establish gestational age. Ideally, a dating chart is then constructed by measuring this variable on a regular basis in a sample of pregnant women in whom the date of conception is accurately known. As determining the date of conception is impossible in most women, data are usually derived from women with a menstrual history that fits the above criteria. In order to evaluate the available charts sufficient detail should be given to determine a) that the sample of women chosen does not differ in important ways from the local population and b) that the statistical analysis was correctly performed.

a) Assessing the sample used to construct the chart Fetal size at birth is known to be affected by multiple factors but fortunately most of the factors only appear to act in the second half of pregnancy. There is, for example, little or no evidence that fetal size in early pregnancy is affected by race.[5–7] Factors such as socio-economic group, parity and maternal age have not been systematically evaluated but the charts that are available for determining gestational age are widely applicable. The similarity is remarkable despite the differences in sample. There are few statistical guidelines on how many patients should be used to construct such charts but for cross-sectional studies (see below) a minimum of 100 patients would seem reasonable.

b) Statistical analysis When a series of ultrasound measurements of a structure that varies with increasing gestational age is recorded, these measurements have to be summarised and a data reference range produced. In its simplest form the data may be described by a mean (and standard deviation) for each week of gestation. This does not use all the available information, and it is usual to employ regression analysis. The details of this method are beyond the scope of this chapter, but the following questions should be asked before using published tables:

a) Does the study contain longitudinal or cross-sectional data?
Many charts employ serial data on a small group of patients (longitudinal studies). This does not meet the strict criteria of independence that is a requirement for regression

analysis. Single measurements on a large series of patients (cross-sectional data) is the most suitable method to construct the chart.

b) Is the chart a growth curve or a dating chart?
In regression analysis two variables are employed with the independent variable being plotted on the x axis (abscissa). This is commonly post-menstrual age. The subsequent curve then describes the change in the dependent variable (for example BPD) with post-menstrual age and is known as a growth curve. If the ultrasonic measurement is made to be the independent variable then a dating curve may be constructed. This curve is often different to the growth curve, not only in shape but also in the variance about the regression line.

c) Are the distribution assumptions correct?
Figure 1 illustrates a calculated regression line that has been superimposed upon the original data. The line does not pass exactly through the data points and the differences between the data points and the line are known as residuals. If the regression line is appropriate then the residuals should have the following properties:

i) They should be normally distributed in a unimodal fashion and the authors should provide evidence to this fact. If the residuals are not normally distributed then the line is a poor representation of the data and the data confidence intervals will be incorrect.

ii) A plot of the residuals against the independent variable should yield a straight line centred on zero. If the line is curved a more complex regression model may be appropriate.

Finally it is important to determine that the scatter (variance) of the data points is similar across the whole range of the independent variable and the results of such an homogeneity test should be reported.

(d) Have the data confidence intervals been correctly constructed?

These lines usually contain 95% of the data and, for sound statistical reasons, should diverge at each end.

More detailed statistical information is available in the standard references.[8]

Gestation sac volume

Introduction   The gestation sac is demonstrated as a circular echo-free area enclosed by a reflective ring within the uterine cavity. It is visible from 5 to 6 weeks post-menstrual age by transabdominal scanning or a week earlier using trans-vaginal scanning (Fig. 2). Gestational age may be established by estimating the sac volume, but the method is inaccurate. For this reason crown-rump length or biparietal diameter measurements are preferred.

Method
Transabdominal scanning   The patient should have a full bladder in order to displace the uterus out of the pelvis and to provide a good acoustic window. A 3.5 or 5 MHz transducer is suitable and the patient is scanned suprapubically in the midline in the sagittal plane until a longitudinal view of the uterus is obtained. Slight lateral movements of the transducer are then made until the longest diameter of the gestation sac is visualised. The image is then frozen and the longitudinal diameter (L) and the anteroposterior diameter (AP) are measured (Fig. 3). The transducer is then rotated through 90° and small adjustments are made until the largest sac diameter is again visualised and then the transverse diameter (T) is measured (Fig. 3). The gestation sac volume (GSV) can then be de-

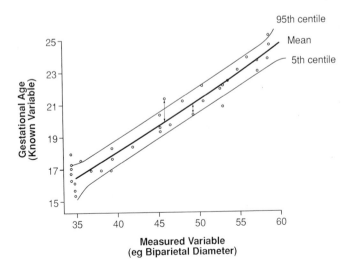

Fig. 1   An illustration of a regression line (with data confidence limits) superimposed on the raw data. Two of the residuals are indicated by arrows.

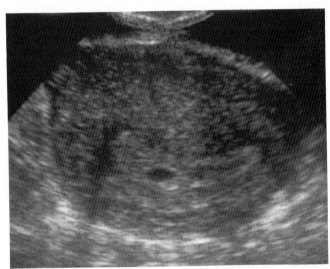

Fig. 2   Trans-vaginal demonstration of early sac. A trans-vaginal scan showing an intra-uterine gestation sac at 5 weeks post-menstrual age.

termined from the following formula: GSV (ml^3) = L(cm) × AP(cm) × T(cm) × 0.5.

Trans-vaginal scanning   In this case the bladder is emptied and a high resolution 7 or 7.5 MHz transducer used. The probe is orientated in the sagittal plane and then slight lateral movements of the transducer handle are made until the full length of the gestation sac is visualised. The longitudinal (L) and anteroposterior (AP) diameters are then measured. A true transverse section cannot usually be obtained with the vaginal probe so a coronal section has to be used. Keeping the gestation sac in view twist the transducer handle through 90°. The maximum diameter of the sac is then obtained by a combination of gentle panning movements across the vagina with slight anteroposterior rocking movements. The maximum diameter is measured and the GSV is derived from the above formula by including this latter measurement as T.

Problems   The gestation sac may change shape between the acquisition of the two frozen images leading to errors in both directions. Using the transabdominal approach the gestation sac may not be visualised in its transverse section if the uterus is retroverted. With an acutely anteflexed or retroflexed uterus, only oblique views of the gestation sac may be possible with trans-vaginal scanning and if these are used, an overestimate of the GSV will occur.

Choice of charts   All of the available charts of GSV are of the growth curve type and therefore cannot be recommended for the purposes of establishing gestational age.

Clinical use of GSV   Routine use of GSV for establishing/confirming gestational age is rarely used because of the inherent errors, the lack of dating charts and because a further scan is necessary in later pregnancy in order to confirm the presence of a viable fetus. Its major use is in establishing the diagnosis of a missed abortion. An embryo and cardiac activity should always be visible when the GSV is 2.5 ml^3 or more.[9]

Crown-rump length

Introduction   The embryo can be visualised from 6 weeks post-menstrual age with a standard transabdominal approach and from 5 weeks trans-vaginally. Cardiac activity can usually be detected about a week before the embryo is resolved. Correctly performed measurements of crown-rump length (CRL) are the most accurate means of estimating gestational age, because the embryo grows very rapidly in the early weeks. The ability to obtain an accurate CRL depends solely upon the operator's ability to obtain a true longitudinal section of the unflexed embryo with end points clearly visualised.

Method   Owing to movements of the embryo there can be no standardised technique for obtaining a CRL. Having located a longitudinal section of the gestational sac, if the embryo is not visualised, then slide the transabdominal transducer (or pan the trans-vaginal transducer) slowly

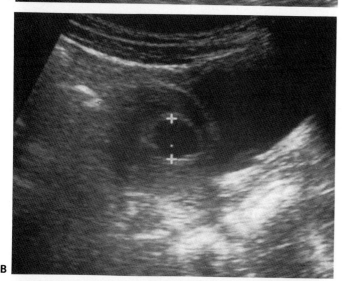

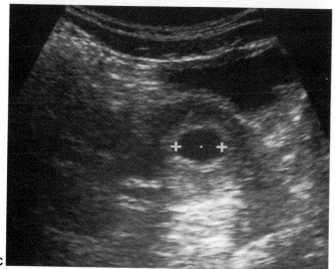

Fig. 3 Gestation sac volume measurement. A longitudinal view of the gestation sac demonstrating measurement of **A**: the longitudinal and **B**: the anteroposterior diameter. **C**: A transverse section of the gestation sac demonstrating measurement of the transverse diameter.

across the gestation sac until part of the embryo becomes visible. Keeping this in view, the transducer is then rotated until the long axis of the embryo is obtained (Fig. 4). From about 9 weeks onwards the spine can be easily identified and this simplifies obtaining a true longitudinal view. Once this is obtained the image is frozen and the measurement is obtained (Fig. 5), from crown to rump.

Problems The yolk sac should not be included in the CRL measurement as this will artefactually increase the gestational age (Fig. 4). The CRL is difficult to measure after 10 weeks gestation when the fetus is often curled (Fig. 5). If the fetus cannot be seen in an extended position then it may be measured by a curved line or by the use of several straight lines (Fig. 6).

Choice of charts Table 1 illustrates the results from the three published charts that have used CRL as the independent variable and meet the statistical criteria detailed above. The charts appear stable with a mean difference of

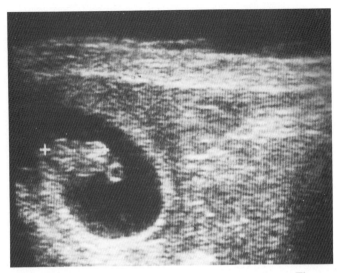

Fig. 4 Measurement of CRL (+. . . .+) in early pregnancy. The yolk sac is visible as a small circular structure.

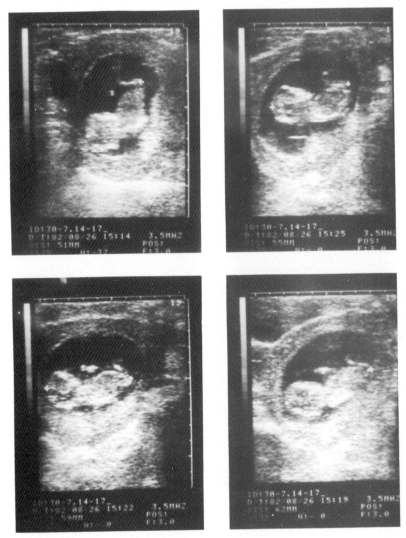

Fig. 5 **Errors in measurement of CRL.** The bottom left hand image is correct with a CRL of 59 mm. The range of 51 to 62 mm is equivalent to 1 weeks error in estimating gestational age.

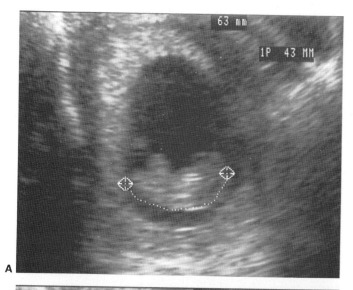

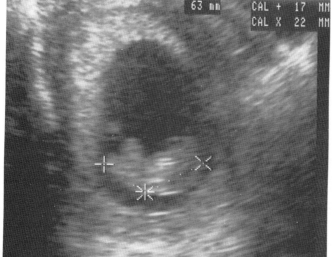

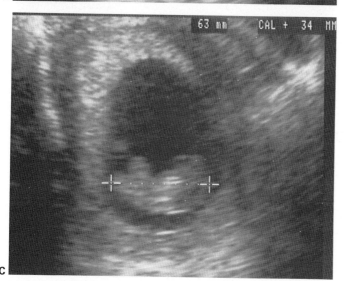

Fig. 6 Technique of CRL measurement on a curled fetus. A: By use of on-screen curvilinear measurement (CRL = 43 mm). **B:** By use of multiple short linear calipers (CRL = 17 + 22 = 39 mm). **C:** Demonstrates that use of linear calipers on a curled fetus gives an underestimate (CRL = 34 mm).

Table 1 Prediction of gestational age in weeks from CRL

CRL (mm)	Drumm[10]	Author Robinson[11]	Nelson[12]
10	6.9	7.0	8.1
12	7.3	7.4	8.3
14	7.6	7.7	8.5
16	7.9	8.0	8.6
18	8.2	8.3	8.8
20	8.5	8.5	9.0
22	8.7	8.8	9.2
24	9.0	9.0	9.3
26	9.2	9.3	9.5
28	9.5	9.5	9.7
30	9.7	9.7	9.9
32	9.9	9.9	10.0
34	10.1	10.1	10.2
36	10.4	10.3	10.4
38	10.6	10.5	10.5
40	10.8	10.7	10.7
42	11.0	10.8	10.9
44	11.2	11.0	11.1
46	11.3	11.2	11.2
48	11.5	11.4	11.4
50	11.7	11.5	11.6

only 0.18 weeks which is unlikely to be clinically significant. All three studies are cross-sectional and the largest study (n = 253)[10] takes into account biological variation as well as potential sources of error.

Biparietal diameter

This measurement has been subject to more studies than any other and is used to confirm/establish gestational age in most pregnancies. The recommendations given in this chapter are based upon those of the British Medical Ultrasound Society Ultrasonic fetal measurement survey.[13]

Method Biparietal diameter measurement is best done with a 3.5 to 5 MHz linear or curved array transducer. Firstly, determine the lie of the fetus and then find the longitudinal axis. This is carried out by sliding the transducer across the maternal abdomen until the fetal heart is found. Keeping the fetal heart in view, the transducer is rotated until the fetal head comes into view. Sliding movements, combined with alterations in the angle of the transducer, bring a longitudinal section of the spine into view and demonstrate the strong midline echo in the fetal head. Keeping the midline in view, rotate the transducer through 90° until a transverse section of the fetal head is obtained. The correct section should demonstrate the following features (Fig. 7):

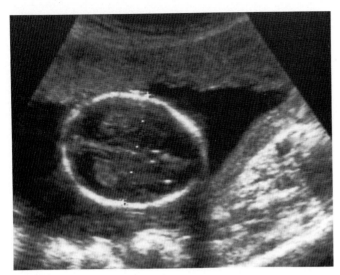

Fig. 7 BPD measurement. A transverse section of the fetal head at the level recommended for measurement of the BPD. The cursors demonstrate the site of measurement.

a) an oval shaped head
b) a short midline in the anterior two thirds of the head
c) the cavum septum pellucidum
d) the basal cisterns.

If the midline is not exactly in the middle of the fetal head, then the angle of asynclytism is wrong and this can be corrected by changing the angle of the transducer to the surface of the maternal abdomen. If the head is not ovoid (rugby ball shaped) then rotation of the transducer is required. Having achieved the correct shape with a central midline echo, the above listed features are sought by small sliding movements of the transducer.

Freeze the image. The biparietal diameter (BPD) is the maximum diameter of the fetal skull at the level of the parietal eminences. It is measured by placing the horizontal component of the on-screen caliper on the outer table of the proximal surface of the fetal skull. The horizontal component of the second caliper is then placed on the inner table of the distal surface of the fetal skull at right angles to the midline and at the widest diameter (Fig. 7).

Problems a) Breech and transverse positions. Measurement of the BPD when the fetus is in either of these positions may lead to an underestimation if the fetal head is dolichocephalic (long and narrow). The fetal head takes on this shape because of the effects of maternal breathing movements and because of pressure from the transducer. If this is suspected then the cephalic index should be determined; if this is less than 75, the measurement of the BPD is unreliable. The cephalic index is the BPD divided by the occipitofrontal diameter (OFD), measured along the length of the midline of the fetal skull (from outer table to outer table) multiplied by 100.[14]

b) Occipito-anterior (OA) and occipitoposterior (OP) positions. Measurement of the BPD can only be made

when the fetal head is in the transverse (OT) position as the landmarks can only be seen when the midline echo from the fetal head is at 90° to the line of the ultrasound beam. When the fetal head is in an OA or OP position, pressure on one end of the transducer may cause the head to rotate; alternatively, tilting the patient slightly head down may move the fetus. If these manoeuvres fail, then estimation of gestational age can be made from femur length but the patient should be rescanned in order to check the intracranial anatomy.

Choice of charts Charts based upon images obtained from static scanners are probably not appropriate for modern real time equipment. The conclusions reached by the BMUS committee were that the data from Hadlock[15] should be used as this was the only published series that met the following criteria:

a) use of a section with well-defined landmarks;
b) use of outer table to inner table measurements with real time apparatus assuming a speed of 1540 m/sec;
c) cross-section data analysed by appropriate regression analysis with the BPD as the independent variable;
d) adequate description of the population sample.
   Hadlock[15] had 533 middle class Caucasian women in his study. The data from this study are shown in Table 2.

Table 2 Prediction of gestational age from BPD (from Hadlock[15])

BPD (mm)	mean (weeks)	95% data confidence limits
35	16.5	15.7–17.3
38	17.4	16.6–18.2
41	18.3	16.4–20.2
44	19.2	17.3–21.1
47	20.2	18.3–22.1
50	21.2	19.3–23.1
54	22.5	20.6–24.4
57	23.5	21.6–25.4
60	24.6	22.7–26.5
63	25.7	23.8–27.6
66	26.8	24.7–28.7
69	28.0	24.7–31.3
73	29.5	26.2–32.8
76	30.8	27.5–34.1
78	31.6	28.3–34.9
81	32.5	29.2–35.8
83	33.8	30.5–37.1
85	34.7	31.4–38.0
87	35.6	32.3–38.9
90	37.0	33.7–40.3
94	38.9	35.6–42.1

Head circumference and abdominal circumference

These measurements are not used to estimate gestational age in the routine situation. They may, however, be included when there is lack of agreement between the post-menstrual age and the gestational age as determined from the BPD and the femur length. The recommended data for these parameters are from the studies of Hadlock[16] and Deter.[17]

Femur length

On a routine basis gestational age can be confirmed or established by the use of the BPD and femur length. Like the BPD, measurement of the femur appears to be highly reproducible, probably because of precisely defined end points.

   The fetal femur is easily located by finding a cross-section of the fetal body and then sliding the transducer caudally along the fetal trunk until a cross-section of the femur is visualised. Keeping the femur in view, the transducer is then rotated until the full length of the bone is displayed. Both ends of the femur should be clearly visualised and neither end should appear to merge with the skin as this produces a foreshortened view. Measurement of the length is made from the centre of the U-shape at each end of the bone (Fig. 8) as this represents the length of the diaphysis.

   Problems   There are few problems with femur length measurements provided the bone can actually be visualised. Ideally the femur should be at 45° to the ultrasound beam because if it is at 90° the bone may be artefactually lengthened by side lobe artefacts (Fig. 9).

   Choice of charts   Table 3 illustrates the prediction of gestational age from femur length by the three studies[18-20]

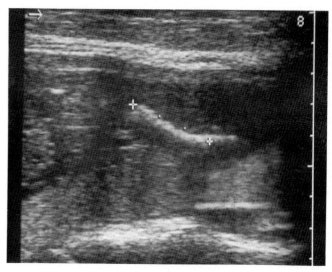

Fig. 9   A femur demonstrating side lobe artefacts. The cursors indicate the true femur length and the artefact can be seen projecting beyond the right hand cursor.

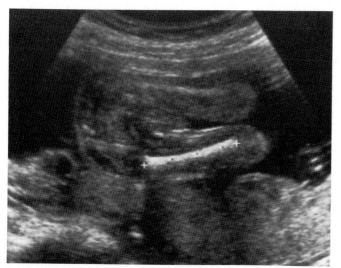

Fig. 8   Measurement of the femur length.

Table 3   Prediction of gestational age in weeks from femur length

Femur length (mm)	Hadlock[18]	Hohler[19]	Jeanty[20]
10	12.8	12.0	12.6
12	13.4	12.6	13.3
14	13.6	13.2	13.9
16	14.5	13.9	14.6
18	15.1	14.5	15.2
20	15.7	15.2	15.9
22	16.3	15.8	16.6
24	16.9	16.5	17.3
26	17.6	17.2	18.0
28	18.2	17.9	18.7
30	18.9	18.6	19.4
32	19.6	19.4	20.1
34	20.3	20.1	20.9
36	21.0	20.9	21.6
38	21.8	21.6	22.4
40	22.5	22.4	23.1
42	23.3	23.2	23.9
44	24.1	24.0	24.7
46	24.9	24.8	25.4
48	25.7	25.7	26.2
50	26.5	26.5	27.0
52	27.4	27.4	27.8
54	28.2	28.3	28.6

Table 4 Variability (2SD) in the prediction of menstrual age (from Hadlock[21])

Gestation interval (weeks)	Variability (weeks)				
	12–18	18–24	24–30	30–36	36–42
Measurement					
BPD	1.19	1.73	2.18	3.08	3.20
HC	1.19	1.48	2.06	2.98	2.70
AC	1.66	2.06	2.18	2.96	3.04
FL	1.38	1.80	2.08	2.96	3.12
BPD, FL	1.08	1.34	1.86	2.52	2.28
BPD, FL, AC	1.20	1.52	1.82	2.50	2.52
BPD, HC, FL, AC	1.08	1.40	1.80	2.44	2.30

Key:
SD – standard deviation of the regression equation representing overall variability
BPD – biparietal diameter
FL – femur length
HC – head circumference
AC – abdominal circumference

that most closely fit the statistical criteria. There is very little difference between the results of these studies.

Multiple parameters

Hadlock et al[21] have examined the use of BPD, head circumference, abdominal circumference and femur length and demonstrated that prior to 18 weeks post-menstrual age the use of multiple variables does not improve the prediction of gestational age obtained by use of the BPD alone. In later pregnancy however, multiple variables do reduce the uncertainty of the prediction, especially when measurements are made for the first time in the third trimester (Table 4).

Choice of measurements for routine ultrasound examinations

In the setting of a routine ultrasound clinic it is recommended that the minimum measurements used to establish gestational age are those of the BPD and the femur length. The following situations may then arise:

a) prediction of the gestational age from measurements of the BPD and femur agree with the post-menstrual age – in this case accept the post-menstrual age as an accurate prediction of gestational age;

b) prediction of gestational age from the measurements of the BPD and femur agree but are outside the data confidence limits for the post-menstrual age. In this case the gestational age should be revised to correspond to the ultrasound measurements if this is less than 18 weeks; if not, the head and abdominal circumferences should be

measured and the gestational age estimated using multiple measurements;

c) the post-menstrual age agrees with the prediction from the BPD but the femur length suggests an earlier gestation: a limb reduction deformity should be considered (see Ch. 20);

d) the post-menstrual age agrees with the prediction from the femur length measurement but the BPD measurement suggests an earlier gestation: the possibility of spina bifida or of microcephaly should be considered (see Ch. 16).

Multiple pregnancy

Measure the BPD and the femur length on all the fetuses. It is rare for fetuses to be different sizes in early pregnancy but if this is the case the pregnancy should be dated on the measurements from the largest fetus.

The evidence for routine ultrasound examination to confirm or establish gestational age

In attempting to determine whether routine ultrasound for the purposes of establishing gestational age is superior to selective ultrasound, two types of studies have been carried out:

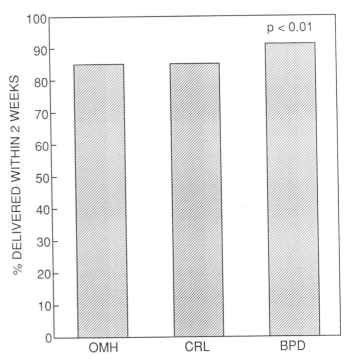

Fig. 10 The accuracy of the prediction of the date of delivery from optimal menstrual history (OMH), the crown-rump length (CRL) and the biparietal diameter (BPD). In a routine clinic only the BPD is significantly better than the OMH.

a) studies that estimate the precision of one or several ultrasound measurements. These studies all use patients with a reliable menstrual history to establish gestational age but, because the date of ovulation is not accurately known, they are inherently flawed;

b) studies that have attempted to demonstrate benefit from a policy of routine scanning. Ideally such studies should be randomised controlled trials comparing the two policies using a reliable outcome measure such as perinatal mortality. Such studies would require extremely large numbers of patients and will probably never be carried out in a developed country. Most studies that have been published have used the date of delivery as the end point (for example see Fig. 10). All have demonstrated that the incidence of pregnancies exceeding 42 weeks gestation is approximately halved (about 6% of patients) when ultrasound is routinely used to establish gestational age. Table 5 illustrates the rates of induction observed in the reported randomised controlled trials. Overall there is a trend to a reduction in the induction rates but only one study has addressed the question of whether this affects the perinatal outcome. Eik-Nes[22] demonstrated that four infants delivered to mothers induced because of post-dates were considered preterm by the paediatricians in the selective scanning group whereas this did not occur in the routine group. In addition infants in the routine scanning groups needed to spend fewer days in the special care unit.

In conclusion there is currently little evidence to justify the routine use of ultrasound solely to confirm gestational age. However, as routine ultrasound in early pregnancy is necessary in order to recognise multiple pregnancies and to exclude major structural abnormalities such examination should include the confirmation of gestational age because of the suggestion of marginal benefit from the reduction in the prevalence of post-dates pregnancies.

Table 5 Induction rates (%) in randomised controlled trials of selective versus routine ultrasound scanning

Author	Routine scanning		Selective scanning
Bennett[1]	19.6	NS	20.2
Bakketeig[23]	6.3	NS	7.6
Eik-Nes[22]	1.9	**	7.8
Waldenstrom[24]	5.9	***	9.1

Key:
** $p < 0.01$
*** $p < 0.001$

REFERENCES

1 Bennett M J, Little G, Dewhurst C J, Chamberlain G V P. Predictive value of ultrasound measurements in early pregnancy: a randomised controlled trial. Br J Obstet Gynaecol 1982; 89: 338–341

2 Warsof S, Pearce J M F, Campbell S. Routine ultrasound screening. Clin Obstet Gynecol 1983; 10: 445–459

3 Grennert L, Persson P H, Gennser G. Benefits of ultrasound screening of a pregnant population. Acta Obstet Gynecol Scand (suppl) 1978; 78: 5–14

4 Robinson H P, Sweet E M, Adam A H. The accuracy of radiological estimates of gestational age using early crown rump length measurements by ultrasound as a basis for comparison. Br J Obstet Gynaecol 1979; 86: 525–528

5 Sabbagha R E, Barton T B, Barton B A. Sonar biparietal diameter. I. Analysis of percentile growth differences in two normal populations using the same methodology. Am J Obstet Gynecol 1976; 126: 479–484

6 Meire H B, Farrant P. Ultrasound demonstration of an unusual fetal growth pattern in Indians. Br J Obstet Gynaecol 1981; 88: 260–263

7 Parker A J, Davies P, Newton J R. Assessments of gestational age of the Asian fetus by sonar measurements of crown-rump length and biparietal diameter. Br J Obstet Gynaecol 1982; 89: 836–838

8 Bland M. An introduction to medical statistics. Oxford: Oxford Medical Publications. 1987

9 Chudleigh P, Pearce J M F. Obstetric ultrasound: how, why and when. Second edition. Edinburgh: Churchill Livingstone. 1990

10 Drumm J E, Clinch J, Mackenzie G. The ultrasonic measurement of fetal crown-rump length as a method of assessing gestational age. Br J Obstet Gynaecol 1976; 83: 417

11 Robinson H P, Fleming J E E. A critical evaluation of sonar 'crown-rump length' measurements. Br J Obstet Gynaecol 1975; 82: 702

12 Nelson L H. Comparison of methods for determining crown-rump length by real time ultrasound. JCU 1981; 9: 67

13 Evans J A, Farrant P, Gowland M, McNay M B. BMUS ultrasonic fetal measurement survey. Br J Radiol 1990; in press

14 Hadlock F P, Deter R L, Carpenter R J, Park S K. Estimating fetal age: effect of head shape on BPD. AJR 1981; 137: 83

15 Hadlock F P, Deter R L, Harrist R B. Fetal biparietal diameter: a critical re-evaluation of the relation to menstrual age by means of realtime ultrasound. J Ultrasound Med 1982; 1: 97–104

16 Hadlock F P, Deter R L, Harrist R B, Park S K. Fetal head circumference: relation to menstrual age. AJR 1982; 138: 649–653

17 Deter R L, Harrist R B, Hadlock F P, Carpenter R J. Fetal head and abdominal circumferences: II. A critical re-evaluation of the relationship to menstrual age. JCU 1982; 10: 365–372

18 Hadlock F P, Harrist R B, Deter R L, Park S K. Fetal femur length as a predictor of menstrual age: sonographically measured. AJR 1982; 138: 875–878

19 Hohler F P, Quetel T A. Fetal femur length: equations for computer calculation of gestational age from ultrasound measurements. Am J Obstet Gynecol 1982; 143: 479–481

20 Jeanty P, Rodesch F, Dekbeke D, et al. Estimation of gestation age from measurements of fetal long bones. J Ultrasound Med 1984; 3: 75–79

21 Hadlock F P, Deter R L, Harrist R B, et al. Estimating fetal age: computer assisted analysis of multiple fetal growth parameters. Radiology 1984; 152: 497–502

22 Eik-Nes S, Okland O, Aure J C, Ulstein M. Ultrasonic screening in pregnancy: a randomised controlled trial. Lancet 1984; 1: 1347

23 Bakketeig L S, Eik-Nes S H, Jacobsen, et al. Randomised controlled trial of ultrasonographic screening in pregnancy. Lancet 1984; 2: 207–211

24 Waldenstrom U, Axelsson O, Nilsson S, et al. Effects of one stage ultrasound screening in pregnancy: a randomised controlled trial. Lancet 1988; 2: 585–588

3D growth

Introduction
Definitions of growth
Normal growth patterns
The gestation sac
Crown-rump length
Fetal abdominal circumference
Biparietal diameter
Other longitudinal studies
Conclusion

Hylton B. Meire

INTRODUCTION

The two chapters which follow are concerned with the application of accepted techniques for the assessment of fetal growth. When evaluating the results and the techniques by which they are obtained it is important for us to be aware of what constitutes growth. Defining the complex processes of growth highlights how incompletely our measurements reflect this.

Growth involves an increase in size of the organism by either an increase in number or size of cells. In the early phase growth is predominantly by cell multiplication (see *Abdominal and General Ultrasound*, Vol. 1, Ch. 17) and, so long as the supplies of oxygen and nutrients to the cells are maintained, this phase of growth continues. For tumour growth this only occurs very early, the lack of structural organisation in a tumour generally leads to the central portion of the tumour outgrowing its blood supply. In the human embryo there is a high degree of organisation and the blood supply is well-maintained to all areas of the developing embryo. This cell multiplication phase of growth therefore continues until at least the end of the first trimester. If we assume that the cell doubling time is constant it will be seen that the total weight or volume of the conceptus should also double during each cell doubling time interval and the rate of increase in the weight of the conceptus will therefore be exponential. However, with ultrasound, we are not able to measure the volume or weight of the conceptus accurately and generally have to confine ourselves to uni-dimensional linear measurements or two-dimensional circumference or area measurements.

Towards the end of pregnancy, in the third trimester, growth is no longer predominantly by cell multiplication with the contribution from cell growth, bone growth etc. increasing. In addition there are complex changes in the relationship between growth of the different components of the fetus, particularly the head and abdomen.

Definitions of growth

When we are assessing the growth of children this is done almost exclusively by measurement of their height and weight. Occasionally head circumference is also monitored. Height is one-dimensional, head circumference two-dimensional and weight three-dimensional and the way in which they reflect the growth of a complex three-dimensional structure is affected by these facts. Similarly when we measure the fetus the crown-rump length and biparietal diameter are one-dimensional, the head and abdomen circumference two-dimensional and the gestation sac volume, fetal weight predictions and total intra-uterine volume estimations are three-dimensional. Not surprisingly the shapes of the growth curves from these different indices of fetal size are not only affected by the growth rate of the fetus itself but also by the mathematical relationship

between the measured value and the growth rate of the three-dimensional structure.[1,2]

There is no universally agreed definition of growth and the 'growth curves' which we customarily use in obstetric measurements reflect the relationship between a linear measurement and the gestational age. The underlying pattern of growth which these charts conceal is not immediately obvious and the subsequent sections of this chapter amplify the relevance of this for measurement of the crown-rump length, biparietal diameter and fetal abdominal circumference.

The concept of 'growth velocity' allows assessment of the rate of change of growth during the gestational age. There is no general agreement about how growth velocity should be assessed and the concepts of both the rate of change of length and rate of change of volume with time are considered.

Normal growth patterns

The gestation sac

The gestation sac is detectable on trans-vaginal ultrasound at 14 days post-conception, and by 18 days its diameters can be measured and its volume calculated. As the pregnancy continues the shape of the gestation sac becomes more asymmetrical and the value of measurement of any single dimension becomes more limited. If normal growth is to be confirmed or the duration of gestation assessed it is essential to compute the volume of the gestation sac by

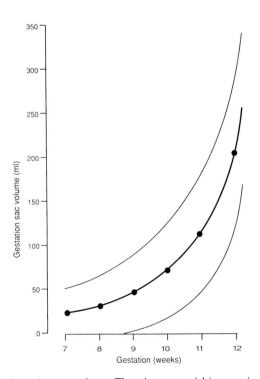

Fig. 1 Gestation sac volume. There is exponential increase in volume during the first 12 weeks of pregnancy.

measurement of three axes at right angles.[3] The graph of gestation sac volume change with increasing gestational age (Fig. 1) is virtually the only instance in current obstetric practice in which volume growth is assessed.

Crown-rump length

The embryo is detectable, on trans-vaginal scanning, at 21 days post-conception when its crown-rump length (CRL) is 4 mm. Using the transabdominal route measurement of the CRL can be made from 6 to 14 post-menstrual weeks. The graphs of Robinson[4] and Drumm[5] (Fig. 2) are a well-accepted method of assessing gestational age, with a high degree of accuracy. It should be noted that this growth shows an upward curve with advancing gestational age, unlike that of the biparietal diameter and abdominal circumference later in pregnancy. The growth of the embryo at this stage in pregnancy is optimal and is predominantly by cell multiplication. There is therefore an exponential increase in the embryonic weight or volume (Fig. 3). The shape of this curve confirms rapid growth at this stage in pregnancy and implies that embryonic growth is occurring at the maximum possible rate.

Crown-rump length growth can alternatively be viewed as the 'growth velocity'; that is the degree by which the CRL increases each week (Fig. 4); the rate of increase in growth velocity is constant, and there is a constant acceleration during this phase of growth. Clearly such growth with constant acceleration cannot continue indefinitely but the mechanisms by which growth is moderated and controlled are, as yet, poorly understood.[6] However, when we look at growth of the other fetal parts throughout the remainder of pregnancy it is clear that

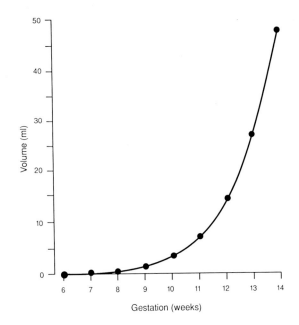

Fig. 3 Embryonic weight or volume. There is exponential growth, probably due to uninhibited cell multiplication at this stage of growth.

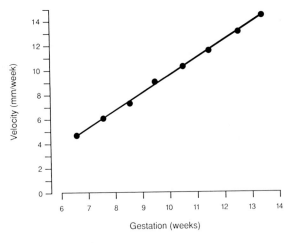

Fig. 4 Growth velocity of crown-rump length. This linear increase in growth velocity (constant acceleration) confirms unrestricted exponential growth.

growth moderation does take place and this affects different components of the fetus to different degrees.

Fetal abdominal circumference

Assessment of fetal trunk growth is generally undertaken by measurement of the abdominal circumference,[7] a two-dimensional index. Typical abdominal circumference growth charts (Fig. 5)[8] do not show straight line growth but an apparent progressive reduction in growth velocity throughout pregnancy. This is a mathematical artefact that results from two-dimensional measurements being taken

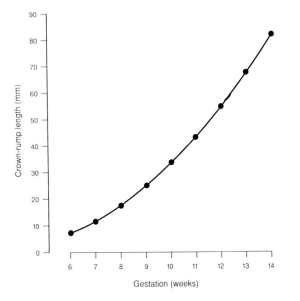

Fig. 2 Crown-rump length. There is a gentle upward curve in the CRL growth during the first trimester.

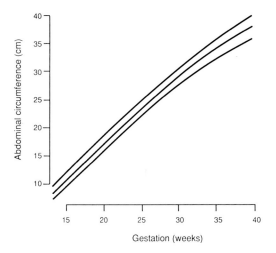

Fig. 5 Abdominal circumference graph. The apparent 'late flattening' in growth is a mathematical artefact.

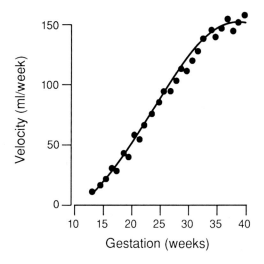

Fig. 7 Abdominal volume growth velocity. The almost linear growth acceleration decreases towards term.

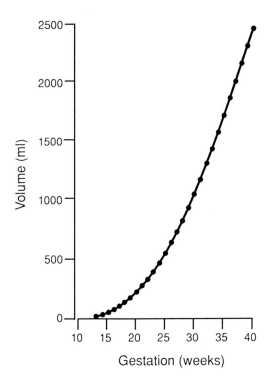

Fig. 6 Fetal trunk volume. The volume growth curve does not show the apparent late flattening.

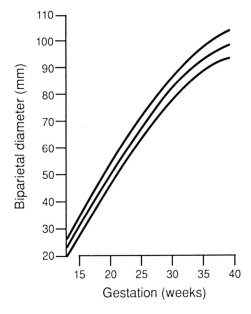

Fig. 8 Biparietal diameter. The apparent 'late flattening' is more noticeable in the head growth curve.

growth acceleration late in pregnancy. It is interesting to compare this with the growth data for the fetal head.

Biparietal diameter

Fetal head growth is customarily monitored by measurement of either the biparietal diameter (BPD)[9] or the head circumference (HC).[7] The growth curves of these two variables are similar and that of the BPD will be considered specifically in this section. The normal curve of BPD against gestational age is generally similar to that of the abdominal circumference (Fig. 8).[8] However, if the head volume is plotted against gestational age a different shaped

from a three-dimensional structure. The growth curve for fetal trunk volume (Fig. 6) shows progressive increase in growth velocity during the first two trimesters and an apparently linear growth velocity thereafter. However, if the abdominal volume growth velocity is plotted in millilitres/week, a progressive fall-off in velocity is seen in the last trimester (Fig. 7). Although abdominal volume continues to increase and the rate of increase (growth velocity) also continues to increase, there is a fall-off in the

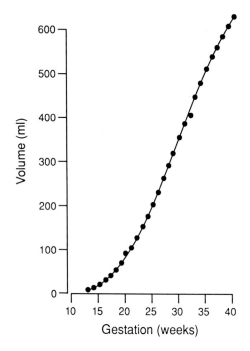

Fig. 9   Fetal head volume. Unlike the abdominal growth (Fig. 6) a slight fall-off in growth rate is evident in the last trimester.

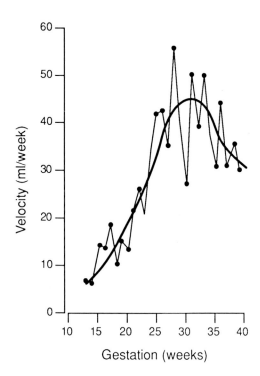

Fig. 11   Serial head measurements on five patients. These pooled measurements suggest that individual fetuses do show late growth deceleration.

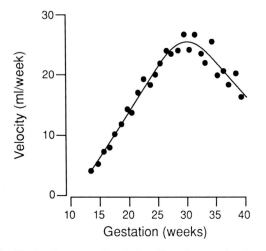

Fig. 10   Head volume growth velocity. There is a genuine 'late flattening' in head growth velocity (compare with Figure 7).

graph results (Fig. 9). Again this is similar to the abdominal volume growth chart but there is a slight decrease in the trajectory in the last trimester. This minor inflection at the upper extremity of the curve conceals a dramatic change in growth velocity (Fig. 10): from approximately 28 weeks gestation onwards there is a progressive reduction in growth velocity which is quite unlike that seen for normal abdominal growth.

It is generally held that fetal growth retardation affects the abdomen preferentially and that brain growth is maintained at the expense of other structures, the 'brain sparing effect'. Figure 10 suggests that there is indeed a normal

reduction in growth velocity of the head towards term and comparative studies suggest that this feature is peculiar to the human. Interestingly there is rapid growth of the head in the first few weeks after birth with apparent neonatal 'catch up growth'. Both of these observations suggest that there is a genuine last trimester reduction in human fetal head growth; the reasons for and the adaptational advantages of this have been the subject of considerable speculation.[10,11]

It is possible that this observation is an artefact arising from the fact that the data are collected from whole populations. If, for example, there was a tendency for babies with larger heads to be born earlier this would result in an apparent reduction in head size of those going to full term. Attempts to clarify this question have centred around the acquisition of 'longitudinal data' involving multiple serial scans on individual patients. Although the inevitable measurement errors on pooled data give rise to large standard deviations (Fig. 11) the continuous line through the mid-points of the data shows the same growth curve as that seen in the cross-sectional studies. This finding supports the observation that there is a genuine reduction in fetal head growth velocity late in pregnancy.

Other longitudinal studies

Post-natal growth studies of children are well-recognised as showing 'growth spurts' and periods of little or no growth.

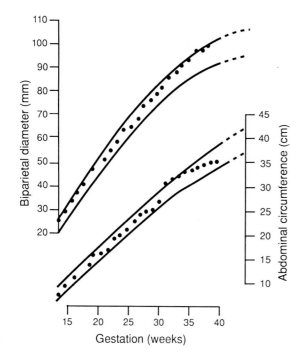

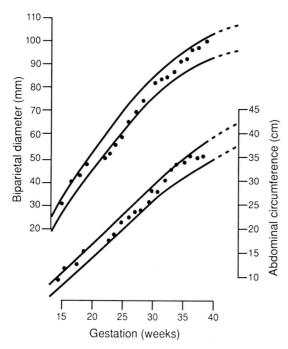

Fig. 12 Longitudinal growth. A and **B:** Serial weekly AC and BPD measurements on two normally growing fetuses. Growth is not linear but appears to be spasmodic (as seen postnatally).

When performing ultrasound examinations we tend to assume that the fetus grows in a continuous uniform fashion throughout the whole of pregnancy, following along a particular centile line. There is no scientific reason for assuming this to be the case and the limited longitudinal patient studies which have been performed suggest that the fetus also shows quite marked variations in growth rate throughout pregnancy (Fig. 12).[1]

Conclusion

The normal patterns of fetal growth are complex and involve differing rates of increase in the volume of the separate components of the fetus throughout pregnancy.

Our relatively simple linear ultrasound measurements give an incomplete estimate of fetal growth and the way in which we customarily plot our data tends to mask the normal growth patterns.

Ideally we should attempt to measure volume and to assess growth velocity. In practice this is currently not feasible as the measurement errors are too large to measure growth velocity accurately and this technique would necessarily require frequent repeat measurements throughout pregnancy.

When performing ultrasound measurements of fetal growth, the factors discussed above should be borne in mind and the limitations of the technique acknowledged.

REFERENCES

1 Meire H B. Ultrasound assessment of fetal growth patterns. Br Med Bull 1981; 37: 253–258
2 Meire H B. Ultrasound measurement of fetal growth. In: Falkner F, Tanner J M. eds. Human growth, a comprehensive treatise. 2nd edition. New York: Plenum Press. 1986: p 275–290
3 Selbing A. Gestational age and ultrasonic measurement of gestational sac, crown-rump length and biparietal diameter during first 15 weeks of pregnancy. Acta Obstet Gynecol Scand 1982; 61: 233–235
4 Robindon H P, Fleming J E E. A critical evaluation of sonar crown-rump length measurements. Br J Obstet Gynaecol 1975; 82: 702–710
5 Drumm J E, Clinch J, MacKenzie G. The ultrasonic measurement of fetal crown-rump length as a method of assessing gestational age. Br J Obstet Gynaecol 1976; 83: 417–421
6 D'Ercole A J, Underwood L E. Regulation of fetal growth by hormones and growth factors. In: Falkner F, Tanner J M. eds. Human growth, a comprehensive treatise. 2nd edition. New York: Plenum Press. 1986: p 327–338
7 Campbell S, Thoms A. Ultrasonic measurement of the fetal head to abdomen circumference ratio in the assessment of growth retardation. Br J Obstet Gynaecol 1977; 84: 165–174
8 Farrant P, Meire H B. A combined biparietal diameter and abdominal circumference graph: using a system velocity of 1540 metres per second. Radiography 1985; 51: 220–221
9 Campbell S, Newman G B. Growth of the fetal biparietal diameter during normal pregnancy. J Obstet Gynaecol Br Cwlth 1978; 78: 513
10 Briend A. Fetal malnutrition – the price of upright posture? BMJ 1979; 2: 317–319
11 Tanner J M. Growth as a target-seeking function. Catch-up and catch-down growth in man. In: Falkner F, Tanner J M. eds. Human growth, a comprehensive treatise. 2nd edition. New York: Plenum Press. 1986: p 167–180

Fetal growth

Martin J. Whittle

INTRODUCTION

Although fetal growth problems are a serious cause of perinatal mortality and morbidity in current obstetric practice, the understanding of the biology of intra-uterine growth remains incomplete. There are both growth promoting and restraining factors, most of which are under some form of genetic control. The issue is, however, complicated by extrinsic factors which may include maternal nutrition, infection and habits such as smoking and alcohol abuse.

Since growth retardation is such an important problem, reliable methods of detection during pregnancy would seem desirable and a number of strategies have been developed, with varying degrees of success. In effect there are two approaches to the problem. The first is screening to identify the pregnancy at risk, and secondly to confirm a clinical suspicion. Unfortunately fetal size alone may not be the most significant factor in the identification of true pathology. The use of other tests such as the biophysical profile (see Ch. 14) and, possibly, new techniques such as Doppler have an important adjunctive role.

Normal intra-uterine growth

Intra-uterine growth is affected by both genetic factors and the supply to the fetus of essential nutrients.

Genetic control

Fetal growth and development goes through three phases:[1]

a) replication or proliferation which may be called hyperplasia;
b) migration, during which process cells move and aggregate to form tissue and organ rudiments;
c) hypertrophy, when the cells increase in size and become part of definitive, functional structures.

These processes are under genomic control but since all embryonic cells have the same 'blueprint'; other influences must cause the differentiation of these early cells into structures with specific function (see Ch. 7). This may be affected by alterations in the DNA or gene arrangement which in turn influence the expression of one gene to alter the response of another. This cascade of genetic activity which controls differentiation and growth is influenced by macromolecules and growth factors which also result from the expression of other genes. The biology of early growth is extremely complex; it forms one of the most challenging and exciting research areas in modern biology.

Growth problems which arise from disorders of the genome itself may be particularly severe. Thus aneuploidy, such as trisomy 18, is often associated with fetal growth disorders and other more subtle abnormalities such as translocations and deletions are also important. Recently there has been particular interest in the concept of genetic imprinting. In this process genes on the male-derived chromosome may produce phenotypic effects, of which differences in growth are just one, to those on the female-derived chromosome.[2]

Infection with certain viruses at a critical stage in embryonic development may interfere with the genomic message and cause either structural abnormalities or reduced growth potential. Rubella and cytomegalovirus are examples of viruses producing these effects.

The genome is also responsible for the production of growth promoting factors such as insulin-like growth factor 1 (IGF-1). The stimulus for genetic expression may relate to nutritional status so that if nutrient supply is diminished IGF-1 manufacture may be reduced. Numerous other growth factors have been isolated and all provide a system which controls growth and differentiation, both from early embryonic existence and throughout life. Although current knowledge is limited, it is expanding rapidly to provide an important insight into the complexities of cellular control.

Nutrient supply

The fetus is uniquely vulnerable since it must rely for its nutritional support on the vascular supply to the uterus[3] and on the function of the placenta.[4] Classical animal experiments indicated the importance of both of these factors in the restriction of fetal growth. Evidence from human pregnancies is also compelling.

The vascular supply is of particular importance; in a normal pregnancy the terminal branches of the uterine arteries, termed 'spiral arteries', become converted into flask-shaped vessels by the removal of the muscularis layer by trophoblasts.[5] This causes them to widen, so allowing an unimpeded flow of maternal blood to the placental bed and thus maximising the exchange potential. Failure of this process seems to be associated with the development of serious complications such as pre-eclampsia and/or fetal growth retardation. It is also known that the mother with vascular disease (e.g. in long standing diabetes or autoimmune diseases such as systemic lupus erythematosus) is much more likely to have a growth retarded baby. Intravascular factors such as sickle cell disease and lupus inhibitor causing coagulopathy are also important.

Placental function is influenced by the maternal vascular supply but it is also possible that humoral factors from the mother control, at a cellular level, certain types of placental activity including its own metabolism. The placental vascular space may well be sensitive to changes in the uterine circulation and an understanding of vascular control within the placenta is only just beginning. Of particular interest are the ways that the placenta may modulate growth in the fetus, not only by changes in nutrient supply but also through the secretion of growth controlling substances.[6] It is possible that there is considerable metabolic 'cross-talk' between the fetus and the placenta.

Abnormal intra-uterine growth

Definition

Considerable confusion surrounds the term 'small for dates' and 'intra-uterine growth retardation' such that they are often erroneously used interchangeably.

i) Small for dates The term 'small for dates' is merely a statistical definition relating to a group of babies found at or below the tenth, fifth or third centile for weight (depending on the chosen centile) of a normally distributed population (Fig. 1).

Although the definition of a 'small for dates fetus' seems simple, difficulty is caused by the variation between birthweight charts; a baby defined as normal by one standard may be small by another. For many years the Lubchenko birthweight charts were used as the 'gold standard' but they may not always be appropriate since they were derived from a population in Denver, Colorado some 5000 feet above sea level. It has become obvious that different populations show considerable variations in their birthweight characteristics. The Aberdeen birthweight data (the most commonly used in the UK) when applied to the

Glasgow population for example, suggest that substantially more babies are small for dates than if local, Glasgow-derived, figures are used.[7]

Whether standard deviation or centiles should be used on birthweight charts depends on the nature of the weight distributions around the mean. Standard deviations are more appropriate when the distribution is symmetrical. Early studies suggested a non-symmetrical distribution, hence the frequent use of centiles. In fact, however, adjustment of the data with accurate knowledge of the gestational age normalises the distribution, making standard deviation the more appropriate measure.[8] In practical terms it probably matters little and other factors such as ethnic origin and the baby's sex may be much more relevant.

ii) Intra-uterine growth retardation (IUGR) The definition of fetal growth retardation is inexact but may be diagnosed when the growth rate deviates significantly from an established norm. IUGR may be implied from the presence of markers such as reduced amounts of amniotic fluid, diminished fetal activity and, more recently, abnormal Doppler waveforms in the umbilical artery. Alternatively the diagnosis of growth retardation can be made retrospectively from the appearances and condition of the newborn. The rapid growth observed in most of these babies once released from the in utero restraints also suggests the diagnosis.

Clinical significance

The risk of being either small for dates or growth retarded is not easy to discern from the literature which relates most often to only birthweight.

Perinatal loss in babies born weighing less than 2.5 kg represents just under 30% of the total perinatal mortality[9] and probably about a fifth of these babies are small for dates. How many of them are actually growth retarded is impossible to discern and, in addition, the proportion of babies weighing 2.5 kg and more who are also growth retarded is unknown. However, the importance of establishing the diagnosis of small for dates is underlined by the fact that when perinatal loss occurs in this group it is much more likely to result in a stillbirth rather than a neonatal death.[10]

Small for dates fetuses who survive to the neonatal period may have problems including the development of hypoglycaemia, hypothermia and birth asphyxia while the preterm, small for dates baby appears to have an excess mortality compared with the one which is of an appropriate weight for dates.[11] In a Scottish study the small for dates babies born alive before 37 weeks had a mortality rate of 12.4% in contrast to babies of appropriate weight of 5%.[12]

Long-term morbidity for the small for dates or IUGR baby is also difficult to assess but there are indications of a statistically significant excess of learning and

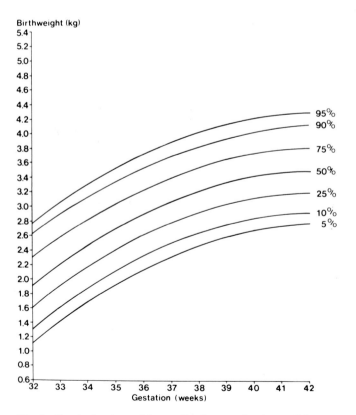

Fig. 1 Graph showing weight centiles for gestational age. (After Thompson.[36])

psychomotor problems.[13,14] More recently evidence of long-term consequences of intra-uterine growth retardation have emerged with an apparent increase in the risk of subsequent development of hypertension in later life.[15]

It would seem that the identification of the small for dates baby in the antenatal period should have an important impact on perinatal mortality and morbidity in current obstetric practice. Unfortunately the evidence that this is so is not convincing, possibly because of the diverse nature of the aetiological factors.

Aetiology

i) Maternal factors There are numerous maternal factors which may affect fetal growth. These are summarised below:

Small for dates – maternal causes
Constitutional
  i) maternal height/weight
  ii) ethnic group
  iii) socio-economic group/nutritional support
Toxins
  i) smoking
  ii) alcohol abuse
  iii) drugs – both addictive and therapeutic
Illness
  i) hypertensive disease – pre-eclampsia, renal disease etc.
  ii) autoimmune disorders – systemic lupus erythematosus
  iii) cyanotic heart and respiratory disease
  iv) haematological disease – sickle cell etc.
  v) long standing diabetes.

Apart from the problem of defining a normal population important factors which influence birthweight include birth order, parental height (particularly the mother's) and ethnic group. This last has always been difficult to separate from economic and social factors but studies in Singapore, which allow the comparison of three different ethnic groups living under similar circumstances, show clear differences in birthweight distributions.

Social and economic status remain important influences on both perinatal outcome and fetal growth in particular; the reasons for this may be partly nutritional or related to habits such as smoking. The effect of diet is difficult to assess, but the starvation of women during the Dutch famine and the siege of Leningrad in the Second World War caused a significant increase in the number of small for dates babies. Supplementation of nutritional requirements may improve pregnancy outcome and have a small effect on birthweight.

Maternal disease, either pre-existing or coincidental with pregnancy, may interfere with fetal growth, and of particular importance are the vascular changes associated with hypertension and microvascular disease.

ii) Fetal factors The fetal causes for poor fetal growth include the following:

Small for dates – fetal causes
  i) chromosome disorders – especially trisomy 13 and 18
  ii) infections – viral such as rubella, cytomegalovirus etc.
  iii) non-chromosomal syndromes
  iv) multiple pregnancy
  v) fetal sex
  vi) birth order

A variety of pathologies may be responsible which, as discussed above, usually relate to interference with the fetal genome. Severe damage usually results in spontaneous abortion, but occasionally the pregnancy survives to term, when the disturbance may manifest itself as growth retardation.

Fetal size is a particular problem in multiple pregnancy. In about two thirds of twin pregnancies one of the babies is born weighing less than 2.5 kg.[16] This low birthweight partly arises because of preterm delivery, which occurs in almost half of cases compared with the singleton rate of about 5%.[16] Although perinatal loss in twins is often the result of immaturity, intra-uterine death occurs (with a frequency of two to three times the singleton rate) in pregnancies of 37 weeks or more in which the babies weigh less than 2.5 kg. Of particular importance is the situation in which there is discordant growth, when the smaller baby is at considerably greater risk.

Why babies from multiple pregnancy should be smaller than singletons is unclear but good teleological reasons may be suggested, including a biological advantage in keeping the intra-uterine contents to the minimum. However, it is also possible that there is a relative failure of nutrient supply which may explain the higher incidence of intra-uterine death in the more mature babies.

iii) Uteroplacental factors Concepts on the role of the placenta in controlling fetal growth have already been discussed in some detail. This area of study may in fact provide important information concerning the aetiology of currently 'unexplained' fetal growth retardation with or without maternal hypertension.

Methods of growth assessment

Biparietal diameter (BPD)

In early work using ultrasound to assess fetal growth the BPD was measured simply because it was the only measurement which could be made reliably. For it to have any value at all the level in the head at which the measurement had to be taken needs to be carefully defined (Fig. 2) so that the section includes the midline echo with the cavum septum pellucidum in the anterior third and the thalami

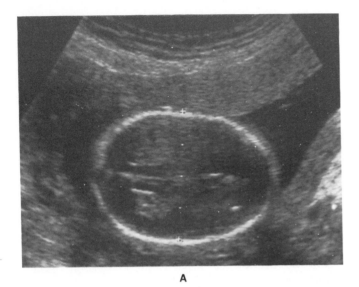

A

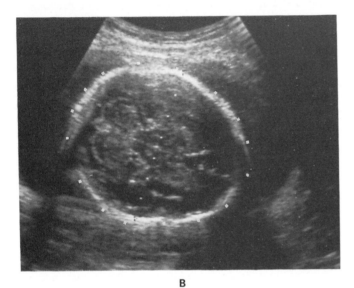

B

Fig. 2 Head measurements. A: Biparietal diameter and **B:** head circumference measurement.

on either side. With great care this is a reproducible measurement with an accuracy of about 1 mm.

Using this technique several workers observed that BPD increased steadily throughout gestation[17,18] but that after about 32 weeks the rate of change decreased and, in fact, the difficulty of accurate measurement increased. Nevertheless it became obvious that up to about 20 weeks the BPD gives an accurate guide to gestational age which in itself formed the basis upon which to judge whether growth retardation was a problem.

The use of BPD as a method of assessing growth has been largely abandoned because the concept that increase in BPD reflects overall fetal growth has been shown to be misplaced. Firstly the increase in head size, which does reflect brain growth, may persist for some time in the face

of quite severe growth retardation. Secondly, although an easy measurement to make, the BPD becomes increasingly inaccurate in the latter weeks of pregnancy, just when an assessment of growth may be most important. Finally the spread of normal BPD size becomes very wide after 32 weeks, again reducing the value of the method as means of identifying the small fetus.

Head circumference (HC)

HC measurements are made at the same level as the BPD but involve a circumference rather than a diameter assessment and this has led to the development of a number of measuring devices including light pen systems, joy sticks and expanding ellipses.

A number of groups have produced charts of HC against gestational age; the two most often used are very similar.[19,20] They both show that changes in HC, like BPD, tend to tail off towards term (Fig. 3) but the standard deviations are much less, so the likelihood of identifying the growth retarded fetus may be higher. In addition, HC is much less dependent on head shape so that the dolichocephalic head, which is narrow but long, has an appropriate circumference for gestational age but a small BPD. However all head measurements become harder to perform in late pregnancy and the brain sparing effect affects both the HC and BPD.

Cerebellar growth

Cerebellar growth has been shown to be reasonably linear from about 14 to 40 weeks[21] with the transverse diameter in millimetres being roughly equivalent to the gestational age in weeks (Fig. 4). The measurement is more difficult to make in the latter weeks of pregnancy but the cerebellar diameter does offer an objective assessment of gestational age throughout pregnancy. Of particular relevance is the

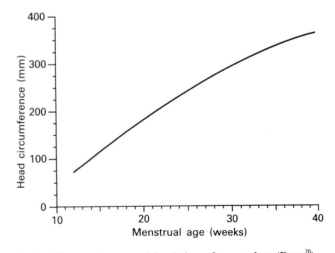

Fig. 3 Ultrasound measured head circumference chart (Deter[20]).

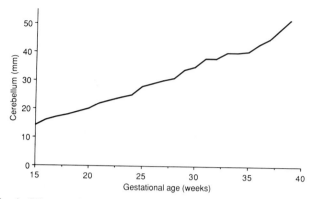

Fig. 4 Ultrasound measured cerebellar diameter. Mean for gestational age (Goldstein[21]).

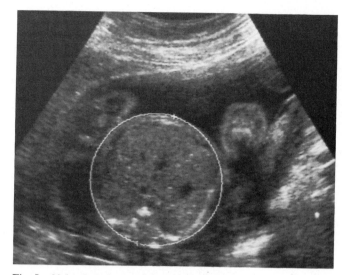

Fig. 5 Abdominal circumference measurement.

fact that the cerebellum does not seem to be affected by intra-uterine growth retardation.

Femur length (FL)

FL is primarily a measurement for the estimation of gestational age with good accuracy from around 15 to 25 weeks.[22] Its use in the estimation of fetal growth is limited, although it has been combined with other measurements to estimate fetal size (see below).

Abdominal circumference (AC)

The AC is undoubtedly the best parameter with which to assess both fetal size and growth because the measurement is taken at the level of the fetal liver which constitutes about 4% of the total fetal weight and which steadily increases in size with gestational age.

Measurement of the AC must be at a carefully defined level in the fetal abdomen if consistency is to be achieved. A British Medical Ultrasound Society Bulletin[23] recommended the Deter tables[20] as the most appropriate. That recommendation has now been altered to the data of Jeanty et al.[24] Figure 5 indicates a cross-sectional view of the fetal trunk with the intrahepatic portion of the umbilical vein situated in the anterior third of the abdominal circumference. This view is best achieved by first aligning the ultrasound transducer with the fetal aorta and then turning it through a right angle.

Tabular data for normal values of fetal growth and gestational age suggest a fairly linear growth throughout (Fig. 6), in contrast to head measurements, although the standard deviations widen towards term. Because of this linear relationship, it has been proposed that a weight estimation taken at, say, 26 weeks may allow the prediction of weight at term.[25] The potential importance of this is found in the philosophy that each baby has its own growth profile which, if not followed, results in growth retardation regardless of absolute weight.

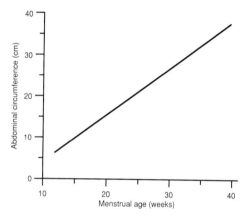

Fig. 6 Ultrasound measured abdominal circumference chart (Jeanty[24]).

Complicated formulae have been devised for estimation of fetal weight but none is very accurate and errors of between 10% and 15% are reported. Attempts to reduce these errors have been made by introducing other measurements such as HC, FL and BPD[26-30] but the best, and probably the most accurate measurement sets are AC and FL, with an absolute error of 7.6%. Other measurements of the fetal abdomen have been used including the area and transabdominal diameters. Although they have their proponents their use seems to confer no additional value to the assessment of fetal growth or size.

Fetal growth dynamics

Normal growth

The original concepts about intra-uterine growth were extrapolated from birthweight data relying on two premises.

The first is that the gestational age at the time of delivery was known accurately, and the second that those babies born prematurely were 'normal' and likely to be of an appropriate weight.

As previously mentioned the sigmoid curve which is usually found for birthweight charts becomes more linear with adjustment of the gestational age but nevertheless the distribution of weights is negatively skewed prior to 36 weeks,[8] implying that babies born prematurely tend to be smaller.

One of the advantages of ultrasound is that it allows repeated examinations of the fetus; both head and abdominal measurements have been used to plot fetal growth and normal patterns have been established for both these components, singly and in combination. Interestingly estimations of weight using such measurements, especially prior to 36 weeks, tend to exceed the weight established from birthweight charts which also suggests that babies born preterm are likely to be smaller than might be expected.

Asymmetrical and symmetrical growth patterns

Considerable debate surrounds the use of the terms 'asymmetrical' and 'symmetrical' growth retardation to describe patterns of growth seen in utero in relation to head and abdominal circumferential measurements. Head size increases because of the progressive growth of the fetal brain and, as mentioned, this is maintained for some time, despite intra-uterine starvation. Fetal liver size, which is the main contributor to the abdominal girth, normally increases steadily throughout pregnancy due to the accumulation of glycogen and storage substances. However, in contrast to the brain, liver growth seems very sensitive to reductions in the supply of nutrients and so provides a potentially useful marker of intra-uterine starvation.

Thus an asymmetrical pattern of growth retardation develops because of continuing head growth with little or no increase in abdominal girth, leading to a high head/abdominal circumference ratio. These changes are probably most often observed when IUGR has a vascular or uteroplacental basis.

In contrast, symmetrical growth retardation, when both head and abdominal size are proportionally small, may be found either with a normal, small for dates fetus or when there has been some serious early insult to the developing embryo, fetus or even possibly the placenta.

From a clinical standpoint the symmetrically small baby has potentially more uncorrectable pathology than the asymmetrical type since intrinsic problems are more likely. However many of these babies are, in fact, just small but normal and in others only the dates are wrong. The latter group is now rare in the UK, although it remains a sig-

nificant obstetric dilemma in countries where early ultrasound dating is not readily available.

Identification of fetal growth retardation

Fetal growth is a dynamic process and yet often only single measurements of the fetus are available to evaluate fetal size at any time. Serial ultrasound measurements are required to measure a growth rate, but they are tedious and time consuming and often not practical clinically. These concerns have led to a search for other methods to identify the pregnancy in which the fetus is growth retarded such as the biophysical profile, and Doppler studies of the umbilical and uterine arteries.

Abdominal measurements

It is apparent that unless serial measurements are taken of any of the indices discussed above it is unlikely that the slowing of growth in an individual fetus could be identified with any degree of certainty. Various strategies have been devised to overcome this difficulty, including the extrapolated growth curve discussed above.[25]

Most groups have used a two stage system, with one early 'dating scan' and one later scan,[31] or just one late scan, in an attempt to identify the fetus at risk. Unfortunately none of the studies demonstrate that in low-risk groups screening in this way has any impact on pregnancy outcome,[32] in spite of the fact that the tests themselves have a reasonable positive predictive power of about 50% to 60%, which is well in excess of the 30% to 40% often quoted for most clinical methods.

HC/AC

One of the weaknesses of a single measurement of AC is that even if it gives some indication of fetal size it does not necessarily help in the identification of pathology. As described above the measurement of both HC and AC allow the independent assessment of head and abdominal growth which tends to differ under circumstances of vascular or placental failure such that head growth is maintained for some time while abdominal growth slows or even ceases. These changes cause the HC/AC ratio (Fig. 7) to rise making it possible to identify the truly growth retarded fetus from a single study. Unfortunately the potential of the HC/AC ratio to assign fetal growth to either an asymmetrical or symmetrical pattern does not run true in practice, although the sensitivity of the ratio for a small for dates baby is about 70%.[33]

Total intra-uterine volume (TIUV)

Since true growth retardation is usually associated with a reduction in size of not only the fetus but also the placenta

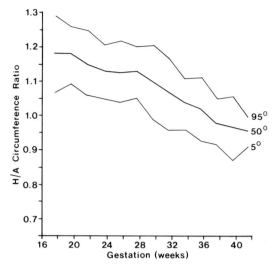

Fig. 7   **Ultrasound measured head/trunk circumference ratio chart** (Campbell and Thoms[33]).

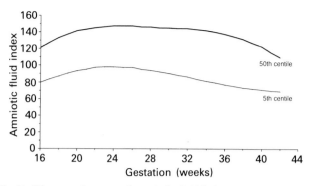

Fig. 8   **Ultrasound measured amniotic fluid index and gestational age** (Moore and Cayle[36]).

and amniotic fluid volume, it is not surprising that an ultrasound assessment which includes them should provide a sensitive test for IUGR. Early reports seemed to suggest this[34] but subsequent studies were less encouraging,[35] indicating that although the sensitivity was around 60%, the predictive value was low at 30%.

Since the technique itself is complex and its practical value limited it is not generally used. However it should be remembered that the end point chosen to evaluate the test, the small for dates fetus, will include many perfectly normal babies who just happen to be small. In view of this TIUV needs to be re-evaluated in terms of the truly pathological pregnancies.

Amniotic fluid volume (AFV)

The use of amniotic fluid volume in the evaluation of the fetal condition is well-established and has been discussed at length in Chapter 14. A reduction in AFV is an important sign that the fetal condition may be impaired, and perinatal mortality rises sharply in these circumstances. From a strictly technical viewpoint accurate measures of AFV are impossible and a number of strategies have been employed. The volume of single pockets of fluid rarely give a good overall impression and a subjective assessment is probably the most commonly used method. The amniotic fluid index (AFI) may prove to be useful and involves the summing of amniotic fluid depth in the four quadrants of the uterus. Normal values have been produced (Fig. 8)[36] which suggest a minimum acceptable index of about 65 mm.

As for the HC/AC ratio and TIUV the AFV should provide direct evidence of pathological growth retardation,

since production of amniotic fluid is reduced in the presence of either vascular or placental deficiency. Most studies suggest that pregnancy outcome is impaired when the AFV is reduced.

Other methods

More recently, alternative methods of fetal evaluation have been assessed approaching the problem from a different direction. Often the identification of growth problems is 'retrospective' only being noticed once it is present. Using Doppler ultrasound to examine the umbilical and uterine arteries it has been suggested that abnormalities in the flow velocity characteristics may predate the development of growth problems (see Ch. 15). Whether all that has been claimed for this new technique will be ultimately established remains to be seen, but the prospect of an effective screening test for fetal growth problems is exciting.

Conclusion

Fetal growth retardation remains a serious obstetric problem both because of the difficulties of identification and the associated perinatal mortality and morbidity. Unfortunately there is no clear definition of what is meant by growth retardation and most statistics deal largely with babies that are small for dates, or perhaps even just small, rather than truly pathologically affected.

In the assessment of the baby suspected of growth problems a number of techniques need to be employed of which ultrasound is just one. Markers likely to indicate a pregnancy at risk of growth retardation, such as hypertension, renal disease or autoimmune problems, are important together with use of cardiotocography and possibly Doppler studies. The aim is to build an overview of the fetal condition, and what has led to it, and to develop a clinical strategy to ensure the best possible outcome.

REFERENCES

1 Han V K M. Genetic mechanisms of regulation of fetal growth. In: Sharp F, Milner R D G, Fraser R B. eds. Fetal growth. England: Peacock Press. 1989: p 77–81

2 Hall J G. Genomic imprinting: review and relevances to human diseases. Am J Hum Gen 1990; 46: 857–873

3 Clapp J F, Szeto H H, Larrow R, Hewitt J, Mann L I. Umbilical blood flow response to embolization of the uterine circulation. Am J Obstet Gynecol 1980; 138: 60–67

4 Robinson J S, Kingstone J E, Jones C T, Thorburn G D. Studies on experimental growth retardation in sheep. The effect of removal of endometrial caruncles on fetal size and metabolism. J Dev Physiol 1979; 379–398

5 Brosen I A, Dixon H G, Robertson W B. Fetal growth retardation and the vasculature of the placental bed. Br J Obstet Gynaecol 1977; 84: 656–664

6 Hayy W W. Placental control of fetal metabolism. In: Sharp F, Milner R D G, Fraser R B. eds. Fetal growth. England: Peacock Press. 1989: p 33–52

7 Forbes J F, Smalls M J. A comparative analysis of birthweight for gestational age standards. Br J Obstet Gynaecol 1983; 99: 297–303

8 Perrson P H. Fetal growth curves. In: Sharp F, Milner R D G, Fraser R B. eds. Fetal growth. England: Peacock Press. 1989: p 13–26

9 SHHD. Report on maternal and perinatal deaths in Scotland. 1981–1985. Edinburgh: HMSO. 1989

10 Whitfield C R, Smith N C, Cockburn F, Gibson A A M. Perinatally related wastage – a proposed clarification of primary obstetric factors. Br J Obstet Gynaecol 1986; 93: 694196703

11 Stewart A. Fetal growth: mortality and morbidity. In: Sharp F, Milner R D G, Fraser RB. eds. Fetal growth. England: Peacock Press. 1989: p 403–412

12 Dickson D M, Forbes J F. Anthropometric standards and the risk of mortality in preterm infants. Social, paediatric and obstetric research unit. University of Glasgow. 1987

13 Neligan G A, Kolvin I, Scott D Mc I, Garside R F. Born too soon or born too small? A follow up study to seven years of age. Philadelphia: Spastic International Medical Publications. William Heineman Medical Books. 1976: p 66

14 Fitzhardinge F M, Kalman E, Ashby S, Pape K. Present status of the infant of very low birthweight treated in a referral neonatal intensive care unit in 1974. In: Major mental handicap: methods and costs of prevention. Amsterdam: Elsevier Excerpta Medica. 1978: p 139–150

15 Barker D J P, Bull A R, Osmond C, Simmonds S J. Fetal and placental size and risk of hypertension in later life. BMJ 1990; 301: 259–262

16 Scottish twin study. Social, paediatric and obstetric research unit. University of Glasgow. 1983

17 Willocks J, Donald I, Campbell S, Dunsmore I R. Intrauterine growth assessed by ultrasonic fetal cephalometry. J Obstet Gynaecol Br Cwlth 1967; 74: 639–647

18 Campbell S, Dewhurst C J. Diagnosis of the small for dates fetus by serial ultrasonic cephalometry. Lancet 1971; 2: 1002–1006

19 Hadlock F P, Deter R L, Harrist R B, Park S K. Fetal head circumference: relation to menstrual age. AJR 1982; 138: 647–653

20 Deter R L, Harrist R B, Hadlock F P, Carpenter R J. Fetal head and abdominal circumference: II. A critical re-evaluation of the relationship to menstrual age. JCU 1982; 10: 365–372

21 Goldstein I, Reece A, Pilu G, Bovicelli L, Hobbins J C. Cerebellar measurements with ultrasonography in the evaluation of fetal growth and development. Am J Obstet Gynecol 1987; 156: 1065–1069

22 Hadlock F P, Harrist R B, Deter R L, Park S K. Fetal femur length as a predictor of gestational age: sonographically measured. AJR 1982; 138: 875–878

23 Evans J A, Farrant P, Gowland M, McNay M J. BMUS Ultrasonic fetal measurement survey. Br J Radiol 1990

24 Jeanty P D, Cousaert M S, Cantraine F. Normal growth of the abdominal perimeter. Am J Perinatol 1984; 1: 129–135

25 Deter R L, Harrist R B, Hadlock F P, Poindexter A N. Longitudinal studies of fetal growth with the use of dynamic image ultrasonography. Am J Obstet Gynecol 1982; 143: 545–554

26 Campbell S, Wilkin D. Abdominal circumference in the estimation of fetal weight. Br J Obstet Gynaecol 1975; 82: 689–697

27 Warsof S L, Gohari P, Berkowitz R L, Hobbins J C. The estimation of fetal weight by computer-assisted analysis. Am J Obstet Gynecol 1977; 128: 881–892

28 Hill L M, Breckle R, Wolfram K R, O'Brien P C. Evaluation of three methods of estimating fetal weight. JCU 1986; 14: 171–178

29 Simon N V, Levisky J S, Shearer D M, O'Lear M S, Flood J T. Influence of fetal growth patterns as sonographic estimate of fetal weight. JCU 1987; 15: 376–386

30 Hadlock F P, Harrist R B, Sharman R S. Estimation of fetal weight by ultrasound. Am J Obstet Gynecol 1985; 151: 333–337

31 Neilson J P, Whitfield C R, Aitchison T C. Screening for the small for dates fetus: a two stage ultrasonic examination schedule. BMJ 1980; 280: 1203–1206

32 Thacker S B. Quality of controlled clinical trials. The case of imaging ultrasound in obstetrics: a review. Br J Obstet Gynaecol 1985; 92: 437–444

33 Campbell S, Thoms A. Ultrasound measurement of the fetal head to abdomen circumference ratio in the assessment of growth retardation. Br J Obstet Gynaecol 1977; 84: 165–174

34 Ghohari M, Berkowitz R K, Hobbins J C. Prediction of intrauterine growth retardation by determination of total intrauterine volume. Am J Obstet Gynecol 1977; 127: 255–260

35 Geirsson R T, Patel N B, Christie A D. Efficacy of intrauterine volume, fetal abdominal area and biparietal diameter measurements with ultrasound in screening small for dates babies. Br J Obstet Gynaecol 1985; 92: 929–935

36 Moore T R, Cayle J E. The amniotic fluid index in normal human pregnancy. Am J Obstet Gynecol 1990; 162: 1168–1173

The biophysical profile

Martin J. Whittle

INTRODUCTION

One of the major problems for the obstetrician in the assessment of the fetus is its inaccessibility. In contrast, the physician can see his patient and determine, for example, his colour, activity and respiratory movements, such information which has been, until recent years, denied to the fetal specialist. The development of ultrasound, however, has largely overcome these difficulties and allowed closer observation of the fetus and its activity so that considerable information concerning the fetal condition can be obtained from a single examination.

Of course the maternal appreciation of fetal life has been, since ancient times, a traditional indication that the pregnancy is proceeding normally, although attempts to use the observation in a scientific way to identify a group of babies at risk of intra-uterine death has met with mixed success. Ultrasound has broadened the scope of the assessment of fetal activity as a means of determining fetal well-being but nevertheless conflicting data exist as to its value.

This chapter will explore the principles upon which the fetal biophysical profile is based, discuss the methods and indications and consider the value of the test as a method of fetal assessment in current obstetric practice.

PHYSIOLOGICAL CONSIDERATIONS

Fetal movement is the manifestation of central nervous system (CNS) activity and this may be influenced by a number of factors. Clearly, the progressive organisation of the fetal CNS will produce increasingly complex patterns of movement as the pregnancy advances.[1] In late pregnancy these patterns can be classified into defined behavioural groups which although difficult to recognise in the fetus undoubtedly exist and will be discussed later. CNS activity will also be influenced by diurnal rhythm, maternal nutritional state, maternal drug therapy and hypoxia. In addition, however, it should be noted that activity will be altered when the brain has been damaged by intra-uterine infection, malformation or a non-hypoxic vascular catastrophe.

BEHAVIOURAL STATES

Since the various forms of fetal activity appear to be influenced by the particular behavioural state of the fetus at that time, it is important to realise how these are determined. Four states have been described[2] and correspond to those seen in the neonate (Table 1). Only 1F and 2F persist for long enough to be identified with certainty in the fetus and these are characterised in the following way:

State 1F: quiescence which can be regularly interrupted by body movements, absent eye movements and a stable heart rate pattern with a small range of variation;

Table 1 Fetal behavioural activity

	1F	2F	3F	4F
Body movements	Incidental	Periodic	Absent	Continuous
Eye movements	Absent	Present	Present	Present
Heart rate patterns	Stable; few accelerations	Frequent accelerations	Stable; no accelerations	Large accelerations

State 2F: frequent and periodic gross body movements, continuous eye movements and a heart rate with a wide range of variation and frequent accelerations;

States 3F and 4F occur infrequently in the fetus and do not show a developmental course and so are not considered further.

As gestational age advances the various activity patterns occur simultaneously with increasing frequency, so-called coincidence. Thus while at 32 weeks a recognisable State 1F exists only 29% of the time this rises to 67% by 38 weeks.[2] These changes presumably relate to increasing maturation in the central nervous system.

The use of alterations in behavioural state as a method of fetal monitoring does not seem to have been considered practicable. Long periods of observation appear to be necessary and in any case significant periods of coincidence do not develop until later in pregnancy, probably not until after 34 weeks. The problem of data handling is certainly surmountable with the use of suitable computer programs[3] but even so the relevance of the data remains unclear.

ANIMAL EVIDENCE

Evidence that specific types of fetal activity really existed in the normal fetus was disputed for some time. Chest wall movements had been seen in fetal lambs delivered into water baths but in the more mature fetal lamb these were only seen when the fetal cord was clamped and the fetus asphyxiated. The questionable validity of these early observations meant that fetal breathing came to be regarded as abnormal and it was some years later before new technology was available to show that in fact fetal breathing was not only normally present but could be observed throughout pregnancy.[4] Various factors were shown to influence the frequency of chest wall movements including gestational age, diurnal rhythm, maternal nutritional state and, importantly, the blood gases. Thus, it was observed that chest wall movements increased when the fetus was hypercapnic but decreased or disappeared completely when there was hypoxia; in fact in the very hypoxic fetus gasping movements were observed.

Other types of fetal activity included forelimb movements which were observed in the exteriorised fetal lamb.[5] This group also noted that the movements were influenced by a number of factors, including hypoxia, although they were unable to define a diurnal rhythm. These changes could be correlated with the pattern of eye movements and thus to the natural rest/activity cycles which became a feature of a normally functioning central nervous system and increasingly prominent as the fetus develops.

FETAL ACTIVITY

The clinical use of fetal movements as a method of fetal evaluation was described by Sadovsky & Yaffe[6] who used a series of case reports to demonstrate that fetal movements, as perceived by the mother, appeared to become markedly reduced or even cease days or occasionally only hours before fetal death. Pearson & Weaver[7] described the use of a fetal movement count chart, often called the 'kick chart', which allowed the mother to record the time at which she had felt 10 kicks over a 12 hour span. The results suggested that movements seemed to cease about 12 to 48 hours before death. In another fetal movement study[8] it was found that babies with reduced movements had a much poorer outcome and were more likely to be small for dates than those moving vigorously.

These observations led to the view that fetal activity indicated fetal health and further, that a reduction in this activity preceded fetal death by a time span of sufficient length to allow effective action to be taken to prevent an adverse outcome. Some support for this comes from a prospective randomised study involving 2250 patients[9] in which all the eight intra-uterine deaths occurred in the non-counting group who were not monitoring fetal movements. In the counting group there were nine cases with reduced fetal movement and six of these babies were delivered by caesarean section; there were no deaths in this group but two babies developed respiratory distress syndrome. The implication from this study is that these nine cases would have died if they had not been delivered at the appropriate time. However, recent evidence derived from a large randomised study[10] comprising 68 000 patients showed that movement counting by the mother was unhelpful in reducing the risk of pregnancy loss, most babies being dead by the time of admission.

Whilst the maternal appreciation of fetal movement provides a simple method of assessing fetal condition on a day to day basis, it is relatively crude and gives no indication of the individual fetal activities. With the development of real time ultrasound technology it became possible to observe these movements and Manning[11] described a 'biophysical' assessment. Other methods of establishing the biophysical profile have been described[12] and there are now innumerable modifications of the original Manning method.

THE BIOPHYSICAL PROFILE

Technique

The components of this score are shown in Table 2 and include fetal heart reactivity, fetal breathing movements, gross body movements, fetal tone and amniotic fluid pool depth. Each component is assigned an arbitrary value of zero or two, such that the minimum total score is zero and the maximum 10.

Fetal heart rate activity

Antepartum fetal heart rate testing has been used as a primary method of fetal assessment for a number of years since the value of non-stressed testing was first discussed.[13] The concept depends on the inter-relationships between fetal movement and accelerations in fetal heart rate which became disturbed in the presence of fetal hypoxia. Two movement-related accelerations in a 20 minute span are needed to deem the heart rate reactive (Fig. 1) although different criteria are used by some groups.

Table 2 Fetal biophysical score

Variable	Score 2	Score 0
Cardiotocography	At least 2 accelerations of 15 bpm, lasting 15 s in 20 min sessions	No accelerations
Fetal breathing	At least 30 s of sustained breathing in 30 min	< 30 s breathing
Fetal movements	3 or more gross body movements in 30 min	< 3 movements
Fetal tone	At least one motion of limb from flexion to extension and back	No movements
Amniotic fluid volume	A pocket of fluid at least 2 cm in depth	< 1 cm² fluid

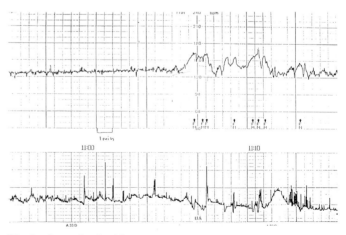

Fig. 1 A reactive fetal heart rate trace. FM indicates the time of fetal movement.

Fetal breathing

The observation of fetal breathing movements is not difficult but requires patience. At least 30 seconds of sustained breathing should be seen in a 30 minute span of observation. It is important to distinguish chest wall from trunk movement and this is best achieved by scanning so that the fetal chest and abdominal walls appear on the screen together (Fig. 2). When the fetus breathes, a see-saw appearance is seen, the chest moving in as the abdomen moves out. A further guide, which may be particularly helpful in cases with reduced amniotic fluid volume, is movement of intra-abdominal structures such as the fetal kidney.

Fetal movements

Gross fetal activity is very easily observed using ultrasound and three or more movements should be seen in 30 minutes. Both limb and trunk movements are counted but it is important to ensure that the limb movements are active and not merely occurring as the result of maternal activity. Trunk movements are usually of a rolling type.

Fetal tone

Although not self-evident it is possible to assess fetal tone most readily by observing the hands and feet, the clenched fist (Fig. 3) being obviously associated with normal tone whilst the same is true for feet undergoing dorsiflexion. In contrast, the fetus with absent tone lies with hands open and feet motionless.

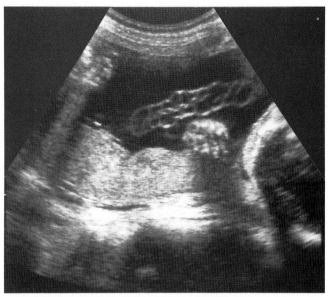

Fig. 3 Fetal hand in clenched posture, below the cord.

Amniotic fluid volume

The measurement of amniotic fluid volume is very subjective but it is important that an empty pool is used, taking care that loops of cord are not mistakenly included in the measurement (Fig. 4). Some consider the original description of a significantly reduced volume as < 1 cm to be too rigorous. Indeed, this criterion probably originated from the use of amniotic fluid measurement in the evaluation of the post-dates pregnancy. Others[12] have considered 2 cm or less to be a more realistic amount (Table 3) although even this degree of oligohydramnios would be considered by many to be profound.

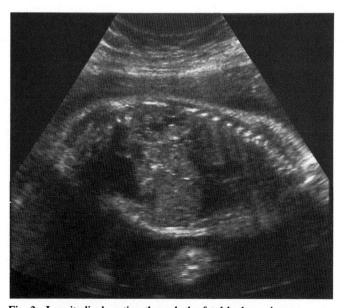

Fig. 2 Longitudinal section through the fetal body to show abdomen and thorax in the same plane.

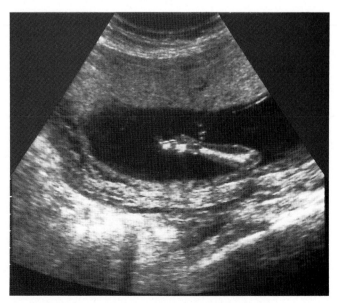

Fig. 4 Fetal forearm showing clear pool of amniotic fluid.

One criticism of much that has been written concerning the biophysical profile relates to a lack of regard for the gestational age at the time of the assessment and this applies particularly for amniotic fluid volume which can change markedly with gestational age. Thus, a 2 cm pool may be acceptable at term but almost certainly is not so at, say 33 weeks. Unpublished data from our own department indicate that 90% of all pregnancies will have a single depth of amniotic fluid of at least 3 cm regardless of gestational age.

A better method of amniotic fluid assessment may be the use of the 'amniotic fluid index',[14] which is the sum of the vertical fluid depth in the four uterine quadrants. A total depth of 5 cm or greater is considered normal but this approach has not, to date, been described as a feature of the biophysical profile technique.

Placental grading

Some systems include placental grading in the biophysical profile score (Table 3) but whether this is a helpful addition is uncertain. Vintzileos and colleagues suggest that a grade III placental score has a significant association with intrapartum distress and placental abruption.

Indications

In Manning's original description, common indications for study were the post-dates pregnancy and maternal diabetes. Since that time larger series have included pregnancies suspected to have a small for dates fetus and pregnancies complicated by hypertension.

Other indications include circumstances in which the cardiotocograph (CTG) is equivocal, altered by drug treatment, e.g. beta-blockers, complicated by the presence of variable decelerations or uninterpretable because of early gestational age. Alternatively, the profile may be indicated because the mother reports reduced fetal movements or as a means of monitoring the fetal condition during treatment, as in rhesus disease.

Method

Using real time ultrasound the fetus may have to be observed for up to half an hour before the criteria are met for a normal result (Table 2). Although it has been proposed that the test interval of a week is adequate this has been disputed,[15] the suggestion being that the test may need to be repeated sooner and should depend upon the underlying clinical problem. Indeed, in circumstances such as growth retardation, daily assessment may be appropriate.

The order in which the tests are performed is not really important and if all four ultrasound components of the profile are normal, fetal heart rate testing may not be necessary and, indeed, the CTG in one series was always reactive.[16] It was found that when any one component was abnormal that 64% of CTGs were normal while if more than two were so, all the CTGs were non-reactive. The one single

Table 3 Criteria for scoring biophysical profiles

Non-stress test (NST)

Score 2 (NST 2): > 5 FHR accelerations of at least 15 bpm in amplitude and at least 15 s duration associated with fetal movements in a 20 min period.

Score 1 (NST 1): 2–4 accelerations of at least 15 bpm in amplitude and at least 15 s duration associated with fetal movements in a 20 min period.

Score 0 (NST 0): < 1 acceleration in a 20 min period.

Fetal movements (FM)

Score 2 (FM 2): At least 3 gross (trunk and limbs) episodes of fetal movements within 30 min. Simultaneous limb and trunk movements were counted as a single movement.

Score 1 (FM 1): 1 or 2 fetal movements within 30 min.

Score 0 (FM 0): Absence of fetal movements within 30 min.

Fetal breathing movements (FBM)

Score 2 (FBM 2): At least 1 episode of fetal breathing of at least 60 s duration within a 30 min observation period.

Score 1 (FBM 1): At least 1 episode of fetal breathing lasting 30–60 s within a 30 min observation period.

Score 0 (FBM 0): Absence of fetal breathing or breathing lasting < 30 s within a 30 min observation period.

Fetal tone (FT)

Score 2 (FT 2): At least 1 episode of extension of extremities with return to position of flexion and also 1 episode of extension of spine with return to position of flexion.

Score 1 (FT 1): At least 1 episode of extension of extremities with return to position of flexion, or 1 episode of extension of spine with return to position of flexion.

Score 0 (FT 0): Extremities in extension. Fetal movements not followed by return. Open hand.

Amniotic fluid volume (AFV)

Score 2 (AFV 2): Fluid evident throughout the uterine cavity. A pocket that measures > 2 cm in vertical diameter.

Score 1 (AFV 1): A pocket that measures < 2 cm but > 1 cm in vertical diameter.

Score 0 (AFV 0): Crowding of fetal small parts. Largest pocket < 1 cm in diameter.

Placental grading (PL)

Score 2 (PL 2): Placental grading 0, I or II.

Score 1 (PL 1): Placenta posterior, difficult to evaluate.

Score 0 (PL 0): Placental grading III.

component most likely to be associated with an abnormal CTG was reduced amniotic fluid volume. The single component most likely to be absent was fetal breathing (72%) with a non-reactive CTG being found in 24% of cases. Very rarely was absent fetal tone or reduced amniotic fluid volume the single missing component.

Conversely, others[15] considered the CTG to be an integral part of the profile which needed to be retained. Although the observation of fetal activity, i.e. breathing, body and limb movement, may take some time, it is important that short cuts are avoided.

The determination of fetal structural normality should be an integral part of the biophysical assessment and this may be especially important when the fetus appears either small for dates or if oligohydramnios is noted.

Results

The results of biophysical testing appear to be remarkably impressive. Table 4 indicates the expected outcome in a large number of high-risk cases referred for evaluation by the profile.[17] It is seen that when the score is 10 the outcome is excellent and this also applies with a score of eight, so long as the two points lost are not because the amniotic fluid is reduced, under which circumstances the perinatal loss rate rises dramatically. Scores that are less than eight are associated with an increasingly high loss, scores four to six demanding a repeat evaluation and two or zero indicating the need to deliver. One important point is the need to establish fetal normality when the profile score is abnormal and particularly if the amniotic fluid volume is reduced – renal agenesis features strongly in one series.[18]

The other approach to the biophysical profile has been the evaluation of each component. It was found[12] that although loss of fetal breathing occurred in many babies with impaired outcome (high sensitivity) it had a low positive predictive value. Conversely, loss of fetal tone was a very good predictor of a poor fetal outcome usually with profound hypoxia, although by the time the fetus has reached this stage salvage may be impossible. Similar observations have been made by other groups[19] who found absent fetal movements to be the most accurate predictor when the end point used was perinatal death.

The association of the various components of the profile with hypoxia demonstrated a high predictive value for the baby with marked acidosis.[20] In this study an abnormal profile score was predictive of a cord pH of < 7.20 in 82% of cases. The fetal activity components of the score all provided a reasonable predictive value for acidosis, the weakest being absent fetal breathing and the strongest absent fetal tone.

The value of the biophysical profile in specific problems such as growth retardation has been addressed.[21] A false negative result occurred more frequently when babies were either probably or definitely growth retarded. The implications of this are unclear and the reasons for the babies to be small for dates are not stated, although fetal abnormality, as such, had been excluded. It may be of significance that in this report all of the losses followed the use of the modified profile (i.e. without CTG) although no comment is made concerning this. Further, the test interval was 7 days in three of the cases and this may be inappropriately long when growth retardation is suspected. The same investigators, using a group of babies with proven neonatal growth retardation, found that the perinatal mortality rate was 27 per 1000 in babies suspected as small for dates and managed prospectively with the profile.[21]

The use of the biophysical profile in the evaluation of pregnancies with premature rupture of the membranes has been described[22] and the test appears to predict those babies in good condition. The specific use of the absence of fetal breathing movements as an indication of intra-uterine infection has also been considered[23] and certainly it appeared that infection was uncommon when breathing was seen. However, both these studies were retrospective, and with few patients, making interpretation difficult.

DISCUSSION

The biophysical profile appears to be more firmly established in the United States of America than in Europe as a method of fetal monitoring. A serious problem with the reported studies is that they use a variety of end points with which to judge the test's value making an objective evaluation difficult. Certainly perinatal death, low cord blood pH values, poor Apgar scores and IUGR have all been used and undoubtedly adverse outcome is associated with an abnormal profile. However, an association alone does not necessarily mean that the test will be an effective predictor of the adverse event, something which can only be assessed from a properly conducted randomised study of sufficient power to distinguish outcome variables between the groups chosen. In fact there appear to be only two randomised studies evaluating the biophysical score.[24,25] Both show some advantage over the CTG alone

Table 4 Expected outcome following biophysical scoring

Score		PNM within a week
10/10		< 1/1000
8/10		< 1/1000
8/10	AFV = 0	89/1000
6/10	AFV = 2	Variable – retest within 24 h
6/10	AFV = 0	89/1000
4/10		91/1000
2/10		125/1000
0/10		600/1000

AFV = amniotic fluid volume
PNM = perinatal mortality

but the studies are small and not particularly well-designed with no attempt to blind results to the clinician. However, in general the method appears to function well at the two extreme results (very bad and very good) and as such may provide helpful clinical information.

To some extent the function of the biophysical profile needs to be defined as well as the end points. Should the test be used primarily as a screening test or as a method of evaluating a preselected group of at-risk pregnancies? Its use as a screening test would seem impracticable since it takes too long to perform and can only be done effectively by staff with reasonable experience in ultrasound technique. Its advantage as a diagnostic test is that it does provide a semiquantitative assessment of fetal condition which at least theoretically allows the progress of the pregnancy to be followed.[26]

If the profile has the ability to identify the deteriorating pregnancy it should provide some evidence about the degree of fetal hypoxia. It has been proposed[15] that the different components of the profile relate to the functioning of various parts of the fetal central nervous system. Thus, brainstem function is considered most sensitive to hypoxia which, if present, would first produce changes in the CTG followed by loss of breathing movements. As hypoxia deepens the higher centres associated with movement and the maintenance of tone cease to function and the baby stops moving – the next stage is death. Although this hypothesis is attractive it does not fully explain observations in the hypoxic adult in whom movement may cease early on in hypoxia but brainstem function is maintained. It would seem likely that what is being observed in the fetus is the effect of progressive hypoxia on the central nervous system as a whole and probably not in the selective way proposed.

If changing fetal activity represents the relatively acute response of the fetus to hypoxia the amniotic fluid volume reflects the effect of chronic hypoxia. Why amniotic fluid volume should decrease in growth retardation is not clear but it has been proposed that it is the result of reduced fetal urine output in the face of a redistributed fetal blood flow. Although this may be the case in some circumstances it cannot be the answer in all since it is a common observation that perfectly adequate fetal activity is seen in oligohydramnios.

One serious criticism of the biophysical profile is that the various components are assigned the same value. This dates back to the origins of the test as an assessment based on the Apgar score but with the evidence now available from a very large experience in the use of the profile perhaps the scoring system should be modified.

The advantages of the biophysical profile are that it provides a non-invasive method of fetal evaluation which, if necessary, can be performed daily or more often if required. Further, it provides a biological assessment of the fetal condition in that it seems reasonable to assume that if the fetus is moving and breathing it will usually be healthy.[15] Although fetal blood sampling by cordocentesis may provide useful information in the growth retarded fetus[27,28] a disadvantage is that it gives information only at one point in time. Further, and perhaps more importantly, it assumes that the growth retarded baby with disordered gases is about to die and needs to be delivered. Whilst there is no doubt that these babies are in serious trouble, lack of knowledge about the aetiology and pathogenesis of fetal growth retardation makes interpretation of these data difficult. For example, it may be that these babies can adjust their metabolism sufficiently to maintain an intrauterine existence even though the gases are deranged. A normal profile under these circumstances would indicate the need to prolong the pregnancy since functionally the baby's condition would be satisfactory.

REFERENCES

1 de Vries J I P, Visser G H A, Prechtl H F R. The emergence of fetal behavior. 1. Qualitative aspects. Early Hum Dev 1982; 7: 301–322

2 Nijuis J G, Prechtl H F R, Martin C B, Bots R S G M. Are there behavioral states in the human fetus? Early Hum Dev 1982; 6: 177–195

3 Rizzo G, Arduini D, Mancuso S, Romanini C. Computer-assisted analysis of fetal behavioural states. Prenat Diagn 1988; 8: 479–484

4 Boddy K. Fetal circulation and breathing movements. In: Beard R W, Nathanielsz P W. eds. Fetal physiology and medicine. London: W B Saunders. 1976: p 302–328

5 Natale R, Clelow F, Dawes G S. Measurement of fetal forelimb movements in the lamb in utero. Am J Obstet Gynecol 1981; 140: 545–551

6 Sadovsky E, Yaffe H. Daily fetal movement recording and fetal progress. Obstet Gynecol 1973; 41: 845–850

7 Pearson J F, Weaver J B. Fetal activity and fetal wellbeing: an evaluation. BMJ 1976; 1: 1305–1307

8 Mathews D D. Maternal assessment of fetal activity in small-for-dates infants. Obstet Gynecol 1975; 45: 488–493

9 Neldum S. Fetal movements as an indicator of fetal wellbeing. Lancet 1980; 1: 1222–1223

10 Grant A, Elbourne D, Valentin L, Alexander S. Routine formal fetal movement counting and risk of antepartum late death in normally formed singletons. Lancet 1989; ii: 345–349

11 Manning F A, Platt L D, Sipos L. Antepartum evaluation: development of a fetal biophysical profile. Am J Obstet Gynecol 1980; 136: 787–795

12 Vintzileos A M, Campbell W A, Ingardia C J, Nochimson D J. The fetal biophysical profile and its predictive value. Obstet Gynecol 1983; 62: 271–278

13 Keegan K A, Paul R H. Antepartum fetal heart rate testing 1V. The non-stress test as a primary approach. Am J Obstet Gynecol 1980; 136: 75–80

14 Phelan J P, Smith C V, Broussard P, Small M. Amniotic fluid assessment with the four quadrant technique at 36 to 42 weeks gestation. J Reprod Med 1987; 32: 540–542

15 Vintzileos A M, Campbell W A, Nochimson D J, Weinbaum P J. The use and abuse of the fetal biophysical profile. Am J Obstet Gynecol 1987; 156: 527–533

16 Manning F A, Morrison I, Lange I R, Harman C R, Chamberlain P F C. Fetal biophysical scoring; selective use of the non-stress test. Am J Obstet Gynecol 1987; 156: 709–712

17 Manning F A, Morrison I, Harman C R, Lange I R, Menticoglou S. Fetal assessment based on fetal biophysical profile scoring: experience in 19 221 referred high risk pregnancies. Am J Obstet Gynecol 1987; 157: 880–884

18 Manning F A, Hill L M, Platt L D. Qualitative amniotic fluid volume determination by ultrasound. Antepartum detection of intra-uterine growth retardation. Am J Obstet Gynecol 1981; 139: 254–258

19 Baskett T F, Allen A C, Gray J H, Young D C, Young L M. Fetal biophysical profile and perinatal death. Obstet Gynecol 1987; 70: 357–360

20 Vintzileos A M, Gaffney S E, Salinger L M, Kontopoulos V G, Campbell W A, Nochimson D J. The relationships among the fetal biophysical profile, umbilical cord pH and Apgar score. Am J Obstet Gynecol 1987; 157: 627–631

21 Manning F A, Menticoglou S, Harman C R, Morrison I, Lange I R. Antepartum fetal risk assessment: the role of the biophysical profile score. In: Whittle M J. ed. Fetal monitoring. London: Balliere's. 1987: p 55–72

22 Vintzileos A M, Feinstein S J, Lodeiro J G, Campbell W A, Weinbaum P J, Nochimson D J. Fetal biophysical profile and the effect of premature rupture of the membranes. Obstet Gynecol 1986; 67: 818–823

23 Vintzileos A M, Campbell W A, Nochimson D J, Weinbaum P J. Fetal breathing as a predictor of infection in premature rupture of the membranes. Obstet Gynecol 1986; 67: 813–817

24 Platt L D, Walla C A, Paul R H, et al. A prospective trial of the biophysical profile verses the non-stress test in the management of high-risk pregnancies. Am J Obstet Gynecol 1985; 153: 624–632

25 Manning F A, Morrison I, Lange I R, Harman C R. Fetal assessment based on fetal biophysical profile scoring: experience 1n 12 620 referred high risk pregnancies. Am J Obstet Gynecol 1985; 151: 342–350

26 Druzin M L, Lockshin M, Edersheim T G, Hutson J M, Krauss A L, Kogut E. Second trimester fetal monitoring and preterm delivery in pregnancies with systemic lupus erythematosis and/or circulating anticoagulant. Am J Obstet Gynecol 1987; 157: 1503–1510

27 Pearce J M, Chamberlain G V P. Ultrasonically guided percutaneous umbilical blood sampling in the management of intra-uterine growth retardation. Br J Obstet Gynaecol 1987; 94: 318–321

28 Cox W L, Daffos F, Forestier F, et al. Physiology and management of intra-uterine growth retardation. A biologic approach with fetal blood sampling. Am J Obstet Gynecol 1988; 159: 36–41

Doppler in obstetrics

Sarah Bower and Stuart Campbell

INTRODUCTION

The Doppler effect has been applied to medical ultrasound for over 30 years,[1] but it is only in the last decade that the technique has become sufficiently refined to be widely applicable.

A variety of invasive procedures have been employed to study the uteroplacental and fetal circulations.[2,3] These methods have poor reproducibility and are unsuitable for serial studies. The advantage of the various clinical applications of Doppler ultrasound is that the technique is fast, reproducible and can be performed on a daily basis.

Basic principles and Doppler physics

When an ultrasound beam is transmitted from a stationary source towards a blood vessel it is reflected and scattered by moving red blood cells and detected by the receiving crystal. The change in frequency, Fd (or Doppler shifted frequency) of the reflected beam is caused by, and directly proportional to, the velocity of the moving blood corpuscles. It is expressed by the formula:

$$fd = \frac{2 \, f \, V \, Cos\theta}{c}$$

where fd is the change in frequency,
  f   is the ultrasound frequency,
  V   is the velocity of the blood cells,
  c   is the velocity of sound in the tissue,
  θ is the angle between the ultrasound beam and the blood vessel (Fig. 1).

When the emitted frequency is between 1 and 10 MHz the Doppler shift for blood flowing in the arteries and veins

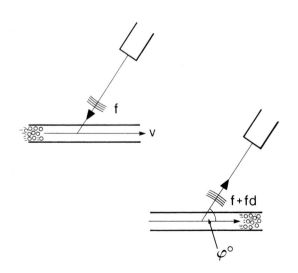

Fig. 1 Doppler ultrasound. The frequency (f) of an ultrasound beam directed at a column of blood moving at a velocity (v) will be increased in proportion to v and the cosine of the angle of intersection of the vessel by the beam.

is within the audible range. Frequencies between 2 and 5 MHz are used for uterine and fetal vessels to compromise between higher frequencies, which are more readily absorbed by the tissues, and lower frequencies which are subject to more scattering.

If the vessel can be visualised and its diameter measured and the angle of insonation of the Doppler beam calculated, then velocity and volume of flow can be assessed. The formula demonstrates the importance of the angle of insonation because when this is 90° relative to the flow the frequency of the shift becomes zero due to the value of Cos 90. Measurements of mean velocity of flow can only be reliably obtained when the angle is less than 60°.[4]

Types of equipment

In clinical practice there are three types of Doppler equipment in use. Probably the most common is continuous wave (cw), which is inexpensive and rapid, but is a blind technique which depends on pattern recognition. The ultrasound beam is emitted and received continuously. The disadvantage of this is that Doppler shifted frequencies can be received from several vessels at once and the resulting waveforms mixed.

Duplex equipment combines conventional real time imaging with pulsed wave Doppler ultrasound. The use of pulsed ultrasound allows the time from emission to reception of a pulse to be measured therefore permitting the depth from which an echo has been reflected to be calculated. The length of time for which the receiver (or range gate) is open determines the length of the sample volume along the beam axis. When used with an imaging system the direction of the Doppler beam can be shown on the screen together with the 'range gate' or area from which the signals are being received. Thus it is possible to measure the angle of insonation and calculate mean or maximum blood velocity. The transmitted ultrasound intensity is often greatly increased when the Doppler function is activated and thus these examinations should only be performed when clinically indicated and the duration of the Doppler procedure should be kept as short as practicable.

Colour flow imaging is one of the more recent advances in Doppler software. It employs two-dimensional flow imaging superimposed on a conventional real time image. The screen is divided into pixels, in each of which the Doppler shifted frequencies are assigned a colour, depending on the direction of movement (towards or away from the transducer), and this is displayed on a time sharing basis with the real time grey scale image. In addition the shades of the assigned colours can be made to represent the degree of Doppler shift. For example, the brighter shades of red represent faster velocities towards the transducer, whilst brighter shades of blue represent faster velocities away from the transducer. This system is useful in two ways.

Firstly, it allows easy visualisation of vessels which can lead to the diagnosis of certain conditions, particularly those involving placement or abnormality of the umbilical cord.[5] Secondly, it permits the repeated study of flow velocity waveforms (FVW) from the same uterine vessel throughout pregnancy and also from small fetal vessels, such as the renal and middle cerebral arteries.[6,7]

Waveform analysis

The Doppler signal is a composite of different frequencies and intensities which change throughout the cardiac cycle. These are processed by a real time spectrum analyser to produce an FVW in which the distribution of frequencies is plotted on the ordinate, with time on the abscissa. The shape of the waveform relates to the changing maximum velocity with time.

Each artery has a fairly characteristic FVW which alters in different physiological and pathological situations. Although the shape of the waveform is influenced by several factors, in particular cardiac contraction force and vessel wall compliance, the end diastolic portion is largely related to downstream resistance or impedance to flow, absent or reversed flow in diastole indicating very high resistance to flow. Impedance is quantified by calculating one of a variety of ratios between peak systolic (A) and end diastolic frequencies (B). Lower end diastolic frequencies produce higher ratios and indicate greater downstream resistance. The A/B ratio[8] is the ratio of peak systole to end diastole, the resistance index, RI,[9] is the ratio of the difference between peak systole and end diastole to peak systole:

$$RI = \frac{A - B}{A}$$

and the pulsatility index, PI,[10] is $\dfrac{A - B}{\text{mean}}$

where mean is the time averaged maximum frequency. The PI is probably the most accurate method of assessing impedance to flow, particularly when end diastolic frequencies are absent.

Uteroplacental circulation

The blood supply to the uterus comes from the uterine and ovarian arteries. These vessels anastomose at the cornu of the uterus and give rise to arcuate arteries that run circumferentially around the uterus. The radial arteries arise from the arcuate vessels and penetrate into the outer third of the myometrium. These vessels then become the spiral arteries which nourish the endometrium and the intervillous space of the placenta during pregnancy. Physiological modification of spiral arteries is required to permit the tenfold increase in uterine blood flow which is necessary to meet the respiratory and nutritional requirements of the fetus

and placenta.[11] This occurs as a result of the second wave of trophoblastic invasion which takes place during the early part of the second trimester of pregnancy.[12]

Pre-eclampsia and some pregnancies complicated by intra-uterine growth retardation (IUGR) are associated with failure of this physiological process.[13,14] The presence of muscular spiral arteries therefore does not permit the necessary increase in intervillous blood flow, and the cascade of pathological events culminating in pre-eclampsia and IUGR can be derived from this basic problem.

The uteroplacental circulation can be studied non-invasively by means of Doppler ultrasound. Most studies have shown an increase in flow impedance associated with proteinuric hypertension and pregnancies with small for gestational age (SGA) fetuses.[15,16] However, the results from various papers have been inconsistent, possibly due to the use of different sampling points in this complex circulation.

Of greater value would be the use of Doppler ultrasound of the uterine artery as a predictive test prior to the development of symptomatology, thus allowing care to be targeted to high risk groups and preventive measures to be undertaken. Unfortunately, when applying the test to unselected populations few large studies have been done and the results are variable.[17–21] We believe that with standardisation and modification of techniques, and the introduction of colour flow imaging, Doppler ultrasound of the uterine artery will be useful as a routine screening test for pre-eclampsia and IUGR.

Background

The uteroplacental arteries are formed as a result of conversion of the maternal spiral arteries by trophoblastic invasion.[22] This is thought to occur in two stages; the first wave of trophoblastic invasion converts the decidual segments of the spiral arteries in the first trimester and the second wave converts the myometrial segments in the second trimester.[12] The arteries dilate progressively towards the intervillous space apparently due to loss of the musculo-elastic structure. These alterations have been described as 'physiological changes'.[23] These vascular changes were found to be restricted to the decidual segments of spiral arteries[13] or to be totally absent[24] in pregnancies complicated by pre-eclampsia and a proportion of those with SGA, thus leaving the segments with intact musculo-elastic walls responsive to vaso-active peptides. This defective maternal response to placentation is thought to be due to failure of the second wave of trophoblastic invasion that normally occurs from about 16 weeks onwards.[25]

Although defective interaction of trophoblast and uterine tissues is well-established in pre-eclampsia and IUGR the reason for failure of trophoblastic invasion is unknown, but it may have an immunological basis.[26] The subsequent pathogenic mechanisms which trigger hypertension and growth retardation are not fully understood, but a possible cascade effect has been described.[27] However, the end result is impaired blood supply to the placenta and this can be assessed using Doppler ultrasound.[28]

Clinical studies

Doppler ultrasound studies of the uteroplacental circulation over a 24 hour period demonstrate that there is no circadian variation in impedance indices and that these are unaffected by eating a meal.[29] Similarly, studies over a 7 day period show no variability of impedance to flow in either normal or complicated pregnancy.[30] Thus the variation that is seen between normal and complicated pregnancy is unlikely to be affected by timing of Doppler examination. However, exercise in the third trimester causes a transient but significant increase in uteroplacental vascular resistance,[31] thus it is important to rest the patient for 10 to 15 minutes prior to performing Doppler studies. Alterations of the uterine artery FVW have also been demonstrated in temporal association with uterine contractions in labour.[32] These alterations consist of a gradual reduction of end diastolic velocities with absence when the intra-uterine pressure exceeds 35 mmHg. Spontaneous low amplitude contractions in the antenatal period have been shown to have the same effect.[33]

Many studies have been carried out using Doppler ultrasound to assess uteroplacental blood flow in women whose pregnancies are complicated by hypertension[28,34–36] or SGA.[37,38] Whilst there is general agreement that there are differences between normal and complicated pregnancies, sensitivities and predictive values differ considerably. There are a variety of reasons for this; different indices of impedance to flow have been used and different cut off limits for abnormality determined. In addition different techniques of obtaining waveforms and different definitions of poor outcome have been used.

Impedance to flow is usually measured by the A/B ratio or resistance index (RI), each group defining their own normal range, often constructed from measurements obtained in small numbers of retrospectively defined normal women followed longitudinally. Some groups also include the presence of a dicrotic or early diastolic notch in the waveform as an indicator of high resistance to flow.[28,34] Different methodology has been used; the first report described the sampling of large uteroplacental vessels in the lateral uterine wall identified with duplex equipment close to the bifurcation of the common iliac artery.[28] Campbell et al called these vessels the arcuate arteries. Schulman used continuous wave apparatus to obtain signals from the main uterine artery low in the lateral uterine wall by directing the transducer medially.[39] Trudinger[40] and Hanretty[18] however both obtained signals from the subplacental vessels. It is likely that studies of the main uterine vessels give

more predictive information on impaired uteroplacental perfusion. This is because not only are the measurements more reproducible, but the major vessels reflect the sum of resistances of the placental bed and therefore are more likely to provide an overall picture of placental perfusion.

A recent study defined landmarks for sampling the uteroplacental circulation (Fig. 2) and found the RI to be lower from placental than non-placental sites and from distal 'arcuate' than proximal 'uterine' sites.[41] Other groups have found that a unilateral placenta is associated with a significant difference in resistance to flow between the two sides of the uterus[42] and that there is an association between a divergent blood supply to the uterus and placenta and the development of pre-eclampsia and fetal growth retardation.[43] Thus fixed standardised sites for sampling would be useful and, in addition, normal ranges should account for variables such as placental site (Fig. 3). Definitions of poor outcome have ranged from severe proteinuric pregnancy induced hypertension (pre-eclampsia) to hypertension alone, with differing cut off points for the definition of hypertension being used. 'Growth retardation' or SGA has variously been defined as a birth weight less than the 2.5th, 5th or 10th centile, sometimes with the inclusion of evidence of fetal hypoxia or neonatal asphyxia at the time of delivery.

Pre-eclampsia is associated with significant maternal and fetal morbidity and mortality and probably has a different pathological basis from pregnancy induced hypertension alone, which may even have a beneficial effect on fetal condition.[44] In the same way the aetiology of fetal smallness is multifactorial and it is the hypoxic SGA or IUGR fetuses who are most at risk of a poor outcome.

Many studies have used Doppler ultrasound of the uterine artery as a screening test to attempt to predict all SGA fetuses and all cases of hypertension.[18] This is illogical

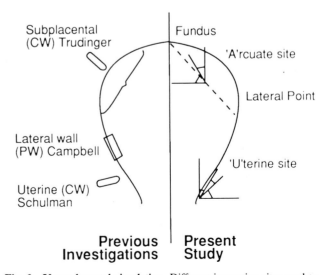

Fig. 2 Uteroplacental circulation. Different insonation sites used to study the uteroplacental circulation.

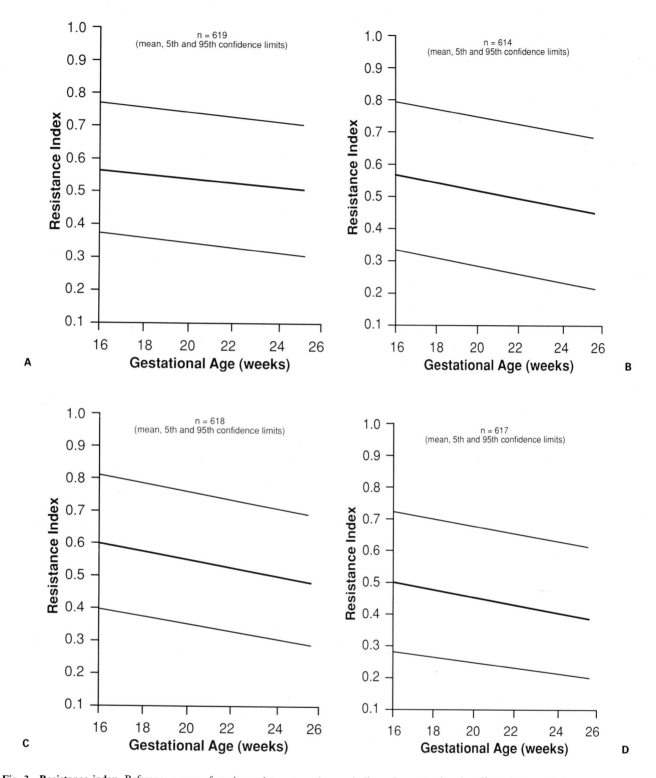

Fig. 3   Resistance index. Reference ranges of uterine and arcuate resistance indices, demonstrating the effect of placental site.
A: Arcuate artery, non-placental side. **B:** Arcuate artery, placental side. **C:** Uterine artery, non-placental side. **D:** Uterine artery, placental side.

and has led to confusion about the usefulness of the test. However, the fact that with all these differences in diagnostic criteria and end points there is still some agreement indicates the potential strength of this test in the detection of pre-eclampsia and IUGR.

Screening studies

The second wave of trophoblastic invasion is complete in most patients by 20 weeks gestation,[45] but the persistence of a diastolic notch can be a normal feature up to 26 weeks gestation[39] suggesting that in some women this wave of invasion may be delayed. Screening studies have been undertaken from 16[21] to 30[18] weeks, but most of them are carried out at 20 weeks when the patient attends for a routine scan. By screening early in the second trimester the false positive rate will be high leading to a low specificity because the process of physiological change is not completed. Screening late in the second trimester may mean that the pathological process is already well-developed and that preventive measures may be less effective.

Screening studies can be divided into examination of selected and unselected populations. Two similar studies on groups of high-risk patients using the same technique of obtaining waveforms and the same definitions of a raised resistance index (albeit with different definitions of hypertension) gave rise to very different results; one showing a significant association between elevated resistance index and the subsequent development of hypertension[15] and the other showing a significant association between abnormal resistance index and the birth of a baby with birthweight less than the tenth centile for gestational age, but no association with hypertension.[16] In the latter paper the authors put the differences down to variations introduced by sampling problems and comment that if sampling could be standardised to a single vessel, such as the main trunk of the uterine artery, results may be more reproducible.

Pre-eclampsia is largely a disease of primigravidae or first pregnancies with a partner. Thus screening preselected groups on the basis of past obstetric history would miss a large number of affected patients. Several screening studies have been carried out in unselected groups of antenatal patients. The results of these vary tremendously as can be seen in Figure 4. The reasons for these different results have already been discussed. Some of the more recent developments in Doppler ultrasound technology may lead to more consistent results.

Current studies at King's College Hospital

In the last 3 years two large screening studies using Doppler ultrasound of the uterine artery have been carried out. The first was done by Bewley et al and she recruited 1014 patients between 16 and 24 weeks gestation attending for the routine booking scan. Continuous wave Doppler ultrasound was used to study both uterine arteries and the

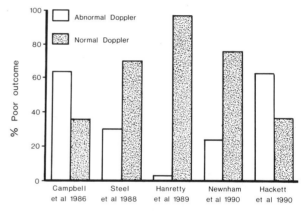

Fig. 4 Doppler screening of the uterine arteries. Unselected screening studies demonstrating the relationship between poor outcome and normal and abnormal Doppler. In Steel's paper all cases of severe pre-eclampsia were detected.

Table 1 The difference in mean resistance index between those patients with a normal outcome and various pregnancy complications

| CW Doppler of the uterine artery in 1014 pregnant women | | | | |
Outcome	n	Mean RI	SD	P
Normals	573	0.50	0.09	
Hypertension				
Non proteinuric	44	0.52	0.11	NS
Proteinuric	40	0.57	0.11	<0.001
Preterm labour (<37)	53	0.51	0.11	NS
Preterm CS	20	0.60	0.11	<0.001
Abruption	8	0.58	0.13	<0.01
Baby to SCBU	36	0.57	0.11	<0.001
SGA < 5th	51	0.57	0.11	<0.001

n = number of patients SD = standard deviation from the mean

Table 2 The value of resistance index > 95th centile in the prediction of poor outcome defined as either SGA < 3rd centile or severe proteinuric pregnancy induced hypertension or abruption or intra-uterine death

CW Doppler of the uterine artery in 1014 pregnant women

Gestation	Sens	Spec	PV+ve*	PV−ve*
	%	%	%	%
16–20 wks	12	95	15	94
20–24 wks	32	95	36	94

*PV = predictive value

RI was measured. Correlations between mean RI and outcome are summarised in Table 1. The highly significant associations of mean RI with proteinuric hypertension, abruption and SGA strongly support the hypothesis that failed trophoblastic invasion is the common underlying pathology of these conditions. The lack of a significant association with non-proteinuric hypertension suggests a different aetiological mechanism between cases of proteinuric hypertension and most cases of non-proteinuric hypertension. The reason for the association of an elevated RI with preterm caesarean section, but not preterm labour, presumably reflects the fact that preterm caesarean sections are usually performed for placental insufficiency, whereas the majority of preterm labours are not associated with this problem.

Table 2 summarises the value of an RI above the 95th centile in predicting severe perinatal complications. There is a marked improvement with increasing gestation, but the sensitivity remains low. However, a positive predictive value of 36% suggests that this may be a clinically useful test for identifying patients at risk of a very poor outcome. In order to try to improve on these results two modifi-

cations were made to the technique; firstly a different analysis of the waveform and secondly the introduction of colour flow imaging of the uterine artery.

It was noted in the previous study that uterine artery flow velocity waveforms (FVW) can vary tremendously in shape. Those associated with hypertension frequently have a steep upward slope to the systolic peak and an early diastolic notch (Fig. 5). We had previously tried to incorporate wave shape information by using the Frequency Index Profile[28] but for this second study we merely noted the presence or absence of a notch.

Colour flow imaging allows direct visualisation of maternal and fetal vessels. By placing the transducer in the lower lateral quadrant of the uterus and angling it medially an apparent cross-over of the external iliac artery and main uterine artery can be identified (Plate 1).[46] This 'cross-over' can be used as a reference point to identify the main uterine artery and is easily reproducible. Thus, by using this point sampling errors are small and the resistance of the whole of the uterine circulation is studied. Direct visualisation of the artery and knowledge of the angle of insonation of the vessel allows mean velocity of flow to be

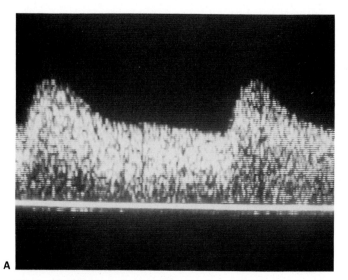 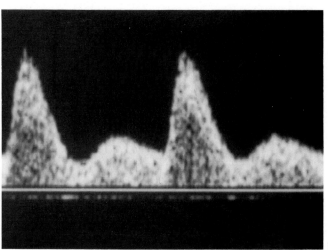

A
B

Fig. 5 Uterine artery flow velocity waveforms. A: Normal pregnancy and **B:** high impedance pattern with well-defined diastolic notch and reduced end diastolic velocity.

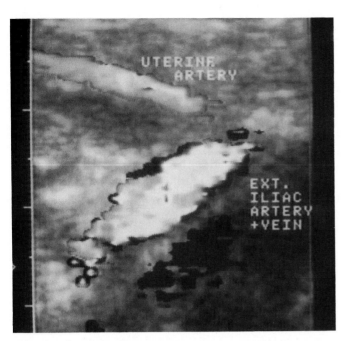

Plate 1 The apparent 'cross-over' of the main uterine artery with the external iliac artery and vein. This figure is reproduced in colour in the colour plate section at the front of this volume.

calculated. By using recent technology a clear image of a length of the artery can be obtained and the diameter of the artery measured. With the knowledge of vessel diameter and mean velocity it is possible to calculate total volume of flow to the uterus in both uterine arteries.

The screening study in progress is being carried out on 2500 women by the authors. A combination of continuous wave Doppler ultrasound and colour flow imaging of the uterine artery is being used to calculate resistance to flow as well as mean velocity and volume flow.

The results are presented of a preliminary analysis of our data: 1300 women recruited from the routine antenatal clinic had continuous wave Doppler ultrasound of both uterine arteries at the 20 week booking scan. This is a rapid procedure which adds only 5 to 10 minutes to the routine scan. If the FVW obtained were found to have either a high resistance index (above 2 standard deviations from the mean of our normal range) or the presence of an early diastolic notch, or both, the patient was asked to return for follow up with colour flow imaging initially at 24 weeks and then at 26 weeks if still abnormal. At 20 weeks 16% of the total study population had abnormal waveforms. At the 24 weeks and 26 weeks follow up scans abnormal waveforms were retained by 4.6% and 3.2% of women respectively. Of the 1300 women studied 19 had severe proteinuric pregnancy induced hypertension/pre-eclampsia (diastolic blood pressure greater than or equal to 110 mmHg on 2 occasions at least 4 hours apart and proteinuria greater than or equal to 500 mg/24 hours) and 15 of these had abnormal uterine artery Doppler studies. The results are summarised in Table 3. We have confirmed the association of abnormal uterine artery flow velocity waveforms and pre-eclampsia and the high sensitivity of 79% at 20 weeks is retained at 24 and 26 weeks, while the specificity and positive predictive value improve progressively on the two subsequent examinations.

Thus, the notch is a much better predictor of poor outcome than RI alone. The presence of a notch was assessed subjectively in this study and it remains for an objective measurement of this to be made. From this study it would appear that 24 to 26 weeks would be the optimum time to screen an unselected population in order to identify a high-risk group.

Good results could probably be produced by an experienced operator using continuous wave Doppler ultrasound alone. However, colour flow imaging does give greater confidence that the main uterine artery has been sampled and that the same point on the artery is sampled in longitudinal studies.

Volume flow is the most direct way to assess perfusion, but has yet to prove clinically valuable due to the significant source of error in measuring the diameter of the vessel. Volume of flow in the uterine artery has been studied by imaging the artery using trans-vaginal ultrasonography.[47] Both the diameter of the vessel and the volume of flow were found to increase with gestation. The results are comparable with our findings in a pilot study using transabdominal colour flow imaging to locate and

Table 3 The value of a resistance index > 95th centile and/or the presence of a diastolic notch in the prediction of severe proteinuric pregnancy induced hypertension

Doppler of the uterine artery in 1300 pregnant women using continuous wave to screen at 20 weeks and colour flow imaging for follow up at 24 and 26 weeks

	Sens	Spec	PV+ve★	PV−ve★
	%	%	%	%
20 wks	79	85	7.6	99.6
24 wks	79	96	25.9	99.7
26 wks	79	98	36.6	99.7

★PV = predictive value

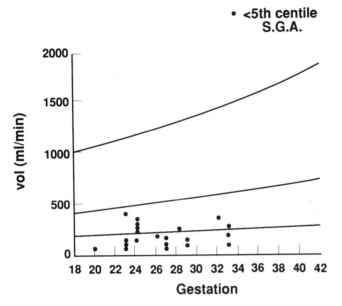

Fig. 6 **Uterine artery flow in growth retardation.** Estimated volume flow in the uterine arteries in 21 women whose pregnancies were complicated by growth retardation. The reference ranges indicate the 5th, 50th and 95th centiles.

measure the uterine artery (Fig. 6). The apparently wide range of normal values is probably attributable to errors in measurement of the vessel diameter on colour flow images. The inherently poor spacial resolution of colour Doppler imaging precludes sufficient accuracy in measurement of vessel diameters.

Conclusion

The purpose of screening unselected pregnancies with Doppler ultrasound of the uterine arteries is to identify a high-risk population for close observation and monitoring. Pre-eclampsia is still a significant cause of maternal and fetal mortality and morbidity whether or not it is associated with hypoxic SGA and the majority of women affected are primigravidae. Screening may also select a group of women suitable for therapy if the CLASP[48] trial demonstrates that low dose aspirin has a role in the prevention of pre-eclampsia and growth retardation.

Fetoplacental circulation

The intervillous space allows free transfer of oxygen and nutrients from the mother to fetus and removal of waste products from the fetus. In order to optimise this an unrestricted flow of fetal blood through the placental villi and maternal blood into the intervillous space is necessary. The maternal side of the circulation can be studied by looking at the uterine FVW, whilst information on the fetal side is provided by studying the FVW of the umbilical artery.

This represents the sum of the resistances to flow in the individual placental villi.

The umbilical artery is readily accessible for Doppler investigation and FVW can be easily obtained by using continuous wave Doppler ultrasound.[8] There is a characteristic saw-tooth appearance of arterial flow in one direction and continuous umbilical venous blood flow in the other. The FVWs may be assessed quantitatively, by calculation of impedance indices, or qualitatively, by noticing the presence or absence of end diastolic frequencies (EDF). Both methods of analysis represent the interaction between the forward compression wave due to cardiac systole and the reflected waves from the peripheral arteriolar bed.

Normal pregnancy

The fetoplacental circulation is characterised by high flow and low resistance. In normal pregnancy there is a progressive increase in end diastolic velocities with advancing gestation,[49] with forward flow being maintained throughout the cardiac cycle from 16 weeks gestation onwards. These changes are reflected in impedance indices which fall with advancing gestation (Fig. 7).[50] These findings presumably reflect the progressive maturation of the placenta and increase in the number of tertiary stem villi.[51]

In contrast to the uterine artery, in normal labour with normal fetal heart rate patterns the umbilical artery FVW is not altered by uterine contractions or amniotomy.[52]

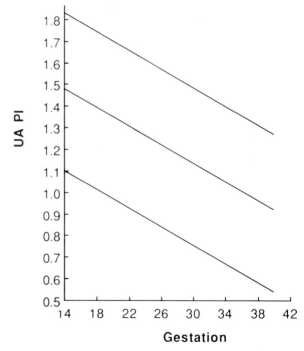

Fig. 7 **Reference range of the umbilical artery pulsatility index, PI,** with gestation.

However, alterations in FVWs have been noted in association with decelerations in the fetal heart rate, although this may be a feature of prolonged diastole leading to an apparent loss of end diastolic frequencies.[53] Thus, the fetal cardiovascular system remains stable throughout contractions allowing uninterrupted gas exchange (on the fetal side), and this helps to explain the ability of the fetus to remain normoxaemic despite frequent and painful uterine contractions.

Complicated pregnancy

Deviations from the low resistance flow pattern of the umbilical artery in normal pregnancy are found in cases of fetal compromise. These consist of a reduction of, or absence of, end diastolic frequencies.[54] These changes represent increasing impedance to flow and are thought to be due to a reduction in the number of arterioles in the tertiary stem villi.[55] Irrespective of the underlying cause this would decrease the surface area available for maternofetal transfer and could lead to fetal hypoxia.

Fetal growth retardation Antenatal detection of growth retarded fetuses at risk of intrapartum hypoxia is important. However, it is difficult to differentiate between suboptimal fetal growth due to intra-uterine 'starvation' and adequate growth of a genetically small infant. Several different studies have confirmed a strong association between abnormal umbilical artery waveforms and the SGA fetus,[56-59] which is surprising in view of the multifactorial aetiology of the SGA infant. However, other studies have found an abnormal umbilical artery FVW to be no better than abdominal circumference in predicting fetal size, but to be a better predictor of the small baby at risk of antenatal fetal compromise.[60,61] Loss of end diastolic flow is associated with fetal hypoxaemia and acidaemia,[62,63] whilst reverse flow in diastole is an indicator of a very poor perinatal outcome (Fig. 8).[64]

The effects of low dose aspirin have been assessed in a group of third trimester patients with abnormal umbilical FVW and described as having placental insufficiency.[65] Aspirin was used because of its inhibitory effect on the formation of thromboxane in maternal and fetal circulations.[66] This may have a causative role in the placental lesions on the fetal side of the circulation found in association with abnormal umbilical FVW.[67] A significant improvement in birth weight, placental weight and head circumference was found in the patients with moderate increase in impedance to flow in the umbilical artery, but not in those with extremely high impedance. While the future role of aspirin in the treatment of growth retardation needs to be elucidated, this paper demonstrates the role of Doppler ultrasound in identifying a high-risk group for therapy.

Studies of umbilical FVW are also useful in the study of pregnancies complicated by oligohydramnios. Only those associated with growth retardation demonstrate abnormal

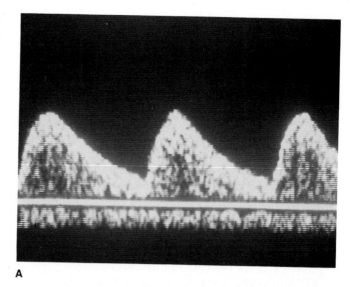

A

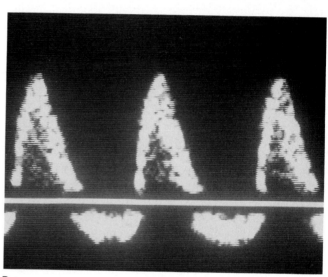

B

Fig. 8 Umbilical arterial waveforms. Examples of normal and abnormal umbilical arterial spectra. **A:** Normal waveform. **B:** Reversed flow in diastole.

umbilical FVW, whereas those with premature rupture of the membranes or renal defects have normal FVW.[68] This is an important distinction as the management is completely different.

Hypertension Severe pre-eclampsia may be associated with abnormal umbilical FVW,[60,69] even when the fetuses subsequently delivered are not growth retarded. This may simply be due to the fact that these pregnancies were delivered for maternal reasons before the fetal growth rate had diminished. In longitudinal studies of the uteroplacental and fetoplacental circulation it appears that uteroplacental ischaemia precedes, and is the determinant of, impaired fetal blood flow in pre-eclamptic patients.[36] The subsequent development of abnormal umbilical FVW is a good indicator of fetal compromise and thus may be helpful in timing delivery. One group disagrees that abnormal umbilical FVWs are secondary to uteroplacental insufficiency and hypothesise that the primary vascular pathology is a placental vascular lesion which deprives the fetus and that maternal hypertension is secondary to this.[69] However, the poor association of abnormal uteroplacental FVW with pre-eclampsia in the studies of this group may be accounted for by the study of subplacental vessels rather than the main uterine artery, which would be expected to give more comprehensive information about this complex circulation.[41] In order to resolve this controversy more longitudinal studies of both sides of the placental circulation are required.

Diabetic pregnancy   Pregnant women with insulin dependent diabetes mellitus are at an increased risk of pre-eclampsia and intra-uterine growth retardation. As these two conditions are associated with abnormal umbilical artery FVWs the use of Doppler ultrasound has been proposed as an additional tool for antenatal surveillance. However, there is a limited amount of information regarding the investigation of this population with Doppler ultrasound.[70,71] From information available at present it would seem that in the absence of maternal vasculopathy most diabetic pregnancies have a normal umbilical artery FVW and that in a well-controlled diabetic population there is no relationship between glycaemic control and impedance to flow. However, umbilical artery FVWS may be useful in patients with vasculopathy in detecting those pregnancies at high-risk of developing growth retardation.

Twin pregnancy   Twin pregnancy is associated with a significant increase in perinatal morbidity and mortality, which is largely due to premature delivery and growth retardation.[72] In uncomplicated twin pregnancies impedance indices of twin fetuses have been compared with those from singletons and found to be identical throughout gestation.[73] Abnormal placentation is a particular problem of twin pregnancy and fistulous communication is unique. Doppler ultrasound has been used to identify these problems. Abnormal umbilical FVWs are found in association with growth retarded twins[74,75] and are able to predict which twins will become discordant in size later on in pregnancy.[76] The degree of discordance in Doppler measurements may be a better predictor of poor outcome than the degree of discordance in fetal abdominal circumference.[77] The situation as regards twin–twin transfusion syndrome is not clearly established, but the simultaneous presence of high and low resistance values has been found.[74]

Other complications   In some chromosomally or anatomically abnormal fetuses the umbilical artery FVWs are abnormal in the presence of a normal uterine waveform.[78] As the placenta is a fetal tissue it is surmised that these are cases of primary fetal effect and that obliteration of the small arteries in the placenta is triggered by the abnormal fetus. In post-term pregnancies increased resistance in the umbilical artery is associated with poor fetal outcome, although there is no correlation between impedance to flow and prolongation of gestation.[79]

Umbilical artery FVWs may be useful in pregnancies which are Lupus anticoagulant-positive to monitor placental vascular insufficiency and to act as an early indicator of developing disease.[80]

Screening studies

There have been a number of screening studies carried out to assess the value of abnormal umbilical artery FVW in the prediction of IUGR. As with the uterine artery screening studies comparison between studies is difficult because of different definitions of what constitutes an abnormal Doppler test and varying definitions of growth retardation. However, there are only two umbilical arteries and they are much easier to study than the uterine circulation. One paper examined a group of 'high-risk' pregnant women at 26 to 28 weeks and found that 60% of those who subsequently delivered a baby with a birthweight less than the tenth centile had abnormal Doppler studies.[81] These results were supported by another study carried out on an unselected population.[82] However, there was a stricter cut off point taken for abnormal impedance index and growth retardation was defined as birthweight less than the 15th centile. However, three other papers studying larger groups of patients have concurred in their conclusion that screening of an unselected population with umbilical artery velocimetry is of limited value.[18,83,84] The largest of these studies[84] found that screening for SGA babies (less than 5th centile) in a three stage programme is of no value regardless of threshold or index chosen. Operative delivery for fetal distress, Apgar scores, cord pH, cord PCV and ponderal index were even less well-predicted than SGA. There were three unexplained stillbirths in the series, in each of which the umbilical FVWs were abnormal, although time of death was not predicted. All the studies agree that the infrequent finding of absent end diastolic flow in an unselected group is associated with an adverse outcome, although the degree of urgency with which these pregnancies should be delivered is still uncertain.

Fetal growth results from the interaction of intrinsic growth potential and placental nutritive and circulatory functions. Doppler ultrasound can only investigate the circulatory component, which may not always be at fault in pregnancies complicated by SGA fetuses. Unlike the uteroplacental circulation there is no obvious gestation at which screening with umbilical artery Doppler would be expected to detect most at risk pregnancies. This combination of factors may account for poor screening results, but in spite of apparent lack of value as a screening tool umbilical artery velocimetry is still a useful diagnostic and monitoring aid in high-risk pregnancies.

The fetal circulation

The major fetal vessels are best studied using pulsed wave Doppler ultrasound. FVWs from fetal vessels are analysed using impedance indices as well as the time averaged mean velocity. It is also possible to calculate volume flow per unit time and fetal weight,[4] but this is limited by the inability to perform accurate diameter measurements on small fetal vessels and errors in fetal weight estimates. Thus, volume flow studies have largely been abandoned.

Doppler ultrasound studies of selected fetal organs are valuable in detecting the haemodynamic rearrangements which occur in response to hypoxia. Animal work has demonstrated that during hypoxia there is preferential perfusion of the fetal brain, heart and adrenals at the expense of the abdominal viscera and limbs. This phenomenon is termed the brain sparing effect.[85] An alteration in the head/abdomen circumference ratio in favour of head growth has been demonstrated by ultrasound biometric measurements in some SGA fetuses.[86] More recently Doppler ultrasound has allowed non-invasive confirmation of the brain sparing effect in human fetuses.

Descending thoracic aorta and common carotid artery

Eik-Nes et al[87] were the first to use pulsed wave Doppler ultrasound to obtain FVWs from the fetal thoracic aorta. The waveform is biphasic, showing continuous forward flow during diastole with no reverse component and is typical of an arterial supply to a low resistance vascular bed (Fig. 9A). The common carotid artery has been studied by Bilardo et al.[88]

In normal pregnancy the impedance indices in the aorta show little change with advancing gestation.[89,90] However, the mean blood velocity increases in the second trimester and this may reflect a progressive increase in cardiac output in step with the demands of the growing fetus (Fig. 10). After 32 weeks gestation, however, the mean aortic blood velocity remains stable, suggesting a possible redistribution of flow. This is supported by the finding that in the common carotid artery the mean blood velocity increases linearly with gestation and there is a decrease in impedance to flow, especially after 32 weeks.[88]

These findings suggest that a greater proportion of the cardiac output is directed to the fetal brain towards the end of pregnancy, presumably to compensate for the progressive fall in fetal blood pO_2 and increase in pCO_2.[91]

Complicated pregnancy The changes in fetal aortic blood flow which occur in intra-uterine growth retardation have been investigated in a number of studies. In growth retarded fetuses changes in the aortic FVW are characterised by an increased PI and decreased or absent end diastolic frequencies (Figs 9B and C), indicating increased vascular resistance.[89,92,93] These changes have been found

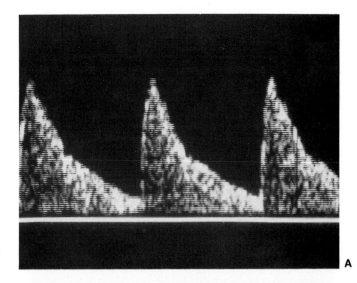

A

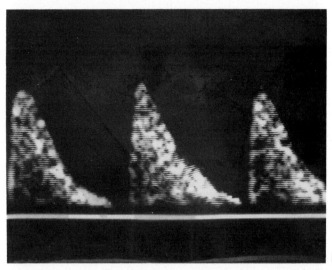

B

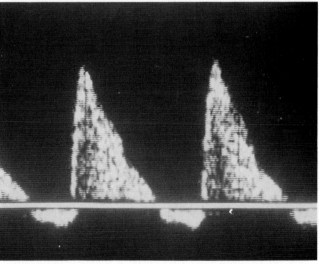

C

Fig. 9 Fetal aortic waveforms. A: Normal FVW from fetal descending thoracic aorta. **B:** Abnormal FVW from fetal descending thoracic aorta demonstrating reduced end diastolic flow. **C:** Reverse flow in diastole.

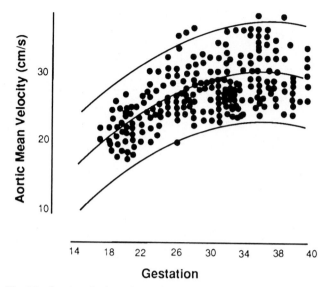

Fig. 10 Aortic velocity reference range (mean and 95% confidence intervals) of mean blood velocity in the fetal descending thoracic aorta with gestation.

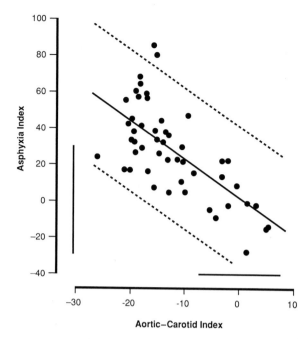

Fig. 11 Doppler versus asphyxia index. Individual values and 95% confidence intervals for the regression line of fetal asphyxia index versus Doppler aortic-carotid index.

to precede the cardiotocograph changes in cases of fetal distress by hours,[92] days[93] or even weeks.[89]

In a study of 29 SGA fetuses[94] where cordocentesis was used to obtain fetal blood samples,[95] a significant negative correlation was found between mean aortic blood velocity and the severity of fetal hypoxia, hypercapnia, acidosis and hyperlacticaemia. This appears to confirm a redistribution of fetal flow in response to hypoxaemia. More recently the mean blood velocity and PI of FVWs from the fetal aorta and common carotid artery in 41 SGA and 10 appropriate for gestational age fetuses were examined.[96] All fetuses also had fetal blood sampling performed by cordocentesis. Blood gases and pH were correlated individually and as an 'asphyxia index' to the Doppler measurements. This index was derived by principal component analysis incorporating pO_2, pH and pCO_2. Although there were significant correlations between the blood gas results and both the PI and mean blood velocity in the individual vessels, better correlations were found with the ratios of common carotid to aortic mean blood velocity and PI. The best predictor of asphyxia, as judged by lowest residual standard deviation and highest correlation coefficient, was an index comprising the aortic mean blood velocity and the PI of FVWs from the common carotid artery. When the aortic-carotid index was abnormal all fetuses had an asphyxia index above the mean; 89% of the fetuses had an asphyxia index one standard deviation above the mean and 60% two standard deviations above the mean. A normal index was always associated with normal blood gases (Fig. 11). Thus the aortic-carotid index appears to be a sensitive indicator of the chemoreceptor response to falling blood oxygen tension. Indeed, since asymmetrical IUGR and a normal pO_2 can coexist, it is possible that alterations in the fetal

circulation can occur before the development of gross fetal hypoxia.

Prediction of neonatal outcome by analysis of the aortic FVWs in IUGR fetuses has been studied.[97] The infants were divided into two groups depending on the presence or absence of aortic EDF at the antenatal Doppler study. There was a significant difference in birthweights between the two groups, although mean gestation at delivery was similar. Necrotising enterocolitis occurred in 27% of the absent EDF group, but in none of positive EDF group. This difference may be due to fetal intestinal hypoxia in utero, a mechanism which has been postulated for the pathogenesis of this condition.[98] With the arrival of colour flow systems it may be possible to visualise the fetal intestinal circulation directly and so perform an accurate study on the predictability of necrotising enterocolitis.

In red cell iso-immunised pregnancies mean aortic blood velocity has been used to predict fetal anaemia.[99] Fetal haemoglobin concentrations were measured in blood samples obtained by cordocentesis. In the non-hydropic fetuses there is an inverse correlation between the haemoglobin concentration and the velocity of blood in the aorta (Fig. 12). This finding is consistent with the hypothesis that in fetal anaemia cardiac output is increased to maintain an adequate delivery of oxygen to the tissues.[100] In hydropic fetuses the correlation is lost.[101]

The fetal cerebral circulation

In normal pregnancy, as already stated, there is apparently

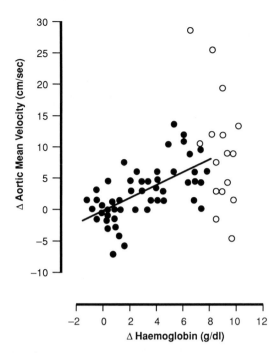

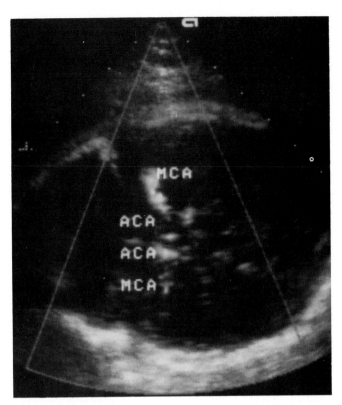

Fig. 12 Aortic velocity versus anaemia. Relation between deviation in aortic mean velocity (observed aortic mean velocity minus normal mean for gestation) and haemoglobin deficit (normal mean haemoglobin for gestational age minus observed value) in non-hydropic (closed circle) and hydropic (open circle) fetuses from red cell iso-immunised pregnancies.

Plate 2 Circle of Willis visualised by colour flow imaging. MCA – middle cerebral artery, ACA – anterior communicating artery. This figure is reproduced in colour in the colour plate section at the front of this volume.

a redistribution of the fetal circulation in favour of the fetal brain with advancing gestation.[88] The common carotid artery supplies the head and neck and, in order to study cerebral perfusion accurately, it is necessary to examine the blood flow in specific intracranial vessels. Pulsed wave Doppler ultrasound has been used to study the intracranial course of the internal carotid artery and continuous forward flow throughout the cardiac cycle has been demonstrated,[102] with a decrease in impedance to flow with increasing gestation.[103]

Complicated pregnancies In hypoxaemic growth retardation low impedance values are found in the internal carotid artery in combination with high impedance in the umbilical artery and thoracic aorta,[102,104] suggesting a redistribution of fetal blood flow. The same reduction of impedance to flow in growth retardation has been demonstrated in the middle cerebral artery[105] and all major intracranial arteries,[103] suggesting their participation in the brain sparing effect. However, when all the intracranial vessels are studied in the same fetus the PI is found to be significantly higher in the middle cerebral artery than in other vessels.[106] This indicates the importance of knowing exactly which cerebral vessel is being insonated in order to interpret the FVW correctly, particularly in longitudinal studies. FVWs from the middle cerebral artery appear to be easier to obtain than from the other intracranial vessels[103] and this may be the vessel of choice in the study

of the fetal cerebral circulation. In addition, the sensitivity of the PI in the internal carotid artery in the prediction of intra-uterine growth retardation is poor[107] and the PI of the middle cerebral artery seems to be a better indicator of fetal compromise.[103]

Further investigation of the intracranial vasculature has been greatly assisted by the advent of colour flow imaging. This allows visualisation of the fetal circle of Willis and the intracranial arteries (Plate 2).[108] The middle cerebral artery is easily and accurately identified, which minimises sampling errors and allows reproducibility in longitudinal studies. Colour flow imaging has been used to study the middle cerebral artery in normal pregnancies at 20 to 40 weeks gestation.[7] With advancing gestation the PI of FVWs from the middle cerebral artery fell and the mean blood velocity increased (Figs 13 and 14). In a group of hypoxic SGA fetuses the PI of FVWs from the middle cerebral artery was significantly lower and the mean blood velocity significantly higher than the normal mean for gestation, again illustrating the brain sparing effect.

In pulsed wave Doppler studies of the internal carotid artery in oligohydramnios due to renal agenesis end diastolic frequencies were found to be reduced, absent or even reversed.[109] From this it was concluded that oligohydramnios hampered cerebral blood flow through fetal head

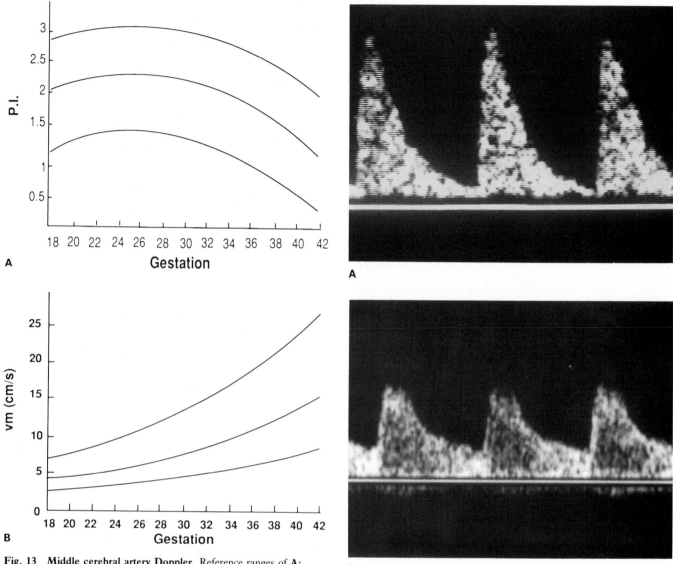

Fig. 13 Middle cerebral artery Doppler. Reference ranges of **A:** Middle cerebral artery pulsatility index (PI) with gestation and **B:** mean blood velocity (vm) in the middle cerebral artery with gestation.

Fig. 14 Middle cerebral artery spectral tracings. A: Normal FVW from the middle cerebral artery at 20 weeks gestation and **B:** at 36 weeks gestation.

compression. However, a study of the middle cerebral artery, internal carotid artery and aorta with colour flow imaging demonstrated that maternal abdominal compression with the ultrasound transducer increased the PI in the cerebral vessels.[110] This is thought to be due to the fetal brain being a compressible structure within a confined space and the application of external pressure leading to an increase in intracranial pressure, resulting in an increase in impedance to flow. Since IUGR is associated with oligohydramnios, and therefore difficulty in imaging, care should be taken to minimise compression of the fetal head during Doppler studies of intracranial vessels. Indeed, undue compression of the fetal head by the ultrasound transducer may be the cause of the findings in the previous paper.[109] This is particularly important when studying intracranial vessels in IUGR in order to avoid artificially increasing impedance values which may truly be low in the presence of hypoxia and leading to a high false negative rate.

In red cell iso-immunised pregnancies there is an inverse correlation between mean velocity of blood in the middle cerebral artery and haemoglobin concentration, measured by cordocentesis. The blood velocity was not related to fetal hypoxaemia and the relationship of increased velocity to anaemia was not affected by PI.[111] Thus, it is suggested that the hyperdynamic circulation is a consequence of decreased blood viscosity.

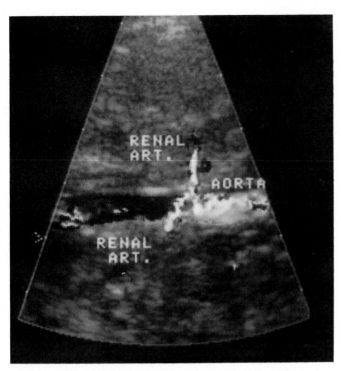

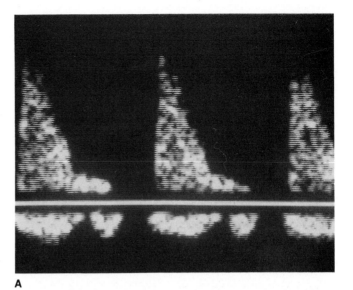

A

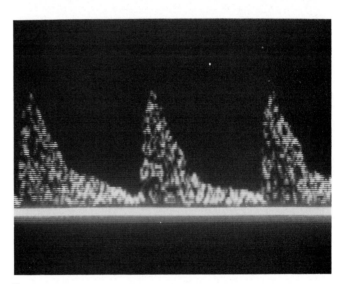

B

Plate 3 **Fetal aorta and renal artery** visualised by colour flow imaging. This figure is reproduced in colour in the colour plate section at the front of this volume.

Fig. 15 **Renal artery spectral tracings.** FVW from the fetal renal artery at **A**: 20 weeks and **B**: 36 weeks.

The fetal renal artery

The renal artery has been studied with colour flow imaging in normal fetuses (Plate 3) and the pulsatility index has been found to decrease with gestation (Fig. 15), presumably reflecting an increase in renal perfusion.[112] The PI of FVWs from the fetal renal artery has also been studied in SGA fetuses and found to be higher than the expected mean for gestation. In all cases cordocentesis was performed and a significant correlation was found between blood oxygen deficit and increased renal artery PI.

Conclusion

At the present time the principal value of uteroplacental vascular studies is as a long-term predictor of the risk of pre-eclampsia and growth retardation. Failure of the fetoplacental circulation is usually secondary to utero-placental insufficiency, but can occur as a primary event. Study of the umbilical artery with continuous wave Doppler ultrasound is a simple bedside technique which is useful in predicting fetal hypoxaemia in the 'at risk' pregnancy. Study of the fetal circulation demands greater expertise and more expensive equipment, but is valuable as a more precise indicator of the degree of hypoxaemia than study of the umbilical artery. Indeed, the present evidence indicates that of all the tests of fetal condition it is the earliest indicator of hypoxaemia and may therefore allow the delivery of a baby in a better condition with less chance of developing neonatal complications. However, the redistribution of flow appears to occur when the degree of hypoxaemia is not very severe and action taken on the Doppler alone could mean the delivery of a baby at unnecessary risk of prematurity. These risks are finely balanced and further refinement of the techniques is needed to optimise the timing of delivery in these high-risk cases.

REFERENCES

1 Satomura A. Study of flow patterns in peripheral arteries by ultrasonics. J Acoust Soc Jpn 1959; 15: 151–159

2 Rekonen A, Lutola H, Pitkaren M, Kuikka J, Pyorala T. Measurement of intervillous and myometrial blood flow by an intravenous 133Xe method. Br J Obstet Gynaecol 1976; 82: 723–728

3 Stembera Z K, Medr J, Ganz V, Fronek A. Measurement of umbilical cord blood flow by local thermodilution. Am J Obstet Gynecol 1964; 90: 531–536

4 Griffin D R, Cohen-Overbeek T E, Campbell S. Fetal and uteroplacental blood flow. Clin Obstet Gynecol 1983; 10: 565–602

5 Jauniaux E, Campbell S, Vyas S. The use of colour flow imaging for antenatal diagnosis of cord anomalies. Am J Obstet Gynecol 1989; 161: 1195–1197

6 Vyas S, Nicolaides K H, Campbell S. Renal artery flow velocity waveforms. Am J Obstet Gynecol 1989; 161: 168–172

7 Vyas S, Nicolaides K H, Bower S, Campbell S. Middle cerebral artery flow velocity waveforms in fetal hypoxaemia. Br J Obstet Gynecol 1990; 97: 797–803

8 Stuart B, Drumm J, Fitzgerald D, Duignan N M. Fetal blood velocity waveforms in normal pregnancy. Br J Obstet Gynaecol 1980; 88: 865–869

9 Pourcelot L. Applications cliniques de l'examen Doppler transcutane. In: Perroneau P. ed. Velocimetrie Ultrasonore Doppler. INSERM 34. 1974: p 213–240

10 Gosling R G, King D H. Ultrasound angiology. In: Marcus A W, Adamson L. eds. Arteries and veins. Edinburgh: Churchill Livingstone. 1975: p 61–98

11 Maini C L, Galli G, Bellati U, Bonetti M G, Moneta E. Non-invasive radioisotopic evaluation of placental blood flow. Gynecol Obstet Invest 1985; 19: 196

12 Pijnenborg R, Bland J M, Robertson W B, Brosens I. Uteroplacental arterial changes related to interstitial trophoblast migration in early human pregnancy. Placenta 1983; 4: 387–414

13 Brosens I, Robertson W B, Dixon H G. The role of the spiral arteries in the pathogenesis of pre-eclampsia. Obstet Gynecol 1972; 1: 177–191

14 Brosens I, Dixon H G, Robertson W B. Fetal growth retardation and the arteries of the placental bed. Br J Obstet Gynaecol 1977; 84: 656–663

15 Arduini D, Rizzo G, Romanini C, Mancuso S. Uteroplacental blood flow velocity waveforms as predictors of pregnancy-induced hypertension. Eur J Obstet Gynecol Reprod Biol 1987; 26: 335–341

16 Jacobson S L, Imhof R, Manning N, et al. The value of Doppler assessment of the uteroplacental circulation in predicting preeclampsia or intrauterine growth retardation. Am J Obstet Gynecol 1990; 162: 110–114

17 Steel S A, Pearce J M F, Chamberlain G. Doppler ultrasound of the uteroplacental circulation as a screening test for severe pre-eclampsia with intra-uterine growth retardation. Eur J Obstet Gynaecol Reprod Biol 1988; 28: 279–287

18 Hanretty K P, Primrose M H, Neilson J P, Whittle M J. Pregnancy screening by Doppler uteroplacental and umbilical artery waveforms. Br J Obstet Gynaecol 1989; 96: 1163–1167

19 Newnham J P, Patterson L L, James I R, Diepeveen D A, Reid S E. An evaluation of the efficacy of Doppler flow velocity waveform analysis as a screening test in pregnancy. Am J Obstet Gynecol 1990; 162: 403–410

20 Hackett G, Panella M. Campbell S. Continuous wave Doppler assessment of the uteroplacental and umbilical circulations: a screening tool for high risk pregnancies? 1990; submitted

21 Campbell S, Pearce J M F, Hackett G, Cohen-Overbeek T, Hernandez C. Qualitative assessment of uteroplacental blood flow: an early screening test for high risk pregnancies. Obstet Gynecol 1986; 68: 649–653

22 Sheppard B L, Bonnar J. Scanning electron microscopy of the human placenta and decidual spiral arteries in normal pregnancy. J Obstet Gynaecol Br Cwlth 1974; 81: 20–29

23 Brosens I, Robertson W B, Dixon H G. The physiological response of the vessels of the placental bed to normal pregnancy.

J Pathol Bacteriol 1967; 93: 569–579

24 Khong T Y, De Wolf F, Robertson W B, Brosens I. Inadequate maternal vascular response to placentation in pregnancies complicated by pre-eclampsia and by small-for-gestational age infants. Br J Obstet Gynaecol 1986; 93: 1049–1059

25 Robertson W B, Brosens I, Dixon H G. Uteroplacental vascular pathology. Eur J Obstet Gynecol Reprod Biol 1975; 5: 47–65

26 Stirrat G M. The immunology of hypertension in pregnancy. In: Sharp F, Symonds E M. eds. Hypertension in pregnancy. Proceedings of the Sixteenth Study Group of the Royal College of Obstetricians and Gynaecologists. Perinatology Press. 1986: p 249–261

27 Wallenburg H C S. Changes in the coagulation system and platelets in pregnancy-induced hypertension and pre-eclampsia. In: Sharp F, Symonds E M. eds. Hypertension in pregnancy. Proceedings of the Sixteenth Study Group of the Royal College of Obstetricians and Gynaecologists. Perinatology Press. 1986: p 227–248

28 Campbell S, Diaz-Recasens J, Griffin D R, et al. New Doppler technique for assessing uteroplacental blood inflow. Lancet 1983; i: 675–677

29 Pearce J M F, Campbell S, Cohen-Overbeek T, Hackett G, Hernandez J, Royston P. Reference ranges and sources of variation for indices of pulsed Doppler flow velocity waveforms from the uteroplacental and fetal circulation. Br J Obstet Gynaecol 1988; 95: 248–256

30 Hastie S J, Howie C A, Whittle M J, Rubin P C. Daily variability of umbilical and lateral uterine wall artery blood velocity waveform measurements, Br J Obstet Gynaecol 1988; 95: 571–574

31 Morrow R J, Knox Ritchie J W, Bull S B. Fetal and maternal hemodynamic responses to exercise in pregnancy assessed by Doppler ultrasonography. Am J Obstet Gynecol 1989; 160: 138–140

32 Fleischer A, Anyaegbunam A, Schulman H, Farmakides G, Randolph G. Uterine and umbilical artery velocimetry during normal labor. Am J Obstet Gynecol 1987; 157: 40–43

33 Bower S, Vyas S, Campbell S. Contractions in the antenatal period alter uterine artery flow velocity waveforms. In preparation. 1990

34 Fleischer A, Schulman H, Farmakides G, et al. Uterine artery Doppler velocimetry in pregnant women with hypertension. Am J Obstet Gynecol 1986; 154: 806–813

35 Ducey J, Schulman H, Farmakides G, et al. A classification of hypertension in pregnancy based on Doppler velocimetry. Am J Obstet Gynecol 1987; 157: 680–685

36 Campbell S, Hernandez C, Cohen-Overbeek T E, Pearce J M F. Assessment of fetoplacental and uteroplacental blood flow using duplex pulsed Doppler ultrasound in complicated pregnancies. J Perinat Med 1984; 12: 262–265

37 McCowan L M, Ritchie K, Mo L Y, Bascom P A, Sherret H. Uterine artery flow velocity waveforms in normal and growth retarded pregnancies. Am J Obstet Gynecol 1988; 158: 499–504

38 Trudinger B J, Giles W B, Cook C M. Flow velocity waveforms in the maternal uteroplacental and fetal umbilical placental circulations. Am J Obstet Gynecol 1985; 152: 155–163

39 Schulman H, Fleischer A, Farmakides G, Bracero L, Rochelson B, Grunfeld L. Development of uterine artery compliance in pregnancy as detected by Doppler ultrasound. Am J Obstet Gynecol 1989; 161: 1536–1539

40 Trudinger B J, Giles W B, Cook C M. Uteroplacental blood flow velocity-time waveforms in normal and complicated pregnancy. Br J Obstet Gynaecol 1985; 92: 39–45

41 Bewley S, Campbell S, Cooper D. Uteroplacental Doppler flow velocity waveforms in the second trimester. A complex circulation. Br J Obstet Gynaecol 1989; 96: 1040–1046

42 Kofinas A D, Penry M, Swain M, Hatjis C G. Effect of placental laterality on uterine artery resistance and development of preeclampsia and intrauterine growth retardation. Am J Obstet Gynecol 1989; 161: 1536–1539

43 Schulman H, Ducey J, Farmakides G, et al. Uterine artery Doppler velocimetry: the significance of divergent systolic/diastolic ratios. Am J Obstet Gynecol 1987; 157: 1539–1542

44 Symonds E M. Aetiology of pre-eclampsia: A review. J R Soc Med 1980; 73: 871–875

45 Pijnenborg R, Dixon G, Robertson W B, Brosens I. Trophoblastic invasion of human decidua from 8–18 weeks of pregnancy. Placenta 1980; 1: 3–19

46 Campbell S, Bewley S, Cohen-Overbeek T. Investigation of the uteroplacental circulation by Doppler ultrasound. Semin Perinatol 1987; 11: 362–368

47 Thaler I, Manor D, Itskovitz J, et al. Changes in uterine blood flow during human pregnancy. Am J Obstet Gynecol 1990; 162: 121–125

48 Collaborative low dose aspirin study in pregnancy for the prevention and treatment of pre-eclampsia and intrauterine growth retardation.

49 Schulman H, Fleischer A, Stern W, et al. Umbilical velocity wave ratios in human pregnancy. Am J Obstet Gynecol 1984; 148: 985–990

50 Campbell S, Vyas S, Nicolaides K H. Doppler investigation of the fetal circulation. Eur J Perinatol 1990; In press.

51 Kaufman P, Sen D K, Schwiekhart G. Classification of human placental villi. 1. Histology. Cell Tissue Res 1979; 200: 409

52 Stuart B, Drumm J, Fitzgerald D E, Duignan N M. Fetal blood velocity waveforms in uncomplicated labour. Br J Obstet Gynaecol 1981; 88: 865–869

53 Fairlie F M, Lang G D, Sheldon C D. Umbilical artery flow velocity waveforms in labour. Br J Obstet Gynaecol 1989; 96: 151–157

54 Trudinger B J, Giles W B, Cook C M, et al. Fetal umbilical artery flow velocity waveforms and placental resistance: clinical significance. Br J Obstet Gynaecol 1985; 92: 23–30

55 Giles W B, Trudinger B J, Baird P J. Fetal umbilical artery flow velocity waveforms and placental resistance: pathological correlation. Br J Obstet Gynaecol 1985; 92: 31–38

56 Fleischer A, Schulman H, Farmakides G, et al. Umbilical velocity wave ratios in intrauterine growth retardation. Am J Obstet Gynecol 1985; 151: 502–506

57 Rochelson B L, Schulman H, Farmakides G, et al. The significance of absent end diastolic velocity in umbilical artery velocity waveforms. Am J Obstet Gynecol 1987; 156: 1213–1218

58 Reuwer P J H M, Bruinse H W, Stoutenbeek P, et al. Doppler assessment of the feto-placental circulation in normal and growth retarded fetuses. Eur J Obstet Gynecol Reprod Biol 1984; 18: 199–205

59 Trudinger B J, Giles W B, Cook CM. Flow velocity waveforms in the maternal uteroplacental and fetal umbilical placental circulations. Am J Obstet Gynecol 1985; 152: 155–163

60 Chambers S E, Hoskins P R, Haddad N G, Johnstone F D, McDicken W N, Muir B B. A comparison of fetal abdominal circumference measurements and Doppler ultrasound in the prediction of small-for-dates babies and fetal compromise. Br J Obstet Gynaecol 1989; 96: 803–808

61 Dempster J, Mires G J, Patel N, Taylor D J. Umbilical artery velocity waveforms: poor association with small-for-gestational-age babies. Br J Obstet Gynaecol 1989; 96: 692–696

62 Nicolaides K H, Bilardo C M, Soothill P W, Campbell S. Absence of end diastolic frequencies in the umbilical artery: a sign of fetal hypoxia and acidosis. BMJ 1988; 297: 1026–1027

63 Tyrrell S, Obaid A H, Lilford R J. Umbilical artery Doppler velocimetry as a predictor of fetal hypoxia and acidosis at birth. Obstet Gynecol 1989; 74: 332–336

64 Brar H S, Platt L D. Reverse end-diastolic flow velocity on umbilical artery velocimetry in high risk pregnancies: an ominous finding with adverse pregnancy outcome. Am J Obstet Gynecol 1988; 159: 559–561

65 Trudinger B J, Cook C M, Thompson R S, Giles H B, Connelly A. Low dose aspirin therapy improves fetal weight in umbilical placental insufficiency. Am J Obstet Gynecol 1988; 159: 681–685

66 Ylikorkala O, Ulla-Maija M, Kaapa P, Viinikka L. Maternal ingestion of acetylsalicylic acid inhibits fetal and neonatal prostacyclin and thromboxane in humans. Am J Obstet Gynecol 1986; 155: 345–349

67 Trudinger B J, Connelly A J, Giles W B, Hales J R S, Wilcox G. The effects of prostacyclin and thromboxane analogue (U 46619) on the fetal circulation and umbilical artery flow velocity waveforms. J Dev Physiol 11: 179–184

68 Hackett G, Nicolaides K H, Campbell S. Doppler ultrasound assessment of fetal and uteroplacental circulations in second trimester severe oligohydramnios. Br J Obstet Gynaecol 1987; 94: 1074–1077

69 Trudinger B J, Cook C M. Doppler umbilical and uterine flow waveforms in severe pregnancy hypertension. Br J Obstet Gynaecol 1990; 97: 142–148

70 Landon M B, Gabbe S G, Bruner J P, Ludmir J. Doppler umbilical artery velocimetry in pregnancy complicated by insulin-dependent diabetes mellitus. Obstet Gynecol 1989; 73: 961–965

71 Bracero L, Schulman H, Fleischer A, Farmakides G, Rochelson B. Umbilical artery velocimetry in diabetic pregnancy. Obstet Gynecol 1986; 63: 654–658

72 O'Connor M C, Arias E, Royston J P, Dalrymple I J. The merits of special antenatal care for twin pregnancies. Br J Obstet Gynaecol 1981; 88: 220–230

73 Gerson A, Johnson A, Wallace D, Bottalico J, Weiner S, Bolognese R. Umbilical arterial systolic/diastolic values in normal twin gestation. Obstet Gynecol 1988; 72: 205–207

74 Farmakides G, Schulman H, Saldana L R, Bracero L A, Fleischer A, Rochelson B. Surveillance of twin pregnancy with umbilical artery velocimetry. Am J Obstet Gynecol 1985; 153: 789–792

75 Giles W B, Trudinger B J, Cook C M. Fetal umbilical artery flow velocity-time waveforms in twin pregnancies. Br J Obstet Gynaecol 1985; 92: 490–497

76 Gerson A G, Wallace D M, Bridgens N K, et el. Duplex Doppler ultrasound in the evaluation of growth in twin pregnancies. Obstet Gynecol 1987; 70: 419

77 Nimrod C, Davies D, Harder J, et al. Doppler ultrasound prediction of fetal outcome in twin pregnancies. Am J Obstet Gynecol 1987; 156: 402–406

78 Trudinger B J, Cook C M. Umbilical and uterine artery flow velocity waveforms in pregnancy associated with major fetal abnormality. Br J Obstet Gynaecol 1985; 92: 666–670

79 Rightmire D A, Campbell S. Fetal and maternal Doppler blood flow parameters in postterm pregnancies. Obstet Gynecol 1987; 69: 891–894

80 Trudinger B J, Stewart G J, Cook C M, Connelly A, Exner T. Monitoring lupus anticoagulant-positive pregnancies with umbilical artery flow velocity waveforms. Obstet Gynecol 1988; 72: 215–218

81 Arduini D, Rizzo G, Romanini C, Mancuso S. Fetal blood flow velocity waveforms as predictors of growth retardation. Obstet Gynecol 1987; 70: 7–10

82 Schulman H, Winter D, Farmakides G, et al. Pregnancy surveillance with Doppler velocimetry of uterine and umbilical arteries. Am J Obstet Gynecol 1989; 160: 192–196

83 Sijmons E A, Reuwer P J H M, Van Beek E, Bruinse H W. The validity of screening for small-for-gestational age and low-weight-for-length infants by Doppler ultrasound. Br J Obstet Gynaecol 1989; 96: 557–561

84 Beattie R B, Dornan J C. Antenatal screening for intrauterine growth retardation with umbilical artery Doppler ultrasonography. BMJ 1989; 298: 631–635

85 Peeters L L H, Sheldon R E, Jones M D, Makowski E L, Meschisca G. Blood flow to fetal organs as a function of arterial oxygen content. Am J Obstet Gynecol 1979; 135: 637

86 Campbell S, Thoms A. Ultrasound measurement of the fetal head to abdomen ratio in the assessment of growth retardation. Br J Obstet Gynaecol 1977; 84: 165–174

87 Eik-Nes S H, Brubakk A O, Ulstein M K. Measurement of human fetal blood flow. Lancet 1980; i: 283–285

88 Bilardo C M, Campbell S, Nicolaides K H. Mean blood velocities and flow impedance in the descending thoracic aorta and common carotid artery in normal pregnancy. Early Hum Dev 1988; 18: 213–221

89 Griffin D, Bilardo K, Masini L, et al. Doppler blood flow waveforms in the descending thoracic aorta of the human fetus. Br J Obstet Gynaecol 1984; 91: 997–1006

90 Tonge H M, Wladimiroff J W, Noordan M J, et al. Blood flow velocity waveforms in the descending fetal aorta: comparisons between normal and growth retarded pregnancies. Obstet Gynecol 1986; 67: 851–855

91 Nicolaides K H, Economides D, Soothill P W. Blood gases and pH in appropriate and small for gestational age fetuses. Am J Obstet Gynecol 1989; 161: 996–1001

92 Jouppila P, Kirkinen P. Increased vascular resistance in the descending aorta of the human fetus in hypoxia. Br J Obstet Gynaecol 1984; 91: 853–856

93 Lingman G, Laurin J, Marsal K. Circulatory changes in fetuses with imminent asphyxia. Biol Neonate 1986; 49: 66–73

94 Soothill P W, Nicolaides K H, Bilardo C M, Campbell S. Relation of fetal hypoxia in growth retardation to mean blood velocity in the fetal aorta. Lancet 1986; i: 1118–1119

95 Nicolaides K H, Soothill P W, Rodeck C H, Campbell S. Ultrasound guided sampling of umbilical cord and placental blood to assess fetal well-being. Lancet 1986; i: 1065–1067

96 Bilardo C M, Nicolaides K H, Campbell S. Doppler measurements of fetal and uteroplacental circulations; relationship with umbilical venous blood gases measured at cordocentesis. Am J Obstet Gynecol 1990; 162: 115–120

97 Hackett G A, Campbell S, Gamsu H, et al. Doppler studies in the growth retarded fetus and prediction of neonatal necrotising enterocolitis, haemorrhage and neonatal morbidity. BMJ 1987; 294: 13–15

98 Touloukian R J, Posch J N, Spencer R. The pathogenesis of ischaemic gastro-entero-colitis of the neonate; selective gut mucosal ischaemia in asphyxiated neonatal piglets. J Paediatr Surg 1972; 7: 194–205

99 Nicolaides K H, Bilardo C M, Campbell S. Prediction of fetal anaemia by measurement of the mean blood velocity in the fetal aorta. Am J Obstet Gynecol 1988; 162: 209–212

100 Huikeshoven F J, Hope I D, Power G G, Gilbert R D, Longo L D. A comparison of sheep and human fetal oxygen delivery systems with use of a mathematical model. Am J Obstet Gynecol 1985; 151: 449–455

101 Soothill P W, Nicolaides K H, Rodeck C H, Clewell W H, Lingridge J. Relationship of fetal haemoglobin and oxygen content to lactate concentration in Rh isoimmunised pregnancies. Obstet Gynecol 1987; 69: 268–270

102 Wladimiroff J W, Tonge H M, Stewart P A. Doppler ultrasound assessment of cerebral blood flow in the human fetus. Br J Obstet Gynaecol 1986; 93: 471–475

103 Van den Wijngaard J A G W, Groenenberg I A L, Wladimiroff J W, Hop W C. Cerebral Doppler ultrasound of the human fetus. Br J Obstet Gynaecol 1989; 96: 845–849

104 Wladimiroff J W, Van den Wijngaard J A G W, Degani S, Noordam M J, Van Eyck J, Tonge H M. Cerebral and umbilical arterial blood flow velocity waveforms in normal and growth retarded pregnancies. Obstet Gynecol 1987; 69: 705–709

105 Woo J S K, Liang S T, Lo R L S, Chan F Y. Middle cerebral artery Doppler flow velocity waveforms. Obstet Gynecol 1987; 70: 613–616

106 Mari G, Moise K J, Deter R L, Kirshon B, Carpenter R J, Huhta J C. Doppler assessment of the pulsatility index in the cerebral circulation of the human fetus. Am J Obstet Gynecol 1989; 160: 698–703

107 Wladimiroff J W, Noordam M J, Van Den Wijngaard J A G W, Hop W C J. Fetal internal carotid and umbilical artery blood flow as a measure of fetal compromise in intrauterine growth retardation. Pediatr Res 1988; 24: 609–612

108 Arbeille P H, Tranquart F, Berson M, Roncin A, Saliba E, Pourcelot L. Visualization of the fetal circle of Willis and intracerebral arteries by color-coded Doppler. Eur J Obstet Gynecol Reprod Biol 1989; 32: 195–198

109 Van Den Wijngaard J A G W, Wladimiroff J W, Reuss A, Stewart P A. Oligohydramnios and fetal cerebral blood flow. Br J Obstet Gynaecol 1988; 95: 1309–1311

110 Vyas S, Campbell S, Bower S, Nicolaides K H. Maternal abdominal pressure alters fetal cerebral flow. Br J Obstet Gynaecol 1990; 97: 740–747

111 Vyas S, Nicolaides K H, Campbell S. Doppler examination of the middle cerebral artery in anaemic fetuses. Am J Obstet Gynecol 1990; 162: 1066–1068

112 Vyas S, Nicolaides K H, Campbell S. Renal artery flow-velocity waveforms in normal and hypoxaemic fetuses. Am J Obstet Gynecol 1989; 161: 168–172

The central nervous system

Alison Fowlie and Glyn Constantine

INTRODUCTION

In the early days of obstetric ultrasound, in the era of the static B-scanner and before grey scale display, very little detail could be seen of the fetus, the part most easily visualised being the axial skeleton. This led initially to some chance diagnoses of hydrocephalus in the late part of pregnancy when the fetal biparietal diameter was found to be abnormally large, and was followed by the first successful mid-trimester diagnosis of fetal abnormality when, in 1972, Campbell identified an anencephalic fetus of 19 weeks gestation.[1]

Around that time the incidence of anencephaly and spina bifida in England and Wales was particularly high. Thus considerable effort was put into further development of ultrasonic antenatal diagnosis of neural tube defects. This led over the years, particularly with the increasing sophistication of ultrasound technology, to the ability to make many different diagnoses of abnormalities of the central nervous system.

Although the neural tube defects themselves have declined in incidence, defects of the central nervous system (CNS) are amongst the commonest congenital abnormalities overall occurring in one per 200 live births[2] and in 3% to 4% of spontaneous abortions.[3] Whilst alpha-fetoprotein has had some part to play, particularly in identifying the neural tube defects, it has no part to play in identification of the closed defects which make up the bulk of the CNS abnormalities. Ultrasound examination remains the essential tool for the identification of these problems.

In assessing any structure with ultrasound it is important to have a thorough knowledge of the normal developmental anatomy and the appearance at different gestations. (Prior to the development of ultrasound, knowledge of the development of the normal fetus was scanty, and of course based on abortion specimens in which normality could be questioned and trauma may have caused an artefact.) This is particularly true for the fetal head. At about 12 weeks the fetal cerebral ventricles have a simple crescent-like shape and occupy the bulk of the intracranial contents. By about 18 weeks, although the cerebral ventricles have not changed very much in size, the cerebral cortex has grown considerably, thus the proportion of the intracranial contents occupied by the ventricles is now much smaller (see Ch. 7). As pregnancy progresses the structure of the ventricles becomes more complex with development of the posterior and occipital horns. Initially the surface of the brain is very smooth but gyri begin to develop late in the mid-trimester. Thus care must be taken in conditions which rely to a large extent on the size of the ventricles much before 18 weeks, and pure lissencephaly (agyria) clearly could not be diagnosed until the third trimester.

In several European countries including Britain, the majority of antenatal patients are scanned routinely. Most of these scans are in the second trimester when the BPD and probably the head circumference are measured. Central nervous system defects may be detected during the course of making these routine antenatal measurements of the fetal head. In this way most CNS defects are potentially detectable, even in the low-risk population.

Whilst the scan plane for the BPD is being aligned it should be possible to establish:

a) the shape of the head in transverse section, noting whether there are any unusual contours or bulges;

b) the presence of a strong midline echo, the midline structures such as the cavity of the septum pellucidum, third ventricle and the bodies of the thalami;

c) the configuration of the lateral ventricles;

d) the configuration of the cerebellum and cisterna magna.

If any deviation from normal is noted during the course of this scan, or the patient is one at increased risk of fetal abnormality and on whom a detailed scan is being performed, further views should be sought. Most abnormalities to be discussed below can be detected and elucidated from these scan planes but other views may be useful in specific cases, e.g. a sagittal section when assessing facial abnormalities such as in holoprosencephaly.

Using transabdominal real time ultrasound it is possible to detect anencephaly and large encephaloceles from 12 weeks onwards. Occasionally spinal lesions are detected at 14 to 16 weeks but generally it is best to search for CNS abnormalities at around 18 weeks. At this time detailed visualisation of the spine is achieved in the majority of fetuses and cerebral ventricular size is fairly constant. Vaginal scanning allows better visualisation of the fetus at a much earlier stage, and it is already possible to detect anencephaly at around 10 weeks. Because of the developmental changes which occur at about this time, considerable care must be exercised in making early diagnoses of other CNS abnormalities.

Neural tube defects

These include anencephaly, exencephaly, encephalocele, spina bifida and diastematomyelia. These conditions have many features in common, the occurrence of one putting the woman at risk of the others in a future pregnancy.

Epidemiology

Neural tube defects have an incidence which varies over time and with geographical location.

Both long and short-term temporal variations have been reported. A major confounding influence in determining the recent overall incidence, however, is the effect of prenatal diagnosis and termination of affected pregnancies. NTDs, in particular anencephaly, have been noted in the past to be more frequent in winter months.[4] More recent reports have suggested that this seasonal variation has disappeared.[5] However, the experience from the West Midlands Region, England, over the past 6 years has been that of two peaks a year at approximately 6 monthly intervals, the larger peak of mid-trimester problems being apparent in August and September, implying conception in April and May. In addition to this seasonal variation it has been found that there is a significant long-term variability in the incidence of neural tube defects. Data covering the years 1910 to 1970 from the Eastern USA show that in 1930 the rate was 2.5 times the levels in 1910 and 1970.[6] A similar variation in the incidence of anencephaly was reported in Birmingham over the period 1936 to 1964. Here cyclical peaks occurred every 14 years when the incidence was around 1.8 times the minimum incidence.[2,7] Recently the incidence in the UK has fallen considerably.[8–11] Between 1964 and 1986 the birth prevalence of NTDs declined in the UK from 31.5 to 6.2 per 10 000,[12] birth prevalence of anencephaly declining by 94% and spina bifida by 68%. When terminations for affected pregnancies were taken into account, however, the overall incidence of affected pregnancies fell by 50% and 32% respectively.[8] In the light of previous experience it will be a long time before it will be known whether this is to be a permanent fall in the incidence of neural tube defects.

Geographical variations are also widespread, with reported rates for NTDs ranging from 0.8 to 7.6 per 10 000, there being a tenfold difference between areas of highest and lowest incidence.[13] The highest recorded incidence was 10 per 1000 in some Welsh mining valleys.[14] Why the United Kingdom, and particularly the Celtic areas, have the world's highest incidence of NTDs, and the Japanese the lowest, is unclear. It has been suggested that the variation within the UK is secondary to geological conditions, soft water areas having a higher prevalence of NTDs.[15] More intensive study, however, suggests this to be an unlikely cause.[16,17]

As well as an apparent correlation with geographical area, a genetic predisposition amongst the inhabitants of those areas has been suggested. This is borne out by the studies of migrants from high and low-risk areas. Thus those of Irish and Sikh descent tend to retain a higher rate of NTDs on emigration, whilst Negroes and Jews retain a lower rate.[18–21]

The vast majority of NTDs therefore appear to be inherited in a multifactorial manner with some evidence of an additional environmental factor. Other specific associations include the anticonvulsants sodium valproate and carbamazepine.[22,23]

Anencephaly and exencephaly

Anencephaly is a condition in which the cranial vault and much of the brain is absent, the residual brain being grossly malformed. In addition the frontal, parietal and occipital bones are often malformed and deficient. The brain remnants are covered by a vascular membrane, the area cerebrovasculosa. It has been thought for many years that the defect resulted from failure of closure of the anterior neuropore at around 24 days gestation,[24] but a more recent theory suggests that an excess of CSF causes disruption of the normally formed cerebral hemispheres.[25,26]

Exencephaly is characterised by a partial absence of the cranial vault with a large amount of protruding brain tissue. This condition is considered to lie somewhere on the spectrum between anencephaly and encephalocele. It may be an embryological precursor of the more common anencephaly, the exposed brain slowly degenerating through trauma and exposure to amniotic fluid, finally reaching the anencephalic state.[27]

Incidence and aetiology Anencephaly is the commonest of the open neural tube defects and is four times more frequent in females. As in the other neural tube defects, geographical differences in incidence are marked, varying from 0.6 per 1000 in Japan to 3.5 per 1000 in parts of the United Kingdom. There is an increased familial incidence and these regional differences appear to be at least partly genetic in origin. Anencephaly has a multifactorial aetiology as well as genetic and geographical factors, specific teratogens having been implicated, including radiation, salicylates and sulphonamides.

Exencephaly is much less common than anencephaly but it has the same aetiology and recurrence risk as the other neural tube defects.

Diagnosis It was not uncommon for anencephaly to present clinically in the late second and third trimesters of pregnancy with polyhydramnios. Most cases nowadays, however, are detected earlier in pregnancy by a combination of ultrasound and maternal AFP screening.[1,28–32] The ultrasound diagnosis depends on visualising the cephalic pole of the fetus clearly so that the absence of the cranial vault and fetal brain above the level of the orbits can be noted. The fetal face often has a 'frog-like' appearance with prominent orbits due to the deficiency of the frontal bone. The neck is often short and this adds to the frog-like appearance (Fig. 1) The diagnosis is often considered when there is difficulty measuring the fetal biparietal diameter. Anencephaly can be suspected as early as 11 to 12 weeks of gestation and it may be possible to be definite at this stage, particularly with the improved image quality of trans-vaginal scans, though it is more usual for the diagnosis to be confirmed around 15 to 16 weeks. The diagnosis can only be excluded by visualising a normal skull and made by having a good clear view of the cephalic pole (Fig. 2) Inattention to this may lead to both false positive and negative diagnoses, although these are extremely rare. Calvarial bones are very small prior to 13 weeks and angiomatous stroma above the orbits, which can occur in up to 45% of cases[33,34] may be mistaken for a normal head

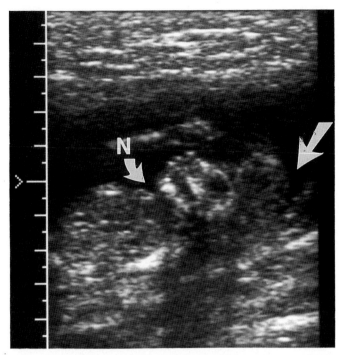

Fig. 1 **Anencephaly.** Longitudinal scan illustrating absence of cranial vault (arrowed), short neck (N) and frog-like face.

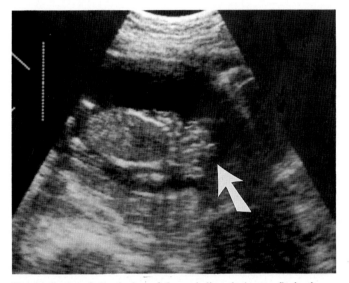

Fig. 2 **Anencephaly.** A view of the cephalic pole (arrowed) clearly illustrates absence of cranial vault and disorganised brain tissue.

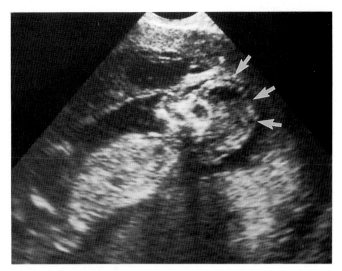

Fig. 3 **Exencephaly.** Calvarial bones are absent from the top of the skull (arrows) and the intracranial anatomy is abnormal.

by the unwary. A head low in the maternal pelvis, particularly in the obese patient, may be so poorly seen that this may be mistaken for anencephaly. If the head is deep in the maternal pelvis and yet there is a strong suspicion that there is anencephaly, then every attempt should be made to obtain a good view, including the use of head down tilt, filling and emptying the bladder, and of trans-vaginal scanning. If these are to no avail, then it must be remembered that an amniocentesis and estimation of the liquor AFP and cholinesterase banding will produce a definitive diagnosis.

For exencephaly, the diagnosis is much the same as for anencephaly and in fact it would be unlikely to be recognised in utero as a different condition in the majority of cases. The most striking feature is the large amount of disorganised cerebral tissue arising from the base of the cranium as well as the non-visualisation of the calvarium (Fig. 3). The residual brain mass is bereft of normal features with convolutions on its surface. The facial structures and base of the cranium are always present.[35,36]

Differential diagnosis In cases in which the fetal head appears small and difficult to visualise the differential diagnosis lies between anencephaly, exencephaly, severe microcephaly, acrania and the amniotic band syndrome. It may be impossible to differentiate between anencephaly and exencephaly, and even acrania antenatally, particularly if the diagnosis is being made very early in the second trimester. Acrania is a developmental abnormality with partial or complete absence of the cranium and nearly complete development of the brain tissue. In principle it should be possible to differentiate this from anencephaly by the presence of the cerebral cortex,[37] but in practice this may be difficult. In later pregnancy the differentiation from microcephaly may be made, not on the size of the head, but on the presence of the skull vault, however small. Amniotic bands may rarely destroy most of the vault and brain.[38] When this occurs, however, the destruction is usually asymmetrical and, unlike anencephaly, associated with oligohydramnios.[33] All these conditions have a very poor prognosis but the recurrence risks and therefore implication for the future differ.

Associated malformations Spina bifida is an associated finding in anencephaly. This may take the form of craniorrhachischisis, complete non-closure of the neural tube or a coexistent sacral spina bifida. Exomphalos, cleft lip and palate and club foot have also been reported.[39] These findings are however of no practical significance as the condition is uniformly fatal. Exencephaly has been reported in association with exomphalos.[36]

Prognosis Around 70% of fetuses with anencephaly will be stillborn, the others surviving for only a matter of hours. Exencephaly is also incompatible with life.

Obstetric management As these conditions are invariably lethal termination of pregnancy at any stage after the diagnosis is made is a reasonable option.[40]

Encephalocele

Encephalocele is a herniation of some of the cranial contents through a defect in the bony skull. Protrusion of the meninges only is strictly a meningocele; when brain tissue itself is extruding through the defect, it is an encephalocele. The lesion is thought to occur because of failed closure of the rostral end of the neural tube during the fourth week of fetal life. This may be due either to primary overgrowth of neural tissue in the line of closure or failure of induction by adjacent neurodermal tissues interrupting this process.[41]

The majority of lesions occur in the midline and vary in size from a few millimetres upwards. The protruded sac can be very small or reach a size larger than the fetal skull. Although usually protruding externally and therefore visible, encephaloceles can occur through the base of the skull and protrude into the orbits, nose or mouth.[42] Sites of occurrence are occipital midline 75%, frontal midline 13%, and parietal 12%, most of the latter being due to amniotic band syndrome. It is thought that in this condition there is early disruption in the formation of the fetal skull. Encephaloceles resulting are atypical and the appearances are very variable. Frontal encephaloceles almost always contain brain tissue[43] and involve the bridge of the nose and nasal cavity in 60% and 30% of cases respectively. In some cases the bulk of the brain is actually situated in the herniated sac.

Incidence and aetiology Encephaloceles are uncommon. In 1984 the incidence in England and Wales was 0.8 per 10 000 births.[44] However it should be noted that the incidence of such disorders is much higher at an earlier stage of pregnancy.

Encephaloceles have a multifactorial aetiology; in common with most neural tube defects, genetic and geographical factors have been implicated and other defects occur with increased frequency in siblings.[43,45] Encephaloceles are commoner in females and have an increased incidence in certain races, e.g. Chinese. They are often found together with other abnormalities in a number of genetic syndromes (Meckel, von Voss, Chemke, Roberts, Knoblock, cryptophthalmos) and non-genetic

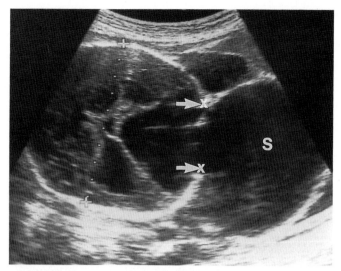

Fig. 4 Encephalocele. There is a large defect in the occipital bone (between arrows) through which protrudes a fluid filled sac (S), a meningocele. The intracranial anatomy is grossly abnormal.

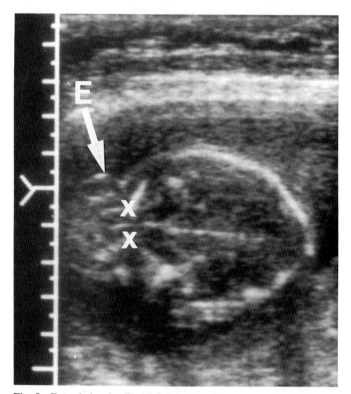

Fig. 5 Encephalocele. The defect is seen (between crosses) and as the herniated sac (E) contains brain tissue, an encephalocele is diagnosed.

syndromes (amniotic bands, warfarin, maternal rubella, diabetes).[46]

Diagnosis The classical ultrasound picture is a mass arising from the occipital or frontal regions of the skull.[47–51] This may appear to be purely fluid filled (Fig. 4), or it can contain echoes from herniated brain tissue (Fig. 5). To make the diagnosis with certainty the bony defect must be demonstrated. This may be difficult, either because of its size, or the presence of artefact due to reflective/refractive shadowing mimicking a defect. Particular problems occur with meningoceles where a large lesion arises from a very small defect that is impossible to visualise.[51,52] The intracranial anatomy should therefore be carefully assessed, as in the majority of cases this is abnormal. Once an encephalocele has been detected a careful search must be made for other associated anomalies.

Differential diagnosis   The chief differential diagnoses lie between cystic hygroma, scalp oedema, branchial cleft cyst, nasal teratoma and clover leaf skull deformity. Of these, encephaloceles are the only ones to be associated with a bony defect, and in the vast majority of cases there is some disorganisation or distortion of the intracranial anatomy including hydrocephalus. Cystic hygromas are usually bilateral in origin and may contain septa; it should also be possible to see that scalp oedema affects the whole skull if scanning is carried on in different planes. Nasal teratomas are often irregular in outline. Haemangiomas can be distinguished by their vascular appearance and confirmed by the demonstration of blood flow with the use of Doppler ultrasound. The clover leaf skull is not a difficult diagnosis when it coexists with a skeletal dysplasia such as thanatophoric dwarfism because the associated abnormalities are obvious. When the head abnormality is isolated careful evaluation of the skull shape is necessary (Fig. 6).

Associated malformations   Other malformations occur commonly. Some are parts of specific syndromes as previously mentioned, the common ones being polycystic kidneys in Meckels syndrome or amputated limbs in the

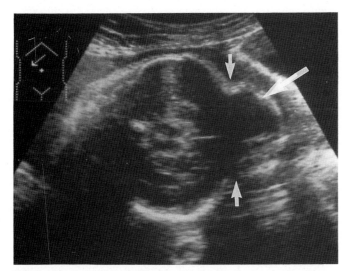

Fig. 6   Craniosynostosis. The frontal bulge (large arrow) caused by the premature fusion of the sutures (small arrows) may easily be mistaken for an encephalocele.

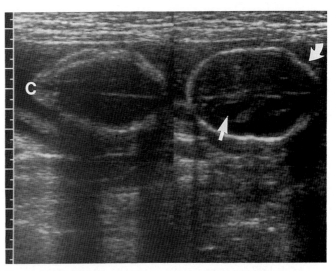

Fig. 7   Encephalocele. Small occipital encephalocele (C) but producing hydrocephalus (straight arrow – dilated posterior horn; curved arrow – 'lemon sign').

amniotic band syndrome. Other malformations such as meningomyeloceles (present in 7% to 33% of cases[47,53]), facial clefts, microcephaly (in 20% of cases[45]), hydrocephalus, Dandy-Walker syndrome and agenesis of the corpus callosum appear to be sporadic. Hydrocephalus occurs in up to 80% of occipital meningoceles and 65% of occipital encephaloceles (Fig. 7),[45] often being secondary to herniation of the cerebellum into the encephalocele and/or aqueduct stenosis.[43] The rarer frontal encephalocele often occurs with the median cleft face syndrome[54] and is associated with hydrocephalus in 15% of cases.[48]

Prognosis   20% of fetuses with an encephalocele will be stillborn. The factors which result in a very poor prognosis, determined from groups of infants which were liveborn, are the coexistence of other abnormalities, the presence of brain in the herniated sac and microcephaly.[55,56] The impact of hydrocephalus is less certain. In general the mortality is lower if that is the only associated problem, but the intellectual impairment is very variable. Meningoceles have the lowest mortality, a 100% survival rate with 60% developing normally having been reported. This compares with a 56% survival rate with 9% normal development for cases where brain tissue is present in an encephalocele.[45] Frontal encephaloceles have a better prognosis than others.

Obstetric management   The prognosis for each encephalocele based on its particular features should be discussed with the parents and in the majority of cases, if detected early enough, termination of pregnancy is chosen. If the abnormality is detected in later pregnancy and there are associated abnormalities which are incompatible with life, termination again may be recommended. If the lesion is extensive and contains brain tissue, or there is microcephaly, the management should be conservative.[47]

Caesarean section may be considered in those cases where neonatal surgery is thought to be appropriate.

Spina bifida

Spina bifida describes a midline bony defect of one or more vertebrae. Usually the defect is in the posterior arch and results in the absence of the arch, broadening of the vertebrae, lateral displacement of the pedicles and a widened spinal canal.[57] Occasionally the defect may be anterior but this is very uncommon. While the term only refers to the bony defect, the problems of the fetus are caused by maldevelopment of the spinal cord and the frequently associated hydrocephalus.

The suggestions concerning the origin of the condition are similar to those for anencephaly. The established theory has been that there is failure of closure of the caudal neuropore[58] but more recently there has been a suggestion of overproduction or underabsorption of CSF in the embryonic period, the excess fluid causing a secondary rupture in the neural tube.[59] In 80% to 90% of cases the lesion affects the lumbar or lumbo-sacral regions; isolated sacral and cervical lesions accounting for most of the remainder. Spina bifida confined to the thoraco-lumbar, thoracic or cervico-thoracic regions is rare.[60] Multiple defects are also unusual, being reported in only 1% of cases.[48]

Spina bifida can be found in a range of severities. At its most severe the lesion is overt and it may be present as a myeloschisis in which the spinal cord is laid wide open, or as a meningomyelocele, a cystic protrusion of meninges containing central nervous system tissue. Meningomyeloceles are typically found in the lower thoraco-lumbar region, lumbar and lumbo-sacral areas. Meningoceles are cystic lesions that may contain peripheral nerves but no central nervous system tissue. These constitute only 5% of the total cases of spina bifida. Meningoceles usually occur in the occipital, cervical or upper thoracic region or lower sacral region. Another form is spina bifida occulta. Here the lesion is usually small and is completely covered by skin. There may be no abnormality on the overlying skin, but a tuft of hair or pigmentation of the skin is a clue in about 50% of cases. They are almost always found at the level of L5 or S1. In the majority of cases lesions such as these are asymptomatic, being picked up incidentally on X-ray examination. Some, however, do result in back pain and neurological disabilities, such as weakness in the lower limbs and poor sphincter control. Coexistent spinal cord abnormalities are common, hydromyelia and/or syringomyelia being present in around 43% of cases.[61]

The vast majority of cases of spina bifida also have the Arnold-Chiari type II malformation.[62] In this the cerebellar vermis herniates within the foramen magnum, leading to a displacement of the fourth ventricle, tentorium and medulla. The return flow of CSF to the intracranial arachnoid granulations is usually subsequently blocked causing obstructive hydrocephalus (> 90% of cases). The lesions without hydrocephalus tend to be meningoceles.

Incidence and aetiology As discussed, the incidence varies with season, geographical area and race. The United Kingdom, and especially Ireland, had a very high incidence of around three per 1000 births but this has declined steadily in the past 15 years, Britain now having one of the lowest instances in Western Europe (0.6 per 1000 births).[63] The condition is commoner in Caucasians than Orientals or Blacks. Spina bifida, like the other neural tube defects, appears to be most commonly inherited in a multifactorial manner. Other associations are with single mutant gene conditions (e.g. Jarco-Levin, Meckel, Robert, and HARDE syndromes) and with teratogens such as sodium valproate and carbamazepine.

Diagnosis The ultrasound appearances of spina bifida can be divided into those of the spinal lesion itself and those of associated findings in the fetal head. Often the latter are much more obvious than the lesion itself and prompt a closer look at the spine.

The fetal vertebrae are composed of three ossification centres, giving rise to the typical view of the fetal spine seen in transverse section. The vertebral body arises from the anterior centre whilst the laminae and neural arches arise from the two posterior centres which develop an inward angulation. In longitudinal section the posterior ossification centres appear as two parallel lines.[64] These normal relationships are the key to diagnosis of the spinal abnormality. Examination of the spine along its entire length should ideally be carried out in the transverse, sagittal and coronal planes. In transverse section of spina bifida the normal appearance of the spine is lost as the posterior ossification centres splay outwards giving a U or V shape rather than the normal closed circle (Fig. 8). In addition the edges of the bones are rather sharp and they are highly reflective. In coronal section the parallel lines of the ossification centres splay out to give a characteristic bulge (Fig. 9), whilst in the sagittal midline section the posterior centres may not be visualised as the posterior arch is absent (Fig. 10). In addition, normal curvature of the spine is often lost, in particular in the sacral region. Kyphoscoliosis may be present. The transverse and sagittal sections are preferable for the identification of the characteristics of the soft tissue component. It should be possible to distinguish between a myeloschisis (Fig. 8) when there is absence of skin or soft tissues over the spinal defect, and the cystic appearance of a meningocele or meningomyelocele (Fig. 11). It may not be easy to distinguish on the ultrasound appearances between a meningocele and a meningomyelocele, although the exact site of the lesion may help with this. Problems in scanning occur when the fetal back is pressed close to maternal tissue or placenta, or when the back is completely posterior and the fetus cannot be persuaded to move. If the spine lies directly at three

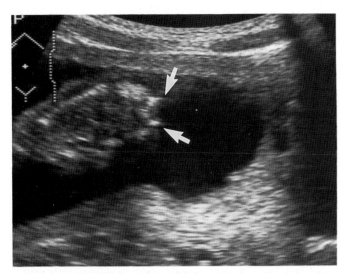

Fig. 8 Spina bifida. A transverse section of the sacral spine (arrowed) is shown. Note the sharpness of the bones producing the typical U-shape and absence of any soft tissue covering, diagnostic of a myeloschisis.

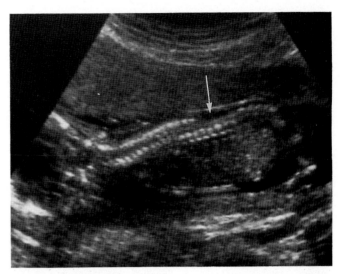

Fig. 10 Lumbo-sacral spina bifida displayed in sagittal section. The posterior arch is absent (arrowed).

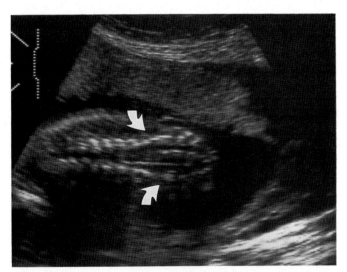

Fig. 9 Large lumbo-sacral spina bifida. The coronal section displays the characteristic bulge (arrowed) caused by the splaying out of the ossification centres.

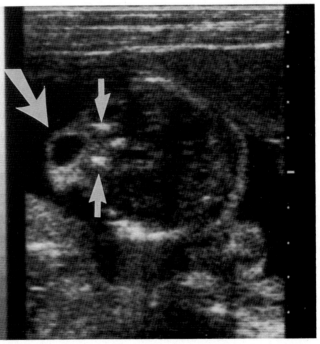

Fig. 11 Meningocele. Transverse scan of meningocele (large arrow) with widening of the posterior vertebral ossification centres (small arrows).

or nine o'clock in the field of view on a transverse scan, the beam spread artefact may cause difficulty in establishing the appearance of a closed ring.

It is very rare for spina bifida to be associated with an overdistended bladder. Study of the lower limb movement has not helped either with the diagnosis or the prognosis of the lesion, apparently normal movements occurring in very severe lesions.

Hydrocephalus associated with the Arnold-Chiari malformation in fetuses with spina bifida is very characteristic, the particular appearances described below are not found

in isolated hydrocephalus. In transverse section the head is irregular with a pointed frontal region,[65] described as the 'lemon' sign (Fig. 12). This is seen at the level used for measuring the biparietal diameter and was present in all 54 of the cases where such a view was available.[66,67] The anterior and the posterior horns of the lateral cerebral

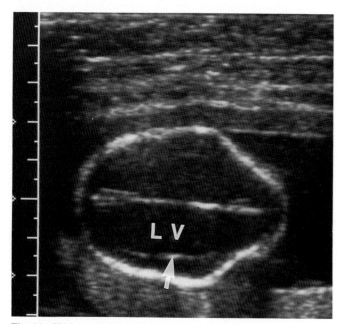

Fig. 12 Hydrocephaly. The characteristic appearances of hydrocephalus associated with spina bifida. Note the lemon shaped head, the pointed end being anterior, and the enlarged lateral ventricles (LV). Arrow – lateral wall of ventricle.

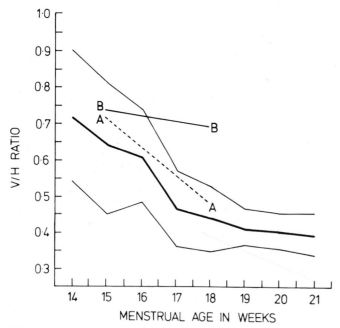

Fig. 13 Graph of the ventricular/hemisphere width ratio for the anterior horns of the lateral ventricles with the ratios of fetus A (normal) and fetus B (spina bifida with hydrocephalus) plotted at 15 and 18 weeks. This illustrates the pitfall of using the ratio before 18 weeks when the normal range is wide.

ventricles are large when compared to the cerebral hemispheres. Ventricular to hemisphere width (V/H) ratios have been established for both anterior and posterior horns (see Appendix).[68]

If these ratios are to be used, and particularly in the case of the anterior horn ratio, care must be taken in making a diagnosis before 18 weeks. Prior to that time the normal range of ventricular size compared to the cerebral hemisphere is large (Fig. 13) so that follow up studies are needed to demonstrate the normal growth of the cerebrum. These ratios were of considerable importance in the earlier days of antenatal diagnosis when the amount of detail visible from the intracranial structures with ultrasound was minimal. With higher resolution imaging however, their use is limited though they are of particular help to the inexperienced scanner. The experienced sonographer with a thorough knowledge of the ultrasound anatomy of the fetal head, can rely on qualitative assessment and readily identify the abnormal.

Another important feature of the hydrocephalus associated with spina bifida is that of an apparently absent or bowed cerebellum.[66] Nicolaides drew attention to abnormalities of the cerebellum in 21 cases.[66] They found it to be absent in eight, or with an anterior concavity (the 'banana' sign) in 12 (Fig. 14). These findings have been generally confirmed in other retrospective and prospective studies, although it seems more usual to have difficulty seeing the cerebellum because of its very low position or hypoplastic state.[69–71] It must be remembered that a normal cerebellum (see Appendix) does not exclude hydrocephalus or spina bifida (Fig. 15).

In addition, in contrast to the normal state, the medial borders of the anterior horns may well be visible and prom-

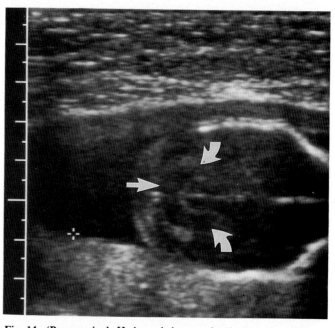

Fig. 14 'Banana sign'. Hydrocephalus associated with spina bifida displaying a bowed cerebellum – the 'banana' sign (curved arrows) – and obliterated cisterna magna (straight arrow).

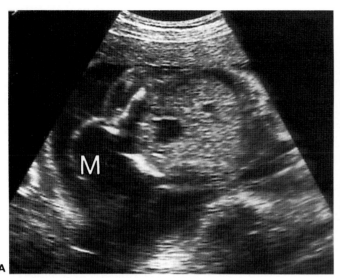

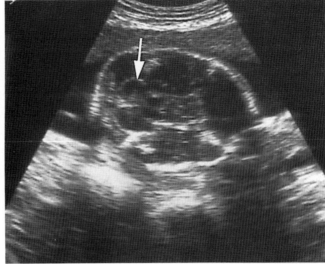

Fig. 15 Sacral meningocele. A: Large sacral meningocele (M) and **B:** normal appearance of cerebellum. The pregnancy proceeded to term and the baby had no neurological deficit.

inent, deviating slightly away from the midline giving a feathered appearance (Fig. 16).

The BPD and head circumference may be small compared to dates or femur length. This applies even in late pregnancy. The abnormally large, fluid filled hydrocephalic head is not found with spina bifida but only with isolated hydrocephalus.

Abnormalities of the head are therefore found in the vast majority of cases of spina bifida. Presence of a normal shape to the head, normal cerebellum and cisterna magna, and normal V/H ratios virtually rules out a serious neural tube defect. A normal appearance is found only in association with a spina bifida where there is a simple meningocele, which for the most part, carries a good prognosis (Fig. 15). This has been borne out in the West Midlands series of 106 cases of spina bifida in which, in 102 (96%), there was obvious hydrocephalus. In one there was dilatation of the third ventricle only and in three there was no abnormality of the head. In these four latter cases the spinal lesions were very low and small with no neurological deficit.

Amniocentesis with measurement of the amniotic fluid alpha-fetoprotein and acetylcholinesterase has been used extensively in the diagnosis of neural tube defects. It is now less widely employed when there is a good ultrasound service, as ultrasound will not only detect the lesion, but indicate its extent and severity to give a guide to prognosis. In addition amniocentesis is subject to errors (Fig. 17) and the incidence of abortion following amniocentesis is up to 1%.[72] Several reports advocate the routine use of amniocentesis in cases where a raised maternal serum AFP is followed by a normal scan.[30,73,74]

Effectiveness of ultrasound in diagnosing spina bifida Ultrasound has been used both as a method of

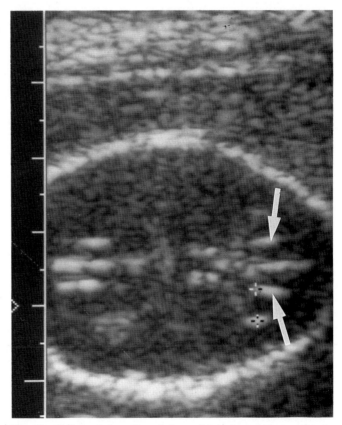

Fig. 16 Hydrocephalus. 15 week fetus with hydrocephalus associated with spina bifida in which the medial borders of the lateral ventricles are clearly seen (arrowed) and deviate away from the midline.

screening for neural tube defects, and to investigate pregnancies singled out as being at high risk, either from the past history or because of raised serum alpha-fetoprotein.

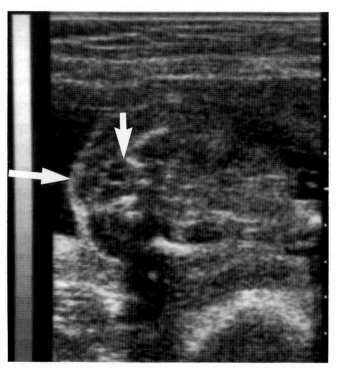

Fig. 17 Closed spina bifida. The skin covering (longer arrow) can be seen over the lesion (short arrow). The serum and liquor AFP were normal.

These different population groups must be borne in mind when evaluating reports as well as experience of the operators and the equipment employed. In addition as knowledge of the appearance of the fetal head, equipment and expertise have all improved during the 1980's earlier reports are unrepresentative. Taking the high-risk group, series dating from the early 1980's show sensitivities ranging from 30% to 87% with specificities of 96% to 99%, positive predictive values of 80% to 92% and negative predictive values of 99%.[31,76] More recent reports show a 91% to 100% sensitivity and 98% specificity in high risk populations for open neural tube defects,[73,75,77,78] but a note of caution was sounded in one series with only a 50% sensitivity.[30] One study has reported the use of the 'lemon' sign and cerebellar abnormalities in the diagnosis of spina bifida in 436 women from an 'at risk' population.[69] The 'lemon' sign was shown to have a 100% sensitivity and 99% specificity with a positive predictive value of 84% and negative predictive value of 100%, whilst cerebellar signs showed figures of 96%, 100%, 100% and 100% respectively. Small sacral lesions, usually particularly difficult to diagnose antenatally with ultrasound were detected by use of these signs in four fetuses.

Only two major population based studies have been reported where all patients were scanned prior to the maternal serum AFP being available.[79,80] In the 1983 study by Persson et al[79] ultrasound detected the only case of anencephaly and 2/3 encephaloceles, but missed 5/5 cases of open spina bifida. Rosendahl & Kivenen[80] reported in 1989 on an 8 year series of 9000 mid-trimester scans performed routinely at 18 weeks. During this time they detected 2/2 anencephalics, 3/4 meningoceles and 2/3 hydrocephalics, a very low instance of NTDs. Between 1984 and 1986 1200 low risk routine 18 to 20 week scans were performed at the Birmingham Maternity Hospital. 5/5 cases of spina bifida associated with hydrocephalus were detected. In this series all the abnormalities were noted in the first instance by recognition of changes in the fetal head. With improvements in technique, training and equipment, experience and knowledge of the important cranial signs, good results should be possible when a low-risk population is screened with ultrasound.

Associated malformations   Other associated malformations are club and rocker bottom feet, both occurring as result of peripheral nerve damage,[81] and single gene disorders such as the Jarco-Levin and Kousseff syndromes.

Prognosis   Figures on prognosis are coloured by the effect of prenatal diagnosis and also preselection of those fetuses referred for treatment. However, before antenatal diagnosis up to 25% of fetuses with spina bifida were stillborn. Untreated, most of the remainder died in the first months of life and even in the treated group, 7 years survival was only 40%.[82] Of these children only 25% had no lower limb disability and only 17% normal continence. In a study of 213 children with spina bifida born between 1965 and 1972, before prenatal diagnosis was introduced, the 5 year survival was 36% for open lesions, 60% for closed lesions and 18% for unclassified lesions.[83] Amongst the survivors with open lesions 84% were severely handicapped, only 6% being normal. These children had spent an average of 6 months in hospital and had an average of six major surgical procedures during their first 5 years of life. In a second study between 1972 and 1979, 154 infants with spina bifida were followed up for 12 months.[84] Survival rates at 12 months were 64%, 73% and 45% for open, closed and unclassified lesions respectively.

It is not possible to predict with certainty which fetuses with spina bifida will die or have a major degree of disability, although certain features are known to be important, such as the level and the extent of the lesion, the presence of kyphoscoliosis and marked hydrocephalus. A large high lesion generally carries a poor prognosis as do marked hydrocephalus and kyphoscoliosis. The presence of CNS tissue within a sac of meninges (Fig. 18) clearly affects the prognosis although it may not be possible to distinguish a meningomyelocele from a meningocele with ultrasound. However, if a lesion is high but small and not causing hydrocephalus, this is likely to be a meningocele with a relatively good prognosis.

Obstetric management   If the diagnosis is made before viability, termination of pregnancy should be considered after appropriate counselling. With widespread adoption of either routine scanning or maternal serum alpha-fetoprotein screening, late diagnosis and the unexpected discovery

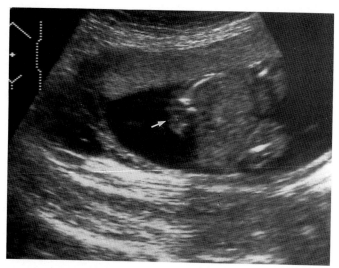

Fig. 18 Spina bifida. A transverse section of a spina bifida. The sac contains soft tissue (arrowed) suggesting that the lesion is a meningomyelocele.

of neural tube defect at birth have become less common. Not all women wish for antenatal diagnosis however, and some women book late in pregnancy. In these groups decisions have to be made about further management if a lesion is found at a late stage. A thorough evaluation of the fetus should be made in order to rule out additional abnormalities. Consultation should take place with the neonatal paediatricians and, if possible, the neurosurgeons. As prediction of which babies will die shortly after birth is not possible, all babies should be delivered in the best condition possible so that they may obtain maximum benefit from whatever post-natal treatment is available. It has been suggested that vaginal delivery could result in traumatising the defect or exposing it to infection[85] and therefore caesarean section is advocated.

Recurrence risks of neural tube defects When a woman has had one pregnancy affected by a neural tube defect she should be carefully counselled about the chances of a recurrence in a subsequent pregnancy. The risk depends on the overall geographic incidence varying from 9% in Northern Ireland to 3% in South East England.[86,87] In Britain overall recurrence risks are generally quoted as being 5% after one neural tube defect, 12% after two and 20% after three. When one of the parents is affected the risk to any pregnancy is of the order of 3%.

Prevention of neural tube defects Major advances have been made in reducing the birth incidence of neural tube defects through antenatal screening and termination of affected fetuses. However the prevention of neural tube defects is also possible in some specific cases such as by altering the anticonvulsant therapy of epileptics who intend to become pregnant. Whether the risk of recurrence can be reduced for those women who have had one or more affected children is controversial. Dietary counselling and

folic acid supplements at the time of conception and in early pregnancy has been shown to reduce the recurrence rate of NTDs in a high risk area.[88,89] Similarly a non-randomised multicentre study using a multivitamin preparation (pregnavite forte F) during the periconceptual period and the first trimester showed a marked decrease in the incidence of recurrent NTDs.[90] This has been confirmed by other workers[91,92] and also by epidemiological data from the USA.[93] Other epidemiological data from an area of low NTD incidence in the USA however suggest periconceptual vitamin supplements to be of less value.[94] At the present time it would seem that multivitamin supplementation for 4 weeks prior to and during the early weeks of pregnancy may be worthwhile in those women with a history of one or more affected fetuses especially as there are no apparent ill effects.

Screening for NTDs with alpha-fetoprotein Because of the high incidence of NTDs and their devastating effects on the fetus leading to death or severe handicap, great efforts have been made to develop efficient screening techniques. These are reviewed thoroughly elsewhere,[53,95] the following being only a brief summary. The first practical technique was developed in the early 1970's when Brock and Sutcliffe[96] measured alpha-fetoprotein (AFP) levels in amniotic fluid and found significantly higher levels in those pregnancies complicated by a NTD. When expressed in multiples of the median for a specific gestation, there is a clear distinction between unaffected pregnancies and those with an open NTD. Around 20% of neural tube defects are missed however in cases where the lesion is closed, whilst other abnormalities such as anterior wall defects and Finnish nephrosis will yield a positive result.

Between 1974 and 1977 a collaborative study using a system of rising cut-offs with increasing gestational age found a sensitivity of 98% for detection of open neural tube defects with a false positive rate of around 0.5%.[96] Subsequently it was found that fetuses with open NTDs secreted acetylcholinesterase (AChE) into the amniotic fluid which could be detected by electrophoresis.[97] This was shown by the presence of a band which could be inhibited by the chemical BW284C51 in addition to the normally occurring pseudocholinesterase. Combining the two techniques eliminates most false positives.[53,95] Amniocentesis is not a technique which can be employed for population screening.

Alpha-fetoprotein is present in maternal serum during pregnancy at about 1/200th the concentration of that in amniotic fluid, and measurement of the maternal serum alpha-fetoprotein only became practical with improved assay techniques. Pregnancies affected with an open NTD were demonstrated to have higher serum AFP levels than controls.[98,99] This finding was tested in a multicentre collaborative study which demonstrated that serum alpha-fetoprotein varied with gestation, was best expressed in multiples of the median for gestation and had a maximum sensitivity between 16 and 18 weeks' gestation.[100] Most laboratories use a cut-off level of between 2.0 and 3.0 multiples of the median; this identifies NTDs with a sensitivity of 80% to 85% and specificity of 96% to 98%.[79,101,102]

The group defined at high risk for NTDs also includes fetuses with other abnormalities, in addition to those with incorrect dates, multiple pregnancies, previous threatened abortion and intra-uterine death. Once these diagnoses have been excluded, only about one in 20 actually have a fetal anomaly,[73] the remainder being at increased risk of abruption, growth retardation and pre-eclampsia. In women with a raised serum alpha-fetoprotein, ultrasound scanning should eliminate many of the possible causes.

Diastematomyelia

This is characterised by the partial or complete clefting of a variable length of the spinal cord into two halves, usually by a midline bony spicule or fibrous band. It occurs most commonly in the lower thoracic and upper lumbar spine and can be found with or without an associated meningomyelocele or neurocutaneous stigmata of spinal dysraphism. It is commoner in females.

Diagnosis and associated malformations Prenatal diagnosis has been reported where a high amplitude central echo was seen running through the spinal canal.[103] In addition there was widening of the posterior ossification centres of the spine. It is commonly associated with spina bifida (Fig. 19).

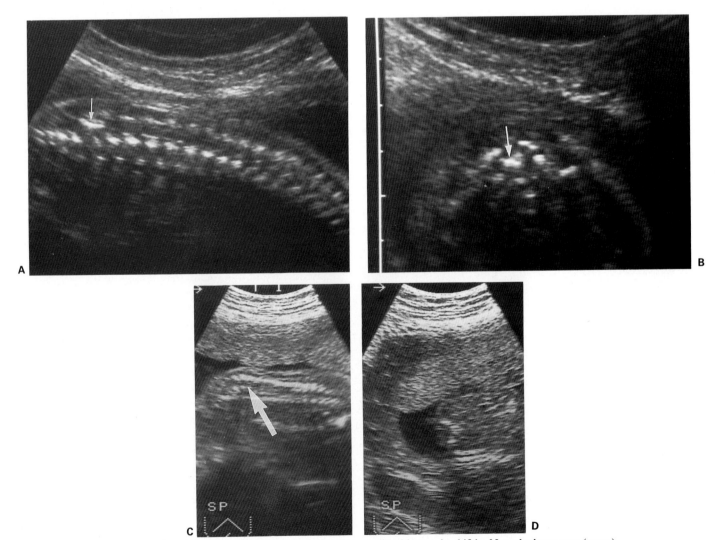

Fig. 19   Diastematomyelia. A and B: A case of lower lumbar diastematomyelia without spina bifida. Note the bony spur (arrow).
C: Longitudinal and **D:** transverse scans of a spine with a large thoraco-lumbar spina bifida. At the lower end the bony spur is seen as a strong echo in the middle of the bulge (arrows).

Prognosis When diastematomyelia occurs in association with a spina bifida the prognosis is the same as for the spina bifida lesion. If it presents as a closed defect the prognosis is variable and may be good. Prognosis for neurological function is enhanced by early surgical removal of the septum dividing the spinal cord.

Hemivertebrae

Hemivertebrae develop when there is aplasia or hypoplasia of one of the two ossification centres which form the vertebral body.

Diagnosis A single hemivertebra may be very difficult to identify. However there is often more than one and they are frequently associated with rib abnormalities and scoliosis, which may be severe. The displacement of the anterior ossification centre from the straight line arrangement of the other centres is apparent on sagittal sections.[104] In coronal sections the normal tramline appearance is lost and a bulge may be present (Fig. 20), easily mistaken for a spina bifida. However in transverse section, although there may be some distortion of the normal closed ring appearance of the spine, the distortion is anterior rather than posterior. In addition, hemivertebrae may be associated with neural tube defects.

Prognosis If there is already marked scoliosis in early pregnancy the deformity of the child will be severe, albeit not life threatening or associated with mental retardation. Multiple surgical procedures are likely to be needed and are seldom entirely successful. Fetuses without significant scoliosis in utero may well develop severe problems after birth. These factors should be borne in mind when counselling the parents.

Caudal regression syndrome

An insult to the developing embryo during the third week of life may result in a wedge-shaped defect in the posterior axis caudal blastema. This may result in fusion of the early lower limb buds and absence or incomplete development of intervening caudal structures. This results in the caudal regression syndrome, a disorder with a wide range of severity; the mildest form is represented by imperforate anus, and the most severe may result in lower limb fusion, sirenomelia, imperforate anus, urological deficits and lower vertebral and pelvic abnormalities, including agenesis (see Ch. 20).

Incidence and aetiology Caudal regression syndrome occurs in about one in 60 000 newborns. It is strongly associated with diabetes mellitus and monozygotic twin pregnancies.[105]

Diagnosis The mildest forms of caudal regression syndrome cannot be diagnosed antenatally. However, sacral agenesis may be recognised. When examining the spine in longitudinal section the normal sacral curve is lost, the spine being somewhat shortened (Fig. 21). The lower limbs may be hypoplastic and a large bladder may be present. In more severe cases the lower thoracic vertebrae may be malformed or absent. The pelvic bones may be absent or rudimentary and the legs may be asymmetrical, grossly shortened or fused.

Associated abnormalities Abdominal wall and genitourinary abnormalities may be present. The prognosis depends on the severity of the lesion: in its severest form it is incompatible with life. In those cases with absent or deformed vertebrae there are likely to be neurological sequelae, such as limb weakness and loss of bladder and bowel sphincter control.

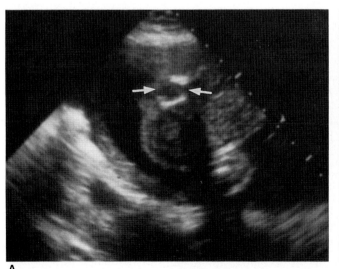
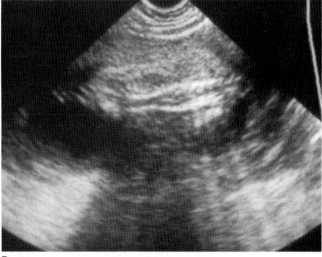

A   B

Fig. 20 Hemivertebrae. The fetus had three consecutive hemivertebrae. **A:** The lesion is seen in transverse section, the normal closed ring appears deficient both anteriorly and posteriorly (arrows) but the ossification centres do not diverge, nor are they sharp. **B:** In a longitudinal section a bulge is noted which is indistinguishable from spina bifida.

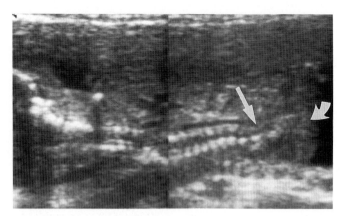

Fig. 21 Caudal regression syndrome. This fetus has sacral agenesis. The spine, shown in longitudinal section, appears to end in the lower lumber region (straight arrow) stopping well short of the caudal pole (curved arrow).

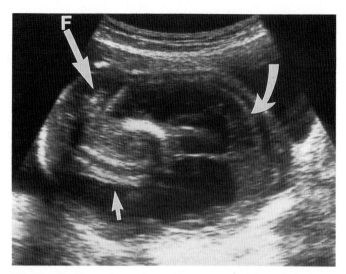

Fig. 22 Acardiac monster. In addition to a normal fetus, in the uterus was a bizarre mass which showed some movement. Part of a spine could be identified (small arrow). At one end, legs could be seen (F). At the other end, was a cystic and solid structure (curved arrow).

Obstetric management   If the abnormality is detected early in pregnancy it is likely that the deformity will be major and termination of pregnancy should be offered.

Acardiac monster

This is a disorder occurring only in monozygotic twin pregnancies when the head and upper part of the thorax of one twin, including the thoracic contents, are absent. Vascular anastomosis between the twins permits the acardiac fetus to survive and grow.

Incidence and aetiology   This rare disorder occurs in one in 35 000 to 48 000 births.[106]

Diagnosis   In addition to the absence of the fetal head, no fetal heart movement can be detected in the abnormal fetus, but lower limb movements may be seen. The spine is short and is found to end abruptly. The lower part of the fetus may also exhibit abnormalities but generally the femora and distal lower limb bones can be identified. The appearance is extremely bizarre (Fig. 22) so that the diagnosis will mostly be made by awareness of the possibility of the condition. Cardiac failure may occur in the normal fetus as it is providing the entire cardiac output for both fetuses, thus the normal fetus may become hydropic. Polyhydramnios may be present.

Obstetric management   The second fetus must be examined carefully for structural abnormalities. If normal, serial examinations are necessary to exclude cardiac failure. Early delivery or digitalisation of the mother[107] may be necessary if hydrops ensues. Platt et al[108] advocated selective ligation of the umbilical artery of the abnormal fetus should hydrops occur. Selective fetocide by other means is not feasible in monozygotic twins. In two cases in which we have been involved one abnormal fetus died in utero at 29 weeks and the other pregnancy developed severe polyhydramnios resulting in preterm labour at 31 weeks.

Iniencephaly

Iniencephaly is an uncommon anomaly, first described in 1887,[109] in which a defect in the occiput resulting in exposure of the brain is combined with dysraphism of the cervical spine. This usually results in fusion of the occiput to the cervical spine and retroflexion of the head with an exaggerated spinal lordosis. The condition is frequently associated with an encephalocele or spina bifida, the spine appearing short and abnormal with pronounced kyphoscoliosis.

Embryologically iniencephaly is thought to be caused by an arrest of the embryo in physiological retroflexion in the third week of gestation or by failure of normal forward bending in the fourth week.[110] Some authors consider that iniencephaly may belong to a group of disorders including Klippel-Feil, Dandy-Walker and Arnold-Chiari syndromes.[110–113]

Incidence and aetiology   Early reports of an incidence of one in 896 seem to be too high.[114] Other estimates in differing populations suggest a frequency varying from one in 1000 to fewer than one in 100 000.[111,115–117] It does not appear to be a familial condition. It is more common in females (male to female ratio 0.28) and in certain geographical areas. In humans it has been found in association with maternal syphilis[118,119] and sedative intake. In animal studies administration of vinblastine,[120] streptonigrin[121] and triparanol[122] have all resulted in iniencephaly.

Diagnosis   Hyperextension of the fetal head with fusion of the occiput to the dorsum of the spine, together with spinal deformities including shortening, lordosis, kyphoscoliosis (Figs 23 and 24) and myelomeningocele are characteristic of iniencephaly.[123–127] Scanning longitudi-

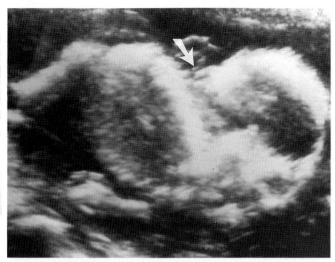

Fig. 23 Iniencephaly. The hyperextension of the fetal head and the fusion of the occiput to the dorsal spine (arrowed) is displayed in this longitudinal section.

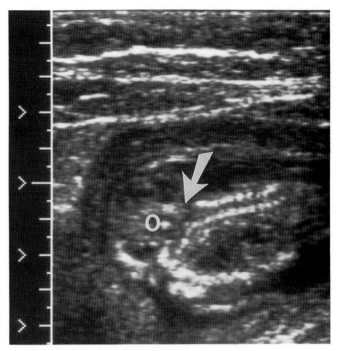

Fig. 25 Iniencephaly. In this scan the entire length of the spine cannot be located in a single plane and the occiput (O) is visualised adjacent to the thoracic spine (arrowed).

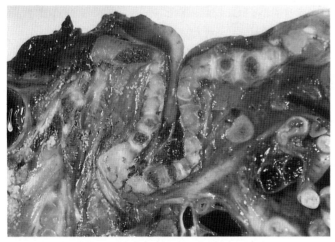

Fig. 24 Iniencephaly. Longitudinal section of an iniencephalic specimen at the level of the cervical spine, displaying its gross curvature. (With thanks to Dr Ian Rushton, Counsultant Perinatal Pathologist, Birmingham Maternity Hospital.)

nally it is difficult to locate the entire fetal spine in a single plane, but on transverse section the head is visualised at the same level as the thorax (Fig. 25).

Associated malformations Iniencephaly is associated with other abnormalities in around 84% of cases.[117,126,128] Morocz et al[126] described 11 cases of iniencephaly diagnosed antenatally, five also having anencephaly and one an encephalocele, one a diaphragmatic hernia, and two lethal pulmonary hypoplasia. Other abnormalities reported were posterior fossa cysts, hydrocephalus, spina bifida, cyclopia, holoprosencephaly, ventricular atresia, polymicrogyria, absence of mandible, facial clefts, cardiac anomalies, exomphalos, gastroschisis, situs inversus, polycystic kid-

neys, arthrogryposis, clubfoot, long upper limbs, thoracic cage deformities, and talipes equinovarus.

Differential diagnosis The main differential diagnosis is that of Klippel-Feil syndrome where fusion of the cervical vertebrae leads to a short neck and deformed spine. It is in fact considered by some that Klippel-Feil syndrome is a mild form of iniencephaly. Other abnormalities which may initially cause confusion include anencephaly and cervical meningomyelocele.

Prognosis Severe iniencephaly is almost invariably fatal in the neonatal period. Out of over 250 cases in the literature, only four cases are reported to have survived; these were cases with a mild abnormality and no associated problems.[113,125]

Obstetric management When diagnosed before viability termination should be offered. Later in pregnancy induction or a non-aggressive approach is justified. Hyperextension of the fetal head may cause obstruction of labour due to a face or brow presentation and these problems should be anticipated. Rarely neonatal surgery has been attempted.[125]

Hydrocephalus

Hydrocephalus is defined as an abnormal increase in the amount of cerebrospinal fluid within the cerebral ventricles. Cerebrospinal fluid (CSF) is formed by the choroid plexuses which occupy much of the fetal ventricular system, flowing through the lateral and third ventricles before escaping into the sub-arachnoid space through the foramina of Luschka and Magendie in the fourth ventricle. After passing through the sub-arachnoid space and cisterna the fluid is reabsorbed by the arachnoid granulations lining the superior sagittal sinus. The system is normally in equilibrium, production being balanced by reabsorption. This increase in the amount of CSF distinguishes true hydrocephalus from conditions in which ventricles appear large secondary to poor cerebral growth, e.g. colpocephaly or destruction/atrophy of the brain tissues such as in hydranencephaly. Hydrocephalus does not necessarily imply a large head, this being a late and inconsistent sign.

Incidence and aetiology Hydrocephalus has an incidence of between 0.1 and 2.5 per 1000 births in various series.[129-131] True hydrocephalus has many associations and causes, but it is almost always secondary to a relative or complete obstruction to the flow of CSF. Rarely it is due to overproduction.[132] If secondary to obstruction it can be further subdivided into communicating and non-communicating varieties, the former being commonly associated with intracranial haemorrhage or meningitis in the neonatal period and consequently rare in fetal life. Non-communicating hydrocephalus implies an obstruction within the ventricular system and is by far the commonest variety presenting in the antenatal period. The majority of cases of non-communicating hydrocephalus or obstructive hydrocephalus are caused by stenosis of the aqueduct of Sylvius which connects the third and fourth ventricles. This is a multifactorial condition in which genetic,[133] infective,[134] teratogenic and neoplastic aetiologies have been postulated. Antenatally, genetic and infective causes predominate, the stenosis being secondary to malformation or gliosis respectively. Malformations include forking, narrowing and septation, narrowing being the most common finding in hereditary cases. In one neonatal autopsy series 50% of cases of aqueduct stenosis were due to gliosis, 46% to forking and 4% to simple narrowing of the canal.[135] Many studies have shown that aqueduct stenosis can be transmitted as an X-linked recessive trait.[136] However it would appear to be inherited in this way in only about 25% of affected male fetuses, while in other families both sexes are affected.[137] Aqueduct stenosis is said to account for about 43% of all cases of congenital hydrocephalus. In other cases obstruction occurs at the foramen of Monro, caused by intracranial cysts, ventriculitis or neoplasms. When obstruction occurs at the foramina of Luschka and Magendie, the Dandy-Walker malformation and other brain cysts and neoplasms are implicated. Obstruction may also occur in the posterior fossa in achondroplasia or clover leaf skull.

Diagnosis Initial attempts at the antenatal ultrasound diagnosis of fetal hydrocephalus relied on measurements of the biparietal diameter. This is a late, crude and totally unreliable sign of hydrocephalus, and has long been superseded by more sophisticated techniques as technology has allowed increasingly detailed imaging. Unlike the hydro-

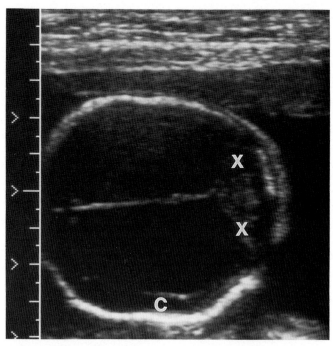

Fig. 26 Isolated hydrocephalus. In transverse section the skull shape is round. Gross dilatation of the lateral ventricle can be seen, the lateral wall being close to the skull, leaving only a rim of cortex (C). The cerebellum (crossed) is normal in shape and clearly seen.

cephalus associated with spina bifida, the head is often rounded in transverse section (Fig. 26). Gross dilatation of the ventricles can easily be demonstrated, the third ventricle being evaluated in addition to the more obvious lateral ventricles (Fig. 27). More subtle degrees of ventricular dilatation, particularly in the second trimester, can be much more difficult to assess. This is partially due to the changing appearance of the ventricular system and choroid plexus during that time.

Assessment of ventricular dilatation has traditionally been performed by measurement of the width of either the anterior horns,[67,138] posterior horns,[68] or the body of the lateral ventricle[139] and comparing these measurements to the hemispheric width (see Appendix). The exact section as used by the authors must be reproduced. In many published graphs there is a large standard deviation making detection of early changes difficult. This is borne out by reports of several false negative diagnoses in early pregnancy.[140-142] In addition, recent work has suggested that the lines previously assumed to be the borders of the anterior horns of the lateral ventricles actually represent reflections from vascular structures in the brain directly above the ventricle.[143] Other authors find the loss of concavity and 'ballooning' of the anterior horns of the lateral ventricles[144] and simultaneous visualisation of both walls of the lateral ventricles[48] useful signs.

A better assessment of ventricular size can be made by studying the choroid plexus and its relationship to the ven-

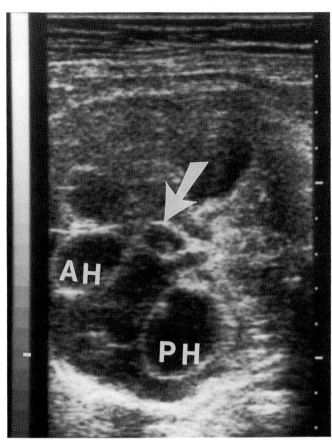

Fig. 27 Isolated hydrocephalus with marked dilatation of the third ventricle (arrowed) as well as the anterior (AH) and posterior (PH) horns of the lateral ventricles. This particular appearance, with a well-formed but ballooned ventricle, is consistent with a late pregnancy insult, rather than a genetic hydrocephalus.

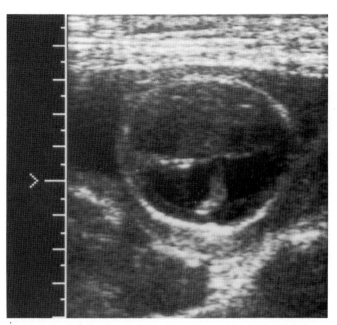

Fig. 28 Isolated hydrocephalus. Large lateral ventricles are displayed and the choroid plexus assumes a long thin appearance and hangs down vertically, leaving a gap between the medial wall of the atrium and its body.

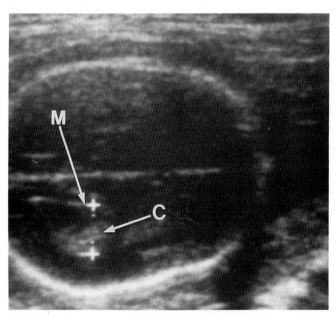

Fig. 29 Mild hydrocephalus. The atrial measurement (marked) is 11 mm, just above the upper limit of normal. The medial wall (M) is separated from the choroid plexus (C). The hydrocephalus was confirmed at autopsy.

tricular system.[144–148] At the start of the second trimester the choroid plexus has a prominent highly reflective 'bat's wing' appearance and proportionally occupies a large part of the fetal cerebral hemispheres. As the head grows the choroid plexus becomes less prominent and on transverse section can be seen to occupy the atrial portion of the lateral ventricles. In the normal fetus the choroid plexus occupies the full width of the atrium. If the ventricular system is enlarged, the choroid plexus becomes compressed to a varying degree and settles to the lowest part of the atrium, leaving a fluid filled gap between the medial walls of the ventricle and the choroid plexus (Fig. 28).[143–145] This has been quantified as a means of detecting mild hydrocephalus.[148] Mild ventricular dilatation has been defined as a separation of 3 to 8 mm between the choroid plexus and the adjacent medial ventricular wall. The effect of gravity on the choroid plexus in cases of hydrocephalus also destroys the usual symmetry of this structure,[144] even causing the superior choroid to 'dangle' through an open septum into the inferior hemisphere.[147]

Measurement of the atria of the lateral ventricles themselves is also useful in the detection of hydrocephaly. In normal fetuses between 14 and 38 weeks gestation it has a constant mean width of 7.6 ± 0.6 mm.[68,149,150] If this measurement exceeds 10 mm (> 4 standard deviations) at any gestational age, ventriculomegaly can be diagnosed with a low false positive rate (Fig. 29).[150] In a retrospective study

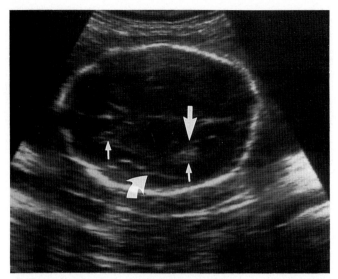

Fig. 30   Normal insula. In this transverse section of a fetal head the straight large arrow points to the medial border of the posterior horn and the curved arrow points to the insula. The insula is commonly mistaken for the lateral wall of the lateral ventricle resulting in the mistaken diagnosis of hydrocephalus. The true lateral wall is indicated by the small arrows.

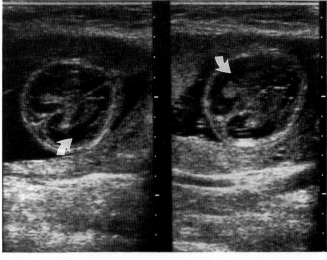

Fig. 31   Osteogenesis imperfecta in which lack of ossification of the bones of the skull results in reduced attenuation so that the cerebral structures (arrow to cortex) are more clearly seen producing the impression of a fluid filled structure and hence the false diagnosis of hydrocephalus.

of 112 fetuses with abnormalities of the CNS 99 (88%) had an atrial width > 10 mm, 81 (72%) exceeding 13 mm.[146] This suggests that measurement of the width of the atrium of the lateral ventricle is a sensitive and specific sign of fetal hydrocephalus with little intra- and inter-observer error.

Not uncommonly artefacts or structures other than the lateral ventricle wall give rise to the appearance of hydrocephalus, especially if insufficient gain has been applied to compensate for attenuation by the fetal skull.[151–153] The insula commonly poses problems (Fig. 30). In such cases studying the position and appearance of the choroid plexus helps avoid a false diagnosis.

It should be noted that in the vast majority of cases of isolated hydrocephalus the cerebellum is seen to be normal in size, in contrast to the hydrocephalus associated with the Arnold-Chiari malformation or neural tube defects (Fig. 26).

Differential diagnosis   The main alternative diagnoses in cases of severe hydrocephalus are holoprosencephaly, hydranencephaly, Dandy-Walker syndrome and porencephalic cysts. In practice genuine hydrocephalus may coexist with, or be secondary to, these conditions. Pseudo-hydrocephalus and colpocephaly (apparent enlargement of the posterior horns secondary to poor development of the surrounding brain substance) may also cause confusion. Another anomaly which may be mistaken for hydrocephalus by the unwary is osteogenesis imperfecta type II where the normal brain structure is seen with remarkable clarity due to the lack of ossification of the cranial vault (Fig. 31) (see Ch. 20).

Associated abnormalities   Around 85% of cases of fetal hydrocephalus diagnosed antenatally are associated with other abnormalities, intracranial abnormalities occurring in 37% and extracranial in 63%.[154] In this series chromosomal abnormalities were present in 11% of cases, including trisomy 21, a balanced translocation and mosaicism. Considering the cases of isolated hydrocephalus without spina bifida, 30% were associated with other abnormalities in one series, 3/30 having chromosomal abnormalities.[51] Other associated intracranial abnormalities include aqueduct stenosis, holoprosencephaly, hydranencephaly, Dandy-Walker malformation, absence of the corpus callosum, encephalocele and a clover leaf skull deformity.

Extracranial anomalies range in frequency from 7% to 15% and include cardiac (VSD, Fallots tetralogy), skeletal (sirenomelia, arthrogryposis, dysplastic phalanges), renal (agenesis, dysplasia), gastrointestinal (colonic and anal agenesis, duodenal atresia, malrotation of the bowel, anterior abdominal wall defects), Meckel's syndrome, gonadal dysgenesis and facial clefting to name but a few.[51,155] Hydrocephalus can be found as part of many uncommon syndromes,[105] to which list may be added Walker-Warburg or HARD(E) syndromes.[156]

The success of ultrasonic diagnosis of hydrocephalus   This depends very much on the aetiology and time of onset and the degree of ventricular dilatation. Clearly if the hydrocephalus is caused by an insult such as infection which occurs some time late in pregnancy, then the condition will not necessarily be detected with ultrasound. If the condition is present at the time of scanning and moderate to severe, then diagnosis should be reliable with no significant errors. The diagnosis of mild hydrocephalus is more difficult. Several authors have documented spontaneous resolution of ventriculomegaly in utero.[157,158] While dilatation of the occipital or temporal horns may be an early sign of hydrocephalus,[142] the diagnosis of ventricular dilatation should not be based solely on these criteria as there is wide variation in this portion of the ventricular system in normal fetuses.[159] The finding of prominent posterior horns has given rise to some problems in our own department. In 12 cases where the posterior horns were described as extremely prominent at 18 to 19 weeks, repeat examination 2 to 3 weeks later showed seven had resolved spontaneously. Of the five that persisted, no other intracranial signs were found. One case was shown to have multiple congenital abnormalities, one a chromosomal abnormality, and three had a normal outcome (Figs 32 and 33). Prominent posterior horns require further evaluation.

Prognosis The prognosis of the hydrocephalic fetus depends on the exact type of concurrent anomalies. Several studies have reported the outcome in a series of hydrocephalic fetuses totalling in excess of 250 cases.[139,155,157,160,161] Although complicated by terminations of pregnancy and destructive operations, quoted survival rates range from 15% to 34%. In one series only 4/41 were terminated, but only 34% survived.[157] Despite neonatal ventricular shunting, only 40% to 60% of those that survived were intellectually normal. In another reported series of 47 cases, 25 were associated with other abnormalities, of which none survived, 19 being terminated.[162] Of the 22 with isolated ventriculomegaly, 14 were developmentally normal, nine required a shunting procedure and of these nine, six were severely handicapped and two mildly delayed. Outcome is strongly affected by the presence of other abnormalities. In one series only 16% of patients with hydrocephalus had no associated abnormality, whilst 56% had extra CNS abnormalities.[155] Some studies have suggested that a cortical thickness of < 1 cm at birth predicts a poor outcome[163] but this association has been questioned.

Recurrence risk If associated with a chromosome abnormality or single gene defect, the recurrence risk is that of the primary condition. Otherwise the empirical recurrence risk has been estimated at 1% to 2%.[137,164,165] If more than one male fetus with hydrocephalus has been born in a family, sex linked recessive aqueduct stenosis is likely. If only one male infant has been affected with aqueduct stenosis, empirical recurrence risks of 4% to 7% are quoted.[136,137,166]

Obstetric management This is thoroughly reviewed elsewhere.[162] Once a firm diagnosis of hydrocephalus has been made a very careful search for other abnormalities is mandatory, specific attention being paid to the fetal spine. The detailed appearance of the hydrocephalus as previously described indicates whether a neural tube defect is likely

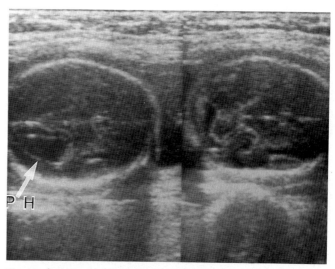

Fig. 32 **Prominent posterior horns** (PH) in a fetus with a chromosomal translocation. The rest of the intracranial anatomy is unremarkable. At autopsy multiple abnormalities were found including mild hydrocephalus.

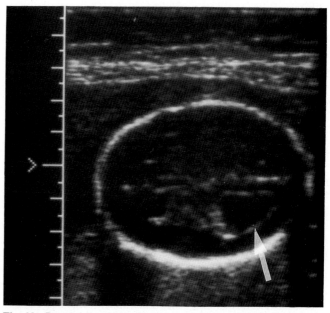

Fig. 33 **Prominent posterior horns** of the lateral ventricle in an otherwise normal head. The pregnancy proceeded to term and an apparently normal baby was delivered. If anything, the horns are more prominent in this normal case than in the abnormal one in Figure 32.

or not. If detected prior to viability, and especially if other abnormalities are found, termination may be offered. If the parents elect to continue with the pregnancy, a karyotyping procedure and viral screen should be performed so that as much information as possible is available when the time comes for delivery. A dilemma is raised by the fetus which appears to have mild hydrocephalus and in which no other abnormality can be visualised.[148] Such cases should be carefully and thoroughly assessed and a guarded prognosis given.[144,148] If parents elect to continue with the pregnancy serial assessments should be performed at regular intervals to detect any significant change.

If hydrocephalus is detected in later pregnancy a thorough search should still be made for other abnormalities, including performing a rapid karyotyping procedure. A decision must be made as to whether intervention for fetal reasons is justified and the mode of delivery that should be attempted. Each case should be assessed on its merits but most obstetricians adopt a conservative approach and aim for a vaginal delivery if the head size permits it. It has been recommended that the fetus should be delivered as soon as lung maturity is demonstrated in order to minimise the potential ill effects of progressive ventricular enlargement.

If there is gross hydrocephalus together with macrocephaly, decompression of the fetal head may be performed abdominally or per-vagina during delivery. This procedure is destructive yet it cannot be guaranteed to be lethal. It may result in a more severely brain damaged child than otherwise would have been the case, therefore in isolated hydrocephalus in utero decompression should be avoided and a caesarean section should be considered if macrocephaly is present.

Intra-uterine treatment with placement of a ventriculo-amniotic shunt has been attempted,[162,167,168] but has not gained widespread acceptance. In one series of 39 treated fetuses the perinatal mortality was 18% with 66% of the survivors having a moderate to severe handicap.[169]

Holoprosencephaly

Holoprosencephaly is a spectrum of disorders resulting from absent or incomplete cleavage of the forebrain or prosencephalon during early embryonic development. The term includes a range of disorders in which a single embryological defect affects the growth of both brain and face.[170] Depending on the degree of division, the condition is classified as alobar, semilobar or lobar.[171] If cleavage is absent alobar holoprosencephaly results with a single ventricular cavity, fusion of the thalami and absence of the corpus callosum, falx cerebri, optic tracts and olfactory bulbs. The thin lining of the ventricular cavity may bulge out to occupy the space between the calvarium and cerebral cortex, forming a cyst filled with CSF known as the dorsal sac. In semilobar holoprosencephaly partial cleavage occurs, the cerebral hemispheres being separated posteriorly with variable degrees of fusion of the thalami and absent olfactory bulbs and corpus callosum. A single ventricle with rudimentary occipital horns is present.

Macrocephaly or microcephaly together with facial defects including cyclopia (fused or nearly fused orbits with supra-orbital proboscis), cebocephaly (hypotelorism, single nostril in nose), ethmocephaly (hypotelorism, high midline proboscis), median cleft and holotelencephaly, can occur with both these forms.[170,172]

In lobar holoprosencephaly the two hemispheres are separated anteriorly and posteriorly with a certain degree of fusion of structures such as the lateral ventricles and cingulate gyrus, and absence of the cavum septum pellucidum.

Incidence and aetiology The incidence of severe holoprosencephaly amongst live births has variously been reported to lie between one in 1660 and one in 16 000,[173,174] whilst cyclopia and cebocephaly occur in one in 40 000 and one in 16 000 births respectively.[171,173] The incidence amongst all pregnancies is considerably greater than this as many abort spontaneously. In one series holoprosencephaly was reported to account for 16% to 19% of all cases of hydrocephalus detected prenatally,[175] but this has not been borne out in other series. Some cases of holoprosencephaly are associated with chromosomal abnormalities. In reported series the incidence of these has been around 55% including trisomies 13, 13/15 and 18, ring chromosomes and deletions.[170,171,175,176] In these cases the recurrence risk is around 1% for a trisomy secondary to non-disjunction, and considerably more if related to the parents carrying a balanced translocation. In other cases the condition appears familial, the mode of inheritance having been reported as both autosomal recessive and autosomal dominant with variable penetrance.[170,171,173,177] Other studies have implicated salicylates,[178] alkaloids and radiation in animals.[171]

Diagnosis Alobar and semilobar holoprosencephaly are both readily amenable to prenatal diagnosis,[175,176,179–184] whilst recently prenatal diagnosis of the lobar variety has been reported.[185]

In alobar and semilobar holoprosencephaly the midline echo of the fetal head generated largely by echoes from the inter-hemispheric fissure, is either completely absent in the former case or incomplete in the latter. The midline echo may also be deficient in hydranencephaly and where there is a large porencephalic cyst. However, in addition in alobar holoprosencephaly a single sickle-shaped ventricle is found occupying the frontal portion of the cerebrum on axial scans. Anterior to this is a thin rim of cortex, shaped like a horseshoe or boomerang (Figs 34 and 35). Posteriorly the ventricle is bounded by the thalami which appear fused. This is an important diagnostic feature. In alobar holoprosencephaly the dorsal sac, if present, can be seen on axial scans at a higher level, and by scanning in the coronal plane it may be possible to demonstrate a connection between the ventricle and the sac (Fig. 36).

Antenatally it may be impossible to distinguish between the alobar and the semilobar forms but this is unimportant as the prognosis is similar (Fig. 37).

In addition to the cerebral features associated facial abnormalities (Fig. 38) including cyclopia,[179,186] cebocephaly, ethmocephaly, hypotelorism,[176,187,188] median cleft and

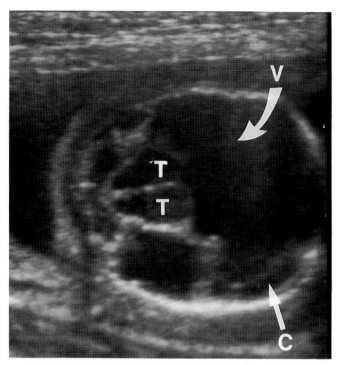

Fig. 34 Alobar holoprosencephaly. There is a large single ventricle (V) surrounded by a rim of cortex (C) anteriorly and the thalami (T) posteriorly. There is no midline echo.

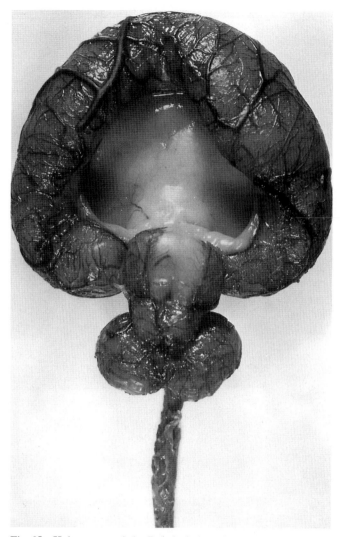

Fig. 35 Holoprosencephaly. Pathological specimen displaying the horseshoe shaped cortex and fused thalami. (With thanks to Dr Ian Rushton, Consultant Perinatal Pathologist, Birmingham Maternity Hospital.)

holotelencephaly may aid diagnosis. If such abnormalities are found fortuitously, a more detailed examination of the fetal brain is indicated. Facial abnormalities almost always predict an abnormal brain,[172] but even in severe alobar holoprosencephaly, may not always be present.[171,175,189]

The lobar form is not so readily diagnosed because the inter-hemispheric fissure is well-formed and the lateral ventricles are only fused anteriorly. The cavum septum pellucidum will be absent and this may alert the sonologist to this diagnosis in cases of apparent hydrocephalus. The antenatal ultrasound findings of two fetuses with lobar holoprosencephaly have been reported,[185] the fusion of the anterior horns of the ventricular system and the central mass were identified.

Associated abnormalities In addition to the facial features described above other abnormalities described in association with holoprosencephaly include polydactyly, exomphalos, renal dysplasia and fetal hydrops.[175] This is to be suspected as many of the cases have abnormal chromosomes.

Differential diagnosis The major differential diagnoses of the more severe forms of holoprosencephaly are severe hydrocephalus and hydranencephaly. Since the prognosis in all these conditions is uniformly poor, the exact prenatal diagnosis is unimportant. Particular features which point to severe forms of holoprosencephaly are facial abnormalities (including reduction in the inter-orbital distances which can be measured and compared to established no-

mograms (see Appendix)) a dorsal sac, fused thalami, an anterior boomerang cortical rim and the absence of a midline echo. In hydrocephalus the thalami may be seen to be separated by a dilated third ventricle, whilst the anterior cortical rim is never seen in hydranencephaly. The presence of a cavum septum pellucidum effectively rules out any form of holoprosencephaly. Semilobar holoprosencephaly can present a similar appearance to complete absence of the corpus callosum with a large inter-hemispheric cyst. Here the presence of a dilated third ventricle and frontal horns may point to the latter. The diagnosis of lobar holoprosencephaly relies mainly on the absence of the cavum septum pellucidum, together with variable enlargement of the lateral ventricles. These features are also seen in absence of the corpus callosum.

Prognosis Alobar and semilobar holoprosencephaly

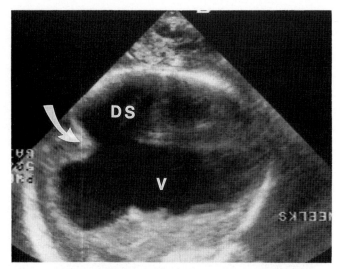

Fig. 36 Alobar holoprosencephaly. Vaginal scan of the head at the level of the dorsal sac (DS). The single ventricle (V) is seen inferiorly and the hippocampal ridge (arrowed) lies between the two. (With thanks to Charles Rodeck.)

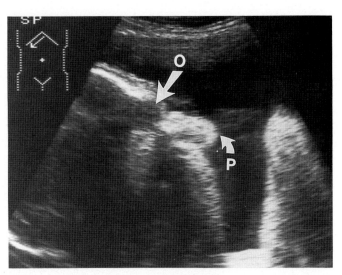

Fig. 38 Holoprosencephaly with anophthalmia and a proboscis. In a profile view of the fetal face the orbits (O) appear to be very shallow and no eye is visible. The nose is long and prominent (P).

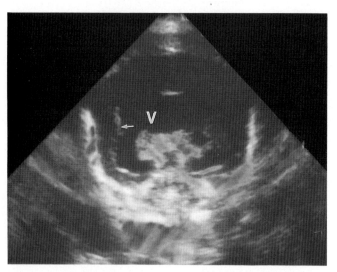

Fig. 37 Semilobar holoprosencephaly. Moderate hydrocephalus was initially diagnosed but the midline was partially deficient anteriorly with no cavum septum pellucidum. In a coronal scan, the single ventricle (V) could be identified surrounded by a thick rim of cortex (arrowed).

have a very poor prognosis, virtually all infants with the more severe form dying in the first year of life. Some with semilobar holoprosencephaly may survive into infancy with amentia.[171] Patients with lobar holoprosencephaly have some degree of mental impairment, but often a normal life expectancy.

Obstetric management If detected before viability and the parents agree, termination of pregnancy is the best management in alobar and semilobar holoprosencephaly. In practice these are the varieties usually recognised prena-

tally. In later pregnancy, or if termination is not an option, conservative management and delivery should be aimed for. Karyotyping should be performed in all cases to aid in management of this and future pregnancies.

Risk of recurrence An empirical risk of recurrence has been reported as 6% in the absence of chromosomal or genetic influences.[170,171,173] In those cases with an autosomal dominant inheritance, the penetrance is reduced such that the risk to first degree relatives is 23% to 35%. If the fetus was chromosomally abnormal then the risk ranges from an assumed 1% if the parents' karyotypes are normal, to a much higher risk if one of the parents is a carrier for a balanced translocation.

Agenesis of the corpus callosum

The corpus callosum consists of bundles of white matter which connect the right and left cerebral hemispheres forming a pathway via which information is exchanged and co-ordinated.[190] Development of the corpus callosum starts later than the majority of the nervous system. The development starts anteriorly at 8 weeks gestation and proceeds posteriorly, complete formation not occurring until after the fifth month.[191-193] Development of the corpus callosum may be arrested leading to complete or partial agenesis. In the latter, the posterior or caudal portion is absent. Postnatal diagnoses of agenesis of the corpus callosum (AGCC) have been made by pneumo-encephalography,[194] ultrasound[195,196] and CT scanning,[192,197] characteristic features being described. These can be extrapolated backwards into the antenatal period.

Incidence and aetiology The true incidence of partial or complete agenesis of the corpus callosum in the general population remains unknown, figures ranging from one in 100 to one in 19 000 being suggested.[198] An autopsy study showed an incidence of 5.3%[198] whilst a study of 6450 pneumo-encephalograms showed an incidence of 0.7%.[199] In mentally retarded persons a frequency of 2.3% has been quoted.[200] All of these series were of highly selected patients and are unlikely to be representative.

Absence of the corpus callosum may occur as an isolated entity. In some cases familial transmission has been described following both autosomal dominant, recessive and sex linked modes of inheritance.[198,201,202] Chromosomal abnormalities (trisomies 18, 13 and 8 and translocations)[200] have been found in association with AGCC. This condition can also occur in a variety of syndromes, examples being the median cleft face syndrome and Andermann's syndrome, and has been reported in association with maternal rubella and toxoplasmosis,[203,204] the fetal alcohol syndrome,[205] tuberous sclerosis,[206] mucopolysaccharidosis[191] and the basal cell naevus syndrome. In many cases, however, no obvious cause is found.

Diagnosis When the corpus callosum is absent the fibres which were destined to develop into it run instead along the medial walls of the lateral ventricles in thick longitudinal bundles[207] setting the ventricles further apart. In addition there is poor development of the white matter surrounding the occipital horns and atria which consequently become enlarged, a condition known as colpocephaly (Fig. 39). As the corpus callosum normally forms the roof of the third ventricle, this is able to enlarge in a cranial direction, sometimes herniating upwards forming a large inter-hemispheric cyst (Fig. 40). The development of the corpus callosum and septum pellucidum are closely related.[193,208] Absence of the latter is an easily noted ultrasound finding which should prompt careful evaluation of the corpus callosum. On routine transverse sections of the fetal head, appearances suggesting AGCC therefore include laterally displaced lateral ventricles, absence of the cavum septum pellucidum, disproportionate enlargement of the occipital horns and variable dilatation of the third ventricle.[209–211] If any of these findings are present, sagittal and coronal views should be obtained to assess the lateral ventricles and any upward extension of the third ventricle. A characteristic 'steerhorn' appearance is seen in frontal coronal sections.[189] A search should always be made for other associated abnormalities.

Associated malformations The defects most commonly associated with this disorder are those of the holoprosencephaly series. Also occurring frequently are hydrocephalus, porencephaly and encephalocele.[200,208,212] In some series up to 88% of cases have other CNS abnormalities while 65% have cardiovascular, gastrointestinal, genitourinary or other extra-CNS lesions.[211,212] When agenesis of the corpus callosum occurs as part of a syndrome it will have the specific abnormalities of that syndrome and condition.

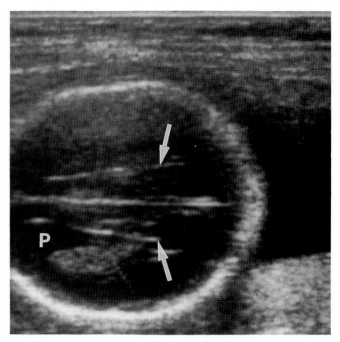

Fig. 39 Agenesis of the corpus callosum. A transverse scan of the head reveals the marked separation of the medial walls (arrows) of the anterior horns of the lateral ventricles which normally nearly touch in the midline. The medial walls are also unusually obvious. Colpocephaly is illustrated by the marginal enlargement of the posterior horns (P).

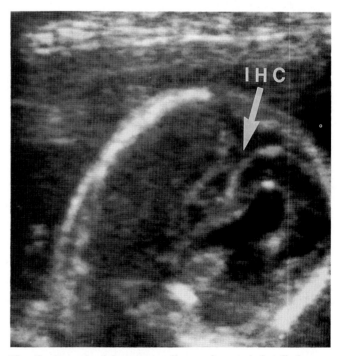

Fig. 40 Agenesis of the corpus callosum. A coronal view displays the inter-hemispheric cyst (IHC).

Differential diagnosis Lobar holoprosencephaly and mild hydrocephalus may be difficult to differentiate. In mild hydrocephalus the cavum septum pellucidum should always be present and only the lateral walls of the lateral ventricles are displaced outwards. This contrasts with AGCC where both walls are displaced outwards. Holoprosencephaly and AGCC are frequently associated. Semilobar holoprosencephaly may be confused with AGCC and a large inter-hemispheric cyst. Determining whether the thalami are fused or separated by the third ventricle clarifies the situation, but this may not be possible.

Prognosis Absence of the corpus callosum may have no or only subtle neurological sequelae,[198] and infants with complete AGCC are often mentally normal and asymptomatic. In one series however low intelligence occurred in 70% and fits in 60%.[208] Associated abnormalities may be the major determinant in prognosis in many cases. Two series of fetuses diagnosed antenatally have been reported with a combined total of 16 infants.[211,213] Of these eight had severe associated abnormalities; of the remainder one suffered from fits whilst seven were developing normally.

Obstetric management Whilst AGCC as an isolated finding may not alter obstetric management, the frequency of other abnormalities should prompt a closer examination of the fetus. Each case should then be managed on its own merits and certainly, in view of the variable prognosis, termination should be considered as an option in early pregnancy.

Recurrence risk In most cases the recurrence risk is very low, the majority of cases being sporadic.[214] A small minority are part of a familial syndrome, chromosomal abnormality or are inherited in a Mendelian fashion.[202]

Lissencephaly

Lissencephaly is a brain malformation where there are essentially no sulci or gyri and a severe arrest of development of grey matter has occurred. The majority of cases of lissencephaly are microcephalic. Other intracranial anomalies may be present, in particular hydrocephalus, agenesis of the corpus callosum and a Dandy-Walker type dilatation of the fourth ventricle with hypoplasia of midline portions of the cerebellum.

Incidence and aetiology This is an extremely rare condition thought to be due to the homozygous state of an uncommon altered cerebral recessive gene.[215,216]

Diagnosis In utero there is commonly polyhydramnios in the second half of pregnancy. The microcephaly or hydrocephalus may be detected, but as yet no case has been reported of a definite diagnosis of lissencephaly based on the absent gyri. The only antenatal diagnosis to date was based on the detection of ventriculomegaly in a patient with a family history of lissencephaly.[213]

Associated abnormalities Commonly in addition to the various intracerebral signs there are other abnormalities such as micromelia, polydactyly, congenital heart disease, renal abnormalities and duodenal atresia. Intra-uterine growth retardation is common.

Prognosis This condition is invariably fatal in infancy or childhood.

Obstetric management In a family at risk of lissencephaly, if there is an indication that the fetus has the condition, termination of pregnancy may be offered.

Hydranencephaly

Hydranencephaly describes a condition where the cerebral cortex and basal ganglia are destroyed, their place being occupied by CSF. The thalami and lower brain centres are usually preserved. The result is a fluid filled skull lined by leptomeninges into which these structures protrude.[51]

Incidence and aetiology Hydranencephaly is a rare central nervous system abnormality. It is said to be present in 0.2% of infant autopsies and approximately 1% of babies who are clinically diagnosed as having hydrocephalus.[217] It is thought to be the result of a destructive process involving the fetal brain early in gestation and therefore could be considered as the extreme end of a spectrum which also includes porencephaly and schizencephaly. Support for the destructive aetiology, which may be secondary to vascular occlusion or a severe infective episode, comes from animal studies, fetal ultrasound changes seen in utero and post-mortem findings. Bilateral occlusion of the internal carotid arteries has been postulated as one mechanism for this destruction. However, this does not account for the occurrence of the anomaly in dyzygotic twins.[200] In studies in monkeys, partial placental abruptions have been shown to be precursors of hydranencephaly[218] whilst changes leading to hydranencephaly have been documented in a fetus followed throughout pregnancy.[219] In post-mortem studies of affected fetuses however the vascular findings are variable. Absence,[220] thrombosis[218] and vasculitis of the cerebral vessels have been reported, but in many fetuses the internal carotid arteries are patent.[221] Hydranencephaly has also been reported to result from toxoplasmosis, probably secondary to vasculitis or local brain destruction.[222]

Diagnosis An intracranial cavity filled with fluid is typical of hydranencephaly, the cerebral tissue and falx usually being totally absent (Fig. 41).[48,223–225] In less severe cases, remnants of the cerebral tissue may remain together with a midline echo from the falx. Close examination shows that there is no rim of cortical tissue, and that the brain stem typically bulges into the cavity giving a characteristic appearance.[51] The head size may be normal or large.[226,227]

Differential diagnosis Other causes of an apparently fluid filled intracranial cavity include gross hydrocephalus and alobar holoprosencephaly. In both cerebral tissue persists, either as a rim lining the vault, or surrounding the

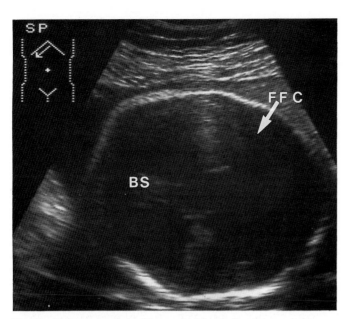

Fig. 41 Hydranencephaly. The cerebral hemispheres are entirely replaced by fluid and the brain stem (BS) protrudes into the fluid filled cavity (FFC). No normal architecture is identified.

brainstem. Other features of these conditions are described in the relevant sections.

Prognosis Not surprisingly, in view of the cerebral destruction, the prognosis for infants with hydranencephaly is very poor. Some die at birth while others initially appear normal, surviving for up to 3 years, but with no intellectual function.[226]

Obstetric management Termination of the pregnancy is recommended once the diagnosis has been confirmed. As the prognosis is so poor cephalocentesis may be indicated if macrocrania develops when the condition is found in late pregnancy.

Recurrence risk As expected, the vast majority of cases represent sporadic events. A handful of case reports have described familial hydranencephaly in association with other findings such as talipes, absent kidneys and arthrogryposis.[226,228]

Porencephaly/schizencephaly

These terms refer to cystic intracerebral structures which if communicating with the ventricular system or subarachnoid space, contain CSF. The nomenclature is confusing, some authorities using the term porencephaly to describe a lesion that follows local destruction of brain substance, others referring to this as pseudo-porencephaly. A similar appearance secondary to a developmental anomaly may be referred to as true porencephaly or schizencephaly when bilateral symmetrical clefts are present in the walls of the lateral ventricles. In the following description, porencephaly is taken to refer to a destructive lesion whilst schizencephaly denotes a developmental origin.

Incidence and aetiology Schizencephaly was found to have an incidence of 2.5% in an autopsy study of infantile brains.[229] The true incidence of porencephaly is unknown, although in one series of 112 CNS abnormalities one case of porencephaly was noted[146] and, in a series of 500 patients with epilepsy, porencephaly was detected in 2%.[230]

Porencephaly is secondary to a destructive process of cerebral tissue which is commonly secondary to infarction or haemorrhage. Post-natally other recognised causes include trauma and infection.[229,231,232] The infarcted area becomes necrotic forming a cystic space which may become confluent with the ventricular system, but may occur in almost any position in the cerebrum and may be single or multiple.

Schizencephaly is a developmental abnormality which arises from a failure of migration of cells destined to form the cerebral cortex. The result is a cleft-like deficiency in the cortex, commonly bilateral, which communicates with the subarachnoid space.[233–235] Such clefts usually occur around the Sylvian fissure in the region supplied by the middle cerebral arteries. Schizencephaly is a severe form of the migration anomaly, less severe forms being manifest as macrogyria or pachygyria (fewer larger cerebral gyri) and lissencephaly (absent gyri).[236]

Diagnosis Both porencephaly and schizencephaly should be considered in the differential diagnosis of cystic lesions in the brain.

Porencephalic cysts are usually unilateral and, because they are caused by destruction of normal tissue, do not create a mass effect.[189] Because there is often ischaemic damage and failure of growth of the surrounding brain tissue, the ipsilateral ventricle may enlarge and appear ragged due to communication with the cyst. Neither of these causes of ventricular enlargement constitutes true hydrocephalus. The midline echo is present, but may be displaced. Some cortical substance should be preserved in each cerebral hemisphere (Fig. 42).

Schizencephaly is usually bilateral although visualisation of the proximal ventricle may be difficult. The appearance is of fluid filled spaces reaching from the skull inwards and communicating with the ventricles (Fig. 43).[235] In some cases shift of the midline may occur.[51] If apparent unilateral 'hydrocephalus' is seen schizencephaly and porencephaly should both be considered.

Differential diagnosis This includes any cystic brain lesion, hydrocephalus, Dandy-Walker cyst, holoprosencephaly, arachnoid cyst, inter-hemispheric cysts in AGCC etc. Each of these has characteristic features described in the appropriate sections.

Prognosis Schizencephaly has a very poor prognosis. In one series of 22 infants, 82% were classified as idiots and 18% as imbeciles, spastic tetraplegia occurring in 95% and blindness in 41%.[229] Porencephaly also has a very poor outcome, not least because ischaemic brain damage is likely to be more widespread than visualised by antenatal ultra-

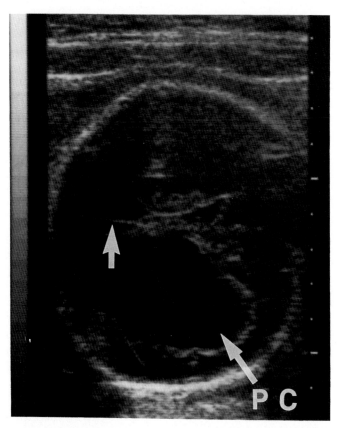

Fig. 42 Porencephaly. A large cystic cavity (PC) occupies most of the inferior hemisphere and the midline (short arrow) is shifted. There is no evidence of a cystic structure in the superior hemisphere.

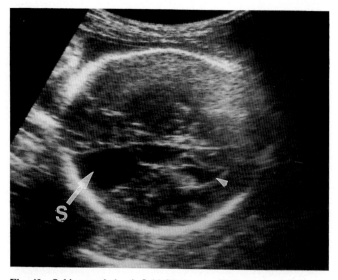

Fig. 43 Schizencephaly. A fluid filled space (S) is seen anteriorly extending through the brain substance to the skull and communicating with the lateral ventricle (arrowhead).

sound scan. Large lesions have a very poor prognosis, although smaller lesions may give rise to lesser degrees of disability.

Obstetric management If diagnosed prior to viability, termination should be offered. If detected at a later stage, non-aggressive management with recourse to caesarean section for maternal reasons only is indicated.

Recurrence risk Both conditions appear to be sporadic, but autosomal dominant and recessive inheritance has been described in one and two families respectively.[237,238]

Dandy-Walker malformation

The Dandy-Walker malformation (DWM) comprises a defect in the cerebellar vermis through which the fourth ventricle communicates with a posterior fossa cyst. After birth it is usually associated with hydrocephalus of variable degree, although this may not be present antenatally. When first described it was thought to be secondary to atresia of the foramina of Luschka and Magendie,[239,240] although this now appears unlikely as they are often patent at post-mortem. A more probable explanation is that the Dandy-Walker malformation is a complex abnormality of midline structures and should be classified together with holoprosencephaly, AGCC etc.[241,242] In support of this an 18% incidence of other midline abnormalities has been reported in association with the Dandy-Walker malformation.[243]

Incidence and aetiology The Dandy-Walker syndrome is reported to occur in approximately one in 25 000 to 35 000 pregnancies.[244] It is thought to represent a non-specific endpoint resulting from a variety of diverse aetiologies.[243] These include such inherited disorders as the Meckel-Gruber, Warburg and Aicardi syndromes and single gene disorders. Inheritance in the different syndromes ranges from dominant to sex linked and recessive. In recent series three out of 40,[244] two out of seven,[245] and four out of 12[246] cases had an abnormal karyotype, including trisomies 13, 18 and 21.

Diagnosis The Dandy-Walker malformation is established early in fetal development and can often be detected on a mid-trimester scan. The finding of a posterior fossa cyst on ultrasound should therefore suggest a Dandy-Walker malformation and initiate a detailed search for further confirmation.[245-248] The specific feature which differentiates this from other causes of a posterior fossa cyst is the cerebellar defect (Fig. 44). The cerebellum should thus be carefully examined. In some cases the cerebellar hemispheres are widely separated and compressed, whilst in others the connection may be small and difficult to visualise (Fig. 45). This is especially true where the superior vermis is intact, the defect occurring in the inferior vermis. In such cases the only finding may be an enlarged cisterna magna.[189] Although the cerebellum may appear

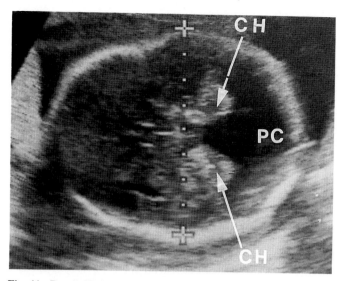

Fig. 44 Dandy-Walker malformation. A large posterior fossa cyst (PC) is seen. The cerebellar hemispheres (CH) are widely separated.

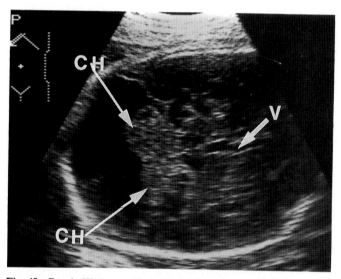

Fig. 45 Dandy-Walker malformation. In this case the cerebellar hemispheres (CH) are not obviously separated, the defect in the vermis being too small to image. Hydrocephalus was present and the dilated third ventricle (V) can be seen.

small, absence of the cerebellum is not typical of the condition. Hydrocephalus is present antenatally in only 20% of cases.[244–246,249] If it occurs care should be taken to differentiate true hydrocephalus, with dilation of the third ventricle, from colpocephaly associated with agenesis of the corpus callosum where this dilatation is absent.

Differential diagnosis Other causes of a cystic structure in the posterior fossa include a prominent cisterna magna, an arachnoid cyst and a dorsal cyst associated with holoprosencephaly. A prominent cisterna magna should never exceed 10 mm in depth,[248] and is associated with a

cerebellum of normal size. An arachnoid cyst is often asymmetrical and again is not associated with cerebellar abnormalities.[250] A dorsal cyst is supratentorial communicating directly with a single ventricle, whilst other features of holoprosencephaly are also present.

Associated malformations Central nervous system abnormalities have been noted at autopsy in 68% of infants and adults with a Dandy-Walker malformation.[251] These include AGCC in 7% to 19% of cases,[244,245,251] lipomas, aqueduct stenosis and non-specific gyral abnormalities. Abnormalities outside the CNS occur in 25% to 60% including polydactyly, cardiac defects, renal malformations and facial anomalies.[242–245,251] The latter includes an association noted with facial haemangiomas.[243,244] In cases where multiple abnormalities are present, an underlying chromosomal problem should be sought.

Prognosis Of cases not detected antenatally, 80% will present with symptoms of hydrocephalus before the age of 12 months,[244] overall mortality being reported as varying from 12% to 67%.[244–246] Many of these are attributable to associated congenital abnormalities. The functional outcome in survivors is variable, with subnormal intelligence (an IQ < 83) in 41% to 71% of survivors.[244,252]

Obstetric management A careful examination for other anomalies should be undertaken, together with a karyotyping procedure. If the diagnosis has been made prior to viability, a termination should be offered. At a later gestation, however, third trimester termination of pregnancy or cephalocentesis cannot be recommended as the survival rate, particularly when the problem is isolated, is greater than 80%.

Recurrence risk Excluding certain autosomal recessive and X linked dominant syndromes the recurrence risk for future pregnancies is between 1% and 5%.[243] There also appears to be a slightly increased risk of 7% that siblings may have other midline abnormalities.

Choroid plexus cysts

The choroid plexus occupies the lateral, the third and the fourth ventricles and is the major source of cerebrospinal fluid. Its size relative to the rest of the brain varies through embryonic life: it appears around 7 weeks gestation, reaches the maximum proportions by the late first/early second trimester and attains its adult appearance by 20 weeks.[253,254] During the early second trimester the size and the reflectivity of the choroid plexus make it one of the most easily recognised parts of the fetal brain. Cysts of the choroid plexus are common and have been reported in up to 50% of all autopsies, occurring in all age groups.[253]

Incidence and aetiology They are thought to represent neuro-epithelial folds that subsequently fill with cerebrospinal fluid and cellular debris.[253,254] The prevalence of choroid plexus cysts has been estimated at between 0.1% to 0.8%.[255–260] This has been noted to vary with the quality

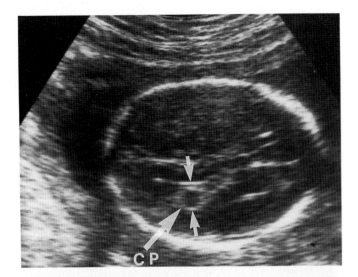

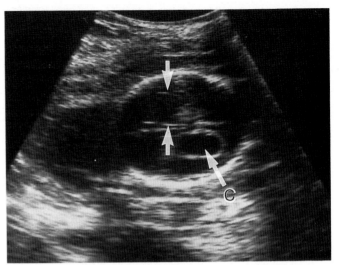

Fig. 47 Choroid plexus cyst causing hydrocephalus. In this case bilateral large cysts (C) caused obstructive hydrocephalus. The enlarged lateral ventricle can be seen between the small arrows.

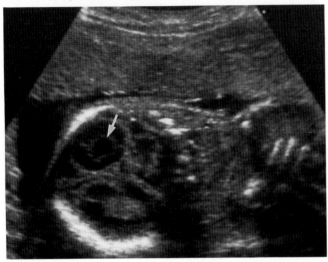

Fig. 46 Choroid plexus cyst. A: This small round cyst can be seen within the substance of the choroid plexus (CP) in the lateral ventricle (arrowed) in the inferior hemisphere. No cyst is seen in the superior hemisphere in the scan but this is probably due to 'reverberation' artefact, when a change in position of the fetal head may reveal another cyst. **B:** When the placenta is anterior, the proximal hemisphere may be better seen. Note the choroid plexus cyst (arrow).

of the ultrasound equipment used, ranging from one in 120 to one in 400.[260]

Diagnosis Choroid plexus cysts are seen as discrete round or oval echo-free structures within the substance of the choroid plexus (Fig. 46), which must be identified as surrounding the cyst, most frequently at the level of the atrium of the lateral ventricle. They are usually detected between 16 and 20 weeks and are typically 3 to 14 mm in diameter. Larger cysts of up to 20 mm have, however, been reported. Unilateral and bilateral cysts have been said to occur with equal frequency, but in fact it is likely that bilateral cysts are the rule, the one present in the nearer hemisphere being difficult to see due to reverberation artefact.[255,260] Generally the cysts decrease in size as the

gestation advances and the majority resolve by 26 weeks,[255,260] although some persist longer.

Associated malformations At least 35 cases of trisomy (31 trisomy 18, one trisomy 21, one trisomy 13, two unspecified) have been reported in association with choroid plexus cysts.[255,257,258,260–264] Population studies suggest that choroid plexus cysts are common in fetuses with trisomy 18, but the incidence of trisomy in fetuses noted to have choroid plexus cysts on a routine mid-trimester scan is not yet determined, being variously quoted as 0% to 10%.[255,257,260] In our own series of 58 cases there were no abnormal karyotypes. In trisomic fetuses the cysts tend to be large, bilateral and persist beyond 22 weeks.[255,260] In addition, in the trisomic fetuses, there are almost certainly other structural abnormalities which can be diagnosed by ultrasound. Other abnormalities reported include obstructive uropathy, hydrocephalus, oesophageal atresia, exomphalos, diaphragmatic hernia, and congenital heart disease.[255,262,264] Large choroid plexus cysts may cause obstructive hydrocephalus (Fig. 47).

Differential diagnosis Porencephalic cysts and hydrocephalus may be confused with choroid plexus cysts at first glance. A closer inspection will always reveal that choroid plexus cysts arise within the choroid plexus, unlike the former.

Prognosis Unless other abnormalities or a trisomy coexist these lesions have an excellent prognosis.

Obstetric management Choroid plexus cysts are common between 16 and 21 weeks gestation and normally resolve spontaneously. When found a careful search must be made for other abnormalities. If these are present then a karyotype procedure is warranted and a termination may be indicated either because of the particular nature of the other abnormalities or because of an abnormal karyotype.

If no other abnormalities are found at that stage a further scan should be performed at about 22 to 23 weeks. At this stage the cysts should be resolving. In addition the growth of the fetus can be checked and a further detailed search made for fine structural abnormalities, such as atrioventricular septal defect, which may be associated with an abnormal karyotype. If the cysts remain large, the growth of the fetus is suspect, or any other abnormality is detected then karyotyping is indicated. If all appears well on the second scan, and the cyst is decreasing in size, no further follow up is needed.

Arachnoid cysts

Arachnoid cysts are fluid filled intracranial cavities lined wholly or partially by arachnoid. As such they enter the differential diagnosis of any cystic intracranial structure, arising at any site within the CNS including the spinal cord, the most frequent sites being the surface of the cerebral hemispheres in the region of the major fissures.[265] Other sites are the anterior and middle fossae[266,267] and the posterior fossa,[268] in the latter closely mimicking a Dandy-Walker malformation (Fig. 48).[250] They may arise either from a localised enlargement of the sub-arachnoid space, a sub-arachnoid cyst, or between the inner and outer layers of arachnoid, an intra-arachnoid cyst.[269] The cyst may grow either as a result of valve-like effect trapping CSF or

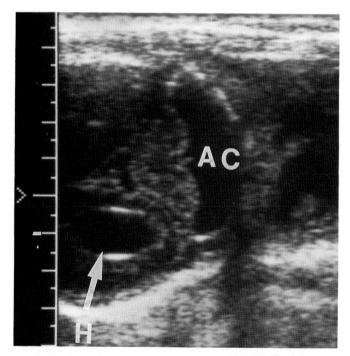

Fig. 48 Arachnoid cyst (AC) in the posterior fossa mimicking a Dandy-Walker malformation although the cerebellar hemispheres are not separated. Hydrocephalus (H) is present. This fetus was affected with CMV and was severely growth retarded.

because of the presence of secreting tissue within the cyst itself.

Incidence and aetiology Arachnoid cysts can be a congenital developmental abnormality or be acquired secondary to infection or haemorrhage.[265,270] The population incidence is unknown. In a series of 112 CNS abnormalities detected by ultrasound, two arachnoid cysts were found.[146] In our experience of over 300 cases of CNS abnormalities we have seen one case secondary to CMV infection.

Diagnosis An arachnoid cyst always presents as a single cystic area within the brain or on its surface.[271] It can easily be confused with other anomalies as described below. However, an arachnoid cyst does not communicate with the ventricular system and causes displacement of other structures rather than being destructive. In the posterior fossa it thus displaces the cerebellum en bloc rather than separating the hemispheres as in the Dandy-Walker malformation.[189] Compression of the ventricular system may lead to hydrocephalus.

Differential diagnosis The differential diagnosis includes any discrete intracranial cystic structure, including choroid plexus cysts, porencephaly, schizencephaly, DWM, inter-hemispheric cysts, aneurysm of the vein of Galen, intracranial neoplasms etc. Often the diagnosis may be clarified by careful attention to detail, in other cases a precise diagnosis may be impossible.[51,272]

Prognosis In the infant period arachnoid cysts may be asymptomatic, or may cause hydrocephalus, epilepsy or mild neurological disturbances.[269,273] No data are available on such lesions discovered antenatally. Some cysts have been successfully resected and, in general, as they cause compression rather than destruction, the prospects for normal growth and development of the infant following treatment are good. However, if the aetiology of the cyst has been infection such as CMV, this may prejudice the prognosis.

Obstetric management and recurrence risk If such lesions are detected in the second trimester, termination should be considered, as an accurate diagnosis may be impossible. In the third trimester, in the absence of hydrocephalus, a normal delivery should be anticipated. Where the diagnosis is moderately certain the labour and delivery should be managed in a normal fashion, but a TORCH screen, either on maternal, but preferably on fetal blood, should be performed, along with a rapid karyotyping procedure.

The recurrence risk is unknown but likely to be very low.

Posterior fossa abnormalities

Some abnormalities of the posterior fossa have been described under the appropriate headings. Some present as a cystic lesion e.g. DWM and arachnoid cysts while others are typified by an absent or abnormal cerebellum, e.g. Arnold-Chiari malformation. Any ultrasound examination of the fetal head should thus include an assessment of both the cerebellum and posterior fossa. This can easily be done by measuring the cerebellum[274] and cisterna magna.[146,248,275] Nomograms for transverse cerebellar diameter can be used (see Appendix)[274] but a useful rule is that between 15 to 25 weeks the mean diameter in millimetres is within 1 mm of the gestational age in weeks. Measurement of the cisterna magna on the same section as that used for cerebellar measurements shows a mean depth of 5 to 7 mm with an upper limit of 10 mm.[146,248,275] Care should be taken that the plane of measurement is not oblique.

Cerebellar abnormalities

The appearance of an absent cerebellum may be caused by the Arnold-Chiari type II malformation in association with spina bifida, when other features should clarify the diagnosis. True cerebellar hypoplasia may also occur, in some cases as an isolated finding in children with mental retardation,[276] while experimentally it has been produced by parvovirus infection.[277] In other cases it occurs as part of a syndrome: in Joubert's syndrome it is in association with a unique respiratory abnormality, whilst in the Walker-Warburg or HARD(E) syndrome it is associated with hydrocephalus, agyria, retinal dysplasia and encephalocele.[278,279] These conditions may be inherited in an autosomal recessive manner. Other rare associations have also been noted.[280] If no definite entity can be found, a recurrence risk of one in eight has been suggested.[281]

An abnormal cerebellar shape is associated both with the Arnold-Chiari malformation and the Dandy-Walker malformation described elsewhere.

Enlarged cisterna magna

An enlarged cisterna magna may be obvious as a large cystic structure, or be detected only by careful measurement. Slight enlargement may be a benign variant of normal,[146] but other causes should be excluded such as Dandy-Walker malformation, arachnoid cyst, communicating hydrocephalus, cerebellar hypoplasia and the dorsal cyst of holoprosencephaly.

Aneurysms of the internal cerebral veins

The cerebral veins may become enlarged as a result of direct arterial fistulae or secondary to adjacent arteriovenous malformations. The great vein of Galen, the major cerebral vein which runs over the thalami to join the inferior sagittal sinus as it runs along the lower edge of the falx, is one such vein which may be affected. In the 20 to 40 mm embryo, fistulous connections may develop between the

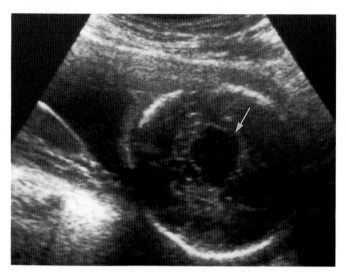

Fig. 49   Aneurysm of the internal cerebral vein displaying the large inter-hemispheric cyst (arrow).

arterial and venous systems near the choroid plexus.[282] This results in a high-flow shunt between the cerebellar arteries and the vein of Galen with progressive dilatation of the vein. The internal cerebral vein has also been reported as affected by aneurysmal dilatation.

Incidence   Around 200 cases in total are recorded in the world literature.[283]

Diagnosis   The antenatal ultrasound diagnosis of an aneurysm of the vein of Galen has been reported on several occasions.[284–286] The salient features are an inter-hemispheric midline cyst of variable size and extending from the thalami to the straight sinus (Fig. 49), from which a characteristic high frequency Doppler signal can be obtained. Aneurysms should be considered if any other unusual cystic structure is identified within the head, and Doppler ultrasound employed.

Associated abnormalities   Increased intracranial venous pressure or direct compression on the ventricular system, particularly the aqueduct of Sylvius, may give rise to hydrocephalus which, with macrocephaly, is frequently seen in the neonatal and infant periods. Ischaemic lesions such as porencephalic cysts may also be present due to the decreased blood supply to the brain, most being shunted away. The size of the shunt may also lead to high output cardiac failure and signs of hydrops fetalis.

Differential diagnosis   This is from other supratentorial cystic lesions including choroid plexus cysts, porencephalic cysts, tumours, inter-hemispheric cysts in AGCC and dorsal cysts in holoprosencephaly. The differential diagnosis may be difficult to make, but a feature unique to an aneurysm is the high frequency Doppler signal.[285]

Prognosis   In paediatric studies the prognosis appears to depend on the age at presentation. In the neonatal period severe high output cardiac failure followed by myocardial ischaemia is the major presenting symptom.[287] In such cases the prognosis is very poor, the few survivors being grossly handicapped.[288] In another series only one out of nine survived with severe handicap after treatment, results no better than without treatment.[289] In the infant and adult periods the results are much better with a survival rate with no handicap of 20% after treatment.[289,290] It would seem likely that cases major enough to be noted and diagnosed in the antenatal period are likely to be at the severe end of the spectrum with a poor prognosis.

Obstetric management If noted before viability then a termination of pregnancy should be offered. If seen in later pregnancy associated hydrops and hydrocephalus should be sought. If either are present the prognosis for the pregnancy is very poor and a non-aggressive approach should be adopted. If these signs are not present the parents should be given a guarded prognosis, especially if the precise diagnosis is in doubt.

Neoplasms

A wide variety of congenital intracranial tumours are recognised in the literature,[291] the vast majority being extremely rare. The commonest tumour is the benign or malignant teratoma, accounting for around 50% of cases,[292] glioblastomas being second in frequency. Even among these 'commoner' lesions only a handful have been diagnosed antenatally.[293,294] In addition to intracranial tumours teratomas of the sacrococcygeal region are found. These comprise over 50% of teratomas found at birth.

Incidence Intracranial neoplasms account for 0.3% of all neonatal deaths before 28 days of life.[295] Some are asymptomatic and are therefore not detected until childhood or later. Sacrococcygeal tumours are the most common tumour encountered in the newborn with an estimated incidence of one in 40 000 births and a high female to male ratio.

Diagnosis The reported intracranial fetal neoplasms presented either with grossly disorganised intracranial contents due to the bulk and mass effect of the tumour (Fig. 50), or distinct lesions which were of different reflectivity to the surrounding brain tissue. Such lesions may be solid or cystic, or contain elements of both.

Diagnosis of the sacrococcygeal tumour is made when a mass is seen to arise from the sacral area and extends around to the perineum. The mass may be cystic, solid or mixed. In cystic cases the initial appearance may be something like a meningomyelocele, but with the sacrococcygeal tumour the spine is found to be intact (Fig. 51). The mass may be extremely large, as big as the fetal head, or even bigger. One rare variety of this tumour does not present externally, occurring as in intra-abdominal mass. It is unlikely that it would be possible to determine the origin of such a mass antenatally. Serum and liquor alpha-

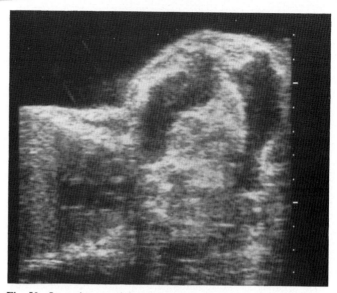

Fig. 50 Large intracranial teratoma expanding the fetal skull in this longitudinal section of a 26 week fetus. There is a complete loss of the normal anatomy, the greater part of the brain being replaced by a complex cystic/solid lesion.

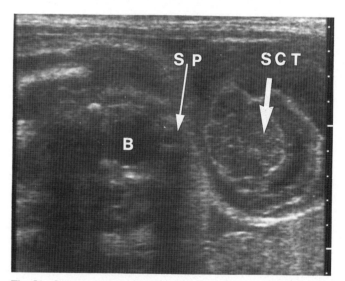

Fig. 51 Sacrococcygeal teratoma. This transverse scan of the lower pole of the fetus at the level of the bladder (B) shows a complex heterogeneous mass (SCT) behind the sacral spine (SP). The spine is intact and the mass does not communicate with the spinal canal.

fetoprotein levels may be elevated as many teratomas contain neural tissue.

Associated abnormalities In intracranial tumours hydrocephalus from the compressive effect of the tumour on the ventricular system is not uncommon.[293] In addition polyhydramnios is often present. The underlying mechanism is not clear but it may be that fetal swallowing is affected by the intracranial mass.

Hydramnios may also be present with sacrococcygeal teratomas. Other anomalies associated with sacrococcygeal teratomas may be of the muscular, skeletal, renal or nervous systems. Overall 18% of neonates with sacrococcygeal teratomas have been reported to have other abnormalities.[296]

Prognosis Cerebral neonatal tumours, benign or malignant, have a poor prognosis, most babies being stillborn or dying in the neonatal period. The size and extent of the tumour and the histological type will have some effect on the outcome.

The prognosis for the sacrococcygeal teratomas is generally very good as the majority are benign. Early surgery is essential.

Obstetric management Because of the poor prognosis of intracranial tumours, termination should be offered if the lesion is detected before viability. If detected at a later stage, management depends very much on the size and extent of the tumour and the appearance of the rest of the brain.

Because of the good prognosis of the majority of sacrococcygeal teratomas, providing other significant abnormalities have been excluded, counselling should be towards continuation of the pregnancy. Serial scans will be useful to detect polyhydramnios and also to measure the size of the tumour towards term to help decide the mode of delivery. With large tumours dystocia is a possibility and caesarean section should be carried out. Care must be taken at the delivery to ensure that the tumour is not damaged as extensive haemorrhage may occur compromising the fetus. Because of the malignant potential of some sacrococcygeal tumours, early surgery is important.

Microcephaly

In paediatric terminology microcephaly is defined as a head which is two[297] or three[298] standard deviations below the mean for age, the quoted incidences varying with the cut-off employed. Three standard deviations below the mean for age is the better definition. If two standard deviations below the mean is used the condition is inconsistently associated with mental retardation, particularly as it includes 2.5% of the general population as opposed to 0.3% when three standard deviations are used. Microcephaly is due to a decrease in brain volume caused by a reduction in telencephalic neurones and, if severe, is associated with gross mental retardation.

Incidence and aetiology The quoted incidence of microcephaly is extremely variable ranging from 1.6 per 1000[130] to 1 in 25 000 to 50 000 births.[298] In one series of microcephalic infants diagnosed by the end of the first year of life, only 14% had been noted at birth.[130] Microcephaly is a heterogeneous entity with many different patterns and aetiologies. The causes can be divided into various non-

genetic insults such as infection, radiation, anoxia etc. and those where there appears to be a genetic component.[298]

Prenatal infections including rubella, cytomegalovirus, herpes, toxoplasmosis and HIV may all lead to microcephaly, as may maternal exposure to excess alcohol, radiation, phenytoin and aminopterin and maternal phenylketonuria. Isolated microcephaly may have a genetic aetiology and be inherited either as an autosomal recessive or dominant condition. It may be found as part of some genetic syndromes such as Fanconi pancytopenia, incontinentia pigmenti, Meckel Gruber syndrome, Smith-Lemli-Opitz syndrome, or be one abnormality in trisomies 13, 18, 21 and 22.[299] In some forms of microcephaly it appears that the cerebellum has continued to develop whilst forebrain development has been impaired. As the growth spurt of the cerebellum is somewhat later than the forebrain it is postulated that a teratogenic insult of short duration might inhibit the growth of one and not the other.[300]

Diagnosis Antenatal diagnosis of microcephaly is for the most part based on the size of the head, its growth and its relative size as compared to some other part of the fetal body. Rarely an intracranial abnormality may be detected such as apparently enlarged ventricles due to cortical atrophy or a brain thought to be featureless, but in the majority of cases the intracranial anatomy is normal and the problem is solely the size of the brain. The diagnosis is made by the head to abdomen circumference ratio (Figs 52 and 53)[123,301,302] or the head perimeter to femur ratio (see Appendix).[77] The biparietal diameter should never be used to make the diagnosis of microcephaly as dolichocephaly and brachicephaly may lead to false positive or false negative diagnoses. Dolichocephalic heads are associated with breech presentations and reduced liquor, or occur for no

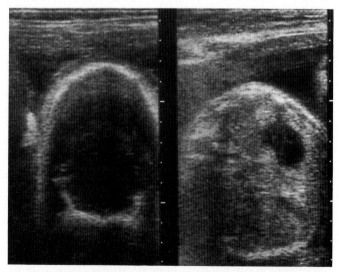

Fig. 52 Microcephaly. The head and abdomen of a severely microcephalic fetus at 26 weeks showing the marked disproportion in size. No intracranial structures are seen.

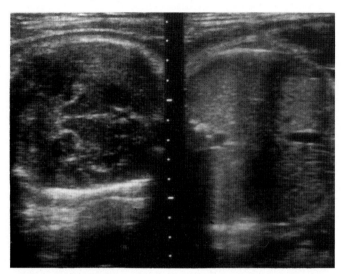

Fig. 53 Microcephaly. In this case of microcephaly at 31 weeks, the head to abdomen circumference ratio is markedly abnormal but the intracranial anatomy is normal.

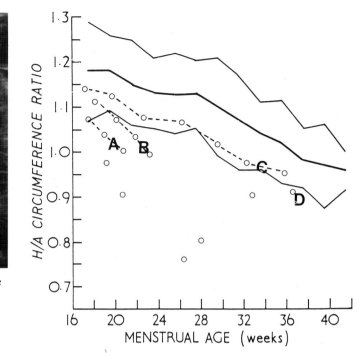

Fig. 54 Head circumference/abdomen circumference ratios. Serial and isolated HC/AC ratios in nine cases of microcephaly. A and B show normal ratios, becoming frankly abnormal by 22 to 24 weeks. C illustrates a case of microcephaly when the HC/AC ratio remained normal throughout pregnancy, the diagnosis not being made till 6 weeks post-partum. The HC/AC ratio D was suggestive but not diagnostic.

apparent reason. Similarly a rounded head shape may lead to false reassurance, thus the head circumference is a better measurement. The head/abdomen circumference ratio is the most reliable but it must be remembered that the abdomen may be affected by intra-uterine growth retardation and this can conceal signs of disproportionate head growth. When using the head/abdomen circumference ratio it must also be remembered that on occasion the head will appear disproportionately small because the abdomen is disproportionately large such as where there is hepatomegaly or macrosomia (which may occur with the Beckwith Wiedemann syndrome, diabetes and early fetal hydrops). Other fetal measurements will be of use in evaluating the situation, in particular the femur length. It is not safe to assume, when using a head circumference/femur chart, that skeletal growth has not been affected.

The diagnosis of microcephaly depends in part on the severity of the condition and in part upon the aetiology. In many cases the diagnosis cannot be made with confidence until beyond 25 weeks. However, occasionally it is apparent at an earlier stage, while others remain undetected until the third trimester[123] and occasional cases go undetected through the antenatal period (Fig. 54); not all microcephalics can be diagnosed at birth.

If there is a family history of the condition it is advisable to date the fetus at an early stage, preferably by CRL in the first trimester, and then to begin making measurements of the head and abdomen circumference from about 18 weeks. A disproportionate decrease in the head/abdomen circumference ratio may well alert one to the presence of the condition. The diagnosis should not be made on a single H/A ratio unless it is well below the lower limit of normal or another abnormality of the brain is seen. How-

ever when serial scans are available, a ratio that falls steadily to just below the normal limits is likely to be significant. Another useful aid to diagnosis is that these fetuses have a characteristic sloping forehead which may be displayed on a profile scan.

Associated abnormalities Because it is associated with a large number of chromosomal defects, gene disorders and syndromes, there are many associated abnormalities. Particular attention should be paid to the presence of encephaloceles, alobar holoprosencephaly and Meckel's syndrome. A thorough examination of the fetus is mandatory.

Differential diagnosis The major diagnostic difficulty is in the exclusion of normal fetuses. Other conditions may rarely be confused including craniosynostosis and anencephaly or acrania.

Prognosis Because of the diversity of the aetiologies and the poor correlation of brain size with the degree of mental retardation, deciding the prognosis of any particular microcephalic fetus poses problems. Clearly if there are other associated abnormalities, and in particular if the microcephaly is part of a particular syndrome or abnormal karyotype, the prognosis will depend on this. Several series have examined the outcome in isolated microcephaly.[297,303,304] Taking a cut off for head size of two standard deviations below the mean, normal intelligence has been variously reported in < 1%,[297] 50%[303] and 82%.[304] Using the cut off of three standard deviations below the mean, a normal intellect was found in 28%.[304] For those with smaller heads the prognosis became increasingly worse. If the head circumference was four to seven standard deviations below the mean the average IQ was 35.6, falling to 20 if the head size was less than seven standard deviations below the mean.[305]

Obstetric management   Sporadic cases of microcephaly often remain undetected until birth, a minority presenting as a chance finding at a routine ultrasound scan. If this diagnosis is suspected a thorough search should be made for other abnormalities and a karyotyping procedure performed. In cases of other associated abnormalities then a termination should be offered. Where the microcephaly appears to be isolated, if the head size is more than four standard deviations below the mean for gestation a termination can be offered as there is an extremely high chance that the infant will be severely mentally retarded. When the head size is not as much reduced as this, the uncertainties regarding the prognosis should be discussed with the parents and termination may be considered as an option, particularly as brain size cannot be directly equated with IQ. In some cases a delay of 2 or 3 weeks to enable serial growth scans to be taken may aid the decision making if the head growth is seen to be falling off further. If there is a past history of microcephaly of genetic origin and if the head size is found to be small and the H/A ratio abnormal, counselling and management is somewhat easier as the previously affected children can be used as guides to the likely prognosis.

Recurrence risk   As microcephaly presents as part of such a large number of chromosomal abnormalities[200] and syndromes,[105] if the index case was associated with such abnormalities, the recurrence risk will be that of the syndrome. Likewise if an infectious aetiology was proven in a previous pregnancy, then the recurrence risk is very low indeed. However, most cases are isolated with no apparent chromosomal or infectious component in which case both autosomal dominant[306] and recessive[307] inheritance patterns have been noted. Widely used recurrence risks for isolated microcephaly are 10% to 20% increasing to 25% if the parents are consanguineous.[308,309]

Conclusions

There is a wide variety of abnormalities of the CNS which can be detected antenatally by ultrasound. Initially only women at high risk of an abnormality were scanned. Increasingly however pregnant women are being scanned routinely between 17 and 19 weeks of gestation in an effort both to date the pregnancy accurately and detect fetal anomalies, including those which cannot normally be detected by maternal serum alpha-fetoprotein testing. Indeed the Royal College of Obstetricians and Gynaecologists of the UK has now recommended that all pregnant women should normally be offered a detailed fetal anomaly scan before 20 weeks gestation. Whether this is practical, or indeed will be successful, will depend on the quality of the equipment available, but much more importantly on the training and quality of the sonographers who perform the routine scanning. They must be experts in the normal appearance of the fetus and have a good knowledge of the possible abnormalities which may be encountered. The time required for a detailed scan in a high-risk patient is not usually available when performing a routine mid-trimester scan; however, considerable progress has been made in the past 4 years in determining key observations which may be made quickly and easily and which, if normal, will rule out major CNS anomaly. These findings are summarised in two key papers[66,146] and are listed below.

a) Shape of the fetal head:
A normal shape virtually rules out spina bifida, anencephaly and encephalocele.

b) Cerebellum and cisterna magna:
A normal cerebellum virtually rules out spina bifida, Dandy-Walker malformation and cerebellar hypoplasia, whilst a cisterna magna of < 10 mm will exclude Dandy-Walker malformation and infratentorial arachnoid cysts.

c) Cavum septum pellucidum:
Presence of a normal cavum rules out AGCC and major degrees of holoprosencephaly.

d) Atria of the lateral ventricles:
A width of < 10 mm rules out hydrocephalus.

e) Choroid plexus:
Inspection of the choroid and their positions relative to the atrium will eliminate choroid plexus cysts and hydrocephalus.

All these observations can be made extremely quickly from the sections required to measure the biparietal diameter and head circumference. Thus the diagnosis of CNS abnormalities in the general population by antenatal ultrasound scanning is potentially extremely successful.

REFERENCES

1 Campbell S, Johnstone F D, Holt E M, May P. Anencephaly: early ultrasonic diagnosis and active management. Lancet 1972; 2: 1226–1227

2 Leck I. Changes in the incidence of neural tube defects. Lancet 1966; 2: 791–792

3 Creasy M R, Alberman E D. Congenital malformations of the central nervous system in spontaneous abortions. J Med Genet 1976; 13: 9–16

4 McKeown T, Record R G. Seasonal incidence of congenital malformations of the CNS. Lancet 1951; 1: 192–196

5 Leck I, Record R G. Seasonal incidence of anencephalus. Br J Prev Soc Med 1966; 20: 67–75

6 MacMahon B, Yen S. Unrecognised epidemic of anencephaly and spina bifida. Lancet 1971; 1: 31–33

7 MacMahon B, Record R G, McKeown T. Secular changes in the incidence of malformations of the central nervous system. Br J Prev Soc Med 1951; 5: 254–258

8 Cuckle H S, Wald N J, Cuckle P M. Prenatal screening and diagnosis of neural tube defects in England and Wales in 1985. Prenat Diagn 1989; 9: 393–400

9 Laurence K M. The apparently declining prevalence of neural tube defects in 2 counties in South Wales over 3 decades illustrating the need for continuing action and vigilance. Z Kinderchir Grenzgeb 1985; 40: 58–60

10 Northern Regional Health Authority. A regional fetal abnormality survey. First progress report. March 1988

11 Carstairs V, Cole S. Spina bifida and anencephaly in Scotland. BMJ 1984; 289: 1182–1184

12 Cuckle H S, Wald N J. The impact of screening for open neural tube defects in England and Wales. Prenat Diagn 1987; 7: 91–99

13 Stevenson A C, Johnson H A, Stewart M I P, Golding D R. Congenital malformations: a report of a series of consecutive births in 24 centres. Bulletin of the World Health Organisation 1966; 34: 1–125

14 Laurence K M, Carter C O, David P A. Major central nervous system malformations in South Wales. 1. Incidence, local variations and geographical factors. Br J Prev Soc Med 1968; 22: 212–222

15 Penrose L S. Genetics of anencephaly. Journal of Mental Deficiency Research 1957; 1: 4–15

16 Fielding D W, Smithells R W. Anencephalus and water hardness in South West Lancashire. Br J Prev Soc Med 1971; 25: 217–219

17 Lowe C R, Roberts C L, Lloyd S. Malformations of the central nervous system and softness of local water supplies. BMJ 1971; 2: 357–361

18 Leck I. Ethnic differences in the incidence of malformations following migration. Br J Prev Soc Med 1969; 23: 166–173

19 Naggan L, MacMahon B. Ethnic differences in the prevalence of anencephaly and spina bifida in Boston. N Engl J Med 1967; 227: 1119–1123

20 Naggan L. Anencephaly and spina bifida in Israel. Pediatrics 1971; 47: 577–586

21 Searle A G. The incidence of anencephaly in a polytypic population. Ann Hum Genet (London) 1959; 23: 279–287

22 Main D M, Mennuti M T. Neural tube defects: issues in prenatal diagnosis and counselling. Obstet Gynecol 1986; 67: 1

23 Lammer E J, Sever L E, Oakley G P. Teratogen update: valproic acid. Teratology 1987; 35: 465–473

24 Moore K L. The nervous system. In: The Developing Human: clinically orientated embryology. 4th ed. Philadelphia: W B Saunders. 1988

25 Gardener W J. The dysraphic states from syringomyelia to anencephaly. Amsterdam: Excerpta Medica. 1973

26 Giroud A. Anencephaly. In: Vinken P J, Bruyn G W. eds. Handbook of Clinical Neurology. Amsterdam: Elsevier/North Holland Biomedical Press. 1977; 30: 173–208

27 Ganchrow D, Ornoy A. Possible evidence for secondary degeneration of central nervous system in the pathogenesis of anencephaly and brain dysraphia: a study in young human fetuses. Virchows Arch (A) 1979; 384: 285–294

28 Skolnick N, Filly R A, Callen P W, Golbus M S. Sonography as a procedure complementary to alpha fetoprotein testing for neural tube defects. J Ultrasound Med 1982; 1: 319–322

29 Hashimoto B E, Mahony B S, Filly R A, Golbus M S, Anderson R L, Callen P W. Sonography: a complementary examination to alpha fetoprotein testing for neural tube defects. J Ultrasound Med 1985; 4: 307–310

30 Lindfors K K, McGahan J P, Tennant F P, Hanson F W, Walter J P. Midtrimester screening for open neural tube defects: Correlation of sonography with amniocentesis results. AJR 1987; 149: 141–145

31 Roberts C J, Hibbard B M, Roberts E E, Evans K T, Laurence K M, Robertson I B. Diagnostic effectiveness of ultrasound in detection of neural tube defect. The South Wales experience of 2509 scans (1977–1982) in high risk mothers. Lancet 1983; 2: 1068–1069

32 Hogge W A, Thiagarajah S, Ferguson J E, Schnatterly P T, Harbert G M. The role of ultrasonography and amniocentesis in the evaluation of pregnancies at risk for neural tube defects. Am J Obstet Gynecol 1989; 161: 520–524

33 Goldstein R B, Filly R A. Prenatal diagnosis of anencephaly: spectrum of sonographic appearances and distinction from the amniotic band syndrome. AJR 1988; 151: 547–550

34 Goldstein R B, Filly R A, Callen P W. Sonography of anencephaly: pitfalls in early diagnosis. JCU 1989; 17: 397–402

35 Cox G C, Rosenthal S J, Holsapple J W. Exencephaly: sonographic findings and the radiologic-pathologic correlation. Radiology 1985; 155: 755–756

36 Hendricks S K, Cyr D R, Nyberg D A, Raabe R, Mack L A. Exencephaly – clinical and ultrasonic correlation to anencephaly. Obstet Gynecol 1988; 72: 898–900

37 Mannes E J, Crelin E S, Hobbins J S, Viscomi G N, Alcebo L. Sonographic demonstration of fetal acrania. AJR 1982; 139: 181–182

38 Mahoney B S, Filly R A, Callen P W, Golbus M S. The amniotic band syndrome: antenatal sonographic diagnosis and potential pitfalls. Am J Obstet Gynecol 1985; 152: 63–68

39 Frezal J, Kelley J, Guillemot M L, Lamy M. Anencephaly in France. Am J Hum Genet 1964; 16: 336–350

40 Chervenak F A, Farley M A, Walters L, Hobbins J C, Mahoney J. When is termination of pregnancy in the first trimester morally justifiable? N Engl J Med 1984; 310: 501–504

41 Leong A S, Shaw C M. The pathology of occipital encephalocele and a discussion of the pathogenesis. Pathology 1979; 11: 223–234

42 Carlan S J, Angel J L, Leo J, Feeney J. Cephalocele involving the oral cavity. Obstet Gynecol 1990; 75: 494–495

43 McLaurin R L. Encephalocele and cranium bifidum. In: Vinken P J, Bruyn G W, Klawans H L. eds. Handbook of clinical neurology. Amsterdam: Elsevier/North Holland Biomedical Press. 1987; 50: 97–111

44 International Clearing House for Birth Defects Monitoring Systems. Annual Report 15; 1983

45 Lorber J. The prognosis of occipital encephalocele. Dev Med Child Neurol (suppl) 1966; 13: 75–86

46 Cohen M M, Lemire R J. Syndromes with cephaloceles. Teratology 1982; 25: 161–172

47 Chervenak F A, Isaacson G, Mahoney M J, Berkowitz R L, Tortora M, Hobbins J C. Diagnosis and management of fetal cephalocele. Obstet Gynecol 1984; 64: 86–91

48 Fiske C E, Filly R A. Ultrasound evaluation of the normal and abnormal fetal neural axis. Radiol Clin North Am 1982; 20: 285–296

49 Graham D, Johnson T R B, Winn K, Sanders R C. The role of sonography in the prenatal diagnosis and management of encephalocele. J Ultrasound Med 1982; 1: 111

50 Chatterjee M J, Bondoc B, Adhate A. Prenatal diagnosis of occipital encephalocele. Am J Obstet Gynecol 1985; 153: 646–647

51 Pilu G, Rizzo N, Orsini L F, Bovicelli L. Antenatal recognition of cerebral anomalies. Ultrasound Med Biol 1986; 12: 319–326

52 Nicolini U, Ferrazzi E, Massa E, et al. Prenatal diagnosis of cranial masses by ultrasound: report of 5 cases. JCU 1983; 11: 170–174

53 Haddow J E. Prenatal diagnosis of neural tube defects. In: Levene M I, Bennett M J, Punt J. eds. Fetal neurology and neurosurgery. Edinburgh: Churchill Livingstone. 1988: p 279–289

54 De Myer W. The median cleft face syndrome: differential diagnosis of cranium bifidum occultum, hypertelorism, and median cleft nose, lip and palate. Neurology 1967; 17: 961–971

55 Field B. The child with an encephalocele. Med J Aust 1974; 1: 700–703

56 Lorber J, Schofield J K. The prognosis of occipital encephalocele. Z Kinderchir Grenzgeb 1979; 28: 347–351

57 Friede R L. Developmental neuropathology. New York: Springer-Verlag. 1975

58 Patten B M. Embryological stages in myeloschisis with spina bifida. Am J Anat 1953; 93: 365–395

59 Gardner W J. Myelomeningocele, the result of rupture of the embryonic neural tube. Cleveland Clin Quart 1960; 27: 88–100

60 Barson A J. Spina bifida: the significance of the level and extent of the defect to the morphogenesis. Dev Med Child Neurol 1970; 12: 129–144

61 Emery J L, Lendon R G. The local cord lesion in neurospinal dysraphism (meningomyelocele). J Pathol 1973; 110: 83–86

62 Lorber J. Systematic ventriculographic studies in infants born with meningomyelocele and encephalocele. The incidence and development of hydrocephalus. Arch Dis Child 1961; 36: 381–389

63 Smithells R W, Sheppard S, Wild J. Prevalence of neural tube defects in the Yorkshire region. Community Med 1989; 11: 163–167

64 Campbell S. Early prenatal diagnosis of neural tube defects by ultrasound. Clin Obstet Gynecol 1977; 20: 351–359

65 Fowlie A. An ultrasonic method of screening for the neural tube defects. Proceedings of the North of England Obstetrics and Gynaecological Society. 1982

66 Nicolaides K H, Gabbe S G, Campbell S, Guidetti R. Ultrasound screening for spina bifida: cranial and cerebellar signs. Lancet 1986; 2: 72–74

67 Thoms A, Campbell S. The diagnosis of spina bifida and intracranial abnormalities. In: Sanders R C, James A E. eds. Principles and practice of ultrasonography in obstetrics and gynaecology. Norwalk: Appleton Century Crofts. 1980: p 179–190

68 Campbell S, Pearce J M. Ultrasound visualisation of congenital malformations. Br Med Bulletin 1983; 39: 322–331

69 Campbell J, Gilbert W M, Nicolaides K H, Campbell S. Ultrasound screening for spina bifida: cranial and cerebellar signs in a high risk population. Obstet Gynecol 1987; 70: 247–250

70 Pilu G, Romero R, Reece E A, Goldstein I, Hobbins J C, Bovicelli L. Subnormal cerebellum in fetuses with spina bifida. Am J Obstet Gynecol 1988; 158: 1052–1056

71 Nyberg D A, Mack L A, Hirsch J, Mahony B S. Abnormalities of the fetal cranial contour in sonographic detection of spina bifida – evaluation of the lemon sign. Radiology 1988; 167: 387–392

72 Tabor A, Madsen M, Obel E B, Philip J, Bang J, Pedersen B N. Randomised controlled trial of genetic amniocentesis in 4606 low risk women. Lancet 1986; 1: 1287–1292

73 Richards D S, Seeds J W, Katz V L, Lingley L H, Albright S G, Cefalo R C. Elevated maternal serum alphafetoprotein with normal ultrasound: is amniocentesis always appropriate? A review of 26 069 screened patients. Obstet Gynecol 1988; 71: 203–207

74 Drugan A, Zador I E, Syner F N, Sokol R J, Sacks A J, Evans M I. A normal ultrasound scan does not obviate the need for amniocentesis in patients with elevated serum alphafetoprotein. Obstet Gynecol 1988; 72: 627–630

75 Hogge W A, Thiagarajah S, Ferguson J E, Schnatterly P T, Harbert G M. The role of ultrasonography and amniocentesis in the evaluation of pregnancies at risk for neural tube defects. Am J Obstet Gynecol 1989; 161: 520–524

76 Allen L C, Doran T A, Miskin M, Rudd N L, Benzie R J, Sheffield L J. Ultrasound and amniotic fluid alpha-fetoprotein in the prenatal diagnosis of spina bifida. Obstet Gynecol 1982; 60: 169–173

77 Romero R, Pilu G, Jeanty P, Ghidini A, Hobbins J C. Prenatal diagnosis of congenital anomalies. Connecticut: Appleton and Lange. 1988

78 Gough J D. In: Wald N J. ed. Ultrasound, antenatal and neonatal screening. Oxford: Oxford University Press. 1984: p 432–433

79 Persson P H, Cullander S, Gennser G, Grennert L, Laurell C B. Screening for fetal malformations using ultrasound and measurements of alpha fetoprotein in maternal serum. BMJ 1983; 286: 747–749

80 Rosendahl H, Kivinen S. Antenatal detection of congenital malformations by routine ultrasonography. Obstet Gynecol 1989; 73: 947–951

81 Sharrard W J W. The mechanism of paralytic deformity in spina bifida. Dev Med Child Neurol 1962; 4: 310–313

82 Lorber J. Results of treatment of myelomeningocele. An analysis of 524 unselected cases, with special reference to possible selection for treatment. Dev Med Child Neurol 1971; 31: 279–303

83 Althouse R, Wald N J. Survival and handicap of infants with spina bifida. Arch Dis Child 1980; 55: 845–850

84 Adams M M, Greenberg F, Khoury M J, Marks J S, Oakley G P. Survival of infants with spina bifida: Atlanta 1972–1979. Am J Dis Child 1985; 139: 514–517

85 Chervenak F A, Duncan C, Ment L R, Tortora M, McClure M, Hobbins J C. Perinatal management of meningomyelocele. Obstet Gynecol 1984; 63: 376–380

86 Nevin N C, Johnstone W P. A family study of spina bifida and anencephalus in Northern Ireland (1964–1968). J Med Genet 1980; 17: 203–211

87 Seller M J. Recurrence risks for neural tube defects in a genetic counselling clinic population. J Med Genet 1981; 18: 245–248

88 Laurence K M, James N, Miller M, Campbell H. Increased risk of recurrence of pregnancies complicated by neural tube defects in mothers receiving poor diets, and possible effects of dietary counselling. BMJ 1980; 281: 1592–1594

89 Laurence K M, James N, Miller M, Tennant G B, Campbell H. Double blind randomised controlled trial of folate treatment before conception to prevent neural tube defects. BMJ 1981; 282: 1509–1511

90 Smithells R W, Nevin N C, Seller M J, et al. Further experience of vitamin supplementation for prevention of neural tube defect recurrences. Lancet 1983; 1: 1027–1031

91 Seller M J, Nevin N C. Periconceptual vitamin supplementation and the prevention of neural tube defects in South East England and Northern Ireland. J Med Genet 1984; 21: 325–330

92 Seller M J. Periconceptual vitamin supplementation to prevent recurrence of neural tube defects. Lancet 1985; 1: 1392–1393

93 Mulinare J, Cordero J F, Erickson J D, Berry R J. Periconceptual use of multivitamins and the occurrence of neural tube defects. JAMA 1988; 260: 3141–3145

94 Mills J L, Rhoads G G, Simpson J L, et al. The absence of a relation between the periconceptual use of vitamins and neural tube defects. N Engl J Med 1989; 321: 430–435

95 Brock D J H. Early diagnosis of fetal defects. Current reviews in obstetrics and gynaecology 2. Edinburgh: Churchill Livingstone. 1982

96 Brock D J H, Sutcliffe R G. Alpha fetoprotein in the antenatal diagnosis of spina bifida and anencephaly. Lancet 1972; 2: 197–199

97 Smith A D, Wald N J, Cuckle H S, Stirrat G M, Bobrow M, Lagercrantz H. Amniotic fluid acetylcholinesterase as a possible diagnostic test for neural tube defects in early pregnancy. Lancet 1979; 1: 685–690

98 Wald N J, Brock D J H, Bonnar J. Prenatal diagnosis of spina bifida and anencephaly by maternal serum alpha fetoprotein measurement. Lancet 1974; 1: 765–767

99 Brock D J H, Bolton A E, Scrimgeour J B. Prenatal diagnosis of spina bifida and anencephaly through maternal plasma alpha-fetoprotein measurement. Lancet 1974; 1: 767–769

100 Wald N J, Cuckle H S. Collaborative study on alpha fetoprotein in relation to neural tube defects. Lancet 1977; 1: 1323–1332

101 Burton B K, Sowers S G, Nelson L H. Maternal serum alpha fetoprotein screening in North Carolina: experience with more than 12 000 pregnancies. Am J Obstet Gynecol 1983; 146: 439

102 Wald N J, Cuckle H S, Boreham T, Turnbull A C. Effect of estimating gestational age by ultrasound cephalometry on the specificity of alpha fetoprotein screening for open neural tube defects. Br J Obstet Gynaecol 1982; 89: 1050–1053

103 Williams R A, Barth R A. In utero sonographic recognition of diastematomyelia. AJR 1985; 144: 87–88

104 Benacerraf B R, Greene M F, Barss V A. Prenatal diagnosis of congenital hemivertebra. J Ultrasound Med 1986; 5: 257–259

105 Smith D W. Recognisable patterns of human malformation. 3rd edn. Philadelphia: WB Saunders. 1982

106 Napolitani F D, Schreiber I. The acardiac monster: a review of the world literature and presentation of 2 cases. Am J Obstet Gynecol 1960; 80: 582–589

107 Simpson P C, Trudinger B J, Walker A, Baird P J. The intrauterine treatment of fetal cardiac failure in a twin pregnancy with an acardiac, acephalic monster. Am J Obstet Gynecol 1983; 147: 842–844

108 Platt L D, Devore G R, Bieniary A, Benner P, Rao R. Antenatal diagnosis of acephalus acardia: a proposed management scheme. Am J Obstet Gynecol 1983; 146: 857–859

109 Lewis H F. Iniencephalus. Am J Obstet Gynecol 1887; 35: 11–53

110 Aleksic S, Budzilovich G, Greco M A, Feigin I, Epstein F, Pearson J. Iniencephaly: neuropathologic study. Clin Neuropathol 1983; 2: 55–61

111 Gunderson C H, Greenspan R H, Glaser G H, Lubs H A. The Klippel-Feil syndrome: genetic and clinical reevaluation of cervical fusion. Medicine 1967; 46: 491–512

112 Gardner W J. Klippel-Feil syndrome, iniencephalus, anencephalus, hindbrain hernia and mirror movements: overdistension of the neural tube. Child's Brain 1979; 5: 361–379

113 Sherk H H, Shut L, Chung S. Iniencephalic deformity of the cervical spine with Klippel-Feil anomalies and congenital elevation of the scapula. J Bone Joint Surg 1974; 1254–1259

114 Paterson S J. Iniencephalus. J Obstet Gynaecol Br Emp 1944; 51: 330

115 Jayant K, Mehta A, Sanghvi L D. A study of congenital malformations in Bombay. J Obstet Gynaecol India 1960; 11: 280

116 Bowden R A, Stephens T D, Le Mire R J. The association of spinal retroflexion with limb anomalies. Teratology 1980; 21: 53–59

117 Lemire R J, Beckwith B, Shepard T H. Iniencephaly and anencephaly with spinal retroflexion, a comparative study of eight human specimens. Teratology 1972; 6: 27–36

118 Abbott M E, Lockhart F A L. Iniencephalus. J Obstet Gynaecol Br Emp 1905; 8: 236

119 Howkins J, Lowrie R S. Iniencephalus. J Obstet Gynaecol Br Emp 1939; 46: 25

120 Cohlan S Q, Kitay D. The teratogenic effect of vincaleukoblastine in the pregnant rat. J Pediatr 1965; 66: 541–544

121 Warkany J, Takacs E. Congenital malformations in rats from streptonigrin. Arch Pathol 1965; 79: 65–79

122 Roux C. Action teratogene du triparanol chez l'animal. Arch Franc Pediatr 1964; 21: 451

123 Campbell S, Allan L D, Griffin D, Little D, Pearce J M, Chudleigh P. The early diagnosis of fetal structural abnormalities. In: Lerski R A, Morley P. eds. Ultrasound '82. Oxford: Pergamon Press. 1983: p 547–563

124 Santos-Ramos R, Duenhoelter J H. Diagnosis of congenital fetal abnormalities by sonography. Obstet Gynecol 1975; 45: 279–283

125 Katz V L, Aylsworth A S, Albright S G. Iniencephaly is not uniformly fatal. Prenat Diagn 1989; 9: 595–598

126 Morocz I, Szeifert G F, Molnar P, Toth Z, Csecsei K, Papp Z. Prenatal diagnosis and pathoanatomy of iniencephaly. Clin Genet 1986; 30: 81–86

127 Foderaro A E, Abu-Yousef M M, Benda J A, Williamson R A, Smith W L. Antenatal ultrasound diagnosis of iniencephaly. JCU 1987; 15: 550–554

128 David T J, Nixon A. Congenital malformations associated with anencephaly and iniencephaly. J Med Genet 1976; 13: 263–265

129 Myrianthopoulos N C, Kurland L T. Present concepts of the epidemiology and genetics of hydrocephalus. In: Fields W J, Desmond M M. eds. Disorders of the developing nervous system. Springfield, Illinois: Charles Thomas. 1961: 187–202

130 Myrianthopoulos N C. Epidemilogy of central nervous system malformations. In: Vinken P J, Bruyn G W, Klawans H L. eds. Handbook of clinical neurology. Amsterdam: Elsevier/North Holland Biomedical Press. 1987; 50: 49–69

131 Habib Z. Genetics and genetic counselling in neonatal hydrocephalus. Obstet Gynecol Surv 1981; 36: 529–534

132 Chuang S. Perinatal and neonatal hydrocephalus. Perinatology 1986; Sept–Oct 8

133 Edwards J H. The syndrome of sex-linked hydrocephalus. Arch Dis Child 1961; 36: 486–493

134 Salam M Z. Stenosis of the aqueduct of Sylvius. In: Vinken P J, Bruyn G W. eds. Handbook of clinical neurology. Amsterdam: Elsevier/North Holland Biomedical Press. 1977; 30: 609–622

135 Milhorat T H. Hydrocephalus and the cerebrospinal fluid. Baltimore: Williams and Wilkins. 1972

136 Halliday J, Chow C W, Wallace D, Danks D M. X-linked hydrocephalus: a survey of a 20 year period in Victoria, Australia. J Med Genet 1986; 23: 23–31

137 Burton B K. Recurrence risks for congenital hydrocephalus. Clin Genet 1979; 16: 47–53

138 Denkhaus H, Winsberg F. Ultrasonic measurement of the fetal ventricular system. Radiology 1979; 131: 781–787

139 Pretorious D H, Drose J A, Manco-Johnson M L. Fetal lateral ventricular determination during the second trimester. J Ultrasound Med 1986; 5: 121–124

140 Chervenak F A, Berkowitz R L, Tortora M, Chitkara U, Hobbins J C. Diagnosis of ventriculomegaly before fetal viability. Obstet Gynecol 1984; 64: 652–656

141 Fiske C E, Filly R A, Callen P W. Sonographic measurement of lateral ventricular width in early ventricular dilation. JCU 1981; 9: 303–307

142 Jeanty P, Dramaix-Wilmet M, Delbeke D, Rodesch F, Struyven J. Ultrasound evaluation of fetal ventricular growth. Neurology 1981; 21: 127–131

143 Hertzberg B S, Bowie J D, Burger P C, Marshburn P B, Djang W T. The three lines: origin of landmarks in the fetal head. AJR 1987; 149: 1009–1012

144 Benacerraf B R, Birnholz J C. The diagnosis of fetal hydrocephalus prior to 22 weeks. JCU 1987; 15: 531–536

145 Chinn D H, Callen P W, Filly R A. The lateral cerebral ventricle in early second trimester. Radiology 1983; 148: 529–531

146 Filly R A, Cardoza J D, Goldstein R B, Barkovich A J. Detection of fetal central nervous system anomalies: a practical level of effort for a routine sonogram. Radiology 1989; 172: 403–408

147 Cardoza J D, Filly R A, Podrasky A E. Exclusion of pseudohydrocephalus by a simple observation: the dangling choroid sign. AJR 1988; 151: 767–770

148 Mahoney B S, Nyberg D A, Hirsch J H, Petty C N, Hendricks S K, Mack L A. Mild idiopathic lateral cerebral ventricular dilatation in-utero: sonographic evaluation. Radiology 1988; 169: 715–721

149 Siedler D E, Filly R A. Relative growth of fetal higher brain structures. J Ultrasound Med 1987; 6: 573–576

150 Cardoza J D, Goldstein R B, Filly R A. Exclusion of ventriculomegaly with a single measurement: the width of the lateral ventricular atrium. Radiology 1988; 169: 711–714

151 Case K J, Hirsch J, Case M J. Simulation of significant pathology by normal hypoechoic white matter in cranial ultrasound. JCU 1983; 11: 281

152 Jeanty P, Chervenak F A, Romero R, Michiels M, Hobbins J C. The Sylvian fissure: a commonly mislabeled cranial landmark. J Ultrasound Med 1984; 3: 15–18

153 Schoenecker S A, Pretorious D H, Manco-Johnson M L. Artifacts seen commonly on ultrasonography of the fetal cranium. J Reprod Med 1985; 30: 541–544

154 Chervenak F A, Berkowitz R L, Romero R, et al. The diagnosis of fetal hydrocephalus. Am J Obstet Gynecol 1983; 147: 703–716

155 Nyberg D A, Mack L A, Hirsch J, Pagon R O, Shepard T H. Fetal hydrocephalus: sonographic detection and clinical significance of associated anomalies. Radiology 1987; 163: 187–191

156 Pagon R A, Clarren S K, Milam D F, Hendrickson A E. Autosomal recessive eye and brain anomalies: Warburg syndrome. J Pediatr 1983; 102: 542–546

157 Cochrane D D, Myles S T, Nimrod C, Still D K, Sugarman R G, Wittman B K. Intrauterine hydrocephalus and ventriculomegaly: associated anomalies and fetal outcome. Can J Neurol Sci 1985; 12: 51–59

158 Glick P L, Harrison M R, Nakayama D K, et al. Management of ventriculomegaly in the fetus. J Pediatr 1984; 105: 97–105

159 Hyndman J, Johri A M, MacLean N E. Diagnosis of fetal hydrocephalus by ultrasound. N Z Med J 1980; 91: 385–386

160 Chervenak F A, Duncan C, Ment L R, et al. Outcome of fetal ventriculomegaly. Lancet 1984; 2: 179–181

161 Serlo W, Kirkinen P, Joupila P, Herva R. Prognostic signs in fetal hydrocephalus. Childs Nervous System 1986; 2: 93–97

162 Hudgins R J, Edwards M S B, Golbus M S. Management of fetal ventriculomegaly. In: Levene M I, Bennett M J, Punt J. eds. Fetal and neonatal neurology and neurosurgery. Edinburgh: Churchill Livingstone. 1988: p 577–585

163 Vintzileos A M, Ingardia C J, Nochimson D J. Congenital hydrocephalus: A review and protocol for perinatal management. Obstet Gynecol 1983; 62: 539–549

164 Carter C O, David P A, Laurence K M. A family study of major central nervous system malformations in South Wales. J Med Genet 1968; 5: 81–106

165 Adams C, Johnston W P, Nevin N C. Family study of congenital hydrocephalus. Dev Med Child Neurol 1982; 24: 493–498

166 Howard F M, Till K, Carter C O. A family study of hydrocephalus resulting from aqueduct stenosis. J Med Genet 1981; 18: 252–255

167 Clewell W H, Johnson M L, Meier P R, et al. A surgical approach to the treatment of fetal hydrocephalus. N Engl J Med 1982; 306: 1320–1325

168 Chervenak F A, Berkowitz R L, Tortora M, Hobbins J C. The management of fetal hydrocephalus. Am J Obstet Gynecol 1985; 151: 933–942

169 Manning F A. International fetal surgery register: 1985 update. Clin Obstet Gynecol 1986; 29: 551–557

170 Cohen M M. An update on the holoprosencephalic disorders. J Pediatr 1982; 101: 865–869

171 DeMyer W. Holoprosencephaly (cyclopia-arhinencephaly). In: Vinken P J, Bruyn G W, Klawans H L. eds. Handbook of clinical neurology. Amsterdam: Elsevier/North Holland Biomedical Press. 1987: p 225–244

172 DeMyer W, Zeman W, Palmer C. The face predicts the brain: diagnostic significance of median facial abnormalities for holoprosencephaly (arhinencephaly). Paediatrics 1964; 34: 256–263

173 Roach E, DeMyer W, Palmer K, Conneally M, Merritt A. Holoprosencephaly: birth data, genetic and demographic analysis of 30 families. Birth Defects 1975; 11: 294–313

174 Saunders E S, Shortland D, Dunn P M. What is the incidence of holoprosencephaly? J Med Genet 1984; 21: 21–26

175 Nyberg D A, Mack L A, Bronstein A, Hirsch J, Pagon R. Holoprosencephaly: prenatal sonographic diagnosis. AJR 1987; 149: 1051–1058

176 Chervenak F A, Isaacson G, Hobbins J C, Chithara U, Tortora M, Berhowitz R C. Diagnosis and management of fetal holoprosencephaly. Obstet Gynecol 1985; 66: 322–326

177 Dallaire L, Clarke Fraser F, Wigglesworth F W. Familial holoprosencephaly. Birth Defects Original Article, series VII, 1971; 7: 136–142

178 Benawra R, Mangurten H H, Duffell D R. Cyclopia and other anomalies following maternal ingestion of salicylates. J Pediatr 1980; 96: 1069–1071

179 Blackwell D E, Spinnato J A, Hirsch G, Giles H R, Sackler J. Antenatal ultrasound diagnosis of holoprosencephaly: a case report. Am J Obstet Gynecol 1982; 143: 848–849

180 Hidalgo H, Bowie J, Rosenberg E R, et al. In utero sonographic diagnosis of fetal cerebral anomalies. AJR 1982; 139: 143–148

181 Hill L M, Breckle R, Bonebrake C R. Ultrasonic findings with holoprosencephaly. J Reprod Med 1982; 27: 172–175

182 Filly R A, Chinn D H, Callen P W. Alobar holoprosencephaly: ultrasonographic prenatal diagnosis. Radiology 1984; 151: 455–459

183 Cayea P D, Balcar I, Alberti O, Jones T B. Prenatal diagnosis of semilobar holoprosencephaly. AJR 1984; 142: 401–402

184 Greene M F, Benacerraf B R, Frigoletto F D. Reliable criteria for the prenatal sonographic diagnosis of alobar holoprosencephaly. Am J Obstet Gynecol 1987; 156: 687–689

185 Hoffman-Tretin J C, Horoupian D S, Koenigsberg M, Schnur M J, Llena J F. Lobar holoprosencephaly with hydrocephalus: Antenatal demonstration and differential diagnosis. J Ultrasound Med 1986; 5: 691–697

186 Benacerraf B R, Frigoletto F D, Bieber F R. The fetal face. Ultrasound examination. Radiology 1984; 153: 495–497

187 Mayden K L, Tortora M, Berkowitz R L, Bracken M, Hobbins J C. Orbital diameters: a new parameter for prenatal diagnosis and dating. Am J Obstet Gynecol 1982; 144: 289–297

188 Pilu G, Romero R, Rizzo N, Jeanty P, Bovicelli L, Hobbins J C. Criteria for the prenatal diagnosis of holoprosencephaly. Am J Perinatol 1987; 4: 41–49

189 Filly R A. Ultrasound evaluation of the fetal neural axis. In: Callen P W. ed. Ultrasonography in obstetrics and gynaecology. Philadelphia: W B Saunders. 1988: p 83–135

190 Sperry R W. Hemispheric disconnection and unity in conscious awareness. Am J Psychol 1968; 23: 723–733

191 Loeser J D, Alvord E C. Agenesis of the corpus callosum. Brain 1968; 91: 553–570

192 Guibert-Tranier F, Piton J, Billerey J, Caille J M. Agenesis of the corpus callosum. J Neuroradiol 1982; 9: 135–160

193 Rakic P, Yakovlev P I. Development of the corpus callosum and cavum septi in man. J Comp Neurol 1968; 132: 45–72

194 Davidoff L M, Dyke C G. Agenesis of the corpus callosum: diagnosis by encephalography. AJR 1934; 32: 1–10

195 Babcock D S. The normal, absent, and abnormal corpus callosum: sonographic findings. Radiology 1984; 151: 449–453

196 Gebarski S S, Gebarski K S, Bowerman R A, Silver T M. Agenesis of the corpus callosum: sonographic features. Radiology 1984; 151: 443–448

197 Byrd S E, Harwood-Nash D C, Fitz C R. Absence of the corpus callosum: computed tomographic evaluation in infants and children. Can Assoc Radiol J 1978; 29: 108–112

198 Ettlinger G, Blakemore C B, Milner A D, Wilson J. Agenesis of the corpus callosum: a further behavioural investigation. Brain 1974; 97: 225–234

199 Grogono J L. Children with agenesis of the corpus callosum. Dev Med Child Neurol 1968; 10: 613–616

200 Warkany J, Lemire R, Cohen M M. Mental retardation and congenital malformations of the nervous system. Chicago: Year Book Medical Publishers. 1981: p 224–243

201 Menkes J H, Philippart M, Clark D B. Hereditary partial agenesis of the corpus callosum. Arch Neurol 1964; 11: 198–208

202 Young I D, Trounce J Q, Levene M I, Fitzsimmons J S, Moore J R. Agenesis of the corpus callosum and macrocephaly in siblings. Clin Genet 1985; 28: 225–230

203 Friedman M, Cohen P. Agenesis of corpus callosum as a possible sequel to maternal rubella during pregnancy. Am J Dis Child 1947; 73: 178–185

204 Bartoleschi B, Cantore G P. Agenesia del corpus calloso in paziente affeto da toxoplasmosi. Riv Neurol 1962; 32: 79

205 Pfeiffer J, Majewski F, Fishback H, Bierich J R, Volk B. Alcohol embryo and fetopathy. J Neuro Sci 1979; 41: 125–137

206 Elliot G B, Wollin D W. Defect of the corpus callosum and congenital occlusion of the fourth ventricle with tuberous sclerosis. AJR 1966; 85: 701–705

207 Probst F P. Congenital defects of the corpus callosum: morphology and encephalographic appearances. Acta Radiol 1973; 331: 1–152

208 Kendall B E. Dysgenesis of the corpus callosum. Neuroradiol 1983; 25: 239–256

209 Comstock C H, Culp D, Gonzalez J, Boal D B. Agenesis of the corpus callosum in the fetus: Its evolution and significance. J Ultrasound Med 1985; 4: 613–616

210 Meizner I, Barki Y, Hertzanu Y. Prenatal sonographic diagnosis of agenesis of corpus callosum. JCU 1987; 15: 262–264

211 Bertino R E, Nyberg D A, Cyr D R, Mack L A. Prenatal diagnosis of agenesis of the corpus callosum. J Ultrasound Med 1988; 7: 251–260

212 Parrish M L, Roessmann U, Levinsohn M W. Agenesis of the corpus callosum: a study of the frequency of associated malformations. Ann Neurol 1979; 6: 349–354

213 Romero R, Pilu G, Jeanty P, Ghidini A, Hobbins J C. In: Prenatal diagnosis of congenital anomalies. Connecticut: Appleton and Lange. 1988

214 Baraitser M. The genetics of neurological disorders. Oxford: Oxford University Press. 1982

215 Dieker H, Edwards R H, Zurhein G, Chou S M, Hartman H A, Opitz J M. The lissencephaly syndrome. Birth Defects 1969; 5: 53–64

216 Garcia C A, Dunn D, Trevor R. The lissencephaly (agyria) syndrome in siblings. Computerized tomographic and neuropathologic findings. Arch Neurol 1978; 35: 608–611

217 Halsey J H. Hydranencephaly. In: Vinken P J, Bruyn G W, Klawans H L. eds. Handbook of clinical neurology. Amsterdam: Elsevier/North Holland Biomedical Press. 1987; 50: 337–353

218 Myers R E. Brain pathology following fetal vascular occlusion: an experimental study. Invest Opthalmol 1969; 8: 41–50

219 Green M F, Benacerraf B, Crawford J M. Hydranencephaly: US appearance during in-utero evolution. Radiology 1985; 156: 779–780

220 Johnson E E, Warner M, Simonds J P. Total absence of the cerebral hemispheres. J Pediatr 1951; 38: 69–79

221 Muir C S. Hydranencephaly and related disorders. Am J Dis Child 1959; 34: 231

222 Altshuler G. Toxoplasmosis as a cause of hydranencephaly. Am J Dis Child 1973; 125: 251–252

223 Carrasco C R, Stierman E D, Harnsberger H R, Lee T G. An algorithm for prenatal ultrasound diagnosis of congenital central nervous system abnormalities. J Ultrasound Med 1985; 4: 163–168

224 Lee T G, Warren B H. Antenatal diagnosis of hydranencephaly by ultrasound: correlation with ventriculography and computed tomography. JCU 1977; 5: 271–273

225 Strauss S, Bouzouki M, Goldfarb H, Uppal V, Costales F. Antenatal ultrasound diagnosis of an unusual case of hydranencephaly. JCU 1984; 12: 420–422

226 Hambey W B, Krauss R F, Beswick W F. Hydranencephaly: clinical diagnosis. Presentation of seven cases. Pediatrics 1950; 6: 371–383

227 Sutton L N, Bruce D A, Schut L. Hydranencephaly versus maximal hydrocephalus: an important clinical distinction. Neurosurgery 1980; 6: 34–38

228 Siber M. X linked recessive microcencephaly, micropthalmia with corneal opacities, spastic quadriplegia, hypospadias and cryptorchidism. Clin Genet 1984; 26: 453–456

229 Gross H, Jellinger K. Morphologische aspekte cerebraler midbildungen. Wien Z Nervenheilk 1969; 27: 9–37

230 Gastaut H, Gastaut J L. Demonstration of a little known cause of infantile epilepsy, occipital porencephaly, by computerised tomography (CT). Computerised Tomography 1977; 1: 323–330

231 Benda C E. The late effects of cerebral birth injuries. Medicine 1945; 24: 71–110

232 Cantu R C, Le May M. Porencephaly caused by intracerebral haemorrhage. Radiology 1967; 88: 526–530

233 Page L K, Brown S B, Gargano F P, Shortz R W. Schizencephaly: a clinical study and review. Childs Brain 1975; 1: 348–358

234 Miller G M, Stears J C, Guggenheim M A, Wilkening G F. Schizencephaly: a clinical and CT study. Neurology 1984; 34: 997–1001

235 Klingensmith W C, Cioffi-Ragan D T. Schizencephaly: diagnosis and progression in-utero. Radiology 1986; 159: 617–618

236 Larroche J C. Cytoarchitectonic abnormalities (abnormalities of cell migration). In: Vinken P J, Bruyn G W. eds: Handbook of clinical neurology. Amsterdam: Elsevier/North Holland Biomedical Press. 1977; 30: 479–506

237 Berg R A, Aleck K A, Kaplan A M. Familial porencephaly. Arch Neurol 1983; 40: 567–569

238 Airaksinen E M. Familial porencephaly. Clin Genet 1984; 26: 236–238

239 Dandy W E, Blackfan K D. Internal hydrocephalus. An experimental, clinical and pathological study. Am J Dis Child 1914; 8: 406–482

240 Taggart J K, Walker A E. Congenital atresia of the foramens of Luschka and Magendie. Arch Neurol Psychiatry 1942; 48: 583–612

241 Benda C E. The Dandy-Walker syndrome or so-called atresia of the foramen Magendie. J Neuropathol Exp Neurol 1954; 13: 14–29

242 Gardner E, O'Rahilly R, Prolo D. The Dandy-Walker and the Arnold-Chiari malformations. Clinical, developmental and teratological considerations. Arch Neurol 1975; 32: 393–407

243 Murray J C, Johnson J A, Bird T D. Dandy-Walker malformation: etiologic heterogeneity and empiric recurrence risks. Genetics 1985; 28: 272–283

244 Hirsch J F, Pierrekahn A, Renier D, Sainterose C, Hoppehirsch E. The Dandy-Walker malformation: a review of 40 cases. J Neurosurg 1984; 61: 515–522

245 Nyberg D A, Cyr D R, Mack L A, Fitzsimmons J, Hickok D, Mahony B S. The Dandy-Walker malformation: prenatal sonographic diagnosis and its clinical significance. J Ultrasound Med 1988; 7: 65–71

246 Russ P D, Pretorius D H, Johnson M J. Dandy-Walker syndrome: a review of 15 cases evaluated by prenatal sonography. Am J Obstet Gynecol 1989; 161: 401–406

247 Hatjis C G, Horbar J D, Anderson G G. The in utero diagnosis of a posterior fossa intracranial cyst (Dandy-Walker cyst). Am J Obstet Gynecol 1981; 140: 473–475

248 Mahony B S, Callen P W, Filly R A, Hoddick W K. The fetal cisterna magna. Radiology 1984; 153: 773–776

249 Pilu G, Romero R, DePalma L, et al. Antenatal diagnosis and obstetrical management of Dandy-Walker syndrome. J Reprod Med 1986; 31: 1017–1022

250 Dempsey P J, Kock H J. In utero diagnosis of the Dandy Walker syndrome: differentiation from extra-axial posterior fossa cyst. JCU 1981; 9: 403–405

251 Hart M N, Malamud N, Ellis W G. The Dandy-Walker syndrome: clinicopathological study based on 28 cases. Neurology 1972; 22: 771–780

252 Sawaya R, McLaurin A L. Dandy-Walker syndrome: clinical analysis of 23 cases. J Neurosurg 1981; 55: 89–98

253 Shuangshoti S, Netsky M G. Neuroepithelial (colloid) cysts of the nervous system: further observations on pathogenesis, location, incidence and histochemistry. Neurology 1966; 16: 887–903

254 Shuangshoti S, Netsky M G. Histogenesis of choroid plexus in man. Am J Anat 1966; 118: 283–316

255 Chitkara U, Cogswell C, Norton K, Wilkins I A, Mehalek K, Berkowitz R L. Choroid plexus cysts in the fetus: a benign anatomic variant or pathological entity? Report of 41 cases and review of the literature. Obstet Gynecol 1988; 72: 185–189

256 Clark S L, DeVore G R, Sabey P L. Prenatal diagnosis of cysts of the fetal choroid plexus. Obstet Gynecol 1988; 72: 585–587

257 Twining P, Zuccollo J, Swallow J, Clewes J. Choroid plexus cysts – a marker for trisomy 18. A prospective study and review of the literature. Br J Radiol 1989; 63: 385

258 Furness M E. Choroid plexus cysts and trisomy 18. Lancet 1987; 2: 693

259 DeRoo T R, Harris R D, Sargent S K, Denholm T A, Crow H C. Fetal choroid plexus cysts: prevalence, clinical significance and sonographic appearance. AJR 1988; 151: 1179–1181

260 Ostelere S J, Irving H C, Lilford R J. Chorioid plexus cysts in the fetus. Lancet 1987; 1: 1491

261 Bundy A L, Saltzman D H, Pober B, Fine C, Emerson D, Doubilet P M. Antenatal sonographic findings in trisomy 18. J Ultrasound Med 1986; 5: 361–364

262 Nicolaides K H, Rodeck C H, Gosden C M. Rapid karyotyping in non-lethal fetal malformations. Lancet 1986; 1: 283–287

263 Benacerraf B R. Asymptomatic cysts of the fetal choroid plexus in the second trimester. J Ultrasound Med 1987; 6: 475–478

264 Thorpe-Beeston J G, Gosden C M, Nicolaides K H. Is karyotyping for choroid plexus cysts necessary? Br J Radiol; 1990: 385

265 Starkman S P, Brown T C, Linell E A. Cerebral arachnoid cysts. J Neuropathol Exp Neurol 1958; 17: 484

266 Geissinger J D, Kohler W C, Robinson B W, Davis F M. Arachnoid cysts of the middle cranial fossa: surgical considerations. Surg Neurol 1978; 10: 27–33

267 Smith R A, Smith W A. Arachnoid cysts of the middle cranial fossa. Surg Neurol 1976; 5: 246–252

268 Roach E S, Laster D W, Sumner T E, Volberg F M. Posterior fossa arachnoid cyst demonstrated by ultrasound. JCU 1982; 10: 88–90

269 Shaw C M, Alvord E C. Congenital arachnoid cysts and their differential diagnosis. In: Vinken G W, Bruyn P W. eds. Handbook of clinical neurology. Amsterdam: Elsevier/North Holland Biomedical Press. 1977; 31: 75–135

270 Oliver L C. Primary arachnoid cysts. BMJ 1958; 1: 1147

271 Diakoumakis E E, Weinberg B, Mollin J. Prenatal sonographic diagnosis of a suprasellar arachnoid cyst. J Ultrasound Med 1986; 5: 529

272 Sauerbrei E E, Cooperberg P L. Cystic tumours of the fetal and neonatal cerebrum: ultrasound and computed tomographic evaluation. Radiology 1983; 147: 689–692

273 Anderson F M, Landing B H. Cerebral arachnoid cysts in infants. J Pediatr 1966; 69: 88–96

274 Goldstein I, Reece E A, Pilu G, Bovicelli L, Hobbins J C. Cerebellar measurements with ultrasonography in the evaluation of fetal growth and development. Am J Obstet Gynecol 1987; 156: 1065–1069

275 Comstock C H, Boal D B. Enlarged fetal cisterna magna: appearance and significance. Obstet Gynecol 1985; 66: 25–27

276 Lyon G, Beaugerie A. Congenital developmental malformations. In: Levene M I, Bennett M J, Punt J. eds. Fetal and neonatal neurology and neurosurgery. Edinburgh: Churchill Livingstone. 1988: p 231–248

277 Kilham L, Margolis G. Cerebellar ataxia in hamsters inoculated with rat virus. Science 1964; 143: 1047–1048

278 Walker A E. Lissencephaly. Arch Neurol Psych 1942; 48: 13–29

279 Dobyns W B, Kirkpatrick J B, Hittner H M, Roberts R M, Kretzer F L. Walker-Warburg and cerebro-ocular-muscular syndromes and a new syndrome with type II lissencephaly. Am J Med Genet 1985; 22: 157–195

280 Young I D. Genetics of neurodevelopmental disorders. In: Levene M I, Bennett M J, Punt J. eds. Fetal and neonatal neurology and neurosurgery. Edinburgh: Churchill Livingstone. 1988: p 249–257

281 Bundy S. Genetics and neurology. Edinburgh: Churchill Livingstone. 1985

282 Padget D H. The cranial venous system in man with reference to the development, adult configuration and relation to the arteries. Am J Anat 1956; 98: 307–355

283 Vintzileos A M, Eisenfeld L I, Campbell W A, Herson V C, DiLeo P E, Chameides L. Prenatal ultrasonic diagnosis of arteriovenous malformation of the vein of Galen. Am J Perinatol 1986; 3: 209–211

284 Reiter A A, Huhta J C, Carpenter R J, Segall G K, Hawkins E P. Prenatal diagnosis of arteriovenous malformation of the vein of Galen. JCU 1986; 14: 623–628

285 Hirsch J H, Cyr D, Eberhardt H, Zunkel D. Ultrasonographic diagnosis of an aneurysm of the vein of Galen in utero by duplex scanning. J Ultrasound Med 1983; 2: 231–233

286 Mao K, Adams J. Antenatal diagnosis of intracranial arteriovenous fistula by ultrasonography: case report. Br J Obstet Gynaecol 1983; 90: 872–873

287 Silverman B K, Brekzt T, Craig J, Nadas A S. Congestive failure in the newborn caused by cerebral arteriovenous fistula. Am J Dis Child 1959; 89: 539–543

288 Norman M G, Becker L E. Cerebral damage in neonates resulting from arteriovenous malformation of vein of Galen. J Neurol Neurosurg Pschy 1974; 37: 252–258

289 Hoffman H J, Chuang S, Hendrick E B, Humphreys R P. Aneurysms of the vein of Galen. Experience at the Hospital for Sick Children, Toronto. J Neurosurg 1982; 57: 316–322

290 Amacher A L, Shillito J. The syndromes and surgical treatment of aneurysms of the great vein of Galen. J Neurosurg 1973; 39: 88–98

297 O'Connell E J, Feldt R H, Stickler G B. Head circumference, mental retardation and growth failure. Pediatrics 1965; 36: 62–66

291 Mori K. Anomalies of the central nervous system. Neuroradiology and neurosurgery. New York: Thieme-Stratton. 1985

292 Koos W, Miller M H. Intracranial tumours of infants and children. Stuttgart: G Thieme. 1971

293 Lipman S P, Pretorious D H, Rumack C M, Manco-Johnson M L. Fetal intracranial teratoma: US diagnosis of 3 cases and a review of the literature. Radiology 1985; 157: 491–494

294 Kirkinen P, Suramo I, Joupila P, et al. Combined use of ultrasound and computed tomography in the evaluation of fetal intracranial abnormality. J Perinat Med 1982; 10: 257–265

295 Fraumeni J F, Miller R W. Cancer deaths in the newborn. Am J Dis Child 1969; 117: 186–189

296 Altman R P, Randolph J G, Lilly J R. Sacrococcygeal teratoma: American Academy of Pediatrics Surgical Section Survey – 1973. J Pediatr Surg 1974; 9: 389–398

297 O'Connell E J, Feldt R H, Stickler G B. Head circumference, mental retardation and growth failure. Pediatrics 1965; 36: 62–66

298 Book J A, Schut J W, Reed S C. A clinical and genetical study of microcephaly. Am J Ment Def 1953; 57: 637–660

299 Haslam R H A. Microcephaly. In: Vinken P J, Bruyn G W, Klawans H L. eds. Handbook of clinical neurology. Amsterdam: Elsevier/North Holland Biomedical Press. 1987; 50: 267–284

300 Dobbing J, Sands J. Quantitative growth and development of human brain. Arch Dis Child 1973; 48: 757–767

301 Thoms A, Campbell S. Ultrasound measurement of the fetal head and abdomen circumference ratio in the assessment of growth retardation. Br J Obstet Gynaecol 1977; 84: 165–174

302 Kurtz A B, Wapner R J, Rubin C S, Cole-Beuglet C, Ross R D, Goldberg B B. Ultrasound criteria for in utero diagnosis of microcephaly. JCU 1980; 8: 11–16

303 Avery G B, Meneses L, Lodge A. The clinical significance of 'measurement microcephaly'. Am J Dis Child 1972; 123: 214–217

304 Martin H P. Microcephaly and mental retardation. Am J Dis Child 1970; 119: 128–131

305 Pryor H B, Thelander H. Abnormally small head size and intellect in children. J Pediatr 1968; 73: 593–598

306 Haslam R H A, Smith D W. Autosomal dominant microcephaly. J Pediatr 1979; 95: 701–705

307 Quazi Q H, Reed T E. A problem in diagnosis of primary versus secondary microcephaly. Clin Genet 1973; 4: 46–52

308 Bartley J A, Hall B D. Mental retardation and multiple congenital abnormalities of unknown etiology: frequency of occurrence in similarly affected sibs of the proband. Birth Defects Original Article Series XIV 1978; 6B: 127–137

309 Opitz J M, Kaveggia E G, Durkin-Stamm M V, Pendleton E. Diagnostic/genetic studies in severe mental retardation. Birth Defects Original Article Series XVI 1978; 6B: 1–38

The urinary tract

Alison Fowlie and Josephine McHugo

INTRODUCTION

One of the earliest congenital abnormalities diagnosed in utero was that of polycystic kidneys reported by Garrett in 1970.[1] Later, in 1975, obstructive nephropathy was recognised in a fetus.[2] These were both gross pathologies found in late pregnancies but, over the last 15 to 20 years improvement in ultrasound technology and techniques, and in the understanding of fetal anatomy and physiology as revealed by ultrasound, has led to increasingly early diagnoses of abnormalities of the urinary tract, even at 12 to 15 weeks[3–7] and the recognition on ultrasound of virtually every possible pathology.

Congenital abnormalities of the urinary tract are common,[8–10] but the true incidence is uncertain. Although exceeded only by malformations of the central nervous system and cardiovascular system as causes of death in infancy from congenital malformation, the majority (approximately 70%) are not lethal.[11] This makes assessment of the true incidence very difficult; it is approximately two or three per thousand live births.[11,12]

As with other organs, the use of routine ultrasound scanning in low-risk pregnancies has resulted in early detection of many cases of urinary tract abnormalities. Lethal conditions may thus be terminated. Forewarning is given of moderate to severe pathologies, allowing planned delivery and post-natal treatment, counselling and preparation of the parents for the problems their baby will have, and opening up avenues for prenatal treatment.[13] Particularly importantly, clinicians are alerted to the presence of asymptomatic and clinically silent lesions (about 65% of abnormalities in live births[8]) which otherwise would be missed in the neonatal period and perhaps remain unrecognised until late presentation with renal failure and chronic infection.

As with all developing fields, problems have occurred with the ultrasonic diagnosis and subsequent management of urinary tract problems. Its accuracy in prenatal diagnosis has been reported to be between 60% and 96%.[14,15] There have been errors such as the large fetal adrenal mistaken for a fetal kidney[16] and confusion between pelvi-ureteric junction obstruction and duodenal atresia.[17,18] There may be difficulty differentiating multicystic dysplasia and an obstructed kidney,[17] but these problems are now well-recognised and mistakes are now few.

However the differentiation of physiological dilatation of the urinary tract from minor degrees of obstructive pathology remains difficult[19] and this is an area which is still incompletely resolved. In addition, even when obstructive uropathy is present, the degree of urinary tract dilation as visualised on ultrasound does not correlate well with the pathological state of the renal tissue or its function.

Attempts have been made to evaluate the presence or degree of dysplasia of the renal tissue and thus infer something about renal function. Increased renal reflectivity together with cortical cysts in the presence of hydronephrosis is strongly suggestive of renal dysplasia.[20] However increased reflectivity has been found in 20% of normal fetal kidneys, and 25% of those with dysplasia were not detected,[20,21] casting doubts on the reliability of ultrasound for this.

One method of evaluating renal function is the assessment of amniotic fluid volume – a useful but fairly crude measure. Although severe oligohydramnios is associated with poor renal function, Glick et al 1984[21] found that one third of pregnancies with only mild reduction in amniotic fluid resulted in infants with severe reduction in renal function and one third with moderately severe oligohydramnios actually had a reasonable outcome.

Attempts to correlate renal function with urine production are made difficult because of several factors:[21–23] polyuria, not oliguria, is the usual response to renal damage; reflux often coexists with obstruction making accurate assessment of flow impossible; while maternal dehydration can severely affect the rate of fetal urine production.[24]

More recently direct measurement of electrolytes, urea and creatinine in aspirated fetal urine have been used to evaluate renal function.[21] Whilst this correlates better with outcome, single or repeated aspiration of fetal urine is not always feasible or acceptable and procedure-related complications are not uncommon.

Despite these problems ultrasonic antenatal diagnosis of fetal urinary tract abnormalities has been useful in the prevention of serious renal damage in the child or young adult and its role here is likely to increase.

Normal urinary tract

Urine production begins at 11 to 13 weeks gestation.[25] Prior to this amniotic fluid is primarily a dialysate of fetal blood across the skin which is permeable.[26] About the time urine production begins, the skin starts to keratinise, making it less permeable to water. Thus, between 13 and 20 weeks menstrual age, there is a gradual change from fetal dialysate to urine as the main component of amniotic fluid.[27] Hence by 16 to 18 weeks absent or non-functioning kidneys are invariably associated with oligohydramnios.

The fetal kidneys may be imaged as early as 9 weeks menstrual age[28] but with transabdominal ultrasound are more usually seen from 14 weeks onwards[29] and reliably visualised in 90% of cases between 17 and 22 weeks.[30] In the first part of the second trimester they are seen in transverse section, usually as areas of low reflectivity (Fig. 1), either side of the spine just inferior to the level where measurements for the abdominal circumference are made. On longitudinal section a bean-shaped structure is seen with very little internal architecture visible (Fig. 2). Later, as renal fat is laid down around the renal fascia and in the central renal sinus, the fetal kidney is more easily

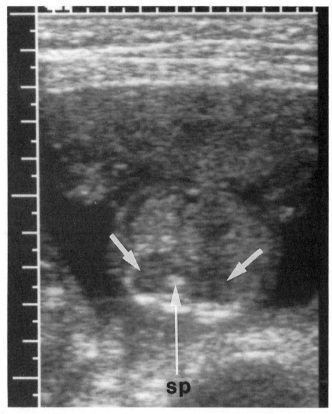

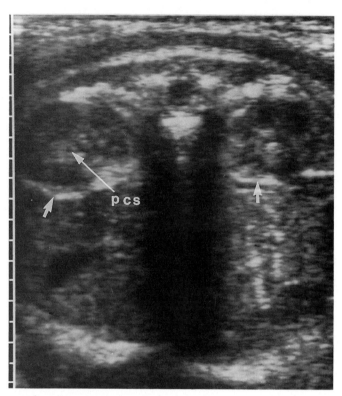

Fig. 1 Normal kidneys – 18 weeks. Transverse section of the fetal abdomen at 18 weeks. The kidneys (arrows) are seen as two echo-poor areas posteriorly within the fetal abdomen and touching the spine (sp) medially. The renal pelvis are not visible.

Fig. 3 Normal kidney – 22 weeks. Transverse section of the fetal abdomen at 22 weeks. The renal capsule (arrows) is well-delineated and the pelvicalyceal system (pcs) can be seen.

seen and its appearance correlates well with that seen in the neonatal period (Fig. 3). The marked cortico-medullary differentiation and lobulated outline that are normal for this age group may confuse the inexperienced operator into mistaking the pyramids for dilated calyces or renal cysts (Fig. 4). However, in hydronephrosis the dilated calyces communicate with the renal pelvis and renal cysts do not surround the renal pelvis so uniformly.

The normal growth pattern of the fetal kidney has been well-established by several workers in dead fetuses,[31,32] and in utero using ultrasound,[30,33–35] Standard measurements for renal circumference, volume, thickness, width and length related to menstrual age are available. Renal width, thickness (AP diameter) and circumference are measured in a transverse section of the fetal kidney. Length is measured from the upper to the lower pole on a longitudinal scan, care being taken to avoid including the adrenal gland in the measurement, particularly in early pregnancy. The ratio of the transverse renal circumference to the abdominal circumference is a simple screening measurement for conditions affecting renal size[34] being fairly constant from 17 weeks to term at 0.27 to 0.30. These measurements however have limited value as improved ultrasound equipment has allowed diagnoses of polycystic kidneys to be made on the appearances alone in the

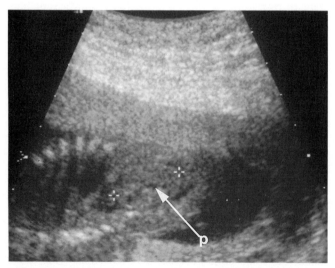

Fig. 2 Normal kidney – 18 weeks. Longitudinal section of a fetal abdomen at 18 weeks. The kidney is seen in longitudinal section. The cortex and medulla cannot be differentiated. A normal 'slit-like' renal pelvis (p) is seen.

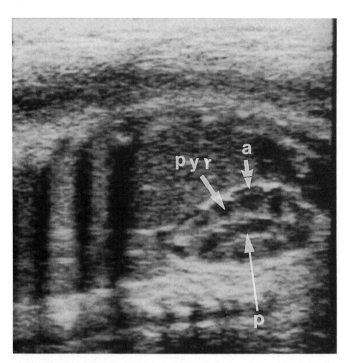

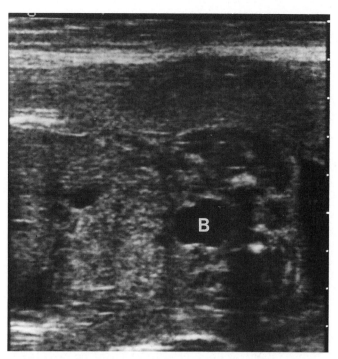

Fig. 4 Normal kidney – 22 weeks. Longitudinal section of the fetal abdomen at 22 weeks displaying the kidney. The cortico-medullary differentiation is well-shown with the arcuate vessels (a) seen at the base of the echo-poor medulla or pyramids (pyr). The renal pelvis (p) is seen centrally.

Fig. 5 Fetal bladder. Longitudinal section showing a normally filled fetal bladder (B).

majority of cases but do occasionally have a place in the diagnosis of renal hypoplasia.

The normal fetal ureters are never visualised but the bladder can be seen as early as 13 weeks and is consistently identified from 16 weeks onwards when it may be observed to fill and empty regularly (Fig. 5). Failure to identify a fetal bladder in the course of an ultrasound examination may be because the fetus has just voided (voiding occurring at least once an hour).[22] If the urinary tract is otherwise unremarkable and the liquor volume is normal, it is not essential to demonstrate the bladder. Urine production increases with menstrual age.[36]

Renal agenesis

Renal agenesis occurs because of failure of development of the ureteric buds of the mesonephros. It may be complete or partial, unilateral or bilateral. Ureteric remnants may be present.

Incidence and aetiology The birth frequency of bilateral renal agenesis was estimated to be 1.2 per 10 000 in England and Wales between 1974 to 1977. Of these, 75% were isolated malformations in that only the kidney and embryologically related tissues were involved. The sex ratio was 3:1 male to female.[37] Almost identical figures were obtained in British Columbia.[38] The incidence of unilateral renal agenesis is more difficult to establish as many cases

are probably never identified. The British Columbia series identified an incidence of 0.15 per 1000 births with a sex ratio of 1:1.[38]

Renal agenesis is an isolated anomaly in approximately 33% to 50% of cases. The aetiology is unclear. Families containing many members with renal agenesis or dysgenesis have been reported; postulated patterns of inheritance include autosomal recessive,[39,40] x-linked recessive,[41] autosomal dominant[42] and multifactorial inheritance.[42,43]

Chromosomal abnormalities have been described as producing bilateral renal agenesis as well as other abnormalities, but are rare. Trisomy 7 has been noted more than once.[44] Familial marker chromosome involving the presence of a small extra chromosome, possibly a segment of 22, has been reported[45] as has renal agenesis in 4p syndrome.[46]

Bilateral renal agenesis may accompany cardiac and other abnormalities. A number of autosomal recessive syndromes include bilateral renal agenesis, namely cerebro-oculo-facial skeletal syndrome, a syndrome with microcephaly, spinal and renal abnormalities[47] and acro-renal mandibular syndrome comprising of severe split extremity abnormalities and renal and genital malformations.[48] Renal agenesis is part of the autosomal dominant disorder of branchio-oto-renal syndrome[49] and occurs with Müllerian duct abnormalities.[50]

Only insulin dependent diabetes mellitus has been implicated as a teratogen in renal agenesis.[51]

Diagnosis The most obvious ultrasound finding in bilateral renal agenesis is severe oligohydramnios, the fetus often being curled up and appearing squashed (Fig. 6). No fetal bladder is seen.[16] In the majority of cases the oligohydramnios results in such poor visualisation of the internal structure of the fetus that a definite diagnosis of absent kidneys is virtually impossible.

This combination (severe oligohydramnios with no bladder) is not specific for bilateral renal agenesis. It may occur in many multiple abnormalities and in bilateral multicystic dysplastic kidneys. These, however, also have a poor outcome, differentiation is therefore unnecessary. More importantly, these may be the findings in premature spontaneous rupture of membranes and early intra-uterine growth retardation (IUGR). A very poor prognosis for all such cases of severe oligohydramnios,[52–54] neglects the fact that the outcome in cases of IUGR and premature ruptured membranes may in fact be good in 20%. These cases consist entirely of early IUGR (62% good outcome) and premature spontaneous rupture of membranes (55% good outcome).[55]

Observations of urine production might be expected to prove the presence of functioning kidneys. Because, in the normal situation voiding takes place at least once an hour,[22] failure to demonstrate the bladder in prolonged or serial examinations half hourly over 2 or 3 hours suggests renal agenesis. In order to speed up the process frusemide may be administered intravenously to the mother.[23] The fetus is then scanned at half hourly intervals over a period of 2 hours, a filling bladder clearly ruling out bilateral renal agenesis. However, several authors have reported failure of diuresis even when renal tissue is present, particularly in early intra-uterine growth retardation.[56,57] There is some controversy as to whether frusemide does in fact cross the placenta consistently, or in high enough doses to be effective and, in fact, whether the kidneys of the early mid-trimester fetus will respond to it.[23,56,58,59] Urine production, assisted or unassisted, is less useful than might be expected in the diagnosis of bilateral renal agenesis.

Attempts to visualise the fetal kidneys directly are also fraught with difficulty. The fetal adrenal gland may be mistaken for the kidney, particularly in renal agenesis[16,60] as it is a surprisingly large organ in the second trimester of pregnancy and, in renal agenesis, does not conform to the usual shape, but forms an oval disc lying against the posterior abdominal wall, presumably due to the absence of the compressive effect of the kidney (Fig. 7).[61] Positive identification of the kidneys therefore depends on a well-defined renal pelvis, capsule and early pyramid structure which can be identified in many cases at 18 to 20 weeks. For more confident identification of the kidneys, visualisation may be improved by instillation of normal saline into the amnion or fetal intraperitoneal space; this may not be useful and is dangerous, often causing uterine discomfort and contraction. The improved imaging of modern equipment usually enables a confident diagnosis of renal agenesis using either the abdominal or the trans-vaginal route (if the fetus is presenting by the breech low down in the pelvis).

The diagnosis of isolated unilateral renal agenesis may well be missed unless the ultrasonographer painstakingly attempts to obtain ideal views of both kidneys in every case. Associated abnormalities may lead to the diagnosis. Aplastic aplasia may be mistaken as unilateral renal agenesis, the aplastic kidney consisting of a nodule of tissue which microscopically represents dysplastic metanephric elements; however, renal agenesis and aplasia may represent a continuum and the differentiation between these two

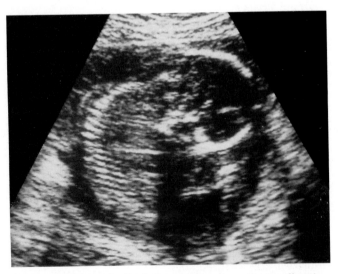

Fig. 6 Renal agenesis. Typical appearance of a pregnancy affected by renal agenesis. Anhydramnios with a curled up, poorly visualised fetus.

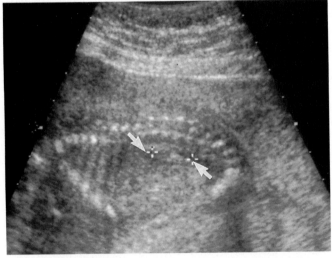

Fig. 7 Renal agenesis. In this longitudinal section of a fetus with renal agenesis, the fetal adrenal (arrows) is seen. It was considered at the time to be either the adrenal gland or a hypoplastic kidney.

conditions on morphological and genetic grounds is probably not valid.[62]

Associated abnormalities In 1946 Edith Potter described infants with characteristic facial abnormalities, limb deformities and lethal pulmonary hypoplasia associated with bilateral renal agenesis.[63] This subsequently became known as the 'Potter syndrome'. It is now recognised that these appearances and the lung hypoplasia are a consequence of any condition leading to severe oligohydramnios[64,65] and that a better term to use is that of Potter sequence.[42] In the Potter sequence lungs often weigh less than one half that expected from the fetal weight, there being a reduction in both the number of alveoli and conducting airways. This suggests that the responsible insult occurs before the sixteenth conceptual week.[66] In Potter sequence the ears are low set, the skin is redundant, the nose is shaped like a parrot's beak and the chin recedes. There is abnormal hand and foot positioning with bowed legs, clubbed feet and congenital dislocation of the hip.

The true associated abnormalities are divided into those involving the other genitourinary organs and those involving other systems. Abnormalities involving the genital organs are common (50% to 60% of cases[67]) including absence of the vas deferens and seminal vesicles, or absence of the uterus and upper vagina. Anomalies of other organ systems have been reported in 44% of patients.[67] Major deformities of the lower half of the body or limbs are common, occurring in about 40% of cases,[38] including lumbar hemivertebrae, sacral agenesis, caudal regression or absent radius and fibula and digital abnormalities. Gastrointestinal abnormalities are common (19% of cases[38]), including anal atresia, absent sigmoid and rectum, oesophageal and duodenal atresia. Cardiovascular malformations occur[38] in about 14% of cases including septal defects, hypoplastic left heart, coarctation of the aorta, transposition of the great vessels, total anomalous pulmonary venous drainage and tetralogy of Fallot. Central nervous system malformations including hydrocephaly, microcephaly, holoprosencephaly, spina bifida and iniencephaly are found in some 10%.[38]

Prognosis Bilateral renal agenesis is incompatible with life. About 40% of these infants are stillborn; the majority of those born alive die within 4 hours. Very rarely an infant will survive for more than 2 days. The cause of death in utero is not certain but other associated congenital abnormalities may be implicated.

Nearly 50% of infants with bilateral renal agenesis are growth retarded,[68] the incidence seeming to be higher in later pregnancy. Unilateral renal agenesis is no longer regarded as a relatively innocuous anomaly compensated for by enlargement of the contralateral kidney. Significantly higher frequencies of renal infection and calculus formation with resulting renal failure occur.[69] However, associated congenital abnormalities are similar to those found in bilateral renal agenesis and these therefore have a bearing on the prognosis.[38]

Obstetric management If a positive diagnosis of renal agenesis has been made prior to viability, termination should be offered. If the diagnosis is made confidently later, management should be conservative with a non-interventional policy if growth retardation or fetal distress ensues.

In the majority of cases however, for reasons already discussed, the diagnosis of renal agenesis is in doubt. The conditions which may initially mimic renal agenesis, but which potentially carry a reasonable prognosis, are premature rupture of membranes and early intra-uterine growth retardation. Careful history taking to elicit any evidence of leaking liquor, speculum examination of the patient, the testing of any secretion found with nitrazine indicator sticks and serial observations of the amniotic fluid volume over about 2 weeks, will in most cases indicate whether or not the membranes have ruptured. The fluid either continues to leak or serial scans show it to be reaccumulating. In early intra-uterine growth retardation, serial scans may be of help, looking for growth increments and also any change in amniotic fluid volume as this may well vary in IUGR. Doppler studies may be helpful.[70] Thus, study of the pregnancy over 2 to 3 weeks should rule out the more benign causes of severe oligohydramnios.

Recurrence risk In bilateral renal agenesis there is an increased risk of a subsequent severely affected child (3.5% to 4.4%[43,67]). In addition, the parents and their unaffected children are at increased risk of having silent genitourinary malformations; all first degree relatives (the parents and siblings) of affected infants should be screened for asymptomatic malformations using ultrasound.[67] Part of the justification for this is the finding that unilateral renal agenesis has medical importance for the affected person as it may be associated with abnormalities such as bicornuate uterus and absence of vas deferens. Patients with unilateral renal agenesis should also be monitored more closely for infection and stone formation in the solitary kidney.

Renal cystic disease

Renal cystic disease encompasses a number of diverse hereditary and non-hereditary disorders. The original Potter[71–74] classification of type I infantile polycystic disease, type II multicystic dysplastic kidney, type III adult polycystic disease and type IV obstructive cystic dysplasia, although useful, is inadequate to cover the range of disorders and thus has largely fallen out of use. The main problems which concern the antenatal ultrasonographer are renal dysplasia and polycystic disease.

Renal dysplasia

Renal dysplasia is defined as abnormal development of nephronic structures resulting in total or partial renal malformations.[75] Formation of the normal kidney is the result of interaction between the metanephric blastema, the metanephric diverticulum or ureteric bud and the egress of urine from a non-obstructive collecting system.[76] The ureteric bud forms the collecting system, the stalk becoming the ureter and the expanded cranial end forming the renal pelvis[25] and the pelvicalyceal system. A crucial function of the cranial end is the induction of nephrons from the metanephric blastema. According to Potter[77] the pathogenesis of dysplasia is failure of this portion of the ureteric bud to divide, resulting in abnormal collecting tubules and nephrons. Dysplasia (excluding hereditary cystic dysplasia) is frequently associated with lower urinary tract malformations, mainly obstructive. The severity of the obstruction and also its site correspond well with the patterns of dysplasia.[75,78]

Multicystic dysplasia

Incidence and aetiology Complete multicystic dysplasia is the most common form. Its precise incidence is unknown but is probably of the order of 1 in 10 000[79] with a male to female ratio of 2:1.[80] It is usually sporadic but has been associated with maternal diabetes. Normal parenchyma cannot usually be identified on histological examination of the dysplastic kidney, only multiple cysts, varying from a few millimetres to 8 centimetres in diameter, being evident (Fig. 8). A unilateral severely dysplastic multicystic kidney is invariably associated with ureteric atresia and profound bilateral maldevelopment is accompanied by bilateral ureteric atresia or urethral atresia.[75,81]

Diagnosis An affected kidney classically appears as a multilobulated mass composed of multiple thin-walled cysts containing clear fluid surrounding a more or less centrally located solid core of fibrous tissue. The reniform shape is totally lost so that the kidney resembles a bunch of grapes.[82] Thus the typical ultrasound appearance is a paraspinal mass with obvious cysts[79] which do not communicate and are randomly distributed with variable sizes.

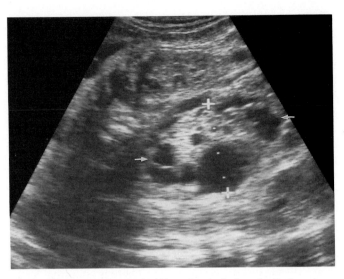

Fig. 9 Multicystic dysplastic kidney (marked). Longitudinal section showing the cysts of varying sizes and fibrous tissue replacing all normal renal substance.

It has an irregular shape and no renal pelvis can be demonstrated. Highly reflective islands of tissue may be seen between the cysts but there is no normal renal tissue (Fig. 9).

The appearances of the kidney may change through the course of the pregnancy, both enlargement and shrinking of the component cysts being reported.[83] This change in size may correlate with the degree of residual renal function. Although the multicystic dysplastic kidney is classically described as being functionless, some nephrons may survive giving partial residual function.[84] As long as the kidney can filter plasma, the overall renal size increases. As the nephrons become fibrotic, the amount of filtrate decreases and growth stops leading eventually to involution.

Many reported cases were diagnosed during the late second and third trimester.[85] In one series the earliest diagnosis made was at 21 weeks despite earlier scans.[86] This late detection may be because the cysts are only macroscopically evident after completion of nephron induction (around 20 weeks) with enough urine production to distend the dysplastic tubules; if so multicystic dysplasia cannot be excluded by a normal mid-trimester scan. Nevertheless, multicystic dysplastic kidney has been diagnosed at 15 weeks[7] and all but one of our 47 cases were manifest by 19 weeks. In that case moderate oligohydramnios was present at 18 weeks but the kidneys were unremarkable. The patient defaulted till 24 weeks, by which time the renal abnormality was obvious.

In bilateral multicystic dysplastic kidney there is severe oligohydramnios and no fetal bladder is seen. If unilateral multicystic dysplastic kidney is diagnosed the rest of the urinary tract must be scanned carefully as the prognosis depends on the state of the other kidney and the rest of

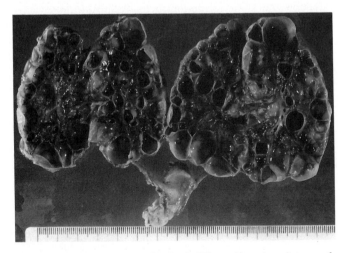

Fig. 8 Bilateral multicystic dysplastic kidney. Note the substance of the kidneys is entirely replaced by cysts of varying sizes. (With grateful thanks to Dr Jane Zuccollo, Queens Medical Centre, Nottingham.)

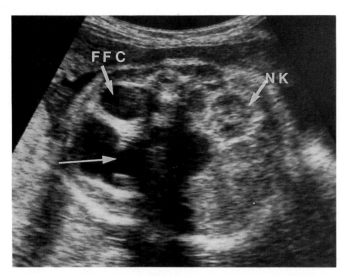

Fig. 10 Multicystic dysplastic kidney. Transverse section at 32 weeks showing one normal kidney (NK) and one fluid filled kidney (FFC) , with a dilated structure below. The appearance of communication (arrow) between the various parts of this led to the incorrect diagnosis of hydronephrosis and hydroureter.

the urinary tract. Contralateral renal abnormalities are present in up to 40% in this condition.[87] The abnormalities include pelvi-ureteric junction obstruction, renal agenesis and renal hypoplasia.

Differential diagnosis The classical multicystic dysplastic kidney may be confused with hydronephrosis.[79] In hydronephrosis the normal reniform shape persists, renal parenchyma is present peripherally and the 'cysts' of calyceal dilatation are orderly and anatomically aligned around and communicate with the renal pelvis.[29] Despite careful attempts using these criteria, it may be impossible to distinguish between the two conditions (Fig. 10),[88] difficulty even occurring in the neonatal period. A necrotic Wilms' tumour or hamartoma producing a large cystic mass can be confused with a multicystic dysplastic kidney. The former conditions are extremely rare and necrotic cystic spaces are unlikely to be as smooth walled as those of cystic dysplasia.

Associated abnormalities Bilateral multicystic dysplasia always leads to the Potter sequence. In addition it may be associated with other multiple abnormalities such as cardiovascular malformations, CNS abnormalities, diaphragmatic hernia, cleft palate, duodenal stenosis and imperforate anus,[77] tracheo-oesophageal fistula and bilateral absence of radius and thumb.[89]

In unilateral multicystic dysplastic kidney other urinary tract abnormalities are common[87] as previously discussed. Anomalies in other systems, similar to those with bilateral disease, are also found.[88,90]

Prognosis Bilateral multicystic dysplastic kidney is a condition incompatible with life. All patients with bilateral multicystic dysplastic kidney have Potter facies at birth and

die within a few days. Isolated unilateral multicystic dysplastic kidney has a good outlook, though it is a usual precaution to follow up such infants at regular intervals. In the majority of cases the kidney shrinks away; in a few cases the mass is large enough to necessitate nephrectomy. Complications resulting from the abnormal renal tissue, such as hypertension, may also necessitate its removal. When unilateral multicystic dysplastic kidney is not isolated, the prognosis depends on the type and severity of the associated conditions.

Obstetric management When bilateral multicystic renal dysplasia is diagnosed early in pregnancy, termination should be offered because of the poor outcome. If the diagnosis is made after the time when termination may be carried out, conservative management should be adopted; growth retardation or fetal distress should not be intervened with. At any age careful examination for other abnormalities should be made and ideally fetal karyotyping should be performed to provide information for counselling in future pregnancies.

In isolated unilateral multicystic disease normal obstetric management should be pursued. If other abnormalities have been detected as well, full assessment of these should be made along with fetal karyotyping; the subsequent management is based on the likely prognosis.

Recurrence risk As the condition is almost always sporadic there is usually no increased risk of recurrence. Rarely familial cases have been reported.[91]

Peripheral cortical cystic dysplasia

Aetiology and incidence Peripheral cortical cystic dysplasia is associated with non-atretic urinary tract abnormalities, most commonly posterior urethral valves. It results from severe but incomplete obstruction of the lower urinary tract and development of the kidney is affected, possibly somewhat later in the embryological period (after the tenth week) than in multicystic dysplasia.[78,79] The later the obstruction the less severe the effect on development. In fetal lambs, obstruction late in gestation produces simple hydronephrosis with no dysplasia.[92] In humans less severe obstructions are rarely associated with dysplasia.[75] Baert[93] suggests that the structural abnormalities of multicystic dysplasia and of peripheral cortical cystic dysplasia are essentially identical, the severity of the changes being the only difference. The cysts are rarely visible macroscopically but histology reveals microscopic cysts sometimes with cartilaginous and increased fibrous tissue intervening. The collecting tubes are dilated and the interstitial tissue is fibrotic and oedematous.

Diagnosis In the presence of urinary tract obstruction (usually by posterior urethral valves or occasionally at the pelvi-ureteric junction level) the kidneys may appear abnormally reflective (Fig. 11); rarely the cortex may be seen to contain small cysts (Fig. 12).[94] The increased reflectivity is due to the multiple microscopic cysts, too small to be imaged clearly by ultrasound, and to the increased fibrous

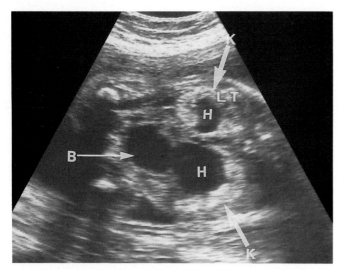

Fig. 11 Peripheral cortical dysplasia. The bladder (B) and both kidneys (K) are seen. There is hydronephrosis (H) and the renal substance (arrows) is extremely reflective.

tissue within the dysplastic kidney. The normal reniform appearance of the kidney is usually undisturbed. Since the majority of dysplastic kidneys do not contain macroscopic cysts and the microscopic cyst and fibrous tissue may not produce a marked increase in reflectivity (which is a subjective finding), the presence of renal cortical dysplasia cannot be predicted accurately.[20] Harrison[95] found that, although renal parenchymal reflectivity did correlate well with moderate to severe dysplasia, mild dysplasia was not easily detectable. Furthermore, not all kidneys which appear of increased reflectivity to the observer are dysplastic.[96]

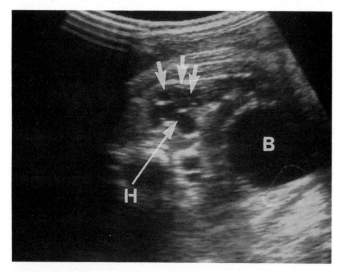

Fig. 12 Peripheral cortical dysplasia. The bladder (B) is dilated secondary to posterior urethral valves. There is hydronephrosis (H) and small cysts (arrows) were seen in the cortex.

Associated malformations These are the associated malformations of obstruction of the urinary tract, namely other genitourinary abnormalities, tracheo-oesophageal fistula, imperforate anus, cardiovascular and skeletal abnormalities.[97,98]

Prognosis The presence of renal dysplasia in urinary tract obstruction worsens prognosis; however if the obstruction is at the pelvi-ureteric junction and the dysplasia unilateral with a normal contralateral kidney the prognosis is better. If the dysplasia is bilateral (as occurs with posterior urethral valves) an accurate prognosis cannot be given as long-term follow up in patients with biopsy-proven peripheral cystic dysplasia is not available.[99] Whilst generally the greater the increase in reflectivity the worse the dysplasia, we have followed at least one case with strikingly high reflectivity secondary to posterior urethral valves and reflux who post-natally had marked dysplasia on biopsy but retained near normal renal function. In an attempt to assess each case the volume of liquor should be graded, oligohydramnios indicating failing renal function, particularly if the urinary tract is not grossly dilated. Aspiration of fetal urine, particularly from the pelves of both the affected kidneys, and catheter measurement of urine production may be useful.[97] A poor prognosis can be predicted for the fetus with bilateral obstructive uropathy and a decreased output of isotonic urine. Conversely a fetus with an output of more than 2 ml per hour of normal hypotonic urine has a good prognosis. Normal hypotonic fetal urine implies intact glomeruli and continued tubular function.[97]

Obstetric management If bilateral cortical dysplasia is suspected in a case of urinary tract obstruction, termination should be considered if the condition is diagnosed before viability. After that normal obstetric management should be given. Decompression of the urinary tract may be considered to prevent further damage to the renal tissue.[100]

Segmental dysplasia

Aetiology and incidence Segmental dysplasia usually involves the upper pole of the kidney and is associated with renal or ureteric duplication with an ectopic ureterocele and ureteric reflux.[101] Cysts, if present, are found in the cortical and medullary remnants and do not reach the dimensions of those of multicystic dysplasia.[99] This condition is also sporadic and the incidence is unknown.

Diagnosis The appearances of segmental dysplasia are not unlike that of cortical dysplasia but small cysts are more common along with increased reflectivity and the changes usually involve the upper pole only (Fig. 13). The kidney retains its shape and dilated calyces and ureter can be identified.[99] The condition is usually unilateral.

Prognosis If the contralateral kidney is normal the prognosis is good but hypertension may occur.[102] In the rare bilateral cases function is maintained by the lower moieties but hypertension may be a problem.

Obstetric management After the exclusion of other ab-

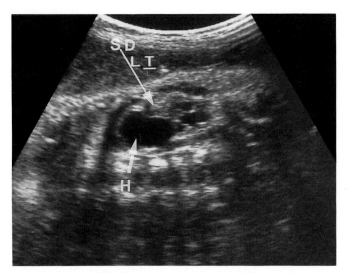

Fig. 13 Segmental dysplasia. In this case of a duplex collecting system and ureter, hydronephrosis (H) of the upper moiety is clearly seen. There appears to be some increased reflectivity (SD) around the dilated system which was more striking post-natally.

normalities an expectant management policy can be pursued.

Heredofamilial cystic dysplasia

Aetiology and incidence Cystic dysplasia occurs in a number of rare inherited syndromes, when it is non-obstructive in origin. In the Meckel-Grüber syndrome, which is autosomal recessive, there is bilateral non-obstructive multicystic dysplastic kidney, a cranio-spinal defect, usually occipital encephalocele, and post-axial polydactyly (Fig. 14). Cystic dysplasia may occur in Jeune syndrome (asphyxiating thoracic dystrophy) short rib polydactyly syndrome and trisomy 18. It also occurs in Zellweger's syndrome (cerebro-hepato-renal dysplasia) in which the appearance of the kidneys is identical to that in obstructive multicystic dysplasia.

Diagnosis The renal abnormalities in these rare syndromes are not constant. The appearance of the kidneys may be identical to multicystic dysplastic kidneys, peripheral cortical dysplasia, or the adult type of polycystic kidney disease. As the kidneys are not obstructed, there is no dilatation of the upper or lower tracts. The ability of these kidneys to function is also variable and therefore the amount of liquor present is variable. Diagnosis depends on the identification of the other abnormalities in the syndrome.

Prognosis These syndromes are all comprised of multiple abnormalities incompatible with sustained existence. The individual prognosis will be that of the particular syndrome.

Obstetric management If diagnosed prior to viability termination should be offered. If diagnosed at a later stage non-interventional management should be practised.

Recurrence risks This is again the individual risk of the

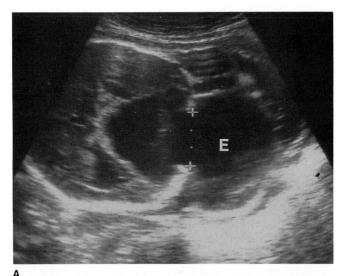

A

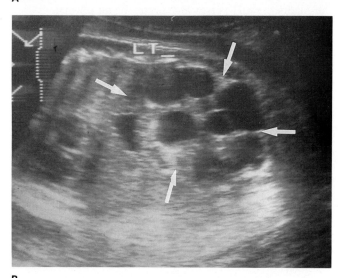

B

Fig. 14 Heredofamilial cystic dysplasia (Meckel's syndrome). **A:** There is a large occipital encephalocele (E). **B:** The kidney (arrows) is enlarged and cystic, the appearance being identical to multicystic dysplastic kidney.

syndrome, these tending to be either autosomal recessive or autosomal dominant carrying a recurrence risk of 25% or 50% respectively.

Polycystic kidney disease

Polycystic kidney disease refers to two familial disorders, infantile polycystic kidney disease (IPCKD) appearing in the first two decades of life with an autosomal recessive inheritance, and adult polycystic kidney disease (APCKD) presenting in adulthood and rarely in children with an autosomal dominant inheritance.

Infantile polycystic disease – congenital hepatic fibrosis complex (type I cystic disease of Potter) In

IPCKD there is bilateral and symmetrical enlargement of both kidneys which retain their reniform appearance. Innumerable cortical and medullary cysts 1 to 3 mm in size are present throughout the kidney (Fig. 15).[99] Microscopically the cysts are radially arranged, fusiform structures located from the pelvis to the capsule in the orientation typical of the renal collecting tubules. Uninvolved nephrons are present in the intervening tissues. Infantile polycystic renal disease is actually a disease spectrum with variable severity of renal and liver involvement.[103,104] The relative severity of the cystic change varies, with the most extensive cyst formation having the worst outcome.[103] Invariably associated with the renal cysts are liver changes including bile duct proliferation with portal fibrosis. In cases demonstrating less severe cystic change of the renal tubules, survival is prolonged with eventual development of more severe portal fibrosis.[82] There is no obstruction, the bladder, renal pelves and ureter being normal.

Aetiology and incidence   The disease is inherited as an autosomal recessive disorder that in its most severe and typical form manifests in the newborn or young infant with renal failure. The pathogenesis has not been fully established. Osathanondh and Potter[71] found fusiform sacculation and cystic diverticula of the collecting tubules which communicated freely with functioning nephrons. The most distal, earliest forming tubules are the most severely affected. They suggested that the changes occurred after induction of the metanephric blastema and attachment of nephrons. Hyperplasia of the interstitial portions of the collecting tubules was the postulated cause and that this hyperplasia began distally and progressed proximally. Thus milder forms of medullary tubular ectasia when IPCKD presents at a later stage would reflect lesser degrees of collecting tubule hyperplasia.

Potter reported an incidence of two cases in 110 000 infants,[105] but rates of 1 in 6000 to 1 in 16 000 live births have been noted subsequently.[106,107]

Diagnosis   The typical ultrasound appearance includes bilaterally enlarged highly reflective kidneys that retain their smooth shape.[108,109] The majority of the innumerable cysts are below the limit of ultrasound resolution and the multiple interfaces produced by these cysts result in the characteristic increased reflectivity (Fig. 16).[96] Some cysts between 1 to 2 mm can be imaged with high resolution scanners (Fig. 17). The enlargement may be assessed by fetal measurement but should not be used as a sole diagnostic criterion since isolated nephromegaly has been reported without any demonstrable pathological significance.[110] The degree of oligohydramnios is variable due to the broad spectrum of renal compromise and the liquor volume may remain within the normal range late into the second, or even the third trimester.[111]

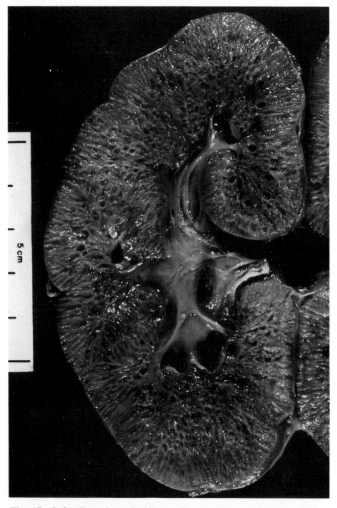

Fig. 15 Infantile polycystic kidney disease. The multiple tiny fairly uniform cysts are seen, along with a normal pelvicalyceal system. (With grateful thanks to Dr Jane Zuccollo, Queens Medical Centre, Nottingham.)

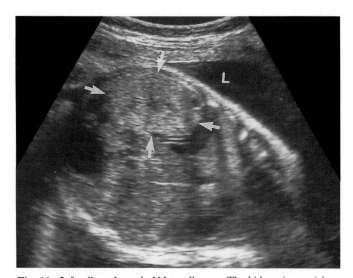

Fig. 16 Infantile polycystic kidney disease. The kidney (arrows) is large and highly reflective due to the multiple tiny cysts. The other kidney was similar in appearance but not well-displayed in this section. Note the normal amount of liquor (L) at 22 weeks.

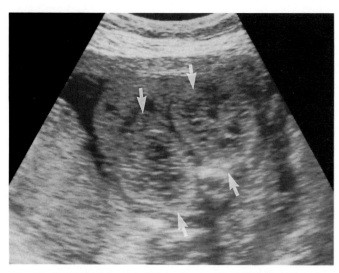

Fig. 17 Infantile polycystic kidney disease. Both kidneys (arrows) are seen to be enlarged and generally highly reflective, but with some small cysts visible.

The presence of smoothly enlarged highly reflective kidneys, with some small cysts scattered throughout, seen in the fetus at risk for IPCKD confirms the diagnosis. This condition has been diagnosed as early as 16 weeks.[96] However, the spectrum of disease is such that accurate diagnosis is not always possible, particularly not as early as the routine 18 to 20 week scan.[108,112] Usually there is evidence of the condition by 24 weeks but occasionally the diagnosis cannot be made until the third trimester.[113,114]

IPCKD is associated with raised maternal serum alpha-fetoprotein levels and must be considered along with many types of renal disease when this is evaluated.[115]

Differential diagnosis The main differential diagnosis is from adult polycystic kidney disease which can also produce large reflective kidneys.[116,117]

Associated abnormalities Apart from the cystic changes in the liver, infants do not have an increased risk of associated abnormalities.[80]

Prognosis Blythe and Ockenden[104] suggested that IPCKD may represent a heterogeneous group of clinical and pathological disorders, and recognised four types:

a) a perinatal form with nephromegaly at birth, absent hepatic symptomatology, probably Potter facies and death in early infancy. The kidneys are massively enlarged with 90% cystic change;
b) a neonatal form with nephromegaly present at birth or noted between 1 week and 1 month of age. The kidneys are somewhat smaller than in the perinatal form with about 60% tissue involved. Death is in the first year of life;
c) an infantile form with hepatomegaly with or without palpable kidneys, there being about 20% renal involvement, recognisable between 3 and 6 months of age and with progressive portal hypertension and renal failure leading to death in the first or second decade of life;

d) a juvenile form presenting between 1 and 5 years of age with hepatomegaly, portal hypertension and variable renal involvement.

The prognosis is therefore generally poor, but the exact nature will depend on the form of the disease. The larger the kidneys and the greater or earlier the onset of oligohydramnios, the more likely the disease will be at the severe end of the spectrum resulting in neonatal death.

Obstetric management In view of the poor prognosis termination should be offered if appropriate or non-interventional management practiced.

Recurrence risks The recurrence risk is 25%.

Adult polycystic kidney disease (type III cystic disease of Potter) APCKD is inherited as an autosomal dominant condition with variable expression and is usually asymptomatic until the fourth or fifth decade of life, when it presents with hypertension or renal failure. The kidneys are bilaterally enlarged with a bosselated outline produced by the innumerable cysts which may be so numerous that normal renal parenchyma is apparent only microscopically in the intervening renal tissue. The cysts vary in size from a few millimetres to several centimetres (in the adult) and are thin walled. The calyceal system may be distended but the pelvis and ureters show no abnormalities.[82]

Aetiology and incidence The disorder is inherited as an autosomal dominant trait, the gene being located on chromosome 16.[118] The pathogenesis remains unknown. Milutinovic[119] examined renal biopsies from a group of patients at risk for APCKD between 11 and 26 years of age and found that individuals who subsequently went on to develop the disease showed focal tubular dilatation and ultrastructure changes of the tubular lumen. (Other means of assessing the kidneys prior to the age of 20 years, including ultrasound, are not sensitive enough to pick up the pre-clinical states of the disease.[120])

One in 1000 people carry the gene for APCKD, it being one of the most common genetic disorders and the third most prevalent cause of chronic renal failure.[119] The expression of the gene is variable, ranging from severe forms which result in neonatal death, to asymptomatic forms found only on autopsy.[121]

Diagnosis Although autosomal dominant polycystic kidney disease is more common in the general population than IPCKD, perinatal presentation of this condition is rare. There have, however, been several documented cases of prenatal diagnosis of this condition,[122–124] the time of diagnosis ranging from 14 weeks[6] to late in the third trimester.[124] In some cases serial examinations have shown normal appearances initially, abnormalities only developing at 30 to 36 weeks.[123] The ultrasound appearance may be similar to IPCKD with enlarged highly reflective kidneys and multiple small cysts (Fig. 18), which tend to be larger than the adult form of the disease; they represent dilated nephrons. The cortico-medullary junction may be accentu-

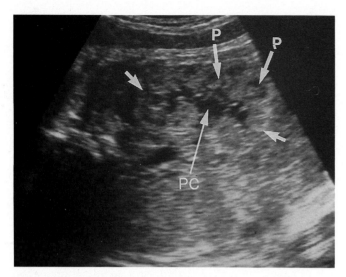

Fig. 18 Adult polycystic kidney disease. The kidney (small arrows) is enlarged, highly reflective with well-demarcated renal pyramids (P). The pelvicalyceal system (PC) (and distal urinary tract) are normal, ruling out cortical dysplasia.

ated in APCKD and this forms a useful differentiating feature from other causes of an enlarged, not grossly cystic, kidney.[125] Initially the abnormality may appear to be unilateral, the lesions often being more prominent in one kidney.

The quantity of amniotic fluid ranges from normal to severely reduced. Examination of the parents may be helpful, one parent at least demonstrating innumerable renal cysts. If however the parents are young, ultrasound examination may be insufficiently sensitive to pick up the pre-cystic form of the abnormal kidneys as ultrasound is only diagnostic in 66% of cases before 20 years of age.[120] APCKD should be suspected when bilateral cystic enlargement of the kidneys is detected in association with a normal amount of amniotic fluid. Diagnosis of the condition has also been made using DNA markers on chromosome 16 after chorionic villus sampling.[126,127]

Differential diagnosis The differential diagnosis (when the kidneys are seen to be bilaterally enlarged) is from the infantile form of the disease. Kidneys in the adult form rarely reach the very large size of the infantile form.[117] The accentuated cortico-medullary junction may be useful.[125] Examination of the parents may prove helpful but as previously mentioned, ultrasound may not be sufficiently sensitive to pick up early forms of these if the full cystic form has not yet become manifest.

Associated abnormalities APCKD is associated with cystic lesions in other organs including the liver, pancreas, spleen and gonads,[121] but these lesions are unlikely to be manifest prenatally. Cardiovascular abnormalities may be prominent in patients with this condition including dilatation of the aortic root, bicuspid aortic valve and coarctation of the aorta.[128] This type of polycystic disease

is also part of some syndromes, namely Meckel's and tuberose-sclerosis.

Prognosis APCKD usually becomes manifest in the fourth or fifth decade of life with hypertension or gradual onset of renal failure; occasionally flank pain attributed to associated renal calculi, haemorrhage into a cyst or ureteric obstruction by a blood clot is reported as the initial presentation. However it is becoming increasingly recognised in the newborn infant,[80] usually as an abdominal mass. Other signs or symptoms of renal disease are rare, although renal failure has been described[129] and hypertension has also been reported. While it is reasonable to assume that cases detected clinically in early childhood are likely to be those detectable antenatally, it is not yet conclusively proven that, in the long-term, these cases carry a worse prognosis than those detected in adulthood. Therefore the prognosis of antenatally detected cases is so far unknown, although it is certain that oligohydramnios carries a very poor prognosis.[130]

Obstetric management If the liquor volume is decreased in the presence of APCKD, termination should be offered. In the presence of normal liquor volume the parents should be counselled that the fetus is suffering from a hereditary kidney disease and that one of the parents must also have the disease. The usual course of the disease should be discussed and termination considered as an option. When the diagnosis is discovered later in pregnancy normal obstetric management should be pursued.

Recurrence risk The condition is autosomal dominant, therefore the recurrence risk is 50%.

Dilatation of the urinary tract

Dilatation of the urinary tract usually results from distal obstruction but dilatation may occur without obstruction.[131-133] Sites of obstruction are at the pelvi-ureteric junction, the uretero-vesical junction and urethra. Obstruction may be complete, partial, unilateral or bilateral. Non-obstructive causes of urinary tract dilatation are vesico-ureteric reflux, neurological lesions, primary (non-refluxing, non-obstructive) megaureter and part of the megacystis-microcolon syndrome.

Whilst moderate to severe examples of urinary tract dilatation are immediately obvious to the ultrasonographer and pose few problems in interpretation, minor changes which nevertheless may have important consequences on prognosis continue to pose problems. To date the criteria developed for differentiating the normal from the dilated renal pelvis are not ideal. Minimal pyelectasis in the fetus is common and unlikely to be significant in every case (Fig. 19). In one study 59% of kidneys in fetuses between 24 and 33 weeks showed demonstrable amounts of fluid in the renal pelves; in 41% the diameter of the renal pelvis measured 1 to 2 mm, in 18% the measurement was 3 mm and over.[134] Although the pathogenesis remains unclear, it

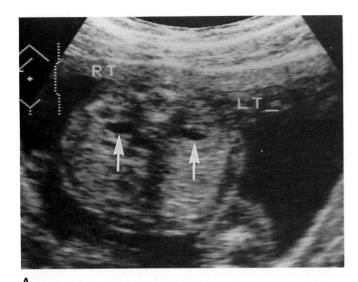

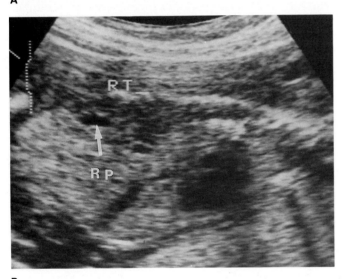

Fig. 19 Filled renal pelvis. A: Transverse section of a fetus at 19 weeks showing prominent (full) renal pelves (arrows). No calyceal dilatation is apparent. **B:** Longitudinal section showing a prominent (full) renal pelvis (RP) but no calyceal dilatation is apparent.

is possible that the fetal urinary tract is responding similarly to the maternal urinary tract to the circulating pregnancy hormones, maternal pelvicalyceal dilatation in pregnancy being well-recognised.

It is firmly established that fetal renal pelves measuring less than 5 mm in the antero-posterior diameter are within the normal range.[131] However, fetal renal pelves measuring greater than 10 mm in diameter[131,132] whilst usually pathological are not always so[135] and the significance of antero-posterior measurements between 5 and 10 mm is problematical.[131,133,135]

It should be noted that in all series to date these cut off points have been chosen on results obtained from groups of fetuses with widely varying gestational ages. A renal

pelvis measuring, for example, 6 mm is of more concern at 18 weeks than at 38 weeks. There is as yet no available data relating renal pelvic size to fetal age.

The ratio of the antero-posterior diameter of the pelvis to the antero-posterior diameter of the kidney has been suggested as another means of differentiating pathological pyelectasis from normal.[131] Hydronephrosis is considered present if this ratio is greater than 0.5.

Calyceal dilatation is much more significant.[87] This indicates hydronephrosis even when the pelvis/kidney ratio is less than 0.5 and always persists into the post-natal period. If rounded calyces are present with a renal pelvic antero-posterior measurement of 10 to 15 mm there is significant hydronephrosis which rarely regresses, often progresses and frequently requires surgical treatment.[136] Grignon et al[136] devised a classification of urinary tract dilatation according to the ultrasound appearances of the pelvicalyceal system and the renal pelvic size. Grades 2 and 3 were defined as renal pelvic measurements of 10 to 15 mm and greater than 15 mm respectively along with normal to slight dilatation of the calyces and resulted in 47% of infants with definite pathology. Grades 4 and 5 with renal pelves greater than 15 mm and moderate to severe dilatation of the calyces were always pathological.

When the pelvis appears prominent at the 18 to 20 week routine scan, there is often uncertainty as to whether or not a mild degree of calyceal dilatation is present (Fig. 20).

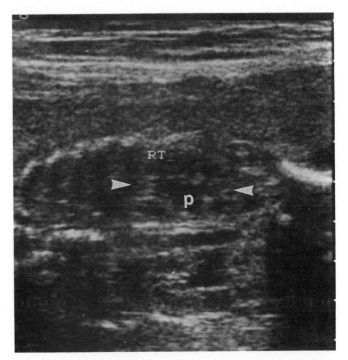

Fig. 20 Filled renal pelvis. A longitudinal section of the fetal kidney (arrowheads) is seen at 18 weeks gestation. A full renal pelvis (p) is seen but calyceal definition is such it is uncertain whether or not they are dilated. A repeat examination at 22 weeks confirmed prominent renal pelves without calyceal dilatation.

It is therefore useful to repeat the examination between 22 and 24 weeks, by which time considerable renal growth has occurred with deposition of fat. The improved renal images at this stage usually allow an accurate definition of calyceal dilatation. One possible source of error is compound upper pole calyces which may simulate calyceal dilatation (Fig. 21).

In order not to miss significant changes cases with more than 5 mm dilatation of the pelvis, as well as those with calyceal dilatation, should be followed up post-natally.

Dilatation of the ureter is always pathological. Gross dilatation of the fetal bladder is easily recognised but less gross degrees are not as easily diagnosed. The fetal bladder fills and empties over the course of an hour[22] so variations in size are normal. Charts of bladder size related to menstrual age have not been developed. In doubtful cases prolonged observation and repeated scanning over 4 to 6 hours to see if the bladder changes in size or empties are useful. Hypertrophy of the bladder wall may also aid diag-

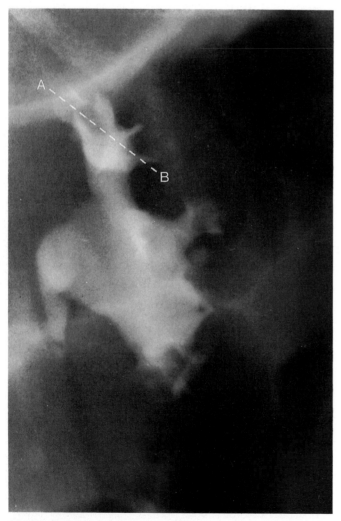

Fig. 21 Compound cystic calyces (IVU). Intravenous urogram showing compound cystic calyces. Ultrasound scanning in the plane A–B results in apparent calyceal dilatation.

nosis, it being pathologically thickened if greater than 2 mm.[96]

Early post-natal diagnosis of urinary tract obstruction or reflux is seldom possible because the clinical signs of an abdominal mass, haematuria or recurrent urinary tract infections (UTIs) are often symptomless until irreversible renal damage has occurred. The timing of surgical correction is thought to be important in reducing chronic renal insufficiency as the best results are achieved in infants operated on in the first year of life.[137] Therefore when pathological dilatation is diagnosed or suspected prenatally, post-natal follow up is essential. Except in severe cases, this is best performed at 5 to 7 days post-partum to avoid the false negative finding of an empty renal pelvis caused by the dehydration that is common in the first 48 to 72 hours after birth.[24,138] Further assessment at 4 to 6 weeks is important if the neonatal scan is negative as it takes that length of time before urine production in the infant has risen back to the levels of a term fetus. A full range of urinary tract investigations may be needed to assess the problems as ultrasound alone may lead to incomplete diagnosis.[139]

A team approach for the care of those mothers with antenatally diagnosed fetal urinary tract abnormalities is best,[140] the team ideally consisting of the ultrasonographer, obstetrician, neonatologist and paediatric nephrologist. This will ensure that parents are correctly and adequately counselled and that the investigations in the post-natal period are planned in advance.

There is a definite association between renal tract dilatation and chromosomal abnormalities. Of 72 cases of obstructive uropathy reported in the Fetal Surgery Registry 1986[100] 8% had karyotypic abnormalities. Nicolaides et al[141] reports an incidence of 24% abnormal karyotypes in a series of 38 cases of obstructive uropathy. However, in the majority of these cases, many of the other multisystem abnormalities which are part of the expression of the abnormal gene are detectable on ultrasound examination, particularly as more subtle markers of chromosomal abnormality can be recognised and confirmed by a rapid karyotyping procedure. The situation in isolated hydronephrosis and, particularly, in mild renal pelvic dilatation is less clear. Nicolaides[142] reports an incidence of 3% abnormal karyotypes in these cases. In our series of 249 cases, where there was more than one structural abnormality an incidence of 3% karyotypic abnormalities was identified.

Thus whilst problems in the interpretation of urinary tract dilatation remain, there seems little doubt that prenatal diagnosis and subsequent follow up improves the management of children with renal tract abnormalities.[9,138,143]

Pelvi-ureteric junction obstruction

Pelvi-ureteric junction obstruction is the most common

cause of neonatal hydronephrosis.[98] It is a stenosis at the junction of the renal pelvis and ureter. Unilateral obstruction is common,[136] more frequently affecting the left side.[144] The condition is bilateral in about 30% of cases, the degree of obstruction usually being different on the two sides. Thinning of the renal parenchyma and kidney enlargement are unusual in the fetus and are signs of severe obstruction.[145] Irreversible parenchymal damage is also unusual as is reduction in or absence of amniotic fluid. Occasionally polyhydramnios is reported, presumably the result of extrinsic compression of the retroperitoneal portion of the duodenum by an enlarged renal pelvis.[146]

Aetiology and incidence The true incidence is unknown. There is an increased frequency in males with a sex ratio of 5:1.[147] The obstruction seems in the majority of cases to be a functional one as the pelvi-ureteric junction is anatomically patent, the abnormality being in the initiation or propagation of the peristaltic activity in the ureter that in the normal results in boluses of urine being passed from the pelvis down the ureter. Histologically the ureter shows signs of chronic inflammation with disruption and disorganisation of the collagen fibres and muscle in the wall. Abnormality of the circular but not the longitudinal layers of muscle has been demonstrated in approximately 70% of cases.[148] Anatomical causes found in a minority of cases are fibrous adhesions, bands, kinks, ureteral valves, aberrant lower pole vessels, abnormal ureteral insertion and odd shapes of the pelvi-ureteric outlet.[149]

Diagnosis Diagnosis depends on the findings of a dilated renal pelvis with or without calyceal dilatation. The criteria for the diagnosis of pathological dilatation have already been discussed. Harrison et al[13] have suggested a semiquantative estimate, mild dilatation showing enlarged renal pelves branching infundibula and calyces; severe dilatation being characterised by a large unilocular fluid collection. We have found a classification of hydronephrosis into mild, moderate and severe, more helpful, the appearances fitting fairly closely to Grignon's gradings.[132] Grade 2 approximates to our mild cases except that we would classify renal dilatation as being 5 mm or greater (Fig. 22). Grades 3 and 4 are equivalent to moderate hydronephrosis (Figs 23 and 24) and grade 5 to severe (Fig. 25).

The rest of the renal tract must be examined carefully particularly looking for evidence of peripheral cortical dysplasia and oligohydramnios. The latter is not usually a feature of this condition and implies a second disease process, (e.g. IUGR) or a misdiagnosis, (e.g. bilateral multicystic dysplastic kidney).[145]

Transient hydronephrosis in utero has occasionally been

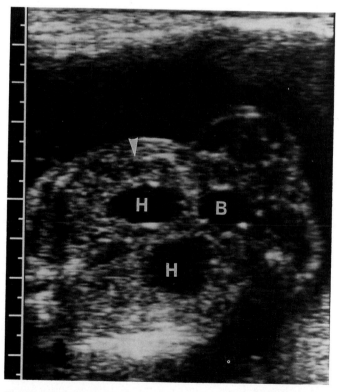

Fig. 22 Mild bilateral hydronephrosis. Oblique scan showing normal bladder (B) and two dilated renal pelves (H) with normal renal tissue (arrow) and no calyceal dilatation. This was a case of pelvi-ureteric junction obstruction.

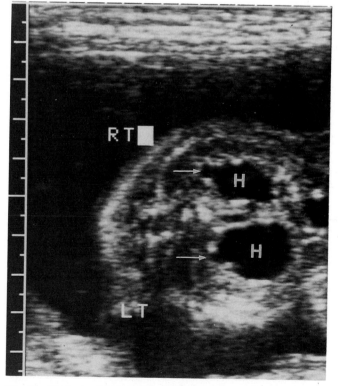

Fig. 23 Moderate bilateral hydronephrosis. Another case of pelvi-ureteric junction obstruction with dilated renal pelves (H) and mild calyceal dilatation (arrows).

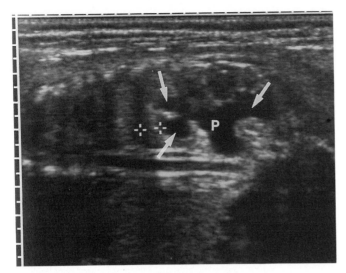

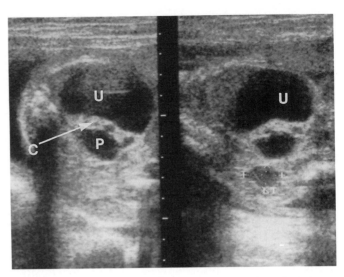

Fig. 24 Moderate bilateral hydronephrosis. This longitudinal scan of a hydronephrotic kidney shows an enlarged renal pelvis (P) and moderately dilated and rounded renal calyces (arrows). There is normal parenchymal thickness and reflectivity.

Fig. 26 Hydronephrosis with urinoma. Oblique sections displaying a hydronephrotic kidney with an enlarged pelvis (P) dysplastic cortex (C) and a retroperitoneal urinoma (U) following spontaneous decompression of pelvi-ureteric junction obstruction.

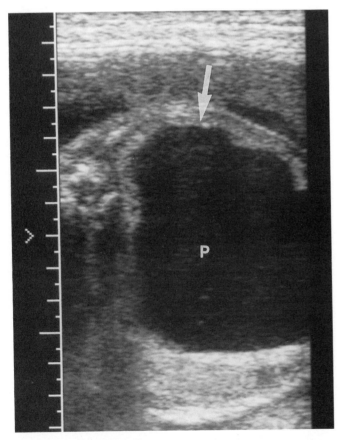

Fig. 25 Severe hydronephrosis. There is massive enlargement of the renal pelvis (P) in this case of unilateral pelvi-ureteric junction obstruction in a Down's syndrome fetus. The calyceal shape is lost and the parenchyma is thin (arrow).

noted; [28,133] its significance is unclear but serial scans are necessary to pick up changes in the condition. If dilatation is identified on only one occasion and is mild, pathology is extremely unlikely. This form of transient dilatation may be due to the state of maternal hydration but this has not been proven.[134] If the dilatation occurs on more than one occasion, post-natal follow up is advised.

The time of onset of the ultrasonic signs of this condition appears to be variable. A significant number of cases have been reported as first recognisable later than 24 weeks,[131] but this is not our experience, nearly all being apparent at the routine mid-trimester scan.

In severe pelvi-ureteric junction obstruction calyceal rupture may occur resulting in only minimal dilatation of the pelvicalyceal system but a large perinephric urinoma (Fig. 26).

Differential diagnosis The main differential diagnosis is multicystic dysplastic kidney.[79] In hydronephrosis the reniform shape is usually present and renal parenchyma is present peripherally. The 'cysts' of calyceal dilatation are orderly and aligned around and communicate with the renal pelvis (Figs 27 and 28). In addition, bilateral reflux may mimic true obstruction and be impossible to distinguish, although in many cases hydroureter will be seen in this condition.

Associated abnormalities The incidence of other renal tract abnormalities, (vesico-ureteric reflux, obstructive mega-ureter and contralateral abnormalities such as multicystic dysplastic kidney) is approximately 27%.[150] Associated extrarenal abnormalities occur in about 19% of

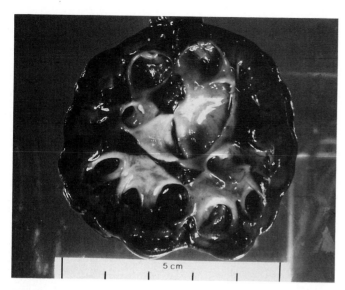

Fig. 27 Moderate hydronephrosis. The dilated calyces are seen to be enlarged in an orderly fashion around the pelvis. (With grateful thanks to Dr Jane Zuccollo, Queens Medical Centre, Nottingham.)

cases.[98] Hirschsprung's disease, cardiovascular abnormalities, neural tube defects, oesophageal atresias and imperforate anus being common. Chromosomal abnormalities also occur.[70]

Prognosis This is generally good for isolated unilateral lesions, even when the degree of dilatation is considerable.[151] Even in bilateral disease, the prognosis appears favourable; in one report following surgical correction of such lesions within 6 months of age there were no postoperative deaths and renal function was generally good.[152]

Obstetric management In unilateral pelvi-ureteric junction obstruction obstetric management should be normal

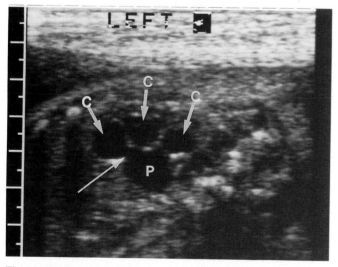

Fig. 28 Moderate hydronephrosis. Longitudinal scan of moderate hydronephrosis. The 'cystic structures' (C) are arranged around, and communicate with (long arrow) the dilated renal pelvis (P).

providing the abnormality appears isolated and the other kidney is normal. In the case of a very large hydronephrosis the pelvis may require decompression antenatally[153] and if polyhydramnios results[146] this may need careful management. There are no data to suggest that early delivery for surgical correction improves outcome.

In bilateral pelvi-ureteric junction obstruction the management depends on the severity of the abnormality and the gestational age. The severity is difficult to quantify. The degree of renal damage is approximately proportional to the severity of the dilatation. However, this is not invariable[154] and hydronephrosis may not be present in a fetus with chronic urinary tract obstruction.[155] Assessment of amniotic fluid volume has been suggested as a helpful guide to prognosis[57] but again is not entirely reliable as polyuria rather than oliguria may occur in failing renal function.[100] As previously discussed peripheral cortical dysplasia poses difficulty in diagnosis.

The best method available to date of assessing renal function is chemical analysis of fetal urine taken from each renal pelvis. Sodium, chloride, urea and creatinine levels have been used to evaluate renal function, the most useful so far being urinary sodium.[97] If the assessment suggests a poor prognosis (urinary sodium greater than 100 mmol/l at 18 weeks) termination must be considered.

In the absence of poor prognostic signs, an expectant management should be pursued. Serial scans are required as occasionally in the third trimester the dilatation may progress markedly (presumably as fetal urinary output increases) and therefore the planned post-natal management may need to be modified.

Prenatal urinary diversion procedures have been developed and may be indicated in cases of bilateral pelvi-ureteric junction obstruction. In the case of pelvi-ureteric junction obstruction the results do not support in utero surgery and such invasive procedures are not without mortality and morbidity. Severe, potentially life-threatening chorioamnionitis, has been reported after diagnostic or therapeutic fetal bladder catheterisation.[145] Until techniques improve management should be expectant.

Recurrence risk The condition is usually sporadic and therefore the recurrence risk is low. However both familial cases[156] and dominant inheritance[157] have been reported.

Ureterovesical junction obstruction

Obstruction at this level has been considered as uncommon for many years[98] being reported in only 8% of cases of urinary tract obstruction. However, a more recent study suggests it accounts for 23% of cases and is the second most common cause of hydronephrosis.[158]

Aetiology and incidence Distal obstruction of the ureter is primarily functional resulting from a narrow segment of the ureter at the lower end which does not transmit the normal peristaltic waves.[159] Less commonly ureteral atresia

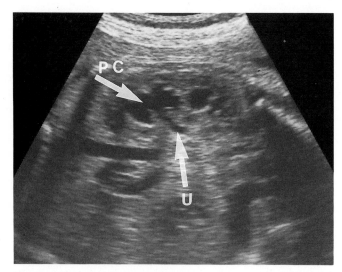

Fig. 29 Uretero-vesical junction obstruction. In this duplex kidney the pelvicalyceal system (PC) of the upper moiety is dilated and the upper part of the dilated ureter (U) can be seen.

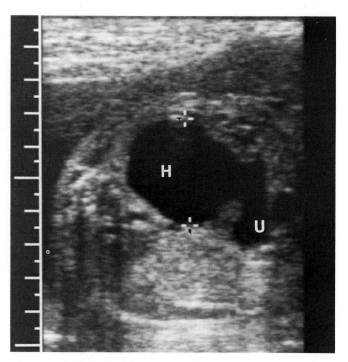

Fig. 31 Dilated ureter. A dilated obstructed ureter (U) can be seen pursuing a serpiginous course, and can be traced back to the hydronephrotic renal pelvis (H).

is responsible. In duplex anomalies obstruction is common, affecting the upper pole moiety, with an ectopic ureterocele (Figs 29 and 30).[160] The incidence is unknown.

Diagnosis The normal fetal ureter is too small to define antenatally with ultrasound and therefore, if it is imaged it is dilated, being seen as an echo-free intra-abdominal tubular structure[161] that can be traced back to the renal pelvis (Fig. 31). If obstruction is the cause, the ureter lengthens and so is more serpiginous than in primary mega-ureter when the course is much straighter. The bladder should be normal in size and the wall not hypertrophic – otherwise urethral outflow obstruction must be considered. In the majority of cases of obstruction, a degree of hydronephrosis is seen.

Associated abnormalities Duplex systems are a common association. Their diagnosis depends on recognition of asymmetrical hydronephrosis between the dilated and non-dilated moieties.[162] Also in this abnormality there is often an element of dysplasia.[160] Other associations are with horseshoe and ectopic kidneys.

Differential diagnosis Uretero-vesical obstruction is easily confused with other causes of mega-ureter and differentiation antenatally is often impossible, though, in the presence of a duplex system, ectopic or horseshoe kidney, obstruction is most likely.

Prognosis In general the prognosis is good provided the condition is isolated.

Obstetric management Normal management should be pursued, with post-natal assessment and follow up planned.

Other causes of mega-ureter

Primary refluxing ureter This is due to an abnormality of the normal anti-reflux mechanisms at the level of the uretero-vesical junction (Fig. 32). This commonly results in hydronephrosis and peripheral cortical dysplasia may occur. The hydronephrosis is usually mild and non-progressive (Fig. 33) but can be severe.[133] Amniotic fluid should be present in normal volumes.[94]

Some investigators have reported spontaneous resolution of apparently significant fetal hydronephrosis;[94] although such cases may represent spontaneous resolution of

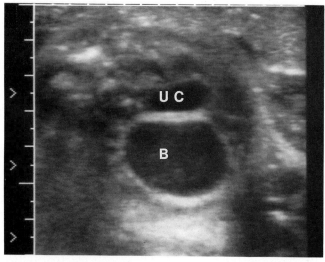

Fig. 30 Uretero-vesical junction obstruction. A ureterocele (UC) is seen adjacent to the bladder (B).

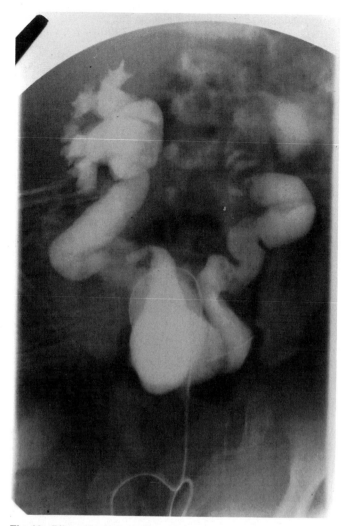

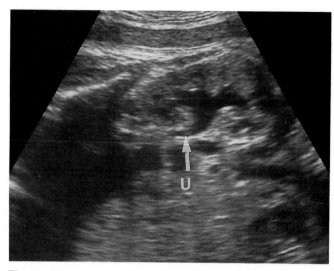

Fig. 33   Primary reflux. The hydronephrosis is commonly mild. Here slightly dilated calyces can be seen along with the upper end of the dilated ureter (U).

there are high rates of urine formation such as in diabetes insipidus or infection and in ureters that remain widened after spontaneous cessation of vesico-ureteric reflux.

Bladder outflow obstruction

The most severe degree of obstructive uropathy is seen with obstruction at urethral level.[164] Bladder outflow obstruction may be partial or complete, the usual cause being posterior urethral valves which have been described as the second most common cause of hydronephrosis (19%). [98] However, more recent data, based on prenatal ultrasound examination, suggest that the urethra is a less

Fig. 32   Bilateral primary reflux. Micturating cystogram showing bilateral ureteric reflux resulting in bilateral hydronephrosis and hydroureter.

obstruction, temporary uretero-vesical reflux would seem a more likely cause. Spontaneous neonatal resolution of congenital reflux may also occur. The degree of reflux decreases and may disappear in more than 50% of affected children.[163] Some boys with reflux have a large, sacculated posterior urethra suggesting that reflux could be secondary to transient obstruction which has been overcome.

Secondary refluxing ureter   This occurs when there is bladder neck obstruction or a neuropathic bladder (Fig. 34). In the former the thick-walled bladder is obvious. A neuropathic bladder may be the result of the vertebro-spinal abnormality of the VACTERL association. This condition should be borne in mind as many of the abnormalities (such as tracheo-oesophageal fistula) are subtle or unlikely to be diagnosed by ultrasound. A dilated ureter may be the only manifestation.

Secondary non-refluxing ureter   Secondary non-refluxing non-obstructive ureteric dilatation is found where

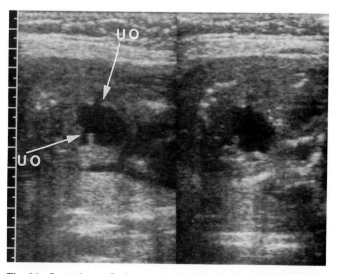

Fig. 34   Secondary refluxing ureter. In this case of the VACTERL association, the bladder was neuropathic due to a sacral spinal abnormality. The wide open ureteric orifices (UO) are demonstrated in the bladder.

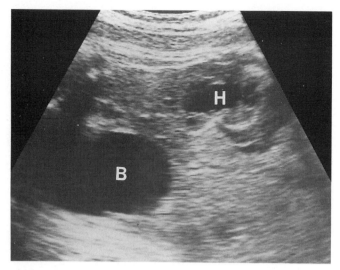

Fig. 35 Posterior urethral valves. The bladder (B) is dilated and there is hydronephrosis (H).

common site of fetal urinary obstruction, accounting for 10% of cases.[158] Posterior urethral valves occur exclusively in males. Urethral obstruction occurring in females is complete, due to urethral atresia or major cloacal abnormalities.

Posterior urethral valves A membranous structure in the posterior urethra constitutes the 'valve'. A classification based on gross anatomical characteristics has been proposed.[165] There are three types, of which types 1 and 3 are clinically significant. In type 1 the valves are folds

that insert into the lateral walls of the urethra. Type 3 valves consist of a diaphragm-like structure with only a small perforation.

Aetiology and incidence The exact incidence is unknown. Type 1 is thought to result from an exaggerated development of persisting urethral/vaginal folds with an abnormal insertion of the distal ends of the Wolffian ducts. Type 3 develops because of abnormal persistence and poor canalisation of the urogenital membrane.

Diagnosis The major features of urethral obstruction by urethral valves are dilatation of the fetal urinary bladder and proximal urethra (Fig. 35) with thickening of the bladder wall (Fig. 36).[166] The urinary bladder fills the true pelvis and frequently also the false pelvis and abdomen and does not empty. A dilated posterior urethra can be visualised as a focal outpouching of the urinary bladder extending towards the perineum. The bladder wall is considered hypertrophied if the wall is thick enough to be measured (Fig. 37).[166] The ureters are usually also dilated

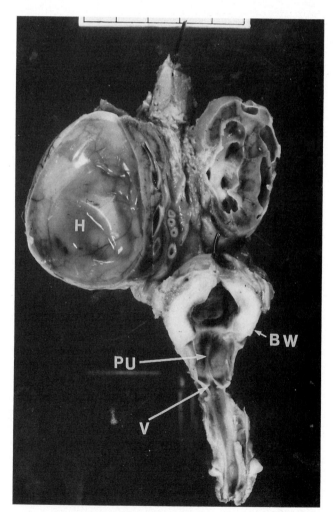

Fig. 37 Posterior urethral valves. Note the severe hydronephrosis (H), the thick bladder wall (BW), the dilated posterior urethra (PU) and the valves (V). (With grateful thanks to Dr Jane Zuccollo, Queens Medical Centre, Nottingham.)

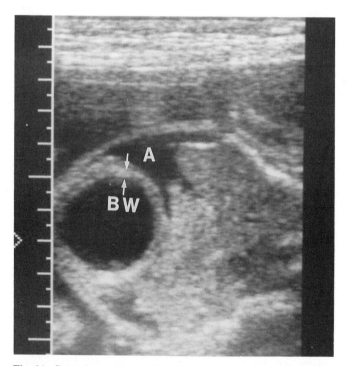

Fig. 36 Posterior urethral valves. Note the thick wall of the bladder (BW). There has been spontaneous decompression resulting in urinary ascites (A).

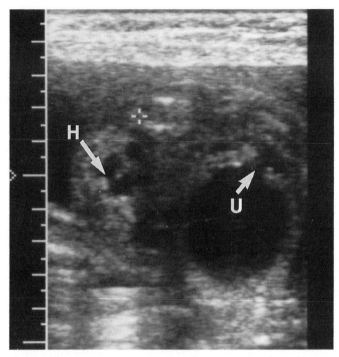

Fig. 38 Posterior urethral valves. The dilated ureter (U) can be seen. There is moderate hydronephrosis (H).

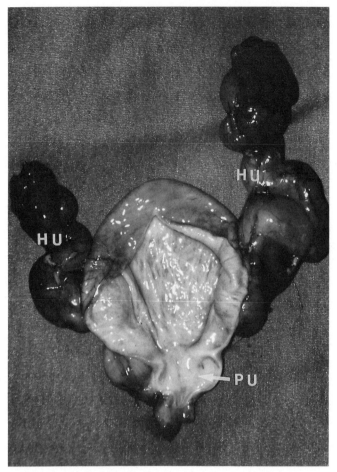

Fig. 39 Posterior urethral valves. There is marked bilateral hydroureter (HU), and a dilated posterior urethra (PU). (With grateful thanks to Dr Jane Zuccollo, Queens Medical Centre, Nottingham.)

and hydronephrosis of variable degrees may be present (Figs 38 and 39), but lack of upper tract dilatation does not exclude urethral valves.[155] Minor degrees of obstruction may not produce much dilatation while severe obstruction may result in dysplasia and therefore diminished urine output.

The urinary tract may be decompressed by bladder rupture and the problem may present as fetal ascites (Fig. 40) or as perinephric urinoma resulting from rupture of the calyces.[155] Examination of the urinary tract reveals the underlying cause. Renal dysplasia gives increased cortical reflectivity and cortical cysts but, as previously discussed, the ultrasound appearance of the kidneys does not correlate well either with the presence of dysplasia or its degree.

The volume of liquor should be noted as oligohydramnios may occur and is related to the severity and duration of the obstruction. Severe oligohydramnios is a poor prognostic sign and, conversely, normal amniotic fluid carries a good prognosis.[1,167]

Differential diagnosis Other obstructive uropathies (namely pelvi-ureteric junction obstruction or uretero-vesical junction obstruction and primary mega-ureter) must be considered, the bladder wall thickening being the distinguishing feature. Massive vesico-ureteric reflux may be difficult to differentiate.[168] Megacystis-microcolon syndrome may be mistaken for posterior urethral valves. In this condition there is usually polyhydramnios and a dilated stomach.

Associated abnormalities Posterior urethral valves are as-

sociated with duplication of the urethra, megalo-urethra, cryptorchidism and hypospadias. Abnormalities outside the urinary tract are tracheo-oesophageal fistula, total anomalous pulmonary venous drainage, mitral stenosis, skeletal abnormalities and imperforate anus.[97,98] Chromosomal abnormalities, including trisomy 13 and 18, have been reported.[141]

Prune belly syndrome, in which there is a hypotonic abdominal wall, a large hypotonic bladder with dilated ureters and cryptorchidism, was originally considered as a separate specific entity[169] but is now considered to be secondary to fetal abdominal distension of various causes, one of the most common being urethral obstruction. This accounts for its male predominance.[170] The condition spans a wide range of severity from death due to pulmonary hypoplasia in the neonatal period, or renal insufficiency in infancy to long-term survival though extensive cosmetic surgery may be required. A case of bladder outflow obstruction where termination was not wanted, apparently resolved (at least ultrasonically) during the remainder of the pregnancy. The liquor volume was slightly reduced.

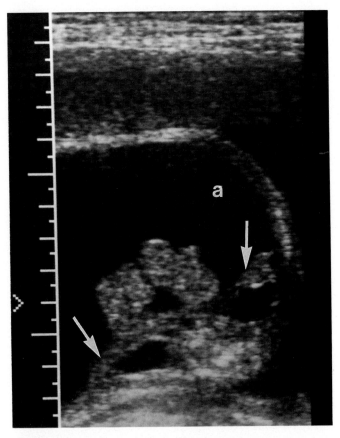

Fig. 40 Posterior urethral valves. The fetal kidneys (arrows) are hydronephrotic. Urinary ascites (a) is present due to rupture of the bladder.

The neonate had prune belly syndrome and died of renal failure within the first few months.

Prognosis Neonates with urethral obstruction have a high mortality, (up to 50%).[171,172] The incidence of chronic renal failure in infants diagnosed in the first 3 months of life is 39%.[173] Most of the data regarding the prognosis, particularly in the long-term, are based on disease diagnosed post-natally and this does not necessarily represent the same spectrum as disease diagnosed antenatally. In general, the prognosis seems much worse when diagnosed in utero. In the majority of survivors, renal function improves following surgery, but this is not always the case. The development of renal failure may be delayed for 9 to 10 years.[174]

Obstetric management When the diagnosis of urethral valves is made, management depends on the presence of other serious abnormality, the gestational age at diagnosis, the parents wishes and renal function. A careful search for other abnormalities must be made and a rapid karyotyping procedure performed. This may prove difficult with oligohydramnios though, as in cases of suspected renal agenesis, warm saline instilled into the intra-uterine cavity may help. In any pregnancy, even in a case of isolated

posterior urethral valves, the prognosis of the condition is such that termination seems a reasonable option if the parents wish it.

Once other abnormalities are excluded, if the parents want to continue with the pregnancy, assessment of the presence of dysplasia and of renal function should be made by careful examination of the kidneys, assessment of amniotic fluid volume and fetal urine aspiration, if possible from both kidneys. One poor prognostic sign is oligohydramnios. Approximately 95% of fetuses with severely reduced liquor will not survive the neonatal period.[166] Other poor prognostic signs are dysplasia of the kidneys present in a high percentage of cases[175] and particularly high urinary sodium, as previously discussed in pelvi-ureteric junction obstruction.

If the prognostic criteria are good, it must still be remembered that these, as yet, cannot be confidently extrapolated from the prenatal period to the long-term outlook. Caution must be exercised when counselling parents. Follow up management of the baby should be planned ahead, probably with delivery in a paediatric surgical centre. If the prognosis is poor, options are termination of pregnancy in the early weeks and non-interventional management later on.

In experiments in fetal lambs, timely decompression of obstructive uropathy has been shown to prevent renal dysplasia[21] and this has led to interest in in utero decompression of the urinary tract with variable success.[13,95,176] Nackayama et al[177] compared a group of neonates in whom posterior valves were diagnosed at birth and active management given, with a similar group treated in utero. There was a significant difference in mortality, 45% in the neonatally diagnosed group compared to 22.8% in the group treated in utero. These data are encouraging but long-term data are awaited and great care must go into the selection of cases to decide suitability for in utero surgery which, as previously discussed, carries a high risk.

Recurrence risks The condition is usually sporadic but familial cases have been reported.[178]

Urethral atresia and cloacal abnormalities In these conditions the bladder outflow obstruction is complete.

Diagnosis Urethral atresia is characterised by anhydramnios. The fetal abdomen is completely filled and distended by an enormous symmetrical cystic structure and the chest circumference is extremely small in relation to the abdominal circumference (Fig. 41). Because of the severity of the oligohydramnios and the massive bladder dilatation, identification of other abnormalities is difficult if not impossible.

If the atresia is due to a persistent cloaca, the cystic structure may be more complex with two or three 'loculations' and some solid content on their posterior wall (Fig. 42). Spontaneous decompression of the urinary tract results in ascites (Fig. 43).

Prognosis This is a lethal condition.

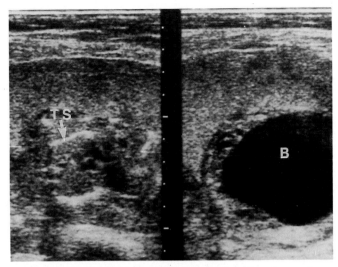

Fig. 41 Urethral atresia. There is anhydramnios. Note the massive centrally placed cystic structure, the completely obstructed bladder (B). The transverse section of the thorax (TS) is very small.

Obstetric management If diagnosed in the early part of pregnancy, termination should be offered.

Megacystis-microcolon-intestinal hypoperistalsis syndrome

This syndrome consists of the association of a distended and unobstructed bladder with a dilated small bowel and distal microcolon. Motility of the stomach and intestine is

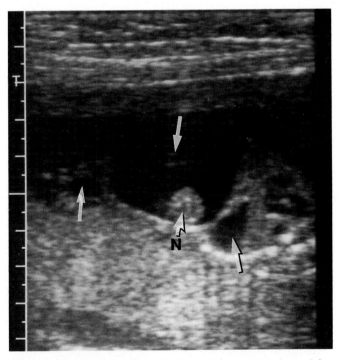

Fig. 42 Cloacal atresia. There are three cystic structures (arrows) in the lower abdomen in this fetus, one containing a solid nodule (N) of embryonic tissue.

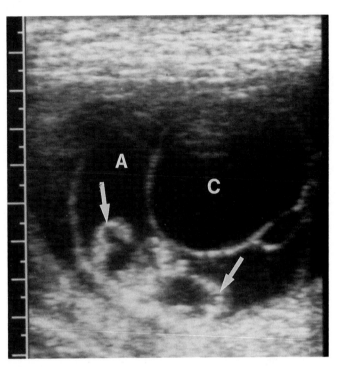

Fig. 43 Cloacal atresia. The kidneys (arrows) are hydronephrotic with highly reflective renal parenchyma indicating dysplasia. (C) indicates the massively dilated persistent cloaca. There is urinary ascites (A).

impaired, leading to malnutrition. The small bowel is short and fixed. The condition is rare, predominantly affecting females.[179,180]

Diagnosis Antenatal visualisation of this syndrome has been reported.[181,182] The condition should be suspected in the presence of a distended bladder with a normal or increased amount of amniotic fluid in a female fetus when no other lower body abnormality can be seen.

Prognosis The condition is usually lethal.

Obstetric management It is unlikely that the diagnosis could be made with certainty antenatally and therefore management must be expectant.

Recurrence risk Whilst usually sporadic, some familial cases have been reported.[179]

Bladder extrophy and extrophy of the cloaca

Bladder extrophy occurs when midline closure of the anterior abdominal wall is incomplete. The defect involves not only the abdomen but also the anterior wall of the urinary bladder. The posterior wall of the bladder is therefore exposed, along with the trigone and ureteric orifices and urine dribbles intermittently from the everted bladder. Bladder extrophy may be isolated or form part of a major maldevelopment: extrophy of the cloaca. In this there may be complete breakdown of the cloacal membrane with extrophy of a persistent cloaca, failure of fusion of the genital tubercles and pubic rami and, often, exomphalos.[183]

Incidence and aetiology Bladder extrophy results from failure of mesenchymal cells to migrate between the ectoderm of the abdomen and cloaca during the fourth week of development.[25] As a result no muscle or connective tissue form in the anterior abdominal wall over the urinary bladder. Later the thin epidermis and the anterior wall of the bladder rupture exposing the mucus membrane of the bladder. Defective development of the mesenchymal cells prior to the fourth week results in the more extensive cloacal extrophy.

Bladder extrophy is a rare condition occurring once in 10 000 to 50 000 births[25] and it is more common in males. Most cases of this condition are sporadic but familial cases have been reported.[184] Extrophy of the cloaca has an incidence of one in 200 000 live births without a sex preponderance.[185] It is sporadic.

Diagnosis Bladder extrophy should be suspected when a solid[186] or a semisolid mass[151] is seen anteriorly in the abdomen or protruding from the lower anterior abdominal wall. No normal bladder is seen even on repeated scans despite the presence of normal amniotic fluid. The penis cannot be identified though the scrotum may be visible.

In cloacal extrophy the most obvious findings may be that of the associated problems, mainly the vertebral abnormalities or the exomphalos. In one case, a severe case examined at 17 weeks gestation, there was a large exomphalos; below this no abdominal wall could be identified. No bladder was seen. Bilateral hydronephrosis was present with moderately reduced liquor. Kyphoscoliosis of the lumbar spine was obvious. In another case of lesser degree, a small exomphalos was present and below this a semisolid mass protruded from the anterior abdominal wall. Again no bladder was present. The liquor was normal. In this case separation of the pubic rami was seen at pathological examination.

Differential diagnosis Other conditions which appear similar to cloacal extrophy are the caudal regression syndrome and body stalk abnormality. In the former, limb abnormalities are likely to be present. In the latter, the short umbilical cord ensures that the anterior part of the fetus touches the placenta.

Associated abnormalities These are rare in bladder extrophy but common in cloacal extrophy,[187] of which the majority of associated problems are a direct result of the underlying maldevelopment process. These are largely skeletal defects which are present in 72% of cases, the majority being incomplete development of the lumbosacral vertebral column, leading to herniation of a grossly dilated central canal of the spinal cord and separation of the pubic bones.[188] Exomphalos, also resulting directly from the maldevelopment, occurs in the majority of cases. Renal abnormalities are common. Some of these, such as urethral tract dilatation, may be secondary to obstruction at the uretero-vesical junction or neurological, due to the spinal cord abnormalities. Renal agenesis and multicystic kidneys

have also been reported. Cardiovascular problems may occur.[187] It should be remembered that, as both these conditions are essentially part of a spectrum, when an apparently isolated bladder extrophy is seen, great care must be taken to exclude other abnormalities, particularly of the sacral spine, before counselling parents.

Prognosis The problems of bladder extrophy are chiefly incontinence of urine and the abdominal wall defect, with maldevelopment of the genitalia. Primary bladder closure or urinary diversion and abdominal wall closure have been performed with reasonable success, although there may be recurrent problems of urinary tract infections, calculi formation and incontinence. Surgical correction of female genitalia is reasonably successful but male genital defects are difficult to correct so sex reassignment is practiced[162] with all its associated problems. Fertility is decreased. Morbidity is generally low and the majority of adults adjust to their problems.[189]

Cloacal extrophy has a mortality rate of 55%.[190] Surgical correction requires a series of operations with variable results. Morbidity in the survivors is very high.

Obstetric management If bladder extrophy is diagnosed in early pregnancy termination should be offered. In late pregnancy normal obstetric management should be pursued. Care must be taken with the exposed bladder mucosa after delivery as it is extremely friable so it should be covered with a non-adherent dressing.[162] Mode or place of delivery seems to have no bearing on outcome.

If cloacal extrophy is diagnosed early in pregnancy termination should be offered. If the problem is encountered later in pregnancy the degree of the abnormality should be assessed as carefully as possible with a view to non-interventional management.

Recurrence risk The majority of cases are sporadic but as familial cases have been reported the risk of recurrence is given as 1%.[184] If the parent has bladder extrophy then the chance of an affected offspring is one in 70.[191]

Renal tumours

Renal tumours in the neonate, and therefore in the antenatal period, are extremely rare. The most common is the mesoblastic nephroma (fetal renal hamartoma) derived from secondary mesenchyme which has a limited capacity to differentiate. The cells are predominantly fibroblasts or intermediate between fibroblast and smooth muscle.[192]

Diagnosis If a solid unilateral mass is seen in the renal area and no normal renal outline can be identified on that side, mesoblastic nephroma should be considered.[193–195] Typically it stretches the kidney and careful imaging may show a rim of normal renal tissue surrounding the tumour. It must be remembered that ultrasound cannot give a histological diagnosis although mesoblastic nephroma is the most likely renal tumour in this age group. The earliest diagnosis has been made at 26 weeks.[193] Polyhydramnios is invariably present, the reason being unknown.[196]

Associated abnormalities 14% of cases are reported as being associated with other abnormalities, chiefly those of the gastrointestinal tract, hydrocephaly and other genitourinary problems.

Prognosis Intra-uterine growth retardation appears to be an associated feature.[196] Nephrectomy is almost always curative[197] though there are isolated reports of local recurrence and a case of malignant mesenchymal nephroma with pulmonary metastases in a 7-month-old child.[198,199]

Obstetric management As the outcome is generally good normal obstetric management may be pursued with careful monitoring and treatment for polyhydramnios.

Renal malposition and abnormalities of shape

Ectopic kidney

Congenital renal ectopia is characterised by an abnormally located kidney supplied by arteries in its immediate vicinity. The ectopic kidney may be located ipsilateral to its normal location (simple ectopia) or contralateral (crossed ectopia). In addition, examples of a simple ectopia with contralateral renal agenesis and crossed ectopia have been reported.[200,201]

Aetiology and incidence The most frequent type of renal ectopia is simple ectopia, found in one per 800 autopsies.[202] All the other types are extremely rare. The majority of all ectopic kidneys, whether simple or crossed, are located more caudally in the fetal abdomen than the normal kidney. The migration of the kidney from its point of origin in the renal pelvis to its usual site, which normally occurs during the second month of gestation, may become arrested at any point. The cause of this migratory inhibition is unknown. Conversely the ascending kidney in rare instances apparently overshoots and migrates into the thorax.[201]

Diagnosis A pelvic kidney has been diagnosed antenatally at 28 weeks.[203] An echo-poor mass was seen above the bladder. In addition on that side the kidney could not be visualised in the renal bed although the kidney on the other side appeared normal in every respect. Post-natally this proved to be a horseshoe kidney.

Considering the apparent commonness of this variant it is surprising it is not more extensively documented in prenatal ultrasound literature.

Differential diagnosis In general echo-poor masses in the pelvis seen on ultrasound represent an abnormality of the urinary tract or bowel, or in the female an ovarian cyst. Most of these can be ruled out by the presence of normal amniotic fluid volume, normality of the rest of the renal tract and the appearance of otherwise normal bowel, the important diagnostic feature being inability to see two kidneys in their correct position.

Associated abnormalities Some types of ectopia, particularly the crossed, are associated with a significant increase of frequency of associated congenital abnormalities of the genitourinary, skeletal and cardiovascular systems.[201]

Prognosis Ectopic kidney, especially a simple one, may be without clinical significance, being detected only at the time of post-mortem as an incidental finding. The clinical significance of ectopia has been reported most commonly with pelvic kidneys and the various forms of crossed ectopia. In addition to the associated abnormalities these are associated with recurrent urinary tract infections, pyelonephritis and renal calculi formation.[201]

Obstetric management Normal obstetric management should be pursued. Knowledge of the presence of an ectopic kidney may aid in prophylaxis against calculus formation and infection in later life.

Horseshoe kidney

Horseshoe kidney is a common congenital anomaly of the kidney. The fusion in 90% of cases involves the lower poles and prevents normal rotation of the kidneys which in turn requires the ureter to rise anterior to it and pass over the fused lower renal poles. The ultimate position of the fused kidneys tends to be lower than normal.[204]

Aetiology and incidence The anomaly results from the fusion of the left and right metanephric blastema during the second month prior to their cephalic migration. The cause is unclear. The frequency has been variously estimated to be from one in 350 to one in 1800.[204] There is a male preponderance.

Diagnosis Sherer et al[205] report the prenatal findings associated with a horseshoe kidney. At the normal level of scanning for kidneys, renal tissue is seen on both sides but, scanning more caudally, the renal tissue could be seen to be continuous across the abdomen. Considering its reported frequency horseshoe kidneys are rarely diagnosed, perhaps because the fused part lies lower than the usual level of scanning for kidneys and the upper poles seen in the usual place are taken to be the kidneys.

Associated abnormalities Horseshoe kidney occurs in a number of chromosome abnormalities, namely Turner's syndrome, trisomy 18 and the 18q syndrome. It is also found in the iris coloboma and anal atresia syndrome. The associated abnormalities are therefore the ones associated with these conditions including IUGR, microcephaly, face dysplasias, hemivertebrae and cardiac abnormalities.

Prognosis Generally the prognosis is good but urinary tract infection and renal calculi formation are common[206] and tumours including renal cell carcinoma, transitional cell carcinomas and Wilms' tumours may develop.[207,208] Another problem is that of pain related to compression of the isthmus of the fused kidneys by the vena cava and aorta accentuated by hypertension and associated with a sensation of fullness and nausea. Surgical procedures are commonly required to treat the complications.[204]

Obstetric management Normal obstetric management should be pursued.

Supernumerary kidney

This term describes a free accessory organ which is distinct, encapsulated and may be large or small and closely related to but not attached to the usual kidney. The majority are in fact smaller and lower than the ipsilateral normal kidney and located on the left side.[209–211] Approximately one third have a completely duplicated ureter but more commonly a bifid ureter is shared with the ipsilateral kidney.

Aetiology and incidence This is an extremely rare abnormality.

Diagnosis to date There is no reported diagnosis of a supernumerary kidney in utero, but the finding of another smaller echo-poor mass just below a kidney should be examined carefully for further typical renal appearances.

Prognosis Prognosis is good but secondary development of hydronephrosis and pyelonephritis are common.[209]

Associated abnormalities When the supernumerary kid-ney has been diagnosed in children multiple non-genitourinary and genitourinary malformations have been observed.[211,212]

Prognosis The presence of other abnormalities alters the prognosis but otherwise in the isolated supernumerary kidney this is good.

Obstetric management In isolated supernumerary kidney management should be normal. When other abnormalities coexist the management should be altered according to the prognosis conferred by the other abnormalities.

Conclusion

Many of the conditions which affect the urinary tract are not clinically obvious at birth. Delay in diagnosis and treatment has been shown to have a deleterious effect on outcome. The fetal urinary tract is very amenable to ultrasound diagnosis and investigation. While the diagnosis and definition of the degree of the disorder are sometimes difficult, much useful information can be gained by a combination of ultrasonic examination and fetal urine sampling, when appropriate. There is little doubt that antenatal ultrasound examination contributes greatly to the management of urinary tract abnormalities.

REFERENCES

1 Garrett W J, Grunwald G, Robinson D E. Prenatal diagnosis of fetal polycystic kidney by ultrasound. Aust NZ J Obstet Gynaecol 1970; 10: 7–9
2 Garrett W J, Kossoff G, Osborn R A. The diagnosis of fetal hydronephrosis, megaureter, and urethral obstruction by ultrasonic echography. Br J Obstet Gynaecol 1975; 82: 115–120
3 Bellinger M F, Cornstock C H, Grosso D, Zaino R. Fetal posterior urethral valves and renal dysplasia at 15 weeks gestational age. J Urol 1983; 129: 1238–1239
4 Diamond D A, Sanders R, Jeffs R D. Fetal hydronephrosis. Consideration regarding urologic intervention. J Urol 1984; 131: 1155–1159
5 Pachi A, Giancotti A, Torcia V, De Prosperi V, Maggi E. Meckel-Gruber syndrome: ultrasonographic diagnosis at 13 weeks gestational age in an at-risk case. Prenat Diagn 1989; 9: 187–190
6 Ceccherini I, Lituania M, Cordone M S, et al. Autosomal dominant polycystic kidney disease: prenatal diagnosis by DNA analysis and sonography at 14 weeks. Prenat Diagn 1989; 9: 751–758
7 Stiller R J, Pinto M, Heller C, Hobbins J C. Oligohydramnios associated with bilateral multicystic dysplastic kidneys: prenatal diagnosis at 15 weeks gestation. JCU 1988; 16: 436–439
8 Watson A R, Readett D, Nelson C S, Kapilar L, Mayell M J. Dilemmas associated with antenatally detected urinary tract abnormalities. Arch Dis Child 1988; 63: 719–722
9 Gunn T R, Mora J D, Pease P. Outcome after antenatal diagnosis of upper tract dilatation by ultrasonography. Arch Dis Child 1988; 63: 1240–1243
10 Livera L N, Brookfield D, Egginton J A, Hawnaur J M. Antenatal ultrasonography to detect fetal renal abnormalities: a prospective screening programme. BMJ 1989; 298: 1421–1423
11 Duval J M, Milon J, Coadou Y. Ultrasonographic anatomy and diagnosis of fetal uropathies affecting the upper urinary tract. I. Obstructive uropathies. Anat Clin 1985; 7: 301
12 Warkany J. The kidney. In: Congenital malformations. Chicago: Year Book Medical Publisher. 1972

13 Harrison M R, Golbus M S, Filly R A. Postpartum evaluation of fetal hydronephrosis: optimal timing for follow-up sonography. Radiology 1984; 152: 423–424
14 Turnock R R, Shawis R. Management of fetal urinary tract anomalies detected by prenatal diagnosis. Arch Dis Child 1984; 59: 962–965
15 Guaderer M W L, Jassan M N, Izant R J. Ultrasonographic antenatal diagnosis: will it change the spectrum of neonatal surgery? J Paed Surg 1984; 19: 404–407
16 Dubbins P A, Kurtz A B, Wapner R J, Goldberg B B. Renal agenesis: spectrum of in utero findings. JCU 1981; 9: 189–193
17 Kramer S A. Current status of fetal intervention for congenital hydronephrosis. J Urol 1983; 130: 641–646
18 Sanders R, Graham D. Twelve cases of hydronephrosis in utero diagnosed by ultrasonography. J Ultrasound Med 1982; 1: 341–348
19 Grupe W E. The dilemma of intrauterine diagnosis of congenital renal dilatation. Pediatr Clin North Am 1987; 34: 629–638
20 Mahoney B S, Filly R A, Callen P W, Hricak H, Golbus M S, Harrison M R. Fetal renal dysplasia: sonographic evaluation. Radiology 1984; 152(1): 143–146
21 Glick P L, Harrison M R, Adzick N S, Noall R A, Villa R L. Correction of congenital hydronephrosis in utero IV: in utero decompression reprevents renal dysplasia. J Pediatr Surg 1984; 19(6): 649–657
22 Wladimiroff J W, Campbell S. Fetal urine-production rates in normal and complicated pregnancy. Lancet 1974; i: 151–154
23 Wladimiroff J W. Effect of frusemide on fetal urine production. Br J Obstet Gynaecol 1975; 82: 221–224
24 Laing F C, Burke V D, Wing V W, Jeffrey R B, Hashimoto B. Postpartum evaluation of fetal hydronephrosis: optimal timing for follow-up sonography. Radiology 1984; 152: 423–424
25 Moore K L. The urogenital system. In: Moore K L. ed. The developing human: clinically orientated embryology. 4th edition. Philadelphia: WB Saunders. 1988: p 246–285
26 Parmley T H, Seeds A E. Fetal skin permeability to isotopic

water (THO) in early pregnancy. Am J Obstet Gynecol 1970; 108: 128–131

27 Fairweather D V I, Eskes T K A B. Amniotic fluid: research and clinical application. Amsterdam: Excerpta Medica. 1978

28 Baker M E, Rosenberg E R, Bowie J D, Gall S. Transient in utero hydronephrosis. J Ultrasound Med 1985; 4(1): 51–53

29 Patten R M, Mack L A, Wang K Y, Cyr D R. The fetal genitourinary tract. Radiol Clin North Am 1990; 28(1): 115–130

30 Lawson T L, Foley W D, Berland L L, Clark K E. Ultrasonic evaluation of fetal kidneys. Radiology 1981; 138: 153–156

31 Gonzales J, Gonzales M, Mary J Y. Size and weight of human kidney growth velocity during the last three months of pregnancy. Eur Urol 1980; 6: 37–44

32 Casey M L, Carr B R. Growth of the kidney in the normal human fetus during early gestation. Early Hum Dev 1982; 6: 11–14

33 Bertagnoli L, Lalatta F, Gallicchio R, et al. Quantitative characterisation of the growth of the fetal kidney. JCU 1983; 11(7): 349–356

34 Grannum P, Bracken M, Silverman R, Hobbins J C. Assessment of fetal kidney size in normal gestation by comparison of ratio of kidney circumference to abdominal circumference. Am J Obstet Gynecol 1980; 136: 249–254

35 Jeanty P, Dramaix-Wilmet M, Elkhazen N, Hubinont C, Van Regemorter N. Measurement of fetal kidney growth on ultrasound. Radiology 1982; 144: 159–162

36 Kurjak A, Kirkinen P, Latin V, Ivankovic D. Ultrasonic assessment of fetal kidney function in normal and complicated pregnancies. Am J Obstet Gynecol 1981; 141(3): 266–269

37 Carter C O, Evans K. Birth frequency of renal agenesis. J Med Genet 1981; 18: 158–159

38 Wilson R D, Baird P A. Renal agenesis in British Columbia. Am J Med Gen 1985; 21: 153–165

39 Hack M, Jaffe J, Blankstein J, Goodman R M, Brish M. Familial aggregation in bilateral renal agenesis. Clin Genet 1974; 5: 173–177

40 Schinzel A, Homberger C, Sigrist T. Renal agenesis in 2 male sibs born to consanguineous parents. J Med Genet 1978; 15: 314–316

41 Pashayan H M, Dowd T, Nigro A V. Bilateral absence of the kidneys and ureters: 3 cases reported in one family. J Med Genet 1977; 14: 205–209

42 Buchta R M, Viseskul C, Gilbert E F, Sarto G E, Opitz J M. Familial bilateral renal agenesis and hereditary renal dysplasia. Z Kinder 1973; 115: 111–129

43 Carter C O, Evans K, Pescia G. A family study of renal agenesis. J Med Genet 1979; 16: 176–188

44 Yunis E, Uribe J G. Full trisomy 7 and Potters syndrome. Hum Genet 1980; 84: 13–18

45 Ferrandez A, Schmid W. Potter syndrom (Nirenagenesie) mit chromosamaler aberation beim patient und mosaik beim vater. Helv Paediatr Acta 1971; 26: 210–214

46 Mikelsaar A V, Lazjuk C J, Lurie J W, et al. A 4p-syndrome. A case report. Humangenetik 1973; 19: 345–347

47 Prevs M, Kaplan P, Kirkham T H. The renal anomalies and oligohydramnios in the cerebro-oculofacio-mandibular syndrome. Am J Dis Child 1977; 131(1): 62–64

48 Halal F, Desgranges M F, Leduc B, Théoré G, Bettez P. Acro-renal-mandibular syndrome. Am J Med Gen 1980; 5(3): 277–284

49 Carmi R, Binshtock M, Abeliovich D, Bar-Ziv J. The brachio-oto-renal (BOR) syndrome: report of bilateral renal agenesis in three sibs. Am J Med Gen 1983; 14(4): 625–627

50 Biedel C W, Pagon R A, Zapata J O. Müllerian anomalies and renal agenesis: autosomal dominant urogenital dysplasia. J Pediatr 1984; 104(6): 861–864

51 Grix A Jr, Curry C, Hall B D. Patterns of multiple malformations in infants of diabetic mothers. Birth Defects 1982; 18: 55–77

52 Balfour R P, Laurence K M. Raised serum AFP levels and fetal renal agenesis. Lancet 1980; i: 317

53 Barss V A, Benacerraf B R, Frigoletto F D Jnr. Second trimester oligohydramnios, a predictor of poor fetal outcome. Obstet Gynecol 1984; 16(5): 608–610

54 Koontz W L, Seeds J W, Adams N J, Johnson A M, Cefalo R C.

55 Mercer L J, Brown L G. Fetal outcome with oligohydramnios in the 2nd trimester. Obstet Gynecol 1986; 67(6): 840–842

56 Raghavendra B N, Young B K, Greco M A, et al. Use of frusemide in pregnancies complicated by oligohydramnios. Radiology 1987; 165: 455–458

57 Hellstrom W J G, Kogan B A, Jeffrey Jnr R B, McAninch J W. The natural history of prenatal hydronephrosis with normal amounts of amniotic fluid. J Urol 1984; 132: 947–950

58 Chamberlain P F, Climming M, Torchia M G, Biehl D, Manning F A. Ovine fetal urine production following maternal intravenous furosemide administration. Am J Obstet Gynecol 1985; 151: 815–819

59 Beerman B, Groschinsky-Grind M, Fahraens L, Lindstrom B. Placental transfer of frusemide. Clin Pharmacol 1978; 24: 560–562

60 Grannum P. Fetal urinary tract anomalies. Diagnosis and management. Clin Diagn Ultrasound 1986; 19: 53–57

61 Potter E L. Bilateral absence of ureters and kidneys: report of 50 cases. Obstet Gynecol 1965; 25: 3–12

62 Curry C J R, Jensen K, Holland J, Miller L, Hall B D. The Potter sequence: a clinical analysis of 80 cases. Am J Med Gen 1984; 19: 679–702

63 Potter E. Facial characteristics of infants with bilateral renal agenesis. Am J Obstet Gynecol 1946; 41: 855–858

64 Thomas I, Smith D W. Oligohydramnios, cause of t̄e non renal features of Potter's syndrome, particularly pulmonary hypoplasia. J Pediatr 1974; 84: 811–814

65 Fantel A, Shepherd T. Potters syndrome – non renal features induced by oligohydramnios. Am J Dis Child 1975; 129: 1346–1347

66 Hislop A, Hey E, Reid L. The lungs in congenital bilateral renal agenesis and dysplasia. Arch Dis Child 1979; 54(1): 32–38

67 Roodhooft A M, Birnholz J C, Holmes L B. Familial nature of congenital absence and severe dysgenesis of both kidneys. N Engl J Med 1984; 310: 1341–1345

68 Ratten J, Beischer N A, Fortune D W. Obstetric complications when the fetus has Potter's syndrome. Am J Obstet Gynecol 1973; 115(7): 890–896

69 Emanuel B, Nachmar R, Aronson N, Weiss H. Congenital solitary kidney: a review of 74 cases. J Urol 1974; 111: 394–397

70 Nicolaides K H, Campbell S. Diagnosis and management of fetal malformations. In: Rodeck C. ed. Fetal diagnosis of genetic defects. London: Bailliere Tindall. 1987

71 Osathanondh V, Potter E L. Pathogenesis of polycystic kidneys. Type I due to hypoplasia of interstitial portions of collecting tubules. Arch Path 1964; 77: 466–473

72 Osathanondh V, Potter E L. Pathogenesis of polycystic kidneys. Type 2 due to inhibition of ampullary activity. Arch Pathol 1964; 77: 474–484

73 Osathanondh V, Potter E L. Pathogenesis of polycystic kidneys. Type 3 due to multiple abnormalities of development. Arch Pathol 1964; 77: 485–501

74 Osathanondh V, Potter E L. Pathogenesis of polycystic kidneys. Type 4 due to urethral obstruction. Arch Pathol 1964; 77: 502–512

75 Bernstein J. The morphogenesis of renal parenchymal maldevelopment. Pediatr Clin North Am 1971; 18(2): 395–407

76 Hartman D S, Davis C J. Multicystic dysplastic kidney. In: Hartman D S. ed. Renal cystic disease. Philadelphia: WB Saunders. 1989: p 127–145

77 Potter E L. Early ampullary inhibition. In: Normal and abnormal development of the kidney. Chicago: Year Book Medical. 1972

78 Felson B, Cussen L J. The hydronephrotic type of unilateral congenital multicystic disease of the kidney. Semin Roentgenol 1975; 10(2): 113–123

79 Sanders R C, Hartman D S. The sonographic distinction between neonatal multicystic kidney and hydronephrosis. Radiology 1984; 151: 621–625

80 Resnick J, Vernier R L. Cystic disease of the kidney in the newborn infant. Clin Perinatol 1981; 8(2): 375–390

81 Griscom N T, Vawter G F, Fellers F X. Pelvicofundibular atresia: the usual form of multicystic kidney: 44 unilateral and two bilateral cases. Semin Roentgenol 1975; 10(2): 125–131

82 Petersen R O. Congenital anomalies. In: Urologic pathology. Philadelphia: Lippincott. 1987

83 Hashimoto B E, Filly R A, Callen P W. Multicystic dysplastic kidney in utero: changing appearances. Radiology 1986; 159: 107–109

84 Sty J R, Babbitt D P, Oechler H W. Evaluating the multicystic kidney. Clin Nucl Med 1980; 5: 457–461

85 Rouse G A, Kaminsky C K, Saaty H P, Grube G L, Fritzsche P J. Current concepts in sonographic diagnosis of fetal disease. Radiographics 1988; 8(1): 119–132

86 Avni E F, Thoua Y, Lalmand B, Didier F, Droulle P, Schulman C C. Multicystic dysplastic kidney: evolving concepts. Natural history from in utero diagnosis and post-natal follow-up. J Urol 1987; 138: 1420–1424

87 Kleiner B, Filly R A, Mack L, Callen P W. Multicystic dysplastic kidney: observations of contralateral disease in the fetal population. Radiology 1986; 161: 27–29

88 Rizzo N, Gabrielli S, Pilu G, et al. Prenatal diagnosis and obstetrical management of multicystic dysplastic renal disease. Prenat Diagn 1987; 7: 109–118

89 D'Alton M, Romero R, Grannum P, De Palma L, Jeanty P, Hobbins J C. Antenatal diagnosis of renal anomalies with ultrasound. IV. Bilateral multicystic kidney disease. Am J Obstet Gynecol 1986; 154(3): 532–537

90 De Klerk D P, Marshall F F, Jeffs R D. Multicystic dysplastic kidneys. J Urol 1977; 118: 306–308

91 Warkany J. Congenital cystic disease of the kidney. Chicago: Year Book Publications. 1981

92 Beck A D. The effect of intra-uterine urinary obstruction upon the development of the fetal kidney. J Urol 1971; 105: 784–789

93 Baert L. Cystic kidneys, renal dysplasia, and microdissection data in 5 children with congenital valvular urethral obstruction. Eur Urol 1978; 4(5): 383–387

94 Sanders R C, Nussbaum A R, Solez K. Renal dysplasia: sonographic findings. Radiology 1988; 167: 623–626

95 Harrison M R, Golbus M S, Filly R A, et al. Management of the fetus with congenital hydronephrosis. J Pediatr Surg 1982; 17(6): 728–742

96 Mahoney B S. The genitourinary system. In: Callen P W. ed. Ultrasonography in obstetrics and gynecology. 2nd edition. Philadelphia: WB Saunders. 1988: p 254–275

97 Glick P L, Harrison M R, Golbus M S, et al. Management of the fetus with congenital hydronephrosis II; prognostic criteria and selection for treatment. J Pediatr Surg 1985; 20(4): 376–387

98 Lebowitz R L, Griscom N T. Neonatal hydronephrosis. Radiol Clin North Am 1977; 15(1): 49–59

99 Sibley R K, Dehener L P. The kidney. In: Dehener L P. ed. Paediatric surgical pathology. 2nd edition. Baltimore: Williams and Williams. 1987: p 589–692

100 Manning F A, Harrison M R, Rodeck C. Members of the International Fetal Medicine and Surgery Society. Catheter shunts for fetal hydronephrosis and hydrocephalus. Report of the International Fetal Surgery Registry. N Engl J Med 1986; 315(5): 336–340

101 Newman L B, McAlister W H, Kissane J. Segmental renal dysplasia associated with ectopic ureteroceles in childhood. Urology 1974; 3: 23–26

102 Fisher C, F S J. Renal dysplasia in nephrectomy specimens from adolescents and adults. J Clin Pathol 1975; 28(11): 879–890

103 Lieberman E, Salinas-Madrical L, Gwinn J L, Brennan L P, Fine R N, Landing E H. Infantile polycystic disease of the kidneys and liver: clinical pathological and radiological correlations and comparison with congenital hepatic fibrosis. Medicine 1971; 50

104 Blythe H, Ockenden B G. Polycystic disease of the kidney and liver. J Med Genet 1971; 8: 257–284

105 Potter E L. Type I cystic kidney: tubular gigantism. In: Normal and abnormal development of the kidney. Chicago: Year Book Publishing. 1972: p 141–153

106 Eggli K D, Hartman D S. Autosomal recessive polycystic kidney disease. In: Hartman D S. ed. Renal cystic disease. Philadelphia: WB Saunders. 1989: p 73–87

107 Grantham J J. Clinical aspects of adult and infantile polycystic kidney disease. Contr Nephrol 1985; 48: 178–188

108 Luthy D A, Hirsch J H. Infantile polycystic kidney disease: observations from attempts at prenatal diagnosis. Am J Med Gen 1985; 20: 505–517

109 Melson G L, Shackelford G D, Cole B R, McClennan B L. The spectrum of sonographic findings in infantile polycystic kidney disease with urographic and clinical correlations. JCU 1985; 13: 113–119

110 Stapleton F B, Hilton S, Wilcox J. Transient nephromegaly simulating infantile polycystic disease of the kidneys. Pediatrics 1982; 67: 554–559

111 Zerres K, Hansmann M, Mallmann R, Gembruch U. Autosomal recessive polycystic kidney disease: problems of prenatal diagnosis. Prenat Diagn 1988; 8: 215–229

112 Simpson J L, Sabbagha R E, Elias S, Talbot C, Tamura R K. Failure to detect polycystic kidneys in utero by second trimester ultrasonography. Hum Genet 1982; 60(3): 295

113 Argubright K F, Wicks J D. Third trimester ultrasonic presentation of infantile polycystic kidney disease. Am J Pediatr 1987; 4(1): 1–4

114 Reuss A, Wladimiroff J W, Niermeijer M E. Prenatal diagnosis of renal tract abnormalities by ultrasound. Prog Clin Biol Res 1989; 305: 13–18

115 Townsend R R, Goldstein R B, Filly R A, Callen P W, Anderson R L, Golbus M. Sonographic identification of autosomal recessive polycystic kidney disease associated with increased maternal serum/amniotic fluid alpha-fetoprotein. Obstet Gynecol 1988; 71(2): 1008–1012

116 Sumner T E, Volberg F M, Martin J F, Resnick M I, Shertzer M E. Real-time sonography of congenital cystic kidney disease. Urology 1982; 20(1): 97–101

117 Romero R, Pilu G, Jeanty P, Ghidini A, Hobbins J C. The urinary tract and adrenal glands. In: Prenatal diagnosis of congenital abnormalities. Norwalk: Appleton and Lange. 1988: p 255–299

118 Reeders S T, Brenning M H, Davies K E, et al. A highly polymorphic DNA marker linked to adult polycystic disease on chromosome 16. Nature 1985; 317: 542–544

119 Milutinovic J, Agodoa L C, Cutler R E, Striker G E. Autosomal dominant polycystic kidney disease: early diagnosis and data for genetic counselling. Lancet 1980; 1: 1203–1206

120 Bear J C, McMannon P, Morgan J, et al. Age at clinical onset and sonographic detection of adult polycystic kidney disease. Am J Med Gen 1984; 18: 45–48

121 Dalgaard O Z. Bilateral polycystic disease of the kidneys: a follow-up study of two hundred and eighty four patients and their families. Acta Med Scand 1957; 158 (Suppl. 328): 1–255

122 Zerres M, Hansmann M, Knupple G, Stephan M. Prenatal diagnosis of genetically determined early manifestation of autosomal dominant polycystic kidney disease. Hum Genet 1985; 71: 368–369

123 Main D, Mennuti M T, Cornfield D, Coleman B. Prenatal diagnosis of adult polycystic kidney disease. Lancet 1983; ii: 337–338

124 Journel H, Guyott C, Barc R M, Belbeoch P, Quemener A, Jouan H. Unexpected ultrasonographic prenatal diagnosis of autosomal dominant polycystic kidney disease. Prenat Diagn 1989; 9: 663–671

125 McHugo J M, Shafi M I, Rowlands D, Weaver J B. Prenatal diagnosis of adult polycystic disease. Br J Radiol 1988; 61: 1072–1074

126 Novelli G, Frontali M, Bladini D, et al. Prenatal diagnosis of adult polycystic kidney disease with DNA markers on chromosome 16 and the genetic heterogeneity problem. Prenat Diagn 1989; 9: 759–767

127 Breuning M H, Verwest A, Ijdo J, et al. Characterization of new probes for diagnosis of polycystic kidney disease. In: Genetics of kidney disorders. Liss. 1989: p 69–75

128 Gabow P A, Ikle D W, Holmes J H. Polycystic kidney disease. Prospective analysis of nonazotemic patients and family members. Ann Intern Med 1984; 101: 238–247

129 Ross D G, Travers H. Infantile presentation of adult-type polycystic kidney disease in a large kindred. J Pediatr 1975; 87(5): 760–763

130 Fryns J P, Vandenberghe K, Moerman F. Mid-trimester ultrasonographic diagnosis of early manifesting 'adult' form of polycystic kidney disease. Hum Genet 1986; 74: 461

131 Arger P H, Coleman B G, Mintz M C, et al. Routine fetal genitourinary tract screening. Radiology 1985; 156: 485–489

132 Grignon A, Filion R, Filiatrault D, et al. Urinary tract dilatation in utero: classification and clinical applications. Radiology 1986; 160: 645–647

133 Blane C E, Koff S A, Bowermann R A, Barr Jr M. Nonobstructive fetal hydronephrosis: sonographic recognition and therapeutic implications. Radiology 1983; 147: 95–99

134 Hoddick W K, Filly R A, Mahony B S, Callen P W. Minimal fetal renal pyelectasis. J Ultrasound Med 1985; 4: 85–89

135 Ghidini A, Sirtori M, Vergani P, Orsenigo E, Tagliabue P, Parravicini E. Ureteropelvic junction obstruction in utero and ex utero. Obstet Gynecol 1990; 75(5): 805–808

136 Grignon A, Filiatrault D, Homsy Y, et al. Ureteropelvic junction stenosis: antenatal ultrasonographic diagnosis, post-natal investigation and follow-up. Radiology 1986; 160: 649–651

137 Mayor G, Genton N, Torrado A, Guignard J. Renal function in obstructive nephropathy: long-term effect of reconstructive surgery. Pediatrics 1975; 56: 740–747

138 Madarikan B A, Hayward C, Roberts G M, Lari J. Clinical outcome of fetal uropathy. Arch Dis Child 1988; 63: 961–963

139 Clarke N W, Gough D C S, Cohen S J. Neonatal urological ultrasound: diagnostic inaccuracies and pitfalls. Arch Dis Child 1989; 64: 578–580

140 Steele B T, De Maria J, Toi A, Stafford A, Hunter D, Caco C. Neonatal outcome of fetuses with urinary tract abnormalities diagnosed by prenatal ultrasonography. CMAJ 1987; 137: 117–120

141 Nicolaides K H, Rodeck C H, Gosden C M. Rapid karyotyping in non-lethal fetal malformations. Lancet 1986; i: 283–287

142 Nicolaides K H. Personal communication. 1991

143 Schwoebl M G, Sacher P, U B H, Hirsig J, Stauffer U G. Prenatal diagnosis improves the prognosis of children with obstructive uropathies. J Pediatr Surg 1984; 19(2): 187–190

144 Kelalis P P, Culp O S, Stickler G B, et al. Ureteropelvic obstruction in children: experience with 109 cases. J Urol 1971; 106: 418–422

145 Manning F A. Common fetal urinary tract anomalies. In: Hobbins J C, Benacerraf B R. eds. Clin Diagn Ultrasound. Edinburgh: Churchill Livingstone. 1989: Vol 25, p 139–161

146 Seeds J W, Mandell J. Congenital obstructive uropathies. Pre- and postnatal treatment. Urol Clin North Am 1986; 13(1): 155–165

147 Johnston J H, Evans J P, Glassberg K I, Shapiro S R. Pelvic hydronephrosis in children: a review of 219 personal cases. J Urol 1977; 117(1): 97–101

148 Antonakopoulos G N, Fuggle W J, Newman J, Considine J, O'Brien J M. Idiopathic hydronephrosis. Arch Pathol Lab Med 1985; 109: 1097–1101

149 Hanna M K, Jeffs R D, Sturgess J M, Barkin M. Urethral structure and ultrastructure. Part II. Congenital ureteropelvic junction obstruction and primary obstructive megaureter. J Urol 1976; 116: 725–730

150 Drake D P, Stevens P S, Eckstein H B. Hydronephrosis secondary to ureteropelvic obstruction in children: a review of 14 years of experience. J Urol 1978; 119: 649–651

151 Jaffe R, Schoenfield A, Ovadia J. Sonographic findings in prenatal diagnosis of bladder extrophy. Am J Obstet Gynecol 1990; 162: 675–678

152 Robson W J, Rudy S M, Johnston J H. Pelviureteric obstruction in infancy. J Pediatr Surg 1976; 11(1): 57–61

153 Jaffe R, Abramovicz J, Feigin M, Ben-Aderet N. Giant fetal abdominal cyst. J Ultrasound Med 1987; 6: 45–47

154 Kleiner B, Callen P W, Filly R A. Sonographic analysis of the fetus with ureteropelvic obstruction. AJR 1987; 148: 359–363

155 Glazer G M, Filly R M, Callen P W. The varied sonographic appearance of the urinary tract in the fetus and newborn with urethral obstruction. Radiology 1982; 144: 563–568

156 Atwell J D. Familial pelviureteric junction hydronephrosis and its association with a duplex pelvicalyceal system and vesicoureteric reflux. A family study. Br J Urol 1985; 57(4): 365–369

157 Buscemi M, Shanske A, Mallet E, Ozoktay S, Hanna M K. Dominantly inherited ureteropelvic junction obstruction. Urology 1985; 26(6): 568–571

158 Brown T, Mandell J, Lebowitz R L. Neonatal hydronephrosis in the era of sonography. AJR 1987; 148: 959–963

159 Tokunaka S, Koyanagi T. Morphologic study of primary non reflux megaureters with particular emphasis on the role of urethral sheath and ureteral dysplasia. J Urol 1982; 128(2): 399–402

160 Share J C, Lebowitz R L. Ectopic ureterocele without ureteral and calyceal dilatation (ureterocele disproportion): findings on urography and sonography. AJR 1989; 152: 567–571

161 Montana M A, Cyr D R, Lenke R R, Shuman W P, Mack L A. Sonographic detection of fetal ureteral obstruction. AJR 1985; 145: 595–596

162 Jeffs R D, Lepor H. Management of the extrophy-hypospadias complex and vulval anomalies. In: Walsh P C. ed. Cambell's urology. 5th edition. Philadelphia: W B Saunders. 1986: p 1882–1921

163 Kessler R M, Altman D H. Real time sonographic detection of vesicoureteral reflux in children. AJR 1982; 138: 1033–1036

164 Mack L A, Davies P F, Cyr D R, et al. Ultrasonic diagnosis of fetal abnormalities. Perinatol Neonatol 1986; 10: 29–31

165 Young H H, Frentz W A, Baldwin J C. Congenital obstruction of the posterior urethra. J Urol 1919; 3: 289–291

166 Mahoney B S, Callen P W, Filly R A. Fetal urethral obstruction: US evaluation. Radiology 1985; 157: 221–224

167 Dean W M, Bordeau E J. Amniotic fluid alpha-fetoprotein in fetal obstructive uropathy. Pediatrics 1980; 66(4): 537–539

168 Reuter K L, Lebowitz R L. Massive vesicoureteral reflux mimicking posterior urethral valves in a fetus. JCU 1985; 13(8): 584–587

169 Bruton O C. Agenesis of abdominal musculature associated with genito-urinary and gastro-intestinal tract anomalies. J Urol 1951; 66(4): 607–611

170 Pagon R A, Smith D W, Shepard T H. Congenital abnormalities of the urinary system. Pediatrics 1979; 94(6): 900–906

171 Tsingoglou S, Dickson J A S. Lower urinary obstruction in infancy. A review of lesions and symptoms in 165 cases. Arch Dis Child 1972; 47: 215–217

172 Egami K, Smith E D. A study of the sequelae of posterior urethral valves. J Urol 1982; 127: 84–87

173 Adzick N S, Harrison M R, Flake A W, deLorimer A A. Urinary extravasation in the fetus with obstructive uropathy. J Pediatr Surg 1985; 20(6): 608–615

174 Warshaw B L, Edelbrock H H, Ettenger R B, et al. Progression to end-stage renal disease in children with obstructive uropathy. J Pediatr 1982; 100(2): 183–187

175 Hayden S A, Russ P D, Pretorius D H, Manco-Johnson M L, Clewell W H. Posterior urethral obstruction. J Ultrasound Med 1988; 7: 371–375

176 Shalev E, Weiner E, Feldman E, Sudarsky M, Shmilowitz L, Zuckerman H. External bladder-amniotic fluid shunt for fetal urinary tract obstruction. Obstet Gynecol 1984; 63(Suppl): 31S–34S

177 Nakayama D K, Harrison M R, de Lorimer A A. Prognosis of posterior urethral valves presenting at birth. J Pediatr Surg 1986; 21(1): 43–45

178 Grajewski R S, Glassberg K I. The variable effect of posterior urethral valves as illustrated in identical twins. J Urol 1983; 130: 1188–1190

179 Berdon W E, Baker D H, Blanc W A, Gay B, Santulli T V, Donovan C. Megacystis-microcolon-intestinal hypoperistalsis syndrome: a new cause of intestinal obstruction in the newborn. Report of radiologic findings in five newborn girls. AJR 1976; 126(5): 957–964

180 Young L W, Yunis E J, Girdany B R, Sieber W K. Megacystis-microcolon-intestinal hypoperistalsis syndrome: additional clinical, radiologic, surgical and histopathologic aspects. AJR 1981; 137(4): 749–755

181 Vezina W C, Morin F R, Winsberg F. Megacystis-microcolon-intestinal hypoperistalsis syndrome: antenatal ultrasound appearance. AJR 1979; 133(4): 749–750

182 Manco L G, Osterdahl P. The antenatal sonographic features of megacystis-microcolon-intestinal hypoperistalsis syndrome. JCU 1984; 12(9): 595–598

183 Verco P W, Khor B H, Barbary J, Enthoven C. Ectopia vesicae in utero. Australas Radiol 1986; 30(2): 117–120

184 Ives E, Coffey R, Carter C O. A family study of bladder extrophy. J Med Genet 1980; 17(2): 139–141

185 Graivier L. Extrophy of the cloaca. Ann Surg 1968; 34: 387–390

186 Mirk P, Calisti A, Fileni A. Prenatal sonographic diagnosis of bladder extrophy. J Ultrasound Med 1986; 5(5): 291–293

187 Muecke E L. Extrophy, epispadias and other anomalies. In: Walsh P C. ed. Cambell's urology. 5th edition. Philadelphia: W B Saunders. 1981: p 1856–1880

188 Soper R T, Kilger K. Vesico-intestinal fissure. J Urol 1964; 92: 490–501

189 Lattimer J K, Beck L, Yeaw S, Puchner P J, Macfarlane M T, Krisiloff M. Long-term follow-up after extrophy closure; late improvement and good quality of life. J Urol 1978; 119(5): 664–666

190 Howell C, Caldamone A, Snyder H, Ziegler M, Duckett J. Optimal management of cloacal extrophy. J Pediatr Surg 1983; 18(4): 365–369

191 Shapiro E, Lepor H, Jeffs R D. The inheritance of the extrophy-epispadias complex. J Urol 1984; 132(2): 308–310

192 Wigger H J. Fetal mesenchymal hamartoma of kidney. A tumour of secondary mesenchyme. Cancer 1975; 36(3): 1002–1008

193 Appuzio J J, Unwin W, Adhate A, Nichols R. Prenatal diagnosis of fetal renal mesoblastic nephroma. Am J Obstet Gynecol 1986; 154: 636–637

194 Ehman R L, Nicholson S F, Machin G A. Prenatal sonographic diagnosis of congenital mesoblastic nephroma in a monozygotic twin pregnancy. J Ultrasound Med 1983; 2(12): 555–557

195 Walter J P, McGahan J P. Mesoblastic nephroma: prenatal sonographic detection. JCU 1985; 13(9): 686–689

196 Blank E, Neerhout R C, Burry K A. Congenital mesoblastic nephroma and polyhydramnios. JAMA 1978; 240(14): 1504–1505

197 Sotelo-Avila C, Gooch W M III. Neoplasms associated with the Beckwith-Wiedemann syndrome. Perspect Pediatr Pathol 1976; 3: 255–272

198 Gonzalez-Crussi F, Sotelo-Avila C, Kidd J M. Malignant mesenchymal nephroma of infancy: report of a case with pulmonary metastases. Am J Surg Pathol 1980; 4(2): 185–190

199 Walker D, Richard G. Fetal hamartoma of the kidney; recurrence and death of patient. J Urol 1973; 110: 352–353

200 Tanenbaum B, Silverman N, Weinberg S R. Solitary crossed renal ectopia. Arch Surg 1970; 101: 616–618

201 Malek R S, Kelalis P P, Burke E C. Ectopic kidney in children and frequency of association with other malformations. Mayo Clin Proc 1971; 46: 461–467

202 Ward J N, Nathanson B, Draper J W. The pelvic kidney. J Urol 1965; 94: 36–39

203 Colley N, Hooker J G. Prenatal diagnosis of pelvic kidney. Prenat Diagn 1989; 9: 361–363

204 Lowsley O S. Surgery of horseshoe kidney. J Urol 1952; 67: 565–578

205 Sherer D M, Cullen J B, Thompson H O, Metlay L A, Woods J R Jnr. Prenatal sonographic findings associated with a fetal horseshoe kidney. J Ultrasound Med 1990; 9(8): 477–479

206 Culp O S, Winterringer J R. Surgical treatment of horseshoe kidney; comparison of results after various types of operations. J Urol 1955; 73: 747–756

207 Ware S M, Shulman Y. Transitional cell carcinoma of renal pelvis in horseshoe kidney. Urology 1983; 21(1): 76–78

208 Weiner M, Sarma D, Rao M. Renal cell carcinoma in a horseshoe kidney. J Surg Oncol 1984; 26: 77–79

209 Carlson H E. Supernumerary kidney; summary of 51 reported cases. J Urol 1950; 64: 224–229

210 Tada Y, Kokado Y, Hashinaka Y, et al. Free supernumerary kidney; a case report and review. J Urol 1981; 126(2): 231–232

211 N'Guessan G, Stephens F D. Supernumerary kidney. J Urol 1983; 130(4): 649–653

212 Antony J. Complete duplication of female urethra with vaginal atresia and supernumerary kidney. J Urol 1977; 118(5): 877–878

The gastrointestinal tract

Lyn S. Chitty and David R. Griffin

INTRODUCTION

Detailed visualisation of the fetal abdominal wall and contents forms part of the routine survey in the second trimester. The liver, gallbladder and spleen are detected in most fetuses from mid-pregnancy onwards in addition to portions of the hollow intestinal organs. Abnormalities of the abdominal wall and the gastrointestinal tract are usually readily demonstrated with ultrasound and form the third largest group of detected anomalies after renal and central nervous system abnormalities.

Anterior abdominal wall defects

Omphalocele

Definition and aetiology Omphalocele is an anterior abdominal wall defect characterised by the herniation of intra-abdominal contents into the base of the umbilical cord. The contents, which may include bowel, liver, spleen and pancreas, are covered with a layer of amnion and peritoneum into which the umbilical cord inserts (Fig. 1). The size of these defects is variable, ranging from a small hernia containing a few loops of bowel to a very large one containing most of the abdominal viscera (see Ch. 7). Omphalocele is estimated to occur between one in 4000 to one in 5800 live births.[1,2]

Associated abnormalities Omphalocele may be an isolated lesion but it is also frequently associated with other abnormalities, syndromes and autosomal trisomies. An overall incidence of associated defects of between 17% and 82% has been reported.[1,3-5] The frequency of abnormal karyotypes varies between 6% and 54%.[1,3,4,6-8] The most common abnormality reported is trisomy 18, but there have been reports of triploidy, 47 XXY, trisomy 13 and trisomy 21. Cardiac anomalies (ventricular and atrial septal defects and tetralogy of Fallot) are found in up to 36% of cases,[1,3,4,6,9] neural tube defects (anencephaly, encephalocele and myelomeningocele) in up to 39%[5,6] and genitourinary abnormalities in up to 40%.[3] Gastrointestinal anomalies, either primary or secondary (e.g. bowel obstruction) are also a frequent association. Intra-uterine growth retardation has been reported in 20% of cases.[2]

Omphalocele may occur as part of a syndrome,[10] the most common being the Beckwith-Wiedemann syndrome where it is associated with organomegaly, gigantism, hemihypertrophy and polyhydramnios.[11,12] This syndrome may account for a significant proportion of all cases of omphalocele.[3,9]

Most cases of omphalocele are sporadic and the recurrence risk for isolated cases appears to be less than 1%. Few familial cases have been reported.[13-15] When an omphalocele is associated with a chromosomal abnormality careful evaluation of the fetal karyotype should exclude the possibility of an unbalanced translocation. This would increase the recurrence risk if one of the parents carries the

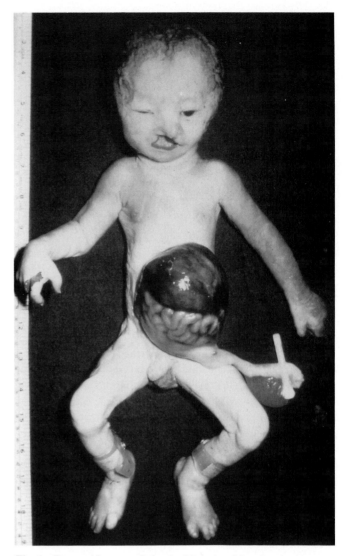

Fig. 1 Fetus with an omphalocele. Note the cleft palate in this case where the underlying pathology was trisomy 18.

balanced form of the translocation. When occurring as part of a syndrome the recurrence risk is that of the syndrome.

Diagnosis The sonographic diagnosis of omphalocele is made by the demonstration of a mass adjacent to the anterior abdominal wall (Figs 2 and 3). The hernia should be in the midline and be covered with a membrane which is continuous with the umbilical cord which inserts into the hernia (Fig. 2B). The main differential diagnosis is gastroschisis which lacks a surrounding membrane and is separate from the cord insertion. These findings permit an accurate diagnosis in most cases, except those rare instances where rupture of the amnioperitoneal sac occurs in utero.[16]

Management and prognosis Any fetus with an omphalocele should undergo careful sonographic examination for associated anomalies, fetal echocardiography and karyotyping. It has been suggested that the ultrasound ap-

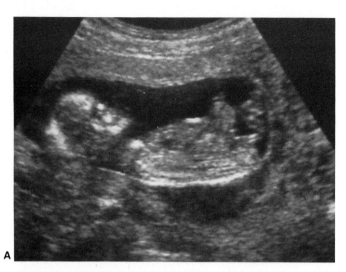
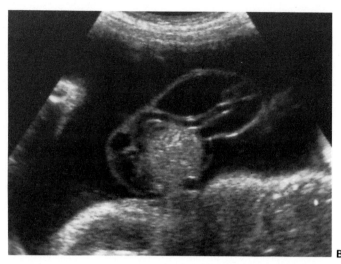

Fig. 2 Omphalocele at 14 and 32 weeks. A: Longitudinal scan showing a small omphalocele at 14 weeks which is about the earliest time the diagnosis can be made because of the physiological herniation seen prior to this. **B:** Same patient at 32 weeks gestation showing detail of the umbilical vessels entering the sac of the omphalocele.

pearances can help determine the risk of a chromosomal anomaly in a fetus with an omphalocele. In most cases with an abnormal karyotype there will be an additional major malformation or markers such as a digital, facial or renal anomaly. The absence of liver from the sac has also been found to be suggestive of an abnormal karyotype. The prognosis, in cases with a normal karyotype but other abnormalities, will depend on the nature of those abnormalities. In all cases where the pregnancy continues serial ultrasonography should be performed to monitor fetal growth.

In cases where the lesion is isolated the prognosis is very good. A small defect can usually be closed in a single operation, larger ones may require a two stage procedure. In a recent unpublished series analysing referrals to the

Hospitals for Sick Children, Great Ormond Street, from 1975 to 1985 (GOS series), 80% of neonates undergoing surgery for omphalocele survived.

The mode of delivery for fetuses with this abnormality is still a subject for debate as there has been no good randomised study comparing the outcome of vaginal versus abdominal delivery. In two retrospective uncontrolled studies there was no obvious benefit gained by delivering these neonates by caesarean section.[2,17]

Gastroschisis

Definition and aetiology Gastroschisis is a prenatal evisceration of abdominal contents through a full thickness, para-umbilical defect in the anterior abdominal wall,

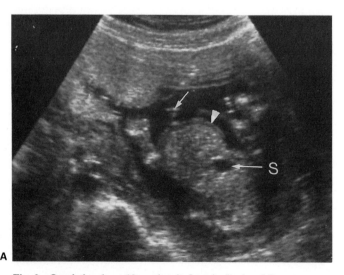
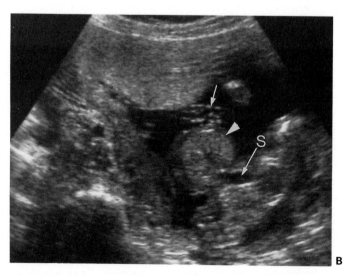

Fig. 3 Omphalocele at 18 weeks. A: Longitudinal and **B:** transverse scans of an omphalocele (arrowhead) at 18 weeks gestation showing the typical features. S – stomach, cord – arrow.

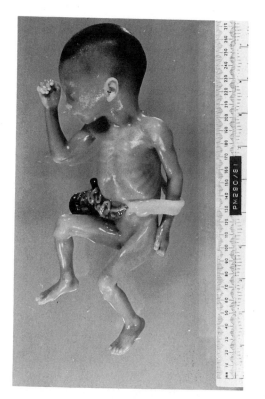

Fig. 4 Fetus with a gastroschisis. Note the cord insertion to the left of the defect in the anterior abdominal wall.

Occasionally stomach or liver may herniate through the defect. Gastroschisis occurs about one in 12 000 live births.[1]

Associated abnormalities Gastroschisis is usually an isolated lesion, reports of associated anomalies (excluding intestinal atresias etc.) varying from 2.5% to 24%.[1,3,4,9] Congenital heart defects have been noted in up to 8.5% of cases.[4] Other malformations associated with gastroschisis include diaphragmatic defects,[1] neural tube defects[6] and mild abnormalities of the renal tract, particularly hydronephrosis and horseshoe kidney.[9,18] It has also been seen as part of the amnion rupture sequence.[18,19] Association with an abnormal karyotype appears to be exceedingly rare, only two such cases being reported in the world literature.[20] However, in up to 25% of cases there may be gastrointestinal problems due to vascular impairment and adhesions. These include bowel malrotation, intestinal atresias and stenosis.[4,21]

Most cases of gastroschisis are sporadic and the recurrence risk is less than 1%.

Diagnosis Sonographically a gastroschisis is characterised by an irregular mass, which has been likened to a cauliflower or a bunch of grapes, in front of the fetal abdomen. It has no membranous covering and frequently loops of bowel may be seen floating outside the abdominal wall attached to mesentery (Figs 5 and 6). The umbilical cord inserts normally, close to and usually to the left of the defect (Fig. 7). False negative and false positive prenatal diagnoses of gastroschisis have been reported.[22] Two false negatives were described, one in which the diagnosis was considered but rejected (the abnormal structure seen was thought to be an oedematous cord) and the other where the diagnosis was missed on a routine scan for fetal growth at 29 weeks. One of two false positive cases was found to have an abruption of the placenta at subsequent caesarean

usually to the right of the umbilical cord, which has a normal insertion (Fig. 4). There is no covering membrane and the defect is usually small. Loops of bowel are most commonly herniated through the defect. These often become thickened and matted together because of inflammation induced by contact with amniotic fluid, or as a result of ischaemia following torsion of the bowel.

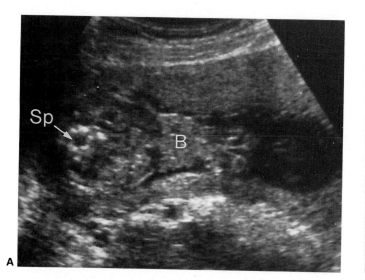

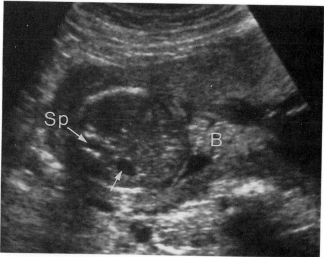

Fig. 5 Gastroschisis. A and **B:** Cross-sectional views of a 17 week fetus with a gastroschisis demonstrating the herniated bowel (B), spine (Sp) and stomach (arrow).

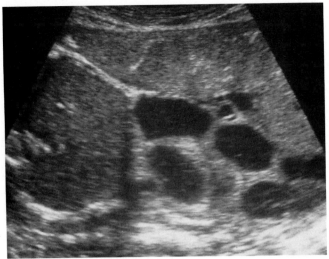

Fig. 6 Gastroschisis with dilated loops of bowel. 37 week fetus with a gastroschisis showing the liver, placenta and dilated loops of herniated bowel with thickened walls.

had multiple congenital abnormalities and two of the others died from sepsis.

The mode of delivery for neonates with a gastroschisis, as with omphalocele, is open to debate with no clear advantage to either abdominal or vaginal delivery.[2,17]

Body stalk anomaly

Definition and aetiology Body stalk anomaly is an extensive defect in the anterior abdominal wall due to failed formation of the body stalk. Absence of the umbilicus and umbilical cord causes adherence of the placenta to the herniated viscera (Fig. 8). The incidence of body stalk anomaly is about one in 14 000 births.[6]

Associated abnormalities Associated abnormalities are common and are generally severe. They include defects of the intestinal and genitourinary tracts, heart, lungs and

section, matted cord and blood clot having caused the confusion. In the other case oligohydramnios following premature rupture of the membranes impaired imaging.

Prognosis and management A fetus found to have a gastroschisis should have a detailed anomaly scan and echocardiography. In cases where the pregnancy continues serial scans should be performed to monitor fetal growth. The prognosis is good where the lesion is isolated, although premature delivery may result in death from respiratory distress syndrome. Sepsis may also be life threatening. In the GOS series 86% of neonates who underwent a surgical repair of a gastroschisis survived. Of the five who died one

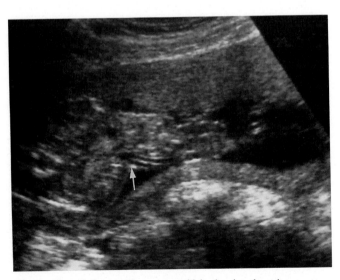

Fig. 7 17 week fetus with a gastroschisis showing the spine, herniated bowel and cord insertion (arrow) to the side of the hernia.

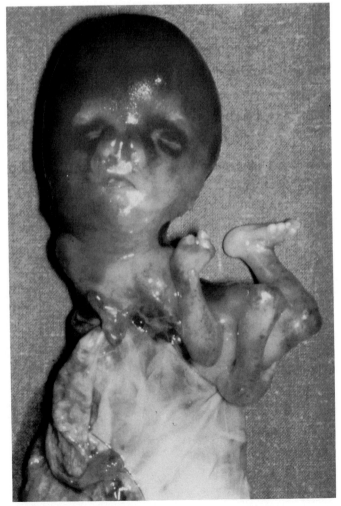

Fig. 8 Fetus with a body stalk anomaly. Note the absence of umbilical cord and membranes adherent to the anterior abdominal wall at the site of the defect. Figure courtesy of D. Donnai.

skeletal system. A marked scoliosis is one of the most frequent and characteristic associations. Neural tube defects are particularly common.[23]

Diagnosis Prenatal diagnosis has been reported using maternal serum alpha-fetoprotein (MSAFP) and ultrasound.[6,24,25] Sonographically the fetus is particularly immobile and apparently attached to the placenta at the site of the abdominal wall defect (Fig. 9). No free loops of umbilical cord are visible.[24,25]

Prognosis and management This condition is invariably fatal[6,23] and, if detected before viability, the option of termination of pregnancy should be discussed.

Anterior abdominal wall defects cause elevation in the MSAFP[6] and therefore examination of the ventral wall is a prerequisite part of the sonographic examination in all pregnancies complicated by raised MSAFP.

Bladder and cloacal extrophy

Definition and aetiology These anomalies are caused by the maldevelopment of the caudal fold of the anterior abdominal wall (see Ch. 7). In bladder extrophy the anterior wall of the bladder is absent, exposing the posterior wall. Cloacal extrophy is a more complex anomaly where the posterior bladder wall protrudes through the anterior abdominal wall as with bladder extrophy, but in addition to the ureters opening into the protruded mucosa, the ileum opens at the umbilical end and the blind-ending colon at the caudal end of the defect. The anus is absent.

Bladder extrophy occurs in between one in 10 000 and one in 50 000 births and is twice as common in males than in females.[26] Extrophy of the cloaca is very rare and only occurs one in 200 000 births.[27] Most cases of extrophy are sporadic and the recurrence risk in a family is 1%.[28,29] However it is much more common in consanguineous Muslim marriages.

Associated abnormalities Associated abnormalities are rare in bladder extrophy but common in cloacal extrophy.[30] Renal anomalies occur in 60%, skeletal defects (spina bifida in particular) in 72%, omphalocele in 87%, cardiovascular abnormalities in 16% and other gastrointestinal abnormalities in 10.5% of cases with cloacal extrophy.[30–32]

Diagnosis Prenatal diagnosis of both forms of extrophy have been reported.[33,34] The diagnosis of bladder extrophy was suspected[33] because of a solid mass in the lower part of the fetal abdomen and the inability to demonstrate a bladder despite the presence of normal amounts of amniotic fluid (Fig. 10). There was excessive mobility of the fetal pelvic girdle when pressure was exerted with the ultrasound transducer because of failed development of the pubic bones. The differential diagnosis of cloacal extrophy includes omphalocele and gastroschisis. The visualisation of a normal bladder and the relationship of the mass to the anterior abdominal wall are helpful features in the precise delineation of the defect.

Management and prognosis The main problems associated with bladder extrophy are urinary incontinence, the anterior abdominal wall defect and variable deformities of the external genitalia which can be serious enough in the male to require sex reassignment in up to 2% of cases.[26] In the female genital defects are more easily repaired, although vaginal dilatation and perineoplasty may be required for satisfactory sexual function. Urinary incontinence can be treated surgically by primary bladder closure and reconstruction of the bladder neck or by urinary diversion and cystectomy.[26] Fertility is decreased in both males and females and the risk of their having an affected offspring is increased to one in 70.[29]

Cloacal extrophy is a much more serious problem, often with a high risk of mortality. However, a recent report has suggested that this can be reduced by optimal surgical management.[32] Untreated infants die from sepsis, short bowel syndrome, renal or central nervous system defects. The surgical approach to repair consists of a series of operations in the first few years of life including early closure of the anterior abdominal wall defect and the bladder, continence surgery in early childhood and vaginal reconstruction as a teenager. There is usually considerable difficulty in creating a functional penis and sex reassignment may be required in affected males.[35] The ultimate prognosis in cases where there is successful surgical repair depends also on the presence of other abnormalities which may confer considerable disability.

If the diagnosis of extrophy is made before viability then termination of pregnancy is an option which should be considered. After this time no alteration in obstetric care

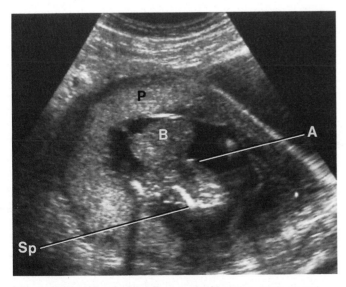

Fig. 9 Fetus with a body stalk anomaly. Note the acutely curved spine (Sp), the defect in the anterior abdominal wall (A) and the herniated contents (B) which are attached to the placenta (P).

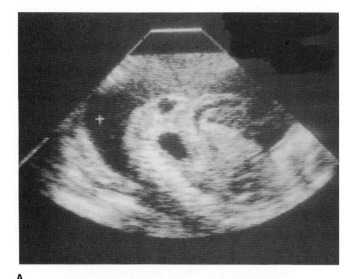

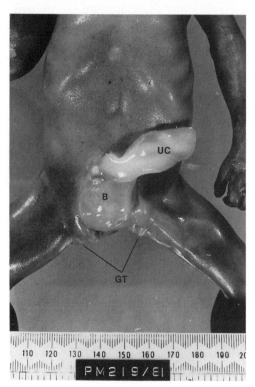

Fig. 10   Bladder extrophy. A: Ultrasound findings in a fetus subsequently shown to have bladder extrophy. **B:** Shows the fetus with bladder (B) exposed, umbilical cord (UC) and the genital tubercles (GT). Note the wide spacing of the pelvic bones.

is required although delivery in a centre with neonatal surgical facilities is advisable. Following delivery the exposed bladder should be covered by an impermeable wrap and fluid and electrolyte balance carefully monitored. Full assessment of the gastrointestinal and urinary systems is needed prior to surgery.

Intestinal obstructions

Oesophageal atresia

Definition and aetiology   Oesophageal atresia is the congenital absence of a segment of the oesophagus. In most cases there is an associated tracheo-oesophageal fistula. The major variations seen in tracheo-oesophageal fistula are shown in Figure 11, the first variant (a) is the most common, occurring in about 80% of cases. Oesophageal atresia (with or without tracheo-oesophageal fistula) occurs in about two in 10 000 live births.[36]

Associated abnormalities   In infants with oesophageal atresia the incidence of associated abnormalities ranges from 40% to 57%.[37] Cardiovascular abnormalities (29%) are the most common association with anorectal (14%), other gastrointestinal and genitourinary problems (14%) also occurring frequently. Several syndromes are associated with oesophageal atresia. These include the VATER (Vertebral defects, Anorectal malformation, Tracheo-oesophageal fistula, Renal anomaly and Radial dysplasia) and Schisis associations (cleft lip and palate, omphalocele and hypogenitalism).[37,38] Oesophageal atresia has been reported in association with Down's syndrome and other karyotypic abnormalities.[37,39] Most cases of isolated oesophageal atresia with or without tracheo-oesophageal fistula are sporadic occurrences and the recurrence risk to sibs is very low.[36]

Diagnosis   The diagnosis of oesophageal atresia is suspected when, in the presence of polyhydramnios, repeated examinations fail to demonstrate a fetal stomach. These signs are almost invariably absent if there is a tracheo-oesophageal fistula as the stomach will fill passively via the trachea. Thus relatively few cases of oesophageal atresia are amenable to prenatal diagnosis. In the few cases reported in the literature prenatal diagnosis of this lesion has been made in the third trimester when ultrasonography has been performed because of polyhydramnios.[40-42] However, it should be possible to make the diagnosis earlier following persistent failure to demonstrate a fetal stomach.

Management and prognosis   In cases where oesophageal atresia is suspected a detailed anomaly scan, echocardiography and fetal karyotyping should be performed to exclude associated anomalies. Survival depends on gestational age at delivery and coexisting anomalies. The prognosis in cases with an isolated lesion born at term is excellent following post-natal surgery. Primary repair or bowel interposition generally result in good long-term survival. In the remainder, where there are other abnormalities or prematurity, the outlook is poorer. Chittmittrapap et al report a survival of 70% in such cases, the major cause of death being cardiac complications.[37] However, other authors report a less favourable prognosis with survival rates as low as 6% in complicated cases.[43]

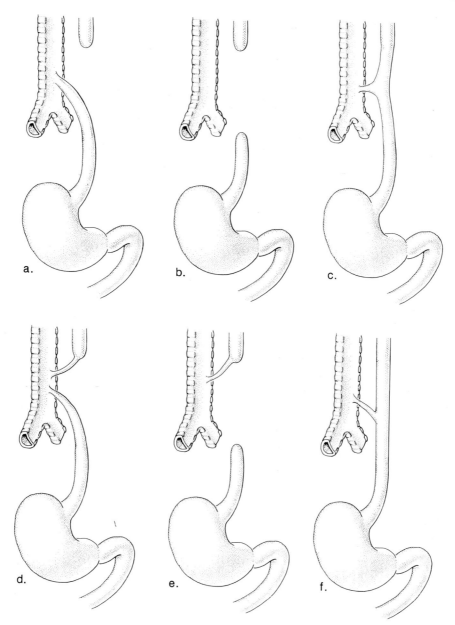

Fig. 11   Oesophageal atresia and tracheo-oesophageal fistula. A diagram showing the major variations seen in tracheo-oesophageal fistula. The first (a) is the most common. Only in types (b) and (e) will ultrasound be able to establish the diagnosis because of an empty stomach.

Duodenal obstruction

Definition and aetiology   Duodenal atresia or stenosis occurs in about two in 10 000 births and is the most common form of small bowel obstruction.[44] The blockage is usually caused by a membrane or web across the lumen of the bowel. Less commonly it results from a blind ending loop of bowel or atresia of large portions of intestine. An annular pancreas coexists in about 20% of cases.[45]

Associated abnormalities   Duodenal obstruction is an isolated abnormality in 30% to 50% of cases.[45,46] In the remainder the condition may be associated with congenital heart disease (8% to 20%), vertebral and skeletal deformities (37%), other intestinal anomalies (26%) and genitourinary malformations (8%). One third of cases of duodenal obstruction are associated with trisomy 21.[44-48]

Diagnosis   Duodenal obstruction may be diagnosed on a transverse abdominal scan by the demonstration of the typical 'double bubble' (Fig. 12) appearance of the dilated stomach and proximal duodenum.[49] A connection between the two structures must be demonstrated at the pylorus

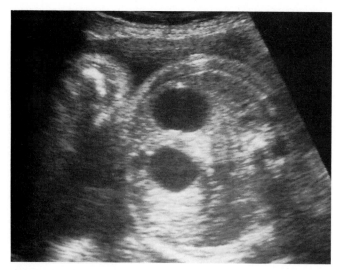

Fig. 12   32 week fetus with duodenal atresia demonstrating the typical 'double bubble' appearance.

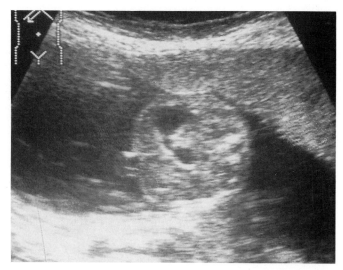

A

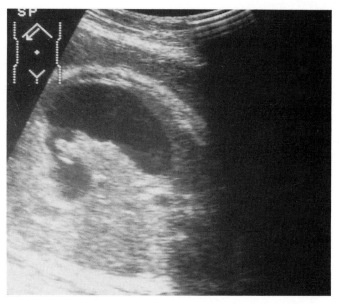

B

Fig. 13   Duodenal atresia at 24 and 36 weeks. A: Fetus at 24 weeks and **B:** again at 36 weeks demonstrating the pylorus connecting the stomach and proximal duodenum. Note the associated polyhydramnios.

(Fig. 13). This abnormality is not usually evident at a routine 18 to 20 week scan but is more often detected later in pregnancy when the patient presents for an anomaly scan because of polyhydramnios. There are however a few reports of the diagnosis being made between 19 and 23 weeks.[20,49] The main differential diagnosis in these cases is that of an abdominal cyst where two fluid structures may also be seen, one corresponding to the normal stomach and the other to the cyst. However in these cases there is not usually polyhydramnios and no connection can be demonstrated between the two fluid filled spaces.

Management and prognosis   The management of any fetus found to have duodenal atresia should include a detailed scan to detect associated abnormalities, echocardiography and karyotyping. When the duodenal atresia is isolated the prognosis is excellent. In the recent GOS series there was a 97% survival. The one death in the 30 cases occurred in a child who had multiple anomalies. Duodenal atresia may be associated with prematurity because of the polyhydramnios which may cause preterm labour and the resultant prematurity may worsen the prognosis. Prenatal diagnosis may decrease morbidity from vomiting, aspiration pneumonia, electrolyte imbalance, and stomach perforation by alerting the neonatologist to the increased risks.[50] Some would argue that delivery in a specialised centre is desirable in order to expedite surgical repair; however, in the series reported here from GOS all infants were ex utero transfers, some may have died before transfer.

Other small bowel obstructions

Incidence and aetiology   Jejunal and ileal atresia and stenosis are less common than duodenal atresia and occur in less than one in 10 000 births. The most common sites are in the distal ileum (36%), proximal jejunum (31%), distal jejunum (20%) and the proximal ileum (13%). They are thought to be due to fibrosis following an intra-uterine vasuclar accident.[38,51] Small bowel obstruction can also result from meconium ileus in which viscid, thick meconium accumulates and obstructs the distal ileum.

Associated abnormalities   Small bowel atresias and stenosis are usually isolated anomalies but may be seen in association with other intestinal anomalies.[52,53] Association with an abnormal karyotype is rare but has been reported.[39,53] Cases secondary to meconium ileus have a

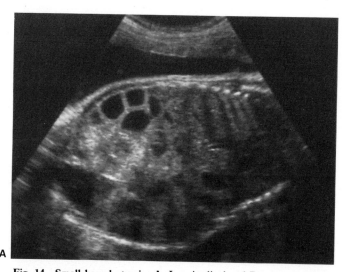

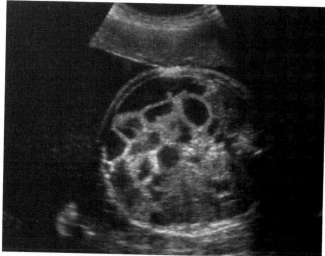

Fig. 14 Small bowel atresia. A: Longitudinal and **B:** cross-sectional views of a fetus with small bowel atresia showing multiple echo-free areas corresponding to loops of dilated bowel. Note the associated polyhydramnios.

significant association with cystic fibrosis and babies who are small for dates because of placental insufficiency.[54,55] Cystic fibrosis is an autosomal recessive disorder and therefore parents who have had one child with this condition have a 25% chance of a recurrence in future pregnancies, although not all recurrences will present with meconium ileus. Prenatal diagnosis for these parents can now be performed in the first trimester using molecular biological techniques.

In uncomplicated cases of small bowel atresia the recurrence risk is small.[56,57]

Diagnosis   Small bowel obstructions may be suspected when multiple fluid filled spaces are seen within the fetal abdomen (Figs 14 and 15). The differential diagnosis includes other conditions capable of causing multiple echo-free areas in the fetal abdomen (duodenal atresia, hydronephrosis, multicystic kidney etc.). Usually the 'cysts' can be recognised as distended loops of bowel be-

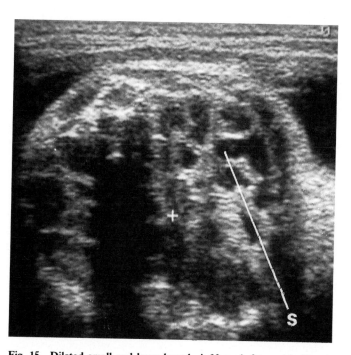

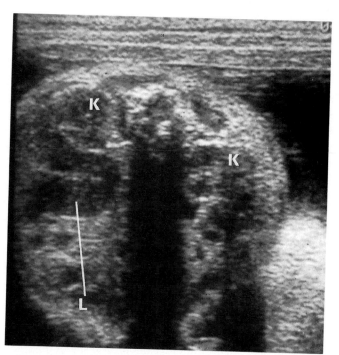

Fig. 15 Dilated small and large bowel. A 32 week fetus with dilated small (S) and large (L) bowel. K – kidneys.

cause of peristaltic activity and floating particles within the lumen.[58] Furthermore, careful examination will demonstrate a normal stomach and renal tract. As with the other intestinal atresias the diagnosis is usually not made until late in the second or third trimester when the fetus is scanned for some obstetric reason. Polyhydramnios may occur in cases of jejunal atresia but is less common when the obstruction is more distal.[58,59] Meconium ileus has been diagnosed at 18 weeks in cases known to be at risk of cystic fibrosis. Increased reflectivity of the intra-abdominal (intestinal) contents is found[54] or, later in pregnancy, classical signs of small bowel obstruction may be observed.[60]

Prognosis and management   The prognosis for infants with isolated intestinal atresia is good. In the GOS series 96% survived. Cases with large areas of affected bowel have a worse prognosis.[53] Neonates with meconium ileus have a variable prognosis depending on the gestational age at delivery and the underlying pathology.

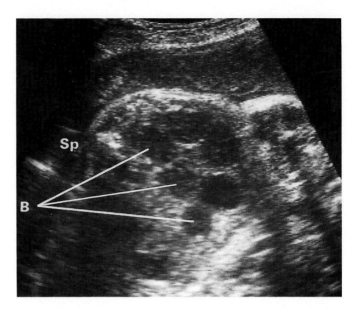

Fig. 16   Normal bowel. A normal 37 week fetus showing the bowel (B) and spine (Sp).

Large bowel obstruction

Incidence and aetiology   Atresia and stenosis of the large bowel occur very rarely and account for less than 10% of all intestinal atresias.[61] Most cases of large bowel atresia are thought to be the result of a vascular accident, volvulus or intussusception.[51] The reported incidences for anal atresia vary from one in 2500 to one in 3300 live births.[62] Hirschsprung's disease, caused by varying lengths of aganglionic bowel, can also give the appearance of bowel obstruction.[63] This condition occurs in one in 8000 births and affects males more commonly than females.[64]

The recurrence risk for large bowel atresia is usually quoted as about 1%. Isolated anal atresia also carries a low risk of recurrence, but where it occurs as part of a syndrome the recurrence risk is as for the syndrome. For Hirschsprung's disease the risk depends on whether the index case was male or female and whether it was long or short segment disease.[64]

Associated abnormalities   Colonic atresias are usually isolated lesions. Up to 70% of anal atresias and stenoses are associated with other anomalies, particularly those involving the vertebrae, trachea, oesophagus and renal tract (VATER association). There are also many syndromes which include anal atresia.[65] Trisomy 21 occurs in 2% of cases of Hirschsprung's disease.

Diagnosis   In contradistinction to small bowel obstruction the diagnosis of large bowel obstruction may be difficult in that, as a result of fluid absorption by the colonic mucosa, there may be little or no proximal dilatation. Furthermore, since obstruction of either small or large intestine may result in grossly enlarged loops of bowel, prenatal identification of the precise site of obstruction may not be possible. In some cases the haustral pattern

may help to localise the obstruction to the large bowel (Fig. 15). Polyhydramnios, on the other hand, usually indicates small bowel obstruction. It must be remembered that there is considerable variability in the appearances of the bowel in the third trimester such that in some cases suspicion of obstruction may arise in a perfectly normal fetus (Fig. 16).

Prenatal diagnosis of anal atresia has been reported in the third trimester.[66] Fluid filled loops of bowel were seen in the lower abdomen in the absence of polyhydramnios. We have recently made the diagnosis in a fetus at 22 weeks gestation (Fig. 17). A fluid filled lesion was seen arising from the perineal region behind the bladder and extending up into the abdomen in the position of the sigmoid colon. Peristalsis could be seen and there was no polyhydramnios.

A precise diagnosis of Hirschsprung's disease in a fetus is difficult in the absence of a positive family history. In a case with progressive dilatation of the large bowel late in the third trimester, the differential diagnosis was between Hirschsprung's disease, colonic atresia and imperforate anus.[63]

Management and prognosis   These abnormalities are rarely detected before viability. A careful search for other abnormalities should be made in order to try to define the prognosis more precisely. However in most cases the definitive diagnosis must await delivery and the results of post-natal investigations. There is not usually any reason to depart from normal obstetric practise, but delivery in a centre where there is easy access to paediatric surgical facilities is advised.

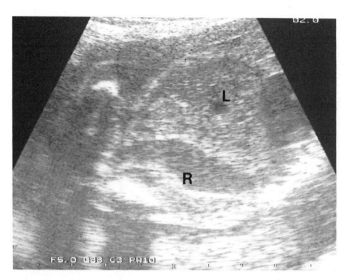

Fig. 17 Anal atresia. A longitudinal view of a 22 week fetus with anal atresia showing liver (L), thorax and dilated rectosigmoid colon (R).

The prognosis for isolated large bowel or anal atresia is excellent. The outcome in cases of imperforate anus associated with other abnormalities or syndromes will depend on the severity of these associations. The prognosis in cases of Hirschsprung's disease depends on the length of bowel involved. Mortality rates of up to 20% in infancy have been reported, however these figures do not include those cases where the diagnosis is suspected prenatally. In these cases some of the complications secondary to delay in diagnosis could be avoided (enterocolitis, caecal perforation, malnutrition etc.) possibly improving prognosis.

Meconium peritonitis

Definition and aetiology Meconium peritonitis occurs as a result of peritoneal inflammation following intra-uterine bowel perforation. Although it is rare, several cases have been diagnosed prenatally.[67,68] In 25% to 40% of cases it is secondary to the meconium ileus of cystic fibrosis.[69,70] In some cases the aetiology is unclear, and in others the perforation occurs proximal to an intestinal atresia or stenosis. Two types of fetal meconium peritonitis have been described: the fibro-adhesive and the cystic varieties. In the former there is an intense inflammatory reaction of the peritoneum which leads to the formation of a dense calcified mass which seals off the perforation. In the other type the perforation is not sealed and loops of bowel become fixed around the perforation site forming a cystic cavity into which meconium continues to leak.

Associated abnormalities The only significant extra-abdominal associations are those of cystic fibrosis.[69,70] The other major associations are the underlying cause of the bowel obstruction which has resulted in perforation, e.g. intestinal atresia, volvulus.

Diagnosis The presence of a highly reflective intra-abdominal mass is suggestive of meconium peritonitis, particularly if associated with ascites and polyhydramnios, though the diagnosis should still be suspected in their absence. The differential diagnosis includes intra-abdominal haemorrhage, early ascites, fetal hypoxia, cystic fibrosis and intra-abdominal tumours (haemangioma, teratoma, ovarian dermoid, hepatoblastoma, metastatic neuroblastoma) and fetal gallstones, but these are not usually associated with polyhydramnios.

Management and prognosis The main diagnosis to be excluded is that of cystic fibrosis. Measurement of amniotic fluid intestinal isoenzymes of alkaline phosphatase can assist in this diagnosis,[71] but with the recent identification of the gene for cystic fibrosis[72] it will probably be more accurate to screen the fetus for a deletion within this gene. Delivery in a tertiary centre is advisable since neonates with meconium peritonitis require immediate surgical care.

Meconium peritonitis is a serious condition with a mortality rate as high as 62% reported for those neonates who undergo surgery.[69] However this figure does not include cases diagnosed prenatally and it is clear that early diagnosis and treatment improves the survival. There are eight prenatally diagnosed cases in the literature and of these five survived, one pregnancy was electively terminated and deaths occurred in two premature neonates.[67,68,73-77]

Intra-abdominal cystic lesions

Abdominal cystic masses are frequent findings at fetal ultrasound examination. Dilated bowel or renal tract anomalies are the most common explanation, although cystic structures may arise from most abdominal or pelvic organs. It may not be possible to make a precise diagnosis prenatally but the most likely diagnosis is usually suggested by the position of the cyst, its relationship to other structures and the normality of other organs.

Choledochal cyst

Definition and aetiology A choledochal cyst is a cystic bile duct dilatation, usually single, but multiple in rare instances. It is usually found in the common bile duct, but can involve the intrahepatic or extrahepatic portions of the biliary tree. It is a rare disorder in the Western world with the majority of cases reported in Japan.[78,79] It is a sporadic occurrence and there are no reported cases of recurrence within a family. The cause of the dilatation is controversial and may be due to weakness in the duct wall, distal obstruction causing increased pressure and hence proximal dilatation or a combination of both factors.

Associated anomalies No specific associations have been described.

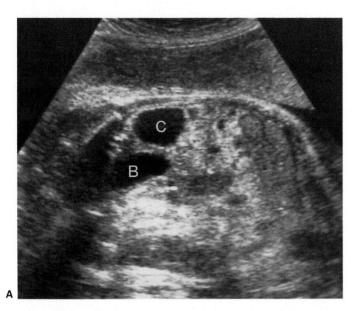

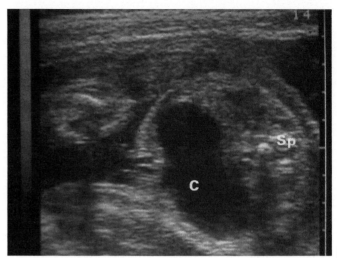

Fig. 18   Ovarian cyst. A: Longitudinal view of a fetus with an ovarian cyst showing normal bladder (B) with a large ovarian cyst (C) arising from the pelvis. **B:** Transverse scan in another case showing a large central lower abdominal cyst. Sp – spine.

Diagnosis   There are several reports of prenatal diagnosis of choledochal cyst.[80-83] The diagnosis was suggested by the visualisation of an echo-free, non-pulsatile area in the right of the fetal abdomen near the portal vein. In two cases the diagnosis was confirmed by defining dilated hepatic ducts near or leading to the cyst.[81,83]

The differential diagnosis includes duodenal atresia and cysts in other intra-abdominal organs such as the liver, mesentery, omentum and ovary. The definition of normal abdominal organs together with the absence of poly-hydramnios, peristalsis in the cyst or a connection with the stomach helps exclude other diagnoses, but a definitive diagnosis is dependent on the visualisation of a tubular structure arising from the cyst passing into the liver parenchyma.

Management and prognosis   Choledochal cysts are usually detected in the third trimester and there seems to be no indication to alter standard obstetric practise. If the findings are confirmed in the neonate then surgery is indicated as untreated cysts can lead to progressive biliary cirrhosis and portal hypertension.[79] A 10% operative mortality is reported.[78]

Ovarian cysts

Definition and aetiology   Ovarian cysts are quite rare with less than 100 neonatal cases reported. They are usually unilateral and vary in size from a few millimetres in diameter to a large cyst which fills the entire abdomen. The majority are benign simple cysts such as theca lutein cysts or corpus luteal cysts, although granulosa cell tumours and teratomas have been reported in neonates.[84]

Associated abnormalities   There is one case reported with associated hydrocephalus and agenesis of the corpus callosum.[85] In other cases hypothyroidism has been diagnosed in the children with ovarian cysts.[86]

Diagnosis   This diagnosis has been reported several times, usually late in the second or third trimester, and may be suspected when a female fetus has an intra-abdominal cystic lesion which is separate from the renal or gastrointestinal tracts.[85,87-90] They may be septate or unilocular and typically arise from the pelvis or lower abdomen. They are usually unilateral, although bilateral cases have been reported, and may measure up to several centimetres in diameter (Fig. 18). Resolution in utero has been reported.[90] The differential diagnosis includes urachal and mesenteric cysts, duodenal atresia and duplication cysts and dilated bowel. Absence of peristaltic movements helps exclude dilated bowel and absence of the typical 'double bubble' makes duodenal atresia an unlikely diagnosis. A urachal cyst is single and lies in the anterior part of the fetal abdomen extending from the bladder to the umbilicus. It may be impossible to exclude the diagnosis of other intra-abdominal cystic lesions prenatally (Fig. 19).

Management and prognosis   Serial ultrasound examinations are recommended to monitor the growth of the cyst. Provided it remains small standard obstetric practise can be followed, but where the cyst grows to very large proportions there is a risk of dystocia or rupture during vaginal delivery. In such a case an elective caesarean section is a reasonable approach. Alternatively, ultrasound guided aspiration of the cyst can be undertaken, despite the remote risk of spillage of an irritant or malignant fluid into the abdominal cavity.

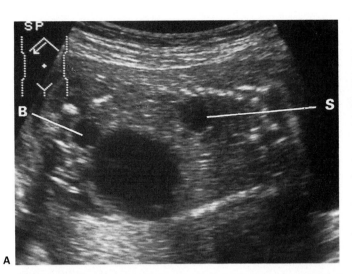
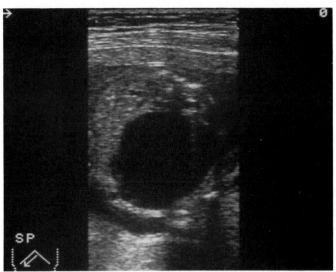

Fig. 19 Duplication cyst. A: Longitudinal and **B:** transverse views of a 20 week female fetus with what was thought prenatally to be an ovarian cyst and which was drained several times during pregnancy. Post-natally at laparotomy this was found to be a duodenal duplication cyst, thus demonstrating the difficulty in correctly identifying some intra-abdominal cystic lesions with ultrasound. Note the normal stomach (S) and bladder (B).

The overall prognosis for a fetus with an ovarian cyst is good since the majority are benign and many will resolve spontaneously. In the neonate large cysts can infarct, undergo torsion, cause ascites, rupture, bleed or cause intestinal obstruction. Torsion in utero has been reported in the case of a large cyst.[90]

Other intra-abdominal cysts

Definition and aetiology These include cysts which are found in the mesentery of the large or small bowel (mesenteric cysts) (Fig. 20), cysts of the omentum (omental cysts) and cysts which are located in the retroperitoneal space (retroperitoneal cysts). They are all rare with mesenteric cysts occurring more commonly than omental cysts which are more frequent than retroperitoneal cysts.[91] The cause of these cysts is unclear, they are generally considered to be lymphatic hamartomas. They are usually single and multilocular and can vary in size from a few millimetres to several centimetres. The fluid they contain may be serous, chlyous or haemorrhagic.

Associated abnormalities There are no recognised associations reported.

Diagnosis These cysts should be considered in the differential diagnosis of any intra-abdominal cystic lesion. Other potential diagnoses include ovarian, pancreatic, choledochal and hepatic cysts and duodenal atresia. In a female the most likely diagnosis is that of an ovarian cyst. Other diagnoses can be excluded by careful delineation of abdominal organs, but it may prove impossible to make a precise diagnosis prenatally. A mesenteric cyst may cause unilateral hydronephrosis by obstructing the ureter (Fig. 20).

Management and prognosis. These cysts are often asymptomatic and found incidentally at surgery for some other indication. The clinical manifestation of the cysts depends on their size and location. Most are benign but malignant degeneration has been described in adulthood.[92] Retroperitoneal cysts have a high tendency to recur as complete excision is difficult due to their close proximity to major blood vessels.[92]

Serial ultrasound examinations should be performed in order to monitor the size of the cysts prenatally. Unless the cysts grow to such proportions that there may be a danger of rupture during a vaginal delivery, standard obstetric practise should be followed. Aspiration may be considered to avoid caesarean section.

Hepatosplenomegaly

Incidence and aetiology Isolated hepatomegaly or splenomegaly are rare and they more commonly occur together in a variety of conditions. Some of the more common causes in the neonate are given in Table 1. They include immune and non-immune hydrops, haemolytic anaemias, congenital infections, metabolic disorders and neoplastic conditions. Hepatosplenomegaly also occurs as part of the Beckwith-Wiedemann and Pearlman syndromes.

Associated abnormalities The associated abnormalities vary according to the underlying pathology.

Diagnosis Hepatosplenomegaly is diagnosed when

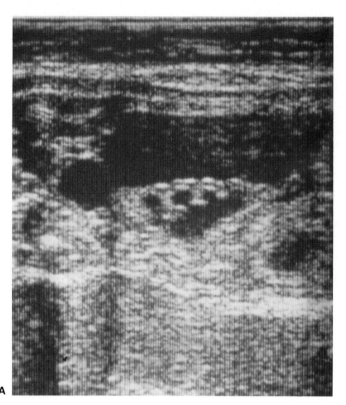

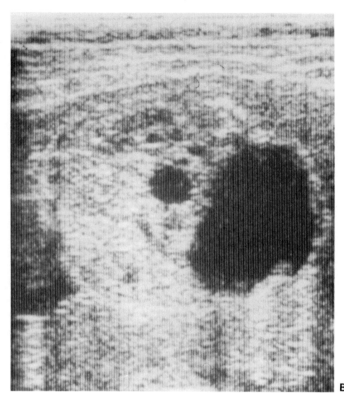

Fig. 20   A and B: Mesenteric cyst causing mild unilateral hydronephrosis.

their sizes lie outside the 95 percentile on the nomograms which exist for evaluation of their size (see Appendix).[93,94]

Tumours can cause diffuse enlargement or a change in the sonographic appearance of all or part of the liver. Calcification within the liver suggests congenital infection or

hepatoblastoma. In the latter case the MSAFP is raised in over 80% of cases. Congenital infections may also cause other structural abnormalities in the fetus (microcephaly, congenital heart defects) which can be detectable with ultrasound. An isolated echo-poor area within the liver may be a solitary cyst or an hepatic haemangioma, a benign tumour which can also give the appearance of a well-circumscribed, homogeneous intrahepatic mass.

Hepatosplenomegaly when found in conjunction with enlarged kidneys, a generally macrosomic fetus and particularly if associated with polyhydramnios, suggests the Beckwith-Wiedemann or Pearlman syndromes. However, in low risk cases it is not possible to make a definite diagnosis based on ultrasound findings alone.

Management and prognosis   Definitive diagnosis will often have to await the results of postnatal investigations. Haemolytic anaemias can be diagnosed either by cordocentesis or by analysis of the bilirubin content of amniotic fluid. Congenital infections can be detected by performing the appropriate tests on maternal serum (VDRL, serum titres for relevant antibodies) or on fetal blood (specific IgM, liver function tests etc.). Where there is a positive family history many of the metabolic disorders can be diagnosed by analysis of amniotic fluid or fetal blood.

The prognosis will depend on the aetiology of the hepatosplenomegaly.

Table 1   Causes of neonatal hepatosplenomegaly

Cause	Hepatomegaly	Splenomegaly
Bacterial infection	+	+
Viral infection	+	+
Toxoplasmosis	+	+
Syphilis	+	+
Congenital haemolytic anaemia	+	+
Isoimmunisation	+	+
Congestive heart failure	+	+
Leukaemia	–	+
Lymphoma	–	+
Haemangioma	+	+
Hamartoma	+	+
Hepatoblastoma	+	–
Metastatic tumour	+	–
Benign cyst	+	+
Galactosaemia	+	+
Zellweger syndrome	+	+
Other metabolic disorders	+	+
Beckwith-Weidemann syndrome	+	+
Pearlman syndrome	+	–

Situs inversus

Situs inversus can be detected in utero if the left and right side of the fetus are established by reference to the positions of the head and spine. If situs inversus abdominis is identified, special attention should be given to the cardiovascular anatomy (see Ch. 19).

REFERENCES

1 Baird P A, MacDonald E C. An epidemiologic study of congenital malformations of the anterior abdominal wall in more than half a million consecutive live births. Am J Hum Genet 1981; 33: 470–478

2. Carpenter M W, Curci M R, Dibbins A W, Haddow. Perinatal management of ventral wall defects. Obstet Gynecol 1984; 64: 646–651

3 Grosfield J L, Dawes L, Weber T R. Congenital abdominal wall defects: current management and survival. Surg Clin North Am 1981; 61: 1037–1049

4 Mayer T, Black R, Matlak M E, Johnson D G. Gastroschisis and omphalocele: an eight-year review. Ann Surg 1980; 192: 783–787

5 Hauge M, Bugge M, Nielson J. Early prenatal diagnosis of omphalocele constitutes indication for amniocentesis. Lancet 1983; ii: 507

6 Mann L, Ferguson-Smith M A, Desai M, Gibson A A M, Raine P A M. Prenatal assessment of anterior abdominal wall defects and their prognosis. Prenat Diagn 1984; 4: 427–435

7 Gilbert W M, Nicolaides K H. Fetal omphalocele: associated malformations and chromosomal defects. Obstet Gynecol 1987; 70: 633–635

8 Nivelon-Chevallier A, Mavel A, Michels R, et al. Familial Beckwith-Wiedemann syndrome: prenatal echography diagnosis and histologic confirmation. J Genet Hum 1983; 5: 397

9 Mabogunje O A, Mahour G H. Omphalocele and gastroschisis. Trends in survival across two decades. Am J Surg 148: 679–686

10 Winter R M, Knowles S A S, Bieber F R, Baraitser M, Body wall defects. In: The malformed fetus and stillbirth: a diagnostic approach. Chichester: John Wiley. 1980: p 134–143

11 Smith D W. Recognizable patterns of human malformation. Genetic, embryologic and clinical aspects. 3rd Edition. Philadelphia: W B Saunders. 1984: p 130–132

12 Koontz W L, Shaw L A, Lavery J P. Antenatal sonographic appearance of Beckwith-Wiedemann syndrome. JCU 1986; 14: 57–59

13 Rott H D, Truckenbrodt H. Familial occurrence of omphalocele. Hum Genet 1974; 24: 259–260

14 Havalad S, Noblett H, Spiedel B D. Familial occurrence of omphalocele, suggesting sex-linked inheritance. Arch Dis Child 1979; 54: 142–151

15 Osuna A, Lindham S. Four cases of omphalocele in two generations of the same family. Clin Genet 1976; 9: 354–356

16 Harrison M R, Golbus M S, Filly R A. Management of the fetus with an abdominal wall defect. In: Orlando F L. ed. The unborn patient. Prenatal diagnosis and treatment. New York: Grune and Stratton. 1984: p 217–234

17 Kirk E P, Wah R M. Obstetric management of the fetus with omphalocele or gastroschisis: a review and report of one hundred and twelve cases. Am J Obstet Gynecol 1983; 146: 512–518

18 Bair J H, Russ P D, Pretoious D H, Manchester D, Manco-Johnson M L. Fetal omphalocele and gastroschisis: a review of 24 cases. AJR 1986; 147: 1047–1051

19 Davidson J M, Johnson T R B, Rigdon D T, Thompson B H. Gastroschisis and omphalocele: prenatal diagnosis and perinatal management. Prenat Diagn 1984; 4: 355–363

20 Romero R, Pilu G, Jeanty P, Ghidini A, Hobbins J C. Prenatal diagnosis of congenital anomalies. Norwalk: Appleton and Lange. 1988

21 Gryboski J, Walker W A. Gastrointestinal problems in the infant. Philadelphia: W B Saunders. 1983: p 284–287

22 Lindfors K K, McGahan J P, Walter J P. Fetal omphalocele and gastroschisis: pitfalls in sonographic diagnosis. AJR 1986; 147: 797–800

23 Potter E L, Craig J M. Diaphragmatic and abdominal hernias. In: Pathology of the fetus and infant. Chicago: Year Book. 1975: p 374–392

24 Lockwood C J, Scioscia A L, Hobbins J C. Congenital absence of the umbilical cord resulting from maldevelopment of the embryonic body folding. Am J Obstet Gynecol 1986; 155: 1049–1051

25 Jauniaux E, Vyas S, Finlayson C, Moscoso G, Driver M, Campbell S. Early sonographic diagnosis of body stalk anomaly. Prenat Diagn 1990; 10: 127–132

26 Jeffs R D, Lepor H. Management of the extrophy-epispadias complex and urachal anomalies. In: Walsh P C. ed. Campbell's Urology. Vol 2. Philadelphia: Saunders. 1986: p 1882–1921

27 Graivier L. Extrophy of the cloaca. Am Surg 1968; 34: 387–390

28 Ives E, Coffey R, Carter C O. A family study of bladder extrophy. J Med Genet 1980; 17: 139–141

29 Shapiro E, Lepor H, Jeffs R D. The inheritance of the extrophy epispadias complex. J Urol 1984; 132: 308–310

30 Muecke E C. Extrophy, epispadias and other anomalies of the bladder. In: Walsh P C. ed. Campbell's Urology. Vol 2. Philadelphia: W B Saunders. 1986: p 1856–1880

31 Soper R T, Kilger K. Vesico-intestinal fissure. J Urol 1964; 92: 490–501

32 Howell C, Caldamone A, Snyder H, Ziegler M, Duckett J. Optimal management of cloacal extrophy. J Pediatr Surg 1983; 18: 365–369

33 Mirk P, Calisti A, Fileni A. Prenatal sonographic diagnosis of bladder extrophy. J Ultrasound Med 1936; 5: 291–293

34 Kutzner D K, Wilson W G, Hogge W A. OEIS complex (cloacal extrophy); prenatal diagnosis in the second trimester. Prenat Diagn 1988; 8: 247–253

35 Tank E S, Lindenauer S M. Principles of management of extrophy of the cloaca. Am J Surg 1980; 119: 95–98

36 David T J, O'Callaghan S E. Oesophageal atresia in the South-West of England. J Med Genet 1975; 12: 1–11

37 Chittmittrapap S, Spitz L, Kiely E M, Brereton R J. Oesophageal atresia and associated anomalies. Arch Dis Child 1989; 64: 364–368

38 Winter R M. Knowles S A S, Bieber F R, Baraitser M. Abnormalities of the gastrointestinal tract. In: The malformed fetus and stillbirth. Chichester: John Wiley. 1988: p 140–143

39 Smith F G, Berg J M. eds. Down's anomaly. Edinburgh: Churchill Livingstone. 1986: p 14–41

40 Eyheremendy E, Pfister M. Antenatal real-time diagnosis of esophageal atresias. JCU 1983; 11: 395–397

41 Zemlyn S. Prenatal detection of esophageal atresia. JCU 1981; 9: 453–454

42 Rahmani M R, Zalev A H. Antenatal detection of esophageal atresia with distal tracheoesophageal fistula. JCU 1986; 14: 143–145

43 Gryboski J, Walker M A. Gastrointestinal problems in the infant. Philadelphia: W B Saunders. 1983: p 151–214

44 Fonkalsrud E W. Duodenal atresia or stenosis. In: Bergsma D. ed. Birth defects compendium. New York: Alan R. Liss. 1979: p 350

45 Fonkalsrud E W, deLorimier A A, Hays D N. Congenital atresia and stenosis of the duodenum. A review compiled from members of the surgical section of the American Academy of Pediatrics. Pediatrics 1969; 43: 79–83

46 Young D G, Wilkinson A W. Abnormalities associated with neonatal duodenal obstruction. Surgery 1968; 63: 832–836

47 Aubrespy P, Derlon S, Seriat-Gautier B. Congenital duodenal obstruction: a review of 82 cases. Prog Pediatr Surg 1982; 11: 109–123

48 Atwell J D, Klijian A M. Vertebral anomalies and duodenal atresia. J Pediatr Surg 1982; 17: 237–240

49 Nicolaides K H, Campbell S. Diagnosis and management of fetal malformations. Baillière's Clinical Obstet Gynaecol 1: 1987; 591–622

50 Romero R, Ghidini A, Costigan K, Touloukian R, Hobbins J C. Prenatal diagnosis of duodenal atresia: does it make any difference? Obstet Gynecol 1988; 71: 739–741

51 Louw J H. Investigations into the etiology of congenital atresia of the colon. Dis Colon Rectum 1964; 7: 471–478

52 Bernstein J, Vawter G, Harris G B C, Young V, Hillman L S. The occurrence of intestinal atresia in newborns with meconium ileus. Am J Dis Child 1960; 99: 804–818

53 De Lorimier A, Fonkalsrud E W, Hays D M. Congenital atresia and stenosis of the jejunum and ileum. Pediatr Surg 1969; 65: 819–827

54 Muller F, Aubry M C, Gasser B, Duchatel F, Boue J, Boue A. Prenatal diagnosis of cystic fibrosis. II. Meconium ileus in affected fetuses. Prenat Diagn 1985; 5: 109–117

55 Blott M, Greenough A, Gamsu H R, Nicolaides K N, Campbell S. Antenatal factors associated with obstruction of the gastrointestinal tract by meconium. BMJ 1988; 296: 250

56 Guttman F M, Braun P, Garance P H, et al. Multiple atresias and a new syndrome of hereditary multiple atresias involving the gastrointestinal tract from stomach to rectum. J Pediatr Surg 1973; 8: 633–640

57 Kao K J, Fleischer R, Bradford W D, Woodward B H. Multiple congenital septal atresias of the intestine: histomorphologic and pathogenic implications. Pediatr Pathol 1983; 1: 443–448

58 Kjoller M, Holm-Nielson G, Meiland H, Mauritzen K, Berget A, Hancke S. Prenatal obstruction of the ileum diagnosed by ultrasound. Prenat Diagn 1985; 5: 427–430

59 Lloyd I R, Chatsworth H W. Hydramnios as an aid to the early diagnosis of congenital obstruction of the alimentary tract. A study of the maternal and fetal factors. Pediatrics 1958; 24: 903–909

60 Shalev J, Navon R, Urbach D, Mashiach S, Goldman B. Intestinal obstruction and cystic fibrosis: antenatal ultrasound appearance. J Med Genet 1983; 20: 229–233

61 Freeman N V. Congenital atresia and stenosis of the colon. Br J Surg 1966; 53: 595–599

62 Ravitch M M, Barton B A. The need for pediatric surgeons as determined by the volume of work and the mode of delivery of surgical care. Surgery 1974; 76: 754–763

63 Vermesch M, Mayden K L, Confino E, Giglia R V, Gleicher N. Prenatal sonographic diagnosis of Hirschprung's disease. J Ultrasound Med 1986; 5: 37–39

64 Carter C O, Evans K, Hickman V. Children of those treated surgically for Hirschsprung's disease. J Med Genet 1981; 18: 87–90

65 Winter R M, Knowles S, Bieber F R, Baraitser M. Genital and anal malformations. In: The malformed fetus and stillbirth: a diagnostic approach. Chichester: John Wiley. 1988: p 160–165

66 Bean W J, Calonje M A, Aprill C N, Geshner J. Anal atresia: a prenatal ultrasound diagnosis. JCU 1978; 6: 111–112

67 Blumenthal D H, Rushovich A M, Williams R K, Rochester D. Prenatal sonographic findings of meconium peritonitis with pathologic correlation. JCU 1982; 10: 350–352

68 Schwimer S R, Vanley G T, Reinke R T. Prenatal diagnosis of cystic meconium peritonitis. JCU 1984; 12: 37–39

69 Bergsmans M G M, Merkus J M W, Baars A M. Obstetrical and neonatal aspects of a child with atresia of the small bowel. J Perinat Med 1984; 12: 325

70 Finkel L I, Solvis T L. Meconium peritonitis, intraperitoneal calcifications and cystic fibrosis. Pediatr Radiol 1982; 12: 92–93

71 Brock D J H, Bedgood D, Barron L, Hayward C. Prospective prenatal diagnosis of cystic fibrosis. Lancet 1985; 1: 1175–1178

72 Riordan J R, Rommens J M, Kaerem B, et al. Identification of the cystic fibrosis gene: cloning and characterisation of complementary DNA. Science 1989; 245: 1066–1072

73 Baxi L V, Yeh M N, Blanc W A, Schillinger J N. Antepartum diagnosis and management of in utero intestinal volvulus with perforation. N Engl J Med 1983; 308: 1519–1521

74 Clair M R, Rosenberg E R, Ram P C, Bowie J D. Prenatal sonographic diagnosis of meconium peritonitis. Prenat Diagn 1983; 3: 65–68

75 Garb M, Rad F F, Riseborough J. Meconium peritonitis presenting as fetal ascites on ultrasound. Br J Radiol 1980; 53: 602–604

76 Lauer J D, Cradock T V. Meconium pseudocyst: prenatal sonographic and radiologic correlation. J Ultrasound Med 1982; 1: 333–335

77 McGahan J P, Hanson F. Meconium peritonitis with accompanying pseudocyst; prenatal sonographic diagnosis. Radiology 1983; 148: 125–126

78 Yamaguchi M. Congenital choledochal cyst. Analysis of 1433 cases in the Japanese literature. Am J Surg 1980; 140: 653–657

79 Gryboski J, Walker W A. Gastrointestinal problems in the infant. Philadelphia: WB Saunders. 1983: p 309–312

80 Dewbury K C, Aluwihare A P R, Chir M, Birch S J, Freeman N V. Case reports. Prenatal ultrasound demonstration of a choledochal cyst. Br J Radiol 1980; 53: 906–907

81 Elrad H, Mayden K L, Ahart S, Giglia R, Gleicher N. Prenatal ultrasound diagnosis of choledochal cyst. J Ultrasound Med 1985; 4: 553–555

82 Frank J L, Hill M C, Chirathivat S, Sfakianakis G N, Marchildon M. Antenatal observation of a choledochal cyst by sonography. AJR 1981; 137: 166–168

83 Howell C G, Templeton J M, Weiner S. Glassman M, Betts J M, Witzleben. Antenatal diagnosis and early surgery for choledochal cyst. J Pediatr Surg 1983; 18: 387–393

84 Carlson D H, Griscom N T. Ovarian cysts in the newborn. AJR 1972; 116: 664–672

85 Sandler M A, Smith S J, Pope S G, Madrazo B L. Prenatal diagnosis of septated ovarian cysts. JCU 1985; 13: 55–57

86 Evers J L, Rolland R. Primary hypothyroidism and ovarian activity: evidence for an overlap in the synthesis of pituitary glycoproteins. Case report. Br J Obstet Gynaecol 1981; 88: 195–202

87 Tabsh K M A. Antenatal sonographic appearance of a fetal ovarian cyst. J Ultrasound Med 1982; 1: 329–331

88 Preziosi P, Fariello G, Maiorana A, Malena S, Ferro F. Antenatal sonographic diagnosis of complicated ovarian cysts. JCU 1986; 14: 196–198

89 Holzgreve W, Winde B, Willital G H, Beller F K. Prenatal diagnosis and perinatal management of a fetal ovarian cyst. Prenat Diagn 1985; 5: 155–158

90 Rizzo N, Gabrielli S, Perolo A, et al. Prenatal diagnosis and management of fetal ovarian cysts. Prenat Diagn 1989; 9: 97–104

91 Vanek V W, Phillips A K. Retroperitoneal, mesenteric and omental cysts. Arch Surg 1984; 119: 838–842

92 Kurtz R J, Heinmann T M, Beck A R, Holt J. Mesenteric and retroperitoneal cysts. Ann Surg 1986; 203: 109–112

93 Schmidt W, Yarkoni S, Jeanty P, et al. Sonographic measurements of the fetal spleen: clinical implications. J Ultrasound Med 1985; 4: 667

94 Vintzileos A M, Neckles S, Campbell W A, et al. Fetal liver ultrasound measurements during normal pregnancy. Obstet Gynecol 1985; 66: 47

19

The heart

Lindsey D. Allan

INTRODUCTION

Cardiac motion has been identified in the fetus by ultrasound for many years, but it was not until 1980 that advances in the resolution of real time equipment were sufficient to allow clear visualisation of the structure of the moving heart. As a result, the cross-sectional appearance of the fetal heart was described by several authors almost simultaneously.[1,2,3] Since then, imaging systems have further improved such that a high degree of diagnostic accuracy in the detection of cardiac disease can be achieved from the mid-trimester of pregnancy onwards.[4] The addition of pulsed and colour flow Doppler adds further information to the cross-sectional images.

Congenital heart disease is now the most common congenital anomaly in children but despite enormous advances in paediatric cardiac surgery over the last 20 years, the outlook for children with many forms of disease remains poor. In addition, although the short-term results for cardiac surgery in children are improving, data on the long-term results are still very incomplete. There are, at present, too few adults with 'corrected' congenital heart disease of the more complex forms to analyse features such as late complications, quality of life and life span. Heart disease affects about 8 in 1000 live births, about three of these eight being severe malformations. A classification of the most important forms of prenatal heart disease is shown in Table 1.

Table 1 Classification of congenital heart disease

Abnormalities of connection	
Right heart	**Left heart**
At the venous-atrial junction	
Interrupted inferior vena cava	Total anomalous pulmonary venous drainage*
At the atrioventricular junction	
Tricuspid atresia*	Mitral atresia*
Atrioventricular septal defect*	
Double inlet ventricle*	
At the ventriculo-arterial junction	
Pulmonary atresia*	Aortic atresia*
Tetralogy of Fallot	
Common arterial trunk	
Transposition of the great arteries	
Double outlet ventricle	
Additional abnormalities	
Pulmonary stenosis (*if severe)	Aortic stenosis (*if severe)
Tricuspid dysplasia*	Interrupted aortic arch*
Ebstein's anomaly*	Coarctation of the aorta*
Tumour*	
Ventricular septal defect (*if large)	
Ectopia cordis*	
Conjoint twins*	

*indicates anomalies in which the four chamber view would be abnormal

The prognosis for survival of children with heart disease can be roughly divided into three groups; good surgical results with less than 20% mortality, a reasonable outlook with successful surgery with about a 30% to 50% mortality, and a mortality with or without surgery of 60% to 100%. In the first group are conditions such as septal defects, coarctation of the aorta, the tetralogy of Fallot and transposition of the great arteries. In the second group are conditions such as atrioventricular septal defects, interrupted aortic arch, double outlet right ventricle and tricuspid atresia. In the last group are severe conditions such as the hypoplastic left ventricle, common arterial trunk, double inlet connection, mitral and pulmonary atresia. Under each diagnostic heading there are also varying grades of severity. Lesions additional to the main abnormality can place the case in a worse category of prognosis. Many, although not all, of the echocardiographic details can be defined prenatally allowing accurate prognosis. However, some forms of heart disease, for example coarctation of the aorta, can progress during gestation to become less amenable to surgery as pregnancy advances.[5]

The most easily obtained view of the fetal heart is the four chamber view. Identifying the normality of this one section will exclude many major defects or alternatively detect abnormality in about 2 in 1000 pregnancies. Including the recognition of this view in a routine ultrasound examination allows for screening the whole pregnant population for major forms of congenital heart disease.[6] Once this section can be reliably obtained in every patient, the ultrasonographer can attempt to recognise the more difficult arterial views.

NORMAL FETAL CARDIAC ANATOMY

Major cardiac malformations affect the connections of the heart. Basically, the heart is made up of six connections, three on each side of the heart. These are: the atria, which receive the venous drainage, the ventricles and the great arteries.

On the right side of the heart, the inferior and superior vena cavae drain to the right atrium, which then connects through the tricuspid valve to the right ventricle. The pulmonary artery then arises from the right ventricle. On the left side of the heart, the left atrium receives the pulmonary veins. The left atrium connects via the mitral valve to the left ventricle which then gives rise to the aorta.

Once the method to image all these connections is learnt, major forms of heart disease can be excluded. Heart defects which do not involve a connection abnormality are usually relatively minor defects with a good chance of successful correction, although many can be recognised prenatally. However, it is mainly the more severe forms of heart disease which are important to diagnose in fetal life.

TECHNIQUE

The four chamber view

Examination of this view will demonstrate the pulmonary veins and atria, the atrioventricular connections and the two ventricles. Thus, in this one view alone, three of the six connections are seen and clues to the normality of the great arteries can be identified. This, therefore, is an important view to master completely and thoroughly. It should be identifiable in every patient from 18 weeks gestation onwards with generally available real time equipment. The operator should become so familiar with this section that failure to obtain a normal appearance of the four chambers of the heart necessitates referral for a specialised heart scan.

The four chambers of the heart are seen in a horizontal section of the fetal thorax just above the level of the diaphragm (Fig. 1). The heart lies mainly in the left chest with the apex pointing out to the left anterior chest wall. The normal position of the heart within the thorax and in

relation to the spine must become absolutely familiar, whatever the fetal position.

The same method of orientation is always used in order to identify the cardiac chambers. In Figure 2 and Plate 1, the first step is to locate the spine. Opposite the spine is the anterior chest wall or sternum. Deep to the sternum is the right ventricle. Returning to the spine, the descending aorta is seen as a circle in the mediastinum lying anterior to the spine. Related to the aorta anteriorly is the left atrium. The remaining intracardiac chambers, the right atrium and left ventricle can then be identified.

The appearance of the four chamber view will vary according to the orientation of the fetus to the ultrasound beam. Figure 2 and Plate 1 illustrate the image obtained when the apex of the heart is closest to the transducer, Plate 1 showing the advantages of colour flow mapping by demonstrating forward flow into the ventricles coloured red. If the view is correctly orientated the flow into each side should appear equal. When the fetus is in this position, the beam is parallel to the inter-ventricular septum. Compare Figure 2 with Figure 3 where the fetus lies with the right chest anterior and the beam is perpendicular to the septum. When the fetus lies with either the left or right back anterior, the view will be less clear but still recognisable (Fig. 4). No matter how the fetus is lying, the important points can always be seen in the normal heart. They are:

1) the heart occupies about a third of the thorax;
2) there are two atria of approximately equal size;
3) there are two ventricles of approximately equal size and thickness. Both show equal contraction in the moving image;

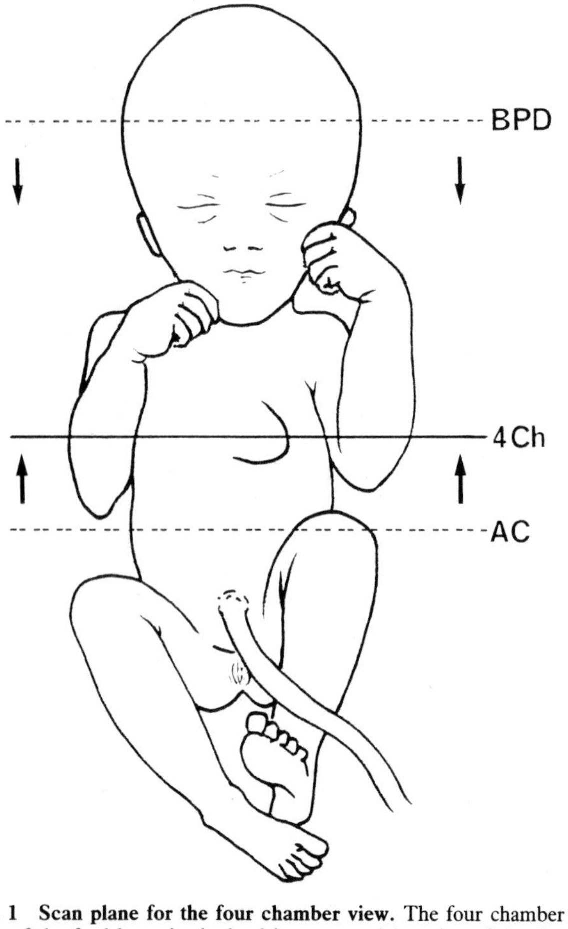

Fig. 1 Scan plane for the four chamber view. The four chamber view of the fetal heart is obtained in a transaxial section of the thorax, just above the diaphragm (4Ch). BPD – biparietal diameter, AC – abdominal circumference.

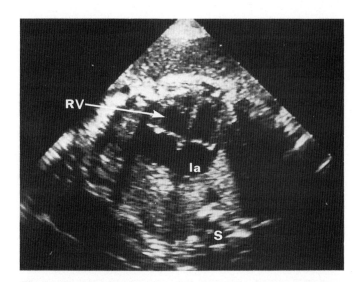

Fig. 2 The four chamber view. This fetus is in an ideal position with the apex of the heart closest to the transducer. The ultrasound beam is parallel to the inter-ventricular septum in this orientation. RV – right ventricle, la – left atrium, S – spine.

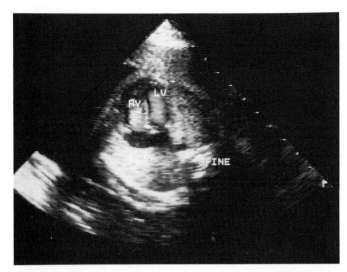

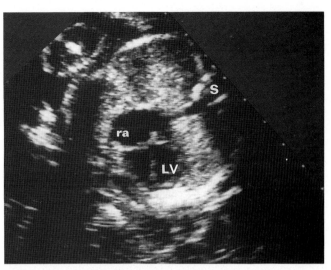

Plate 1   **The four chamber view.** The apex of the heart is closest to the transducer. The colour flow map shows equal forward flow, coded in red, into both ventricles through the mitral and tricuspid values. RV – right ventricle, LV – left ventricle. This figure is reproduced in colour in the colour plate section at the front of this volume.

Fig. 4   The right back of the fetus is lying anteriorly such that the fetal heart is at the opposite side of the chest from the transducer. LV – left ventricle, ra – right atrium, S – spine. The image quality when the fetus is in this position will be at its poorest but the normal features are still recognisable. Note that when the beam is parallel to the septum, as it is here, the thin membranous portion of the septum just below the atrioventricular valves may not be visualised. This should not be mistaken for a ventricular septal defect.

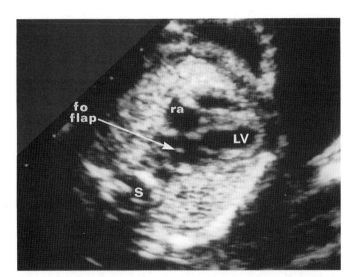

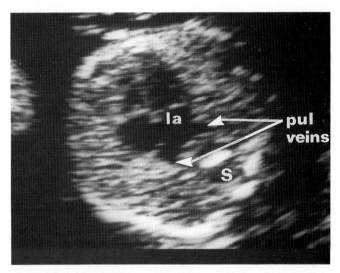

Fig. 3   The fetus is lying with the right anterior thorax nearest the transducer such that the beam is now perpendicular to the septum. LV – left ventricle, ra – right atrium, fo – foramen ovale, S – spine.

Fig. 5   Two of the pulmonary veins are seen entering the back of the left atrium (la). S – spine.

4) the atrial and ventricular septa meet the two atrioventricular valves at the crux of the heart in an offset cross;
5) two opening atrioventricular valves are seen in the moving image.

It should be noted that these rules are true of the fetal heart until about 32 weeks gestation. After this time, the right ventricle may look slightly larger than the left in the normal fetus. The reason the cross at the centre of the heart is not 'straight', is that the septal leaflet of the tricuspid valve inserts slightly lower in the ventricular septum than the mitral valve. Scanning up and down in the four chamber projection will demonstrate the pulmonary veins entering the back of the left atrium (Fig. 5).

Imaging the great arteries

The great arteries can be imaged in a variety of projections[7] but only four of the views will be described here. The transaxial views of the great vessels are usually the easiest to obtain but may be difficult to understand at first. The longitudinal views are more familiar to those used to post-natal cardiac imaging. Moving cranially from the four chamber view, maintaining a horizontal projection, the aorta can be seen arising in the centre of the chest from the left ventricle (Fig. 6). This artery sweeps out to the right of the thorax at its origin. The horizontal section cranial to this plane will visualise the pulmonary artery. This artery arises anteriorly, close to the chest wall and is directed straight back towards the spine. The right ventricular outflow tract, the pulmonary valve, main and right pulmonary artery and the ductal junction with the descending aorta can be seen in this view (Fig. 7). The

ascending aorta is seen in cross-section as a circle. Slightly further cranially, the crest of the arch of the aorta can be seen in the inlet of the thorax (Fig. 8). A diagrammatic

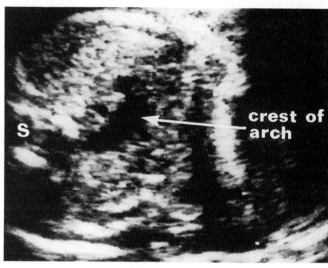

Fig. 8 The crest of the arch of the aorta is seen in front of the spine (S) in the inlet of the thorax.

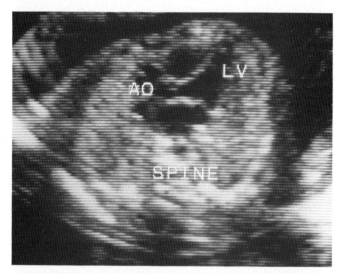

Fig. 6 In a horizontal section above the four chamber view the origin of the aorta (AO) from the left ventricle (LV) can be seen.

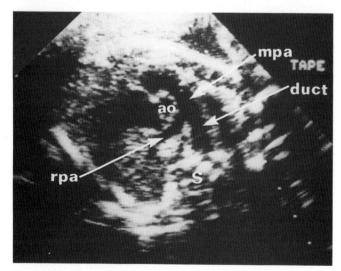

Fig. 7 The main pulmonary artery (mpa) arises from close to the anterior chest wall and divides in front of the spine (S) into the duct and right pulmonary artery (rpa). ao – aorta.

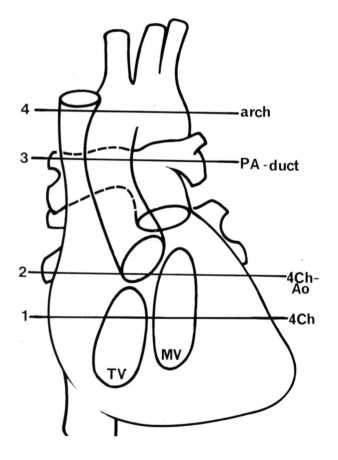

Fig. 9 The cardiac skeleton is illustrated diagrammatically. Section 1 images the four chamber view, section 2 the origin of the aorta, section 3 the origin of the pulmonary artery, section 4 the crest of the arch. TV – tricuspid valve, MV – mitral valve.

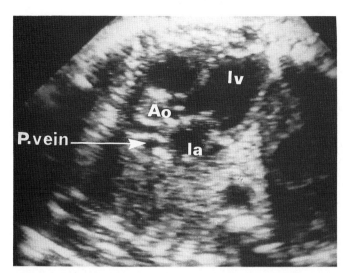

Fig. 10 The long axis view of the left ventricle is seen which illustrates all the left heart connections; the pulmonary vein (P. vein) to left atrium (la), the mitral valve between the left atrium and left ventricle (lv) and the aorta (Ao) arising from the left ventricle.

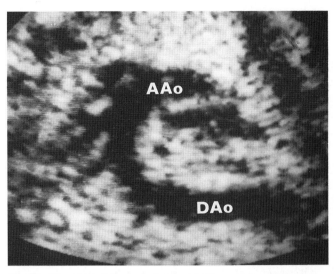

Fig. 12 The arch of the aorta is imaged. The aorta normally arises in the centre of the thorax and forms a tight hook shape with the head and neck vessels arising from the crest of the arch. AAo – ascending aorta, DAo – descending aorta.

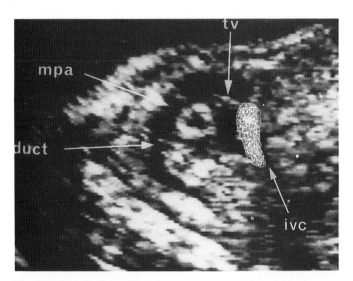

Fig. 11 This section of the fetus demonstrates the right heart connections; the inferior vena cava (ivc) entering the right atrium, the tricuspid valve (tv) between the right atrium and ventricle, the origin of the pulmonary artery (mpa) from the right ventricle and its connection to the duct.

representation of the transducer position relative to the intracardiac structures in these sections is seen in Figure 9. Figure 10 illustrates the long axis view of the left ventricle, which is achieved by tilting the transducer from the horizontal position. Transducer angulation in the other direction will allow the right heart connections to be seen (Fig. 11). The aortic arch can also be imaged in a longitudinal section of the fetus (Fig. 12). The important features to note in these views are:

1) two arterial valves can always be seen;

2) the aorta arises wholly from the left ventricle;
3) the pulmonary artery at the valve ring is slightly bigger than the aorta;
4) the pulmonary valve is anterior and cranial to the aortic valve;
5) at their origins the great arteries lie at right angles to, and cross over, each other;
6) the arch of the aorta is of similar size to the pulmonary artery and duct and is complete.

If all these normal features are seen, major anomalies of the great arteries can be excluded.

CARDIAC MALFORMATIONS

Abnormalities of connection

These can occur at the veno-atrial, the atrioventricular or the ventriculo-arterial connection. Any of the connections may be absent (or atretic), displaced (or inappropriate).

The veno-atrial junction

The venous connection on the right side of the heart, the inferior vena cava, is rarely abnormal. When it is absent, this is usually associated with complex heart disease, which would be recognised from other features. For this reason it is not essential to identify this structure in a normal study.

Total anomalous pulmonary venous drainage Absence of the pulmonary venous connection, however, is important to recognise. In the isolated form it is an uncommon defect constituting about 2% of post-natal cardiac abnormalities.[8] The prenatal features include right ventricular dilatation and failure to identify the normal insertion of the pulmonary veins. There are three possible anatomical sites for anomalous venous drainage, supracardiac, infracardiac or the coronary sinus. The echocardiographic appearance will depend on the site of drainage. Where total anomalous pulmonary venous drainage occurs as an isolated anomaly, there is a good prognosis for corrective surgery if the infant is in good condition at operation. Thus it would be a lesion which would particularly benefit from prenatal diagnosis and immediate post-natal therapy. However, the condition often occurs as part of the asplenia syndrome in combination with other cardiac anomalies where the outlook is poor.

The atrioventricular junction

Tricuspid atresia In tricuspid atresia, there is no patent valve seen in the normal position between the right atrium and ventricle. The right ventricular chamber is small or indiscernible as a consequence of the lack of flow into the ventricle. There is a ventricular septal defect of varying size. An example is seen in Figure 13. The great arteries may be normally connected or transposed. The arterial connection is important to identify as this will influence the prognosis. Tricuspid atresia constitutes about 3% to 4% of both the infant and prenatal cardiac anomalies.[9] This form of heart disease is rarely associated with extracardiac anomalies.

Mitral atresia This is present when the mitral valve is not patent. It occurs in combination with a normally connected but atretic aorta in the hypoplastic left heart syndrome (described with aortic atresia, p. 371) or with double outlet right ventricle. In mitral atresia with double outlet, there is no direct communication between the left

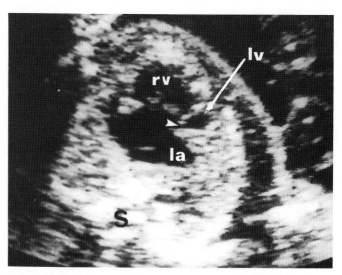

Fig. 14 Mitral atresia. In this fetus the left atrioventricular valve is atretic. There is a small ventricular septal defect (arrowhead). rv – right ventricle, lv – left ventricle, la – left atrium, S – spine.

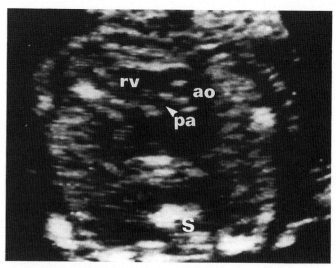

Fig. 15 Mitral atresia. Both great arteries can be seen arising anterior to the inter-ventricular septum, therefore both from the right ventricle (rv). The aorta (ao) proved to be the anterior artery. pa – pulmonary artery, S – spine.

atrium and ventricle, the floor of the left atrium being formed by muscular tissue. There is usually a ventricular septal defect, as in the case illustrated in Figure 14. The great arteries arise from the right ventricle in abnormal parallel orientation as illustrated in Figure 15. It is seen more frequently prenatally than in post-natal series forming 5% of our prenatal cardiac anomalies.

Atrioventricular septal defect A common atrioventricular valve is found when there is a defect in both the atrial and ventricular septa at the crux of the heart at the normal point of insertion of the two atrioventricular valves

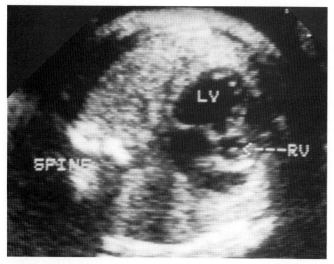

Fig. 13 Tricuspid atresia. The right ventricle (RV) is much smaller than the left (LV) and there was no opening valve in the position of the tricuspid valve.

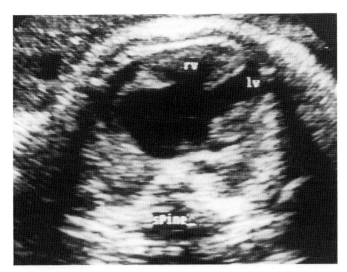

Fig. 16 **Atrioventricular septal defect.** There is a large defect in the atrial and ventricular septum with a common atrioventricular valve seen open in diastole in this frame. rv – right ventricle, lv – left ventricle.

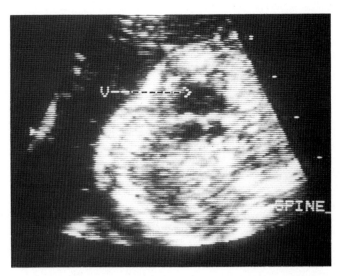

Fig. 17 **Double inlet connection.** There is no ventricular septum seen dividing the single ventricular chamber (V). The two atrioventricular valves drain to this one ventricle.

(Fig. 16). The echocardiographic appearance is of the single valve opening astride the crest of the ventricular septum. It is one of the commonest forms of heart disease seen in prenatal life[10] representing 17% of our prenatal series compared with the expected rate of around 5% found in post-natal life. This type of defect is found in two situations, associated with complex other cardiac anomalies or associated with trisomy 21. An isolated defect in a normal child can occur but is uncommon. Thus, when the diagnosis of an atrioventricular septal defect is made, the fetal chromosomes should be analysed. The prognosis will depend on the presence of associated cardiac or extracardiac lesions.

Double inlet connection. Double inlet connection is an unusual defect where both atrioventricular valves drain to one ventricle. The appearance is of absence of the interventricular septum (Fig. 17). The origin of the great arteries is variable.

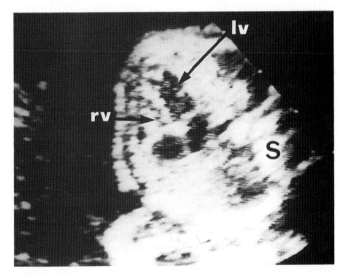

Fig. 18 **Pulmonary atresia.** The right ventricle (rv) is small and thick walled. lv – left ventricle, S – spine.

The ventriculo-arterial junction

Pulmonary atresia In pulmonary atresia, the pulmonary root will not be found in its usual position, or it will be very small in relation to the aorta. It occurs in three settings – with intact ventricular septum, with a ventricular septal defect, or as part of a complex of congenital heart disease. Pulmonary atresia with intact ventricular septum of the form seen most commonly post-natally is characterised by a small and hypertrophied right ventricle (Fig. 18). This form represents about 2% of CHD in both the prenatal and post-natal series. However, pulmonary atresia is commonly found prenatally with a dilated right ventricle and severe tricuspid incompetence. This form is described later in the chapter under tricuspid dysplasia.

Aortic atresia In this fatal condition the aorta is tiny and the left ventricle small. Prenatally the left ventricle can be impossible to find or the left ventricular cavity can be small, thick walled and usually highly reflective. Examples of each form are seen in Figures 19 and 20. The aorta is hypoplastic from its origin to the site of entry of the duct where it becomes larger. Flow in the ascending aorta can be documented as reversed on pulsed or colour Doppler. This is a common form of heart disease representing about 10% of post-natal and up to 20% of the prenatal series. It is rarely associated with extracardiac anomalies.

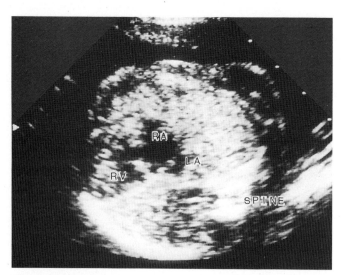

Fig. 19   Aortic atresia. Two atria are seen, with the right atrium (RA) connecting normally to the right ventricle (RV) but no visible left ventricle is found. LA – left atrium.

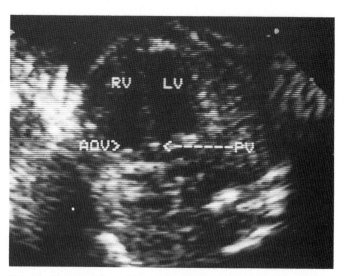

Fig. 21   Transposition of the great arteries. The aorta arises close to the anterior chest wall in parallel orientation to the pulmonary artery. The aorta connects to the right ventricle (RV) and the pulmonary artery to the left (LV) in this case of transposition of the great arteries. AOV – aortic valve, PV – pulmonary valve.

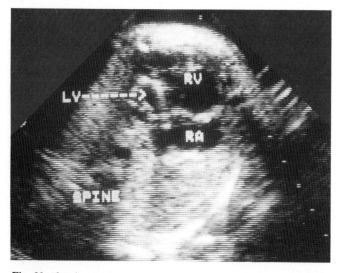

Fig. 20   Aortic atresia. The left ventricle (LV) is seen but it is small, thick walled and highly reflective. RV – right ventricle. RA – right atrium.

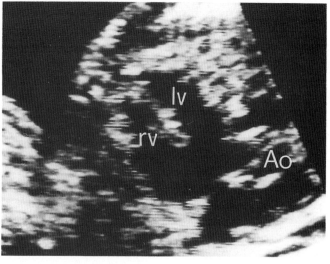

Fig. 22   Aortic over-ride. The aorta (Ao) arises astride the ventricular septum. There is a large ventricular septal defect positioned below the aorta. Examination of the pulmonary outflow tract will differentiate the three possible underlying diagnoses in this condition. rv – right ventricle, lv – left ventricle.

Transposition of the great arteries   In transposed great arteries the normal positional arrangement of the arteries is lost. The aorta will arise anterior to the pulmonary artery and parallel with it, instead of the normal appearance at right angles to the pulmonary artery at its origin (Fig. 21). It constitutes around 10% of infant series although it is infrequent in the prenatal series. This discrepancy is because the lesion will not be detected by the four chamber view alone and it is rarely associated with extracardiac anomalies. It can be a difficult diagnosis to make unless the operator is experienced in the interpretation of both the horizontal and longitudinal views of the fetal heart.[7] However, it is important to recognise prenatally as it has a

relatively good prognosis if early corrective surgery is performed.

Aortic over-ride   In some forms of heart disease the aorta is displaced anteriorly and arises astride the ventricular septum with a subaortic ventricular septal defect (Fig. 22). This finding is seen in Fallot's tetralogy, pulmonary atresia with a ventricular septal defect and with a common arterial trunk. These three conditions are differentiated by examination of the pulmonary outflow tract. The distinction is important as each carries a very different prognosis for corrective surgery. In the tetralogy, the pulmonary outflow is narrowed but patent. It is completely obstructed in pulmonary atresia and arises from the aorta in the common arterial trunk anomaly. The tetralogy of Fallot is much the most common of the three conditions. All are seen prenatally with around the same incidence as is found post-natally but in prenatal life the tetralogy of Fallot is associated in up to 50% of cases with extracardiac anomalies, particularly chromosomal aberrations.

Double outlet right ventricle In double outlet right ventricle both great arteries arise from the right ventricle anterior to the ventricular septum. This anomaly is illustrated in Figure 15 in a case where it was found in association with mitral atresia. Other lesions which can occur in association with double outlet right ventricle include a ventricular septal defect, an atrioventricular septal defect and pulmonary stenosis. The position of the great arteries relative to each other can vary but the normal 'crossing over' of the two is usually lost.

Additional abnormalities

Many other cardiac malformations can occur which do not involve abnormality of the connections of the heart. These tend to be less severe defects and more amenable to correction. Some can, however, be recognised prenatally. They include:

1) valve stenosis;
2) ventricular septal defect;
3) valvular dysplasia or displacement;
4) cardiac tumour;
5) aortic arch abnormalities.

Valve stenosis Any intracardiac valve can be stenosed or partially obstructed but in practice this mainly occurs at the aortic or pulmonary valve. The respective ventricular chamber and the valve itself may appear thickened.

When there is valvular obstruction prenatally, the affected artery will often be disproportionately small relative to the other artery. The Doppler sample volume placed in the stenosed artery sometimes will show a velocity of blood flow above the normal range but this is not such a consistent feature as that produced by a valvular stenosis post-natally. The globular, stiff, highly reflective appearance of the left ventricle characteristic of this lesion is seen in Figure 23. The high left ventricular diastolic pressure in this condition will often lead to secondary left atrial hypertension and left to right shunting across the foramen ovale (Plate 2). In critical aortic stenosis the prognosis is very poor, even if the obstruction is relieved immediately after delivery, as the damage to the left ventricle is usually irreversible. In contrast, in critical pulmonary stenosis, early balloon valvotomy should be associated with a good result.

Ventricular septal defect This is the most frequent

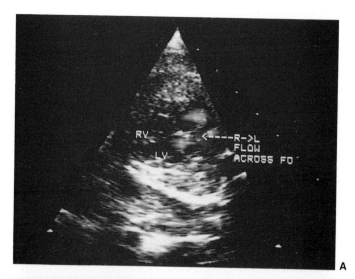

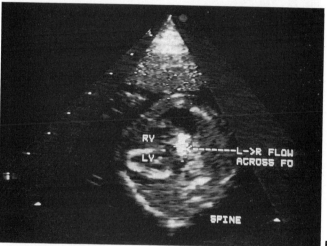

Plate 2 Flow through the foramen ovale. A: This shows a right to left jet coloured blue through the foramen ovale in a normal heart. **B:** Aortic stenosis. The left ventricle is thick walled and highly reflective due to aortic outflow obstruction. There is a left to right jet through the foramen ovale due to raised left atrial pressure. This figure is reproduced in colour in the colour plate section at the front of this volume.

form of heart disease seen in childhood, constituting nearly 20% of cases.[8] However, it is relatively uncommon in the prenatal series and in the fetus it is frequently associated with chromosomal anomalies. Ventricular septal defects (VSDs) can be present in various sizes and positions or be part of more complex anomalies. These factors influence the prognosis. The majority of isolated VSDs close spontaneously post-natally and therefore have an excellent prognosis (Figs 24 and 25). Less than 5% of VSDs will require surgical correction.

Valvular dysplasia Any cardiac valve can be dysplastic but in practice in prenatal life this particularly affects the tricuspid valve (Fig. 26). This valve may also be displaced from its normal position into the body of the right ventricle in Ebstein's anomaly (Fig. 27). Both abnormalities will

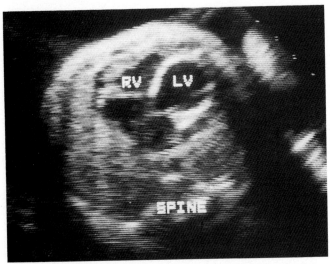

Fig. 23 Aortic stenosis. The left ventricle (LV) is highly reflective, hypertrophied and globular in shape. In the moving image the poor contraction could be appreciated. This was due to critical aortic stenosis. RV – right ventricle.

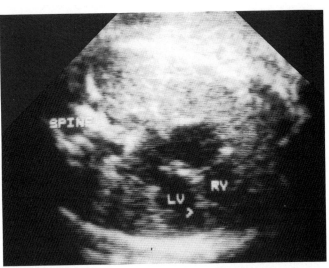

Fig. 25 There is a small ventricular septal defect (arrowhead) in the muscular part of the septum. This closed spontaneously by 1 year of age. LV – left ventricle, RV – right ventricle.

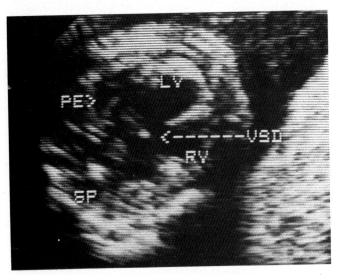

Fig. 24 There is a large ventricular septal defect (VSD) positioned in the inlet septum below the two atrioventricular valves. This is unlikely to close spontaneously. LV – left ventricle, RV – right ventricle, PE – pericardial effusion, SP – spine.

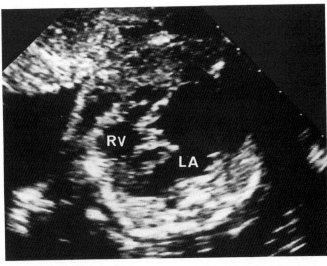

Fig. 26 Tricuspid dysplasia. The right atrium is grossly enlarged due to severe tricuspid incompetence. The valve is dysplastic. RV – right ventricle, LA – left atrium.

produce incompetence of the tricuspid valve and right atrial dilatation which may be severe and lead to secondary lung compression and hypoplasia. These conditions are both rare in paediatric practice but frequent in prenatal series, probably because secondary lung hypoplasia results in early post-natal death. Only two patients survived in our series of 28 such cases where the right atrium was significantly dilated during gestation.

Tumour Cardiac tumours are occasionally seen in prenatal life. They carry a high risk of blood flow obstruction, fetal hydrops and intra-uterine death. The majority of tu-

mours are rhabdomyomas histologically and are associated with tuberose sclerosis.

Aortic arch anomalies The aortic arch can be interrupted completely or partially obstructed, as in coarctation. Coarctation can be a simple shelf at the distal end of the arch or be associated with severe arch hypoplasia. Coarctation is a common form of heart disease comprising about 10% of the total but those cases recognised prenatally constitute the more severe end of the spectrum of this disease. The association of cystic hygroma, fetal hydrops, coarctation and Turner's syndrome is commonly recognised in

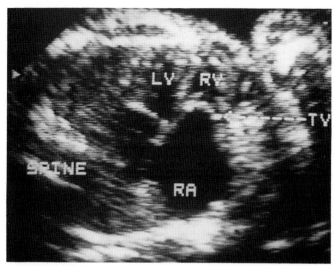

Fig. 27 Ebstein's anomaly. The right atrium (RA) is enlarged and the tricuspid valve (TV) is incompetent but also displaced into the right ventricle (RV). LV – left ventricle.

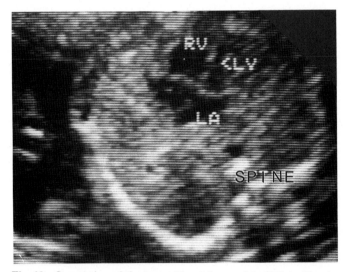

Fig. 28 Coarctation of the aorta. The right ventricle (RV) is dilated relative to the left (LV) in this case of coarctation of the aorta. LA – left atrium.

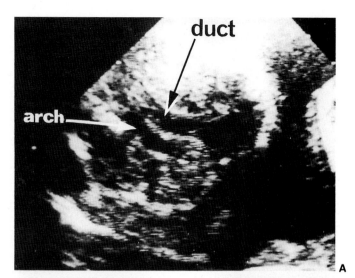

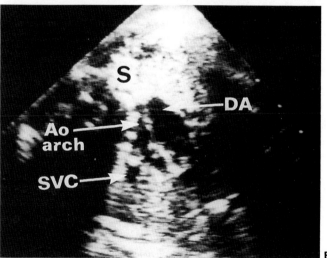

Fig. 29 A: The normal aortic arch and duct in a normal heart.
B: Coarctation of the aorta. The aortic arch (Ao arch) and duct are visualised in the same plane in order to assess their relative size. The arch was severely hypoplastic in this case in association with coarctation. DA – ductus arteriosus, SVC – superior vena cava.

early fetal life. The clues to the diagnosis of arch anomalies include recognition of enlargement of the right ventricle and pulmonary artery relative to the left ventricle and aorta (Fig. 28). A horizontal section of the arch of the aorta will show varying degrees of narrowing in coarctation (Fig. 29) and be incomplete in interruption. Where the coarctation is discrete and there are no other anomalies, the prognosis after early corrective surgery is good. However, complete interruption or severe arch hypoplasia can prove difficult or impossible to reconstruct and the mortality in those cases is high.

Ectopia cordis and conjoint twins These are rare severe defects which involve the fetal heart. In both conditions the majority of fetuses will die spontaneously in utero. In ectopia, the heart lies outside the fetal thorax and is also commonly structurally abnormal. The prognosis, even with a normal cardiac structure, is extremely poor. In conjoint twins where the heart is shared, it is rarely possible to salvage either twin.

Artefacts A common finding which is not an abnormality is a highly reflective mass within the cavity of the left ventricle related to the papillary apparatus of the mitral valve (Fig. 30). It probably represents some degree of fibrous deposition but has no pathological significance. It should not be confused with the appearance of a tumour which can be in any site in the heart, is less reflective, often larger or multiple and obstructive to blood flow.

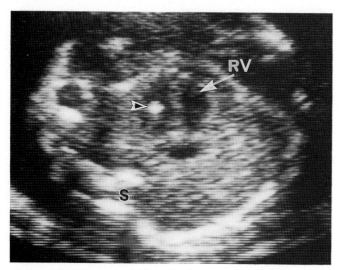

Fig. 30 **There is a very highly reflective structure** (arrowhead) within the left ventricle. This is related to the free wall of the ventricle in the region of the papillary muscle of the mitral valve. It is not of pathological significance. RV – right ventricle, S – spine.

ORGANISATION OF FETAL ECHOCARDIOGRAPHY

Certain groups of pregnancies are at increased risk of congenital heart disease (CHD). These include:

1) a family history of CHD. If one previous child has had CHD the recurrence risk is 1 in 50. Where there have been two affected children the risk increases to 1 in 10. When a parent is affected the risk to the next generation is of the order of 1 in 10;

2) maternal diabetes is associated with a statistical risk of cardiac malformation of about 1 in 50. Good diabetic control in early pregnancy probably diminishes this risk;

3) exposure to teratogens in early pregnancy such as lithium, phenytoin or steroids is reported to be associated with a 1 in 50 risk of heart malformation;

4) the detection of an extracardiac fetal anomaly on ultrasound should lead to a complete examination of the fetal heat as many types of abnormality, for example exomphalos, are often linked with heart disease. Abnormalities in more than one system in the fetus should arouse the suspicion of a chromosome defect and a fetal blood sample or amniocentesis should be performed in order to give an accurate prognosis to the parents;

5) some fetal arrhythmias are associated with structural heart disease, especially complete heart block which produces a sustained bradycardia of less than 100 beats per minute;

6) non-immune fetal hydrops can be due to congenital heart disease and a fetal echocardiogram should be an essential part of the work-up of these patients. Fetal hydrops is cardiac in origin in up to 25% of cases;

7) by far the most important 'high-risk group' seen in the last 2 years are those 'normal' pregnancies where the ultrasonographer notices an abnormality of the four chamber view on a routine scan. In the UK at the present time over 90% of pregnancies have a routine ultrasound examination. The timing and thoroughness of the routine scan varies but those departments where an adequate 'abnormality' scan is performed at about 18 weeks gestation can potentially detect severe cardiac anomalies in up to 2 per 1000 studies. Over 80% of the last 100 anomalies seen in our department have been referred because of the suspicion of CHD from examination of the four chamber view. Ideally ultrasonographers performing a high standard of fetal obstetric ultrasound working in collaboration with a centre specialised in paediatric echocardiography should produce the highest accuracy in fetal cardiac diagnosis. The paediatric specialist must be included in the team to counsel the parents on the prognosis for the child. Some forms of defect will benefit from early diagnosis by preparing medical staff for early neonatal intervention.

Our high-risk patients are booked for a fetal cardiac scan at 18 and 24 to 28 weeks gestation. At 18 weeks all the connections are seen, later more minor defects are sought. Over 6000 such patients have been examined since early 1980 and over 400 anomalies have been accurately detected. In no patient has it proved impossible to visualise the atrioventricular connections and the two great arteries. Some minor defects, such as small ventricular septal defects, secundum atrial septal defects and valve stenosis have been overlooked. No major false positive predictions have been made.

It is apparent from consideration of the forms of CHD seen prenatally that a different spectrum of disease is seen in prenatal life from those who survive to infancy.[11] This is reflected in the outcome of the pregnancies where fetal

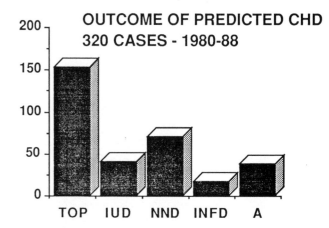

Fig. 31 **Histogram to show outcome of the pregnancies in which fetal heart disease has been detected.** TOP – termination of pregnancy, IUD – intra-uterine death, NND – neonatal death, INFD – infant death, A – alive.

heart disease has been detected (Fig. 31). Malformations detected tend to be the most severe forms of heart disease and defects which are not commonly seen post-natally are frequently recognised, such as tricuspid dysplasia and cardiac tumours. Many of these fetuses do not survive intra-uterine life which partly accounts for the discrepancy between prenatal and post-natal life. Up to 25% of continuing pregnancies with CHD resulted in spontaneous fetal loss. A high proportion of parents, up to 75% where the diagnosis is made in time, will elect termination of pregnancy. Our attitude is that the parents make their own decision concerning termination or continuation of the pregnancy based on the information given by the paediatric cardiologist. A significant proportion (20%) of our detected cardiac abnormalities have had associated chromosome defects. This possibility must be included in the counselling and the karyotype performed where this is appropriate. The presence of multiple congenital anomalies contributes to the high mortality found in our series of prenatally detected heart disease.

SUMMARY

Fetal echocardiography can accurately detect structural heart malformations. Almost all forms of congenital heart disease have been recognised prenatally. The ultrasonographer can learn to recognise the normal cardiac anatomy, first of all the four chamber view in every patient and then the arterial connections. Deviations from the normal appearance or failure to find the standard views will then indicate the need for specialist help (from the paediatric echocardiographer).

REFERENCES

1 Lange L W, Sahn D J, Allen H D, Goldberg S J, Anderson C, Giles H. Qualitative real-time cross-sectional echocardiographic imaging of the human fetus during the second half of pregnancy. Circulation 1980; 62: 799

2 Kleinman C S, Hobbins J C, Jaffe C C, et al. Echocardiographic studies of the human fetus: prenatal diagnosis of congenital heart disease and cardiac dysrhythmias. Pediatrics 1980; 65: 1059

3 Allan L D, Tynan M J, Campbell S, Wilkinson J, Anderson R H. Echocardiographic and anatomical correlates in the fetus. Br Heart J 1980; 44: 444

4 Allan L D, Crawford D C, Anderson R H, Tynan M J. Echocardiographic and anatomical correlates in fetal congenital heart disease. Br Heart J 1984; 52: 542

5 Allan L D, Crawford D C and Tynan M J. Evolution of coarctation of the aorta in intrauterine life. Br Heart J 1984; 52: 271–473

6 Allan L D, Crawford D C, Chita S K and Tynan M J. Prenatal screening for congenital heart disease. BMJ 1986; 292: 1717

7 Allan L D. Manual of Fetal Echocardiography. MTP Press, Lancaster, England. 1986

8 Anderson R H, Macartney F J, Shinebourne E A, Tynan M. eds. In: Paediatric cardiology. London: Churchill Livingstone. 1987

9 Fyler D C, Buckley L P, Hellenbrand W E, Cohn H E. Report of the New England Regional Infant Cardiac Care Program. Pediatrics 1980; 65 (suppl): 376

10 Machado M V L, Crawford D C, Anderson R H, Allan L D. Atrioventricular septal defect in prenatal life. Br Heart J 1988; 59: 352

11 Allan L D, Crawford D C, Anderson R H, Tynan M J. Spectrum of congenital heart disease detected echocardiographically in prenatal life. Br Heart J 1984; 54: 523

The skeleton

David R. Griffin and Lyn S. Chitty

INTRODUCTION

A description of the normal ultrasound examination of the fetal musculoskeletal system is contained in Chapter 10. Figure 1 shows the normal appearances of the fetal limb bones for comparison with the commoner skeletal dysplasias and malformations to be described.

Patient selection for detailed skeletal survey

There are several groups of women who are at increased risk of carrying a fetus with a skeletal abnormality. They can be classified into four main categories:

a) those with a positive family history,
b) women who have been exposed to certain drugs in the first trimester,
c) insulin dependent diabetics and
d) those cases where another fetal abnormality has been detected at ultrasound examination.

a) Family history of deformity

Many of the syndromes described in this chapter are single gene disorders of autosomal dominant (AD) or autosomal recessive (AR) inheritance. Dominantly inherited conditions may either occur as a new mutation or show a typical family history with one parent affected. All affected members may not manifest the disease to the same extent as a result of variable expression of the gene. Examples of conditions showing dominant inheritance are cleidocranial dysostosis, achondroplasia and Holt-Oram syndrome. Lethal dominant conditions will obviously not occur in other

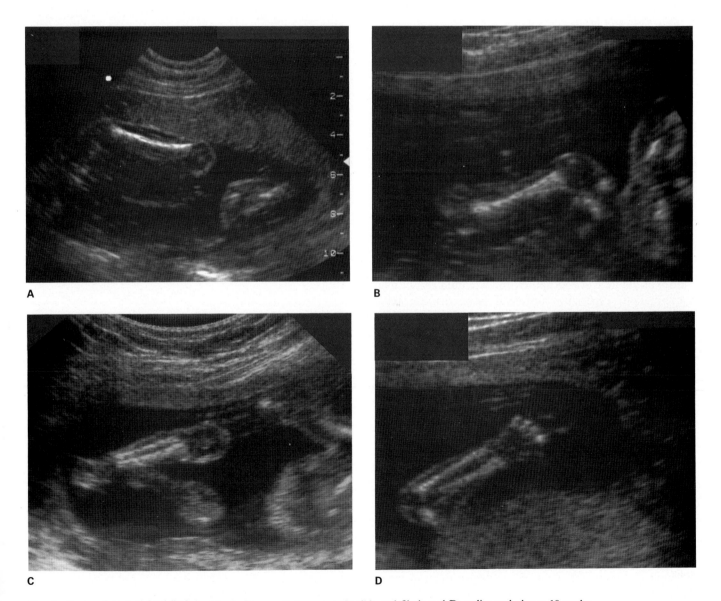

Fig. 1 Scans of normal fetal limb bones. A: Femur, **B:** humerus, **C:** tibia and fibula and **D:** radius and ulna at 18 weeks.

generations and are usually new mutations unlikely to recur in the family. Lethal conditions with recessive inheritance, on the other hand, will only occur in the homozygous offspring of heterozygous unaffected parents. Following the first affected child those parents run a 25% risk of having another and a 67% risk of passing the gene on to their unaffected children. Happily the gene frequency of these conditions is very low and the chance of two carriers meeting is extremely remote. However, if members of the same family (particularly first cousins) marry, the likelihood of two carriers of the same recessive gene meeting is considerably increased. Such consanguineous marriages are common amongst some Muslim communities who should be considered at increased risk of having a child with a recessive syndrome. Many of the lethal and crippling deformities described here are recessive.

b) Drugs in early pregnancy

It is as well to perform a skeletal survey on any patient who has taken significant quantities of medication in the first trimester during this critical time of organogenesis. The devastating effects of the hypnotic thalidomide are well-recorded. Other drugs that have been specifically implicated in skeletal dysmorphism are warfarin, which may produce a syndrome identical to chondrodysplasia punctata, phenytoin (digital hypoplasia), alcohol, known teratogens such as methotrexate and aminopterin and some anaesthetic agents. A comprehensive list of drug associated malformations has been published by Koren et al.[1]

c) Diabetics

Insulin-dependent diabetics, particularly those with poor control at the time of conception, run a tenfold risk of fetal malformation, especially congenital heart disease, renal anomalies and skeletal anomalies (caudal regression syndrome) (Fig. 2).

d) The finding of any fetal anomaly found during scanning

The abnormalities below are particularly associated with skeletal malformations:

- polyhydramnios/oligohydramnios
- fetal hydrops
- small thorax
- facial clefting
- short femur found on routine examination.

Aids to diagnosis of skeletal dysplasias

The skeletal dysplasias are a heterogeneous group of over 100 rare disorders, the distinction between them in many cases being subtle. It is therefore helpful for those particularly interested in the differential diagnosis of these

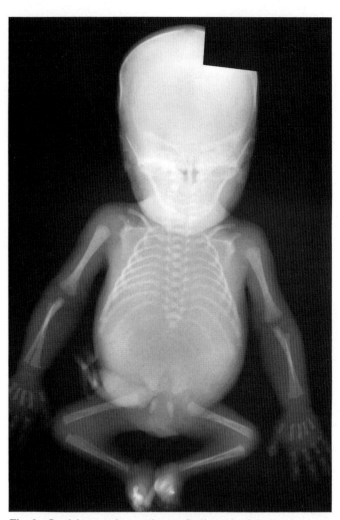

Fig. 2 Caudal regression syndrome. Radiograph of the 26 week fetus of a diabetic mother. It shows agenesis of the lumbar and sacral spine typical of caudal regression syndrome.

conditions to have access to a comprehensive reference of fetal and neonatal pathology.[2] It is also important to collaborate closely with the geneticists who may have access to a dysmorphology computerised database.

Before scanning a patient at known risk of a skeletal dysplasia, request as much information on the affected member(s) of the family as possible. This may include photographs, X-rays, detailed pathology reports and reports of any genetic consultations.

Skeletal malformations

Osteochondrodysplasias

These skeletal dysplasias are rare with an incidence of less than one in 30 000 (Table 1). The list of syndromes and subgroups continues to grow steadily. The degree of limb shortening (Fig. 3) and deformity is variable between (and sometimes within) syndromes.[3]

The diagnosis or exclusion of recurrence of a limb reduction syndrome in a family known to be at risk is an easy matter as the diagnostician is primed in his search by knowledge of the previous malformations. By contrast accurate diagnosis of an unexpected case discovered at routine scanning is a challenge which demands expert knowledge and diligent attention to detail. Some of the features to note before making a diagnosis are listed below.

Long bones   Note the degree of shortening in relation

Table 1   Approximate incidence of 'common' lethal skeletal dysplasias

Thanatophoric dysplasia	1 in 30 000
Osteogenesis imperfecta (type II)	1 in 55 000
Achondrogenesis (all types)	1 in 75 000
Chondrodysplasia punctata	1 in 85 000
Hypophosphatasia (severe form)	1 in 110 000
Campomelic dysplasia	1 in 150 000

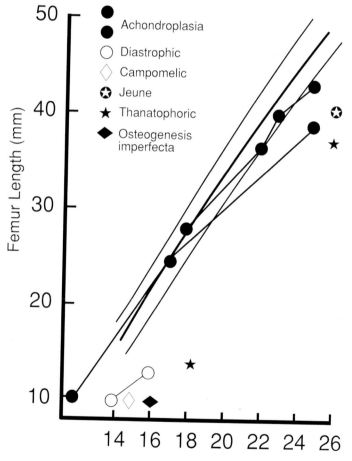

Fig. 3   Nomogram of fetal femur length (O'Brien et al[3]) showing measurements of femur length in fetuses confirmed as having achondrogenesis type II, achondroplasia, osteogenesis imperfecta type IIa, diastrophic dysplasia, campomelic dysplasia, Jeune thoracic dystrophy and thanatophoric dysplasia. Note the late deviation from normal growth in two fetuses with achondroplasia and one with Jeune thoracic dystrophy.

to nomograms (see Appendix). Is the shortening greater in the proximal (rhizomelic) femur and humerus or distal (mesomelic) radius/ulna and tibia/fibula or equal in all? Do the bones appear straight, bowed or crumpled?

Joints   Note attitude and movement of joints with particular attention to lower limbs and talipes equinovarus (Fig. 22).

Spine   Examine the spine for deformities, hemivertebrae, normal ossification of the vertebral bodies and platyspondyly (flattened vertebrae).

Ribs and thorax   The heart should normally fill about one third of the thoracic cavity. If the ribs are short the thorax will be small and narrow and bell-shaped and the abdomen protuberant (champagne cork appearance).

The ribs may appear beaded in osteogenesis imperfecta type II.

Skull   A poorly ossified skull will be virtually echo-free or only weakly reflective casting little or no acoustic shadow. The intracranial contents will be more than usually clear and the cerebral hemispheres echo-free (pseudohydrocephaly) (Fig. 7). In later pregnancy the skull will deform easily if pressed by the transducer (Fig. 9).

Note any brachycephaly, clover leaf deformity or other abnormality.

Hands and feet   Count fingers to exclude polydactyly.

Extra fingers are usually found next to the fifth finger (post-axial) but thumbs or big toes may be split or duplicated (pre-axial). Note the position of wrists and fingers and the length of the fingers.

Limb girdles   There is little data on normal fetal limb girdle dimensions but some osteochondrodystrophies are characterised by short clavicles and hypoplastic ilia and scapulae.

Face   A facial profile (sagittal plane) may show depressed nasal bridge or prominent forehead (frontal bossing) (Fig. 16A) or a receding chin (micrognathia).

A full facial view in the coronal plane (Fig. 4) will show cleft lip.

Non-skeletal features   A full examination of the rest of the fetus including the heart, kidneys, cerebral ventricles and amniotic fluid may uncover further anomalies to narrow down the differential diagnosis.

Table 2 shows syndromes associated with specific malformations. Tables 3 and 4 are rapid diagnostic guides to some of the commoner osteochondrodystrophies. These various skeletal dysplasias will be described in diagnostic groups, but it must be remembered that many conditions will fall into more than one category. The syndromes described below include only those which are more common. A comprehensive list would be impossible to produce as new variants continue to be described. However, the information given below should aid diagnosis but, in cases where there is no positive family history, definitive diagnosis may have to await post-natal radiological and pathological investigations.

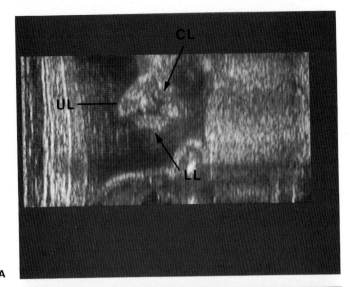

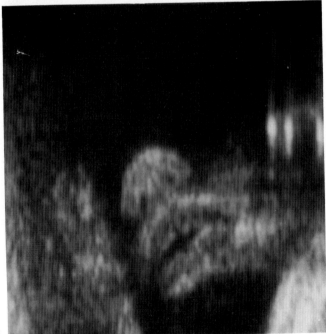

Fig. 4 Cleft lip. A: Coronal scan of the lips to show a paramedian cleft (CL) of the upper lip (UL). LL – lower lip. **B:** Normal for comparison.

Table 2 Clues to the differential ultrasound diagnosis of skeletal dysplasias

Polyhydramnios	Achondrogenesis type I or II Thanatophoric dysplasia Short rib-polydactyly syndrome
Fetal hydrops	Achondrogenesis type I SRP syndromes
Undermineralised skull	Osteogenesis imperfecta (IIa) Achondrogenesis type I Hypophosphatasia
Clover leaf skull	Thanatophoric dysplasia
Small thorax	Achondrogenesis Hypochondrogenesis Thanatophoric dysplasia SRP syndromes Chondroectodermal dysplasia Campomelic dysplasia
Marked femoral bowing	Campomelic dysplasia Osteogenesis imperfecta Hypophosphatasia
Talipes equinovarus	Campomelic dysplasia Diastrophic dysplasia
Polydactyly	Chondroectodermal dysplasia SRP syndromes Grebe syndrome Jeune thoracic dystrophy
Short clavicles	Campomelic dysplasia Cleidocranial dysostosis Kniest syndrome

usually clear. The skull is soft so that the head may be deformed by depressing the transducer on the maternal abdomen.

Achondrogenesis type II (Langer-Saldino) shows micromelia to a lesser degree than in type I.[6–8] The characteristic feature is absent mineralisation of the vertebral bodies. The limb bones may be short (Fig. 5A). The definitive diagnostic feature is the finding of an echo-free column extending from the sacrum to the base of the skull (Fig. 5B) which represents the unossified vertebral bodies (Fig. 5C). The skull appeared normal.

Hypochondrogenesis is another form of neonatally lethal short limb dwarfism which is now thought to be part of the same spectrum of disease as achondrogenesis type II with hypochondrogenesis representing the milder end of the spectrum.[9–12] A case initially diagnosed at 31 weeks as Jeune thoracic dystrophy because of moderately short, straight long bones (femur length 42 mm) with thickened metaphyses and small thorax is illustrated in Figure 6. The diagnosis was revised to hypochondrogenesis after examination of neonatal radiographs. Radiologically the condition is characterised by flared metaphyses and poor mineralisation of the cervical and sacral vertebral bodies.

Osteogenesis imperfecta is subdivided into four main groups. Only types IIa and IIc are characterised by signifi-

Conditions characterised by undermineralisation

Achondrogenesis types I and II are inherited in an autosomal recessive fashion and occur in approximately one in 75 000 births. Both types are lethal and may be complicated by polyhydramnios.

Achondrogenesis type I (Parenti-Fraccaro) is characterised by extreme micromelia (very short limbs), a short poorly mineralised spine, short ribs and almost absent ossification of the calvarium. Glen and Teng[5] noted femur lengths of 10 mm at 19 weeks. As a result of poor skull mineralisation details of the brain structure will be un-

Table 3 Skeletal dysplasias characterised by poor mineralisation

Type & Inheritance		Long bones	Spine	Ribs	Other features	Prognosis	References
Achondrogenesis type I	(AR)	Extreme micromelia	Poorly mineralised Short	Short	Polyhydramnios, hydrops, very poor cranial ossification	Lethal	Golbus et al (1977) Smith et al (1981) Glen & Teng (1985) Muller et al (1985a) Donnenfeld (1987)
Achondrogenesis type II	(AR)	Severe micromelia	Unossified spine and sacrum	Short	Polyhydramnios Micrognathia Good cranial ossification	Lethal	Griffin et al (1985)
Osteogenesis imperfecta (type II)	VAR	V short, crumpled multiple fractures	Vertebrae may be flattened	Beaded +/− short	Polyhydraminos Unossified skull Brachycephaly	Lethal	Hobbins et al (1982) Milsom et al (1982) Shapiro et al (1982) Dinno et al (1982) Elejalde et al (1983) Brons et al (1988)
Hypophosphatasia (lethal form)	(AR)	Short, bowed	May show deformity	Thin +/− short +/− beaded	Poorly ossified skull	Lethal	Wladimiroff et al (1985)

cant undermineralisation. Types I and IV are usually manifest in childhood and are probably rarely amenable to antenatal diagnosis. Individuals affected by osteogenesis imperfecta type III or III/IV are usually born with fractures and there is progressive deformity in childhood. In more severely affected cases these types may be lethal in the perinatal period or early childhood. Diagnosis in utero at 19 weeks has been reported.[12]

The perinatally lethal type II has been the subject of many reports of early antenatal diagnosis with ultrasound.[13–18]

The long bones are short, deformed and crumpled because of multiple intra-uterine fractures (Figs 7B and 9C) (the positional appearance of the lower limbs may be similar to that in campomelic dysplasia and diastrophic dysplasia). Fetal movement is reduced. The ribs appear thin, short and beaded (Fig. 9B) and the thorax may be small. All reported cases have shown marked undermineralisation of the skull (Figs 7A and 8). In later pregnancy the gyri may be seen clearly and the skull can easily be distorted by the pressure of the ultrasound transducer (Fig. 9A). The appearance of the spine is usually normal but the vertebrae may be flattened (Fig. 9D). There may be associated polyhydramnios.

The outlook for fetuses with types IIa and IIc is almost invariably fatal, death usually resulting from pulmonary hypoplasia. A few cases with type IIb (Fig. 10) survive. It is believed that the majority of cases of type IIa are of sporadic occurrence but occasional recurrences have been reported within a family for type IIb.[19,20] The recurrence risk will depend on the type of osteogenesis and parental consanguinity.[19]

Hypophosphatasia presents several different clinical pictures and is classified according to the age of onset. It is the severe lethal form where the bones are undermineralised and which is the main concern of the prenatal diagnostic sonologist. Although its occurrence (one in 100 000) is said to be about half that of osteogenesis imperfecta type II, reports in the literature of ultrasound diagnosis are few.[21,22] Measurement of amniotic fluid alkaline phosphatase is unreliable.[23] There are reports of successful diagnosis from the measurement of cellular alkaline phosphatase from amniocytes or chorionic cells.[24] The gene locus for this condition has now been identified. Identification of heterozygous gene carriers is possible as they have low serum levels of bone alkaline phosphatase and phosphoethanolamine is present in the urine.

The ultrasonographic appearance is of an undermineralised skull, similar to that of osteogenesis imperfecta, and short, bowed long bone diaphyses. In the case reported by Wladimiroff the femur length (14 mm) below the fifth centile at 16 weeks.[22] There was also displacement of the long bones at the elbows and knees. Marked angulation of the femur may also occur (Fig. 11). Inheritance is autosomal recessive. The severe neonatal form of hypophosphatasia is usually lethal, with a high incidence of stillbirths and neonatal death secondary to respiratory insufficiency.

Conditions characterised by a hypoplastic thorax
Achondrogenesis see above. Asphyxiating thoracic dystrophy (Jeune syndrome) is a short-ribbed limb reduction syndrome inherited in an autosomal recessive pattern. There is only minimal to moderate diaphysial shortening and measurements of the long bones may not fall below normal ranges until late in the second trimester, if at all (Fig. 12). There may be severe rib shortening and thoracic reduction (Fig. 13). The diagnosis can be suspected prenatally on finding a hypoplastic thorax with moderately

Table 4 Skeletal dysplasias characterised by short ribs

Type & Inheritance		Long bones	Spine	Other features	Prognosis	References
Achondrogenesis type I	(AR)	Extreme micromelia	Poorly mineralised Short	Polyhydramnios, hydrops, very poor cranial ossification	Lethal	Golbus et al (1977) Smith et al (1981) Glen & Teng (1985) Muller et al (1985a) Donnenfeld (1987)
Achondrogenesis type II	(AR)	Severe micromelia	Unossified spine and sacrum	Polyhydramnios Micrognathia Unossified spine/sacrum	Lethal	Griffin et al (1985)
Hypochondrogenesis (Mainly sporadic)	(?AR)	Moderate shortening Flared metaphyses	Flat vertebral bodies	Poor ossification of cervical and sacral spine	Lethal	Stoll et al (1985) Griffin (1990)
Thanatophoric dysplasia	(sporadic)	Severe micromelia Thick diaphysis +/− bowing	Flat vertebral bodies	Polyhydramnios Megalocephaly Ventriculomegaly +/− Cloverleaf skull Renal & cardiac anomalies Trident hand	Lethal	Chervenak et al (1983) Beetham Reeves (1984) Burrows et al (1984) Camera et al (1984) Elejalde et al (1985) Weiner et al (1986)
Jejune thoracic dystrophy	(AR)	Variable/moderate (especially mesomelic) shortening	Normal	+/− Postaxial polydactyly Hypoplastic lungs Renal dysplasia	70% lethal	Little D (1984) Elejalde et al (1985) Griffin & Chitty (see text)
Short rib-polydactyly syndromes Saldino-Noonan (type I)	(AR)	Moderate shortening Spikey metaphyses	Normal	Postaxial polydactyly Hydrops, anal atresia	Lethal	Wladimiroff et al (1984) Meizner & Bar-Ziv (1985) Gembruch et al (1985)
Majewski (type II)		Tibia hypoplastic		Median cleft lip Cardiac & renal anomalies		
Ellis-Van Creveld syndrome (Chondroectodermal dysplasia)	(AR)	Variable shortening Hypoplastic tibia	Normal	Postaxial polydactyly 50% cardiac anomaly (ASD)	50% lethal Normal IQ	Mahoney & Hobbins (1977) Filly & Golbus (1982) Muller et al (1985)
Campomelic dysplasia	(AR)	Moderate shortening Bowed femur/tibia Hypo/aplastic fibula	Flat vertebrae	Short clavicles, micrognathia, talipes eq. varus Sex reversal	Usually lethal	Fryns et al (1981) Hobbins et al (1982) Redon et al (1984) Winter et al (1985) Griffin (1990)

short long bones.[25,26] Liquor volume is often increased. Post-axial polydactyly is an occasional finding. There is high (70%) perinatal and infant mortality from respiratory failure secondary to pulmonary hypoplasia. Associated renal, liver and pancreatic dysplasia cause complications in survivors and, in many cases, result in death in early childhood.[27]

Campomelic dysplasia. This autosomal recessive syndrome is typified by variable shortening and bowing of the femur and tibia which show angulation in the mid-shaft. The upper limbs are normal or only mildly affected. Associated skeletal deformities include macrocephaly (often with associated ventriculomegaly) micrognathia, short clavicles, talipes and small scapulae and ilia. Most of these features are detectable on careful ultrasonic survey.[13,28–30] The ribs are usually short and the thorax small. Congenital heart disease (VSD, ASD, tetralogy of Fallot) and hydronephrosis each occur in about one third of cases. Phenotypic sex reversal of XY fetuses is common. In about 95% of cases the condition is lethal in the first year of life.

Figure 14 shows a case which was diagnosed on the basis of femoral bowing, short and deformed tibiae and relatively normal upper limbs.

Ellis-van Creveld syndrome (chondro-ectodermal dysplasia) is recessively inherited, being particularly prevalent amongst the inbred Amish community in Pennsylvania. Affected fetuses may show variable degrees of shortening of long bones, which is more pronounced in the forearm

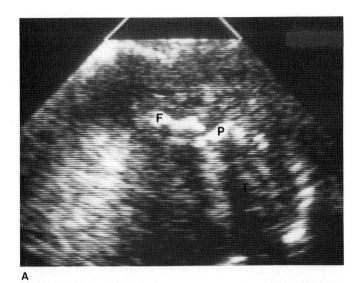

A

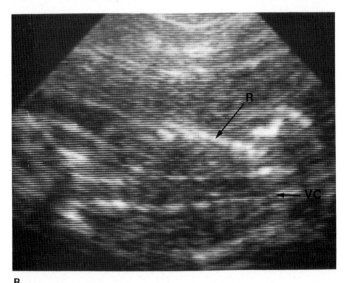

B

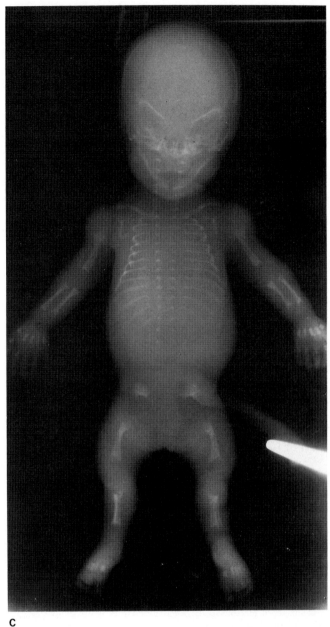

C

Fig. 5 Achondrogenesis. Scans of an 18 week fetus with achondrogenesis type II. **A:** Extremely short but modelled femur (F) with a length of 18 mm. P – pelvis, T – trunk. **B:** Coronal section of the trunk showing cartilaginous, unossified vertebral column (VC). R – ribs. **C:** Radiograph of the fetus showing unossified vertebral bodies and severe micromelia.

and lower leg (mesomelic). There is post-axial polydactyly of hands and feet. The ribs are short and horizontal causing a reduced thoracic cavity and lethal pulmonary hypoplasia in about half of affected infants. 50% of cases have congenital heart disease (ASD). Survivors reach adulthood with moderate to severe short stature (40 to 63 inches) being the major problem. The main differential diagnosis is Jeune syndrome. Prenatal diagnosis has been reported.[8,31,32]

Homozygous achondroplasia can present with severe micromelia and a small thorax.[33] It may be lethal.

Thanatophoric dysplasia is the commonest of the lethal dysplasias occurring about one in 30 000 births. Most cases are sporadic. There is severe micromelia. The femora are extremely short, thickened and bowed and have been likened to a telephone receiver handle (Fig. 15). The ribs are very short and thick (Fig. 16E) and the thoracic cavity constricted. The combination of small chest and normal abdominal size gives the torso a 'champagne cork' appearance in a longitudinal anteroposterior view (Fig. 16). Vertebrae are flat (platyspondyly) making the spine short. The skull tends towards brachycephaly and in some cases

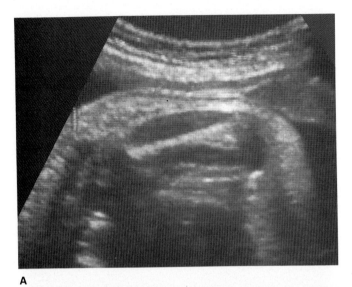

A

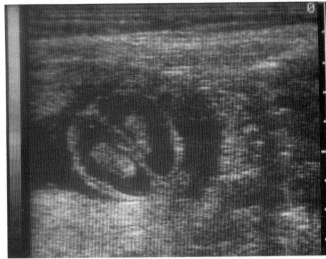

A

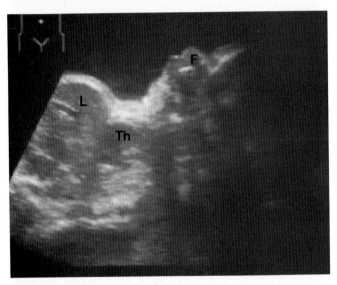

B

Fig. 6 Hypochondrogenesis. Scans of a 31 week fetus found on post-natal radiography to have hypochondrogenesis. **A:** Short femur with thickened metaphysis. **B:** Sagittal section of the trunk and face (F) to show 'champagne cork' appearance due to small thorax (Th) and protuberant liver (L).

may show the clover leaf deformity.[34–39] There may be associated megalencephaly and cerebral ventriculomegaly. Polyhydramnios is a common presenting sign in the late second or early third trimester.

Several authors have reported femur lengths of between 18 mm and 21 mm at 19 to 20 weeks, 23 mm at 22 weeks and only 26 to 27 mm at 32 weeks. It is thus apparent that very little growth of the long bones occurs from the middle of the second trimester onwards. The condition may be associated with cardiac and renal anomalies. In later pregnancy other dysmorphic features of the condition such as frontal bossing, depressed nasal bridge, short splayed

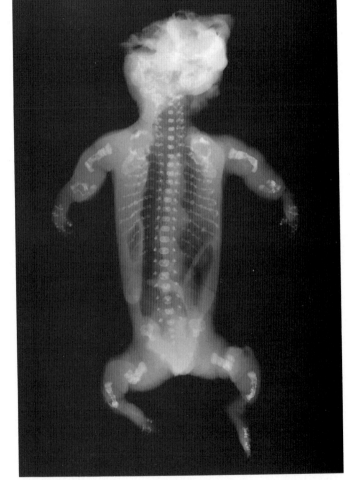

B

Fig. 7 Osteogenesis imperfecta. A: Fetal head in a case of osteogenesis imperfecta type IIa at 17 weeks. The skull shows severe undermineralisation giving the impression of ventriculomegaly. **B:** Radiograph of this case.

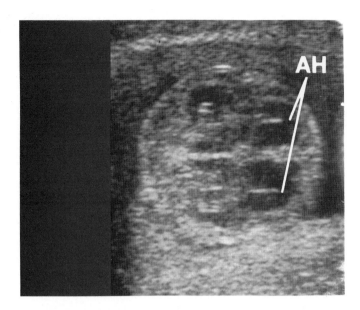

fingers (trident hand) and excessive skin folds may be evident (Fig. 16).

Short rib-polydactyly syndromes (SRPS) are characterised by moderate micromelia, very short ribs and narrow thorax and post-axial polydactyly. They have a recessive pattern of inheritance. Associated anomalies may include anal atresia, renal, cardiac and intestinal deformities and hydrops. SRPS may be classified into two groups, although other variants have been recognised (including some cases with similar dysmorphic features without poly-

Fig. 8   Osteogenesis imperfecta. Axial scan of a 20 week fetus with osteogenesis imperfecta type IIA showing undermineralised skull and echo-poor cerebral hemispheres (pseudohydrocephalus). The normally placed anterior horns (AH) show normal ventricular anatomy.

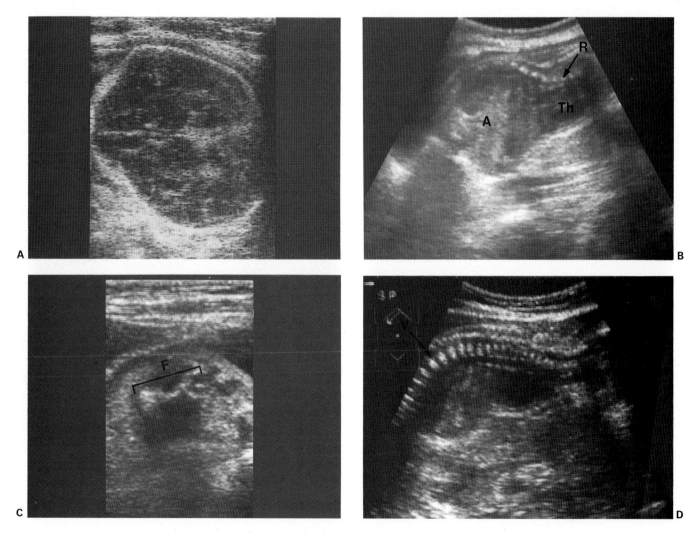

Fig. 9   Scans from a 31 week fetus with osteogenesis imperfecta type IIa. A: The head shows an undermineralised skull distorted by transducer pressure and casting no acoustic shadow. **B:** Coronal section of the trunk showing small thorax (Th) relative to the abdomen (A) ('champagne cork' appearance). R – ribs. **C:** The femur (F) is short, undermineralised and crumpled. **D:** Spine with flattened vertebrae (V).

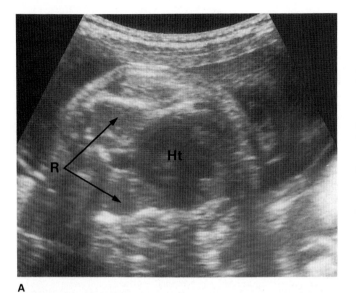

A

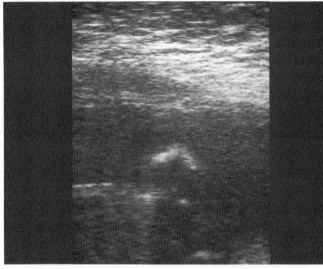

A

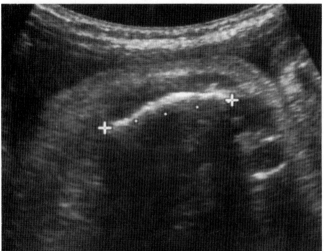

B

Fig. 10   Osteogenesis imperfecta Type IIb at 32 weeks.
A: Small, distorted rib cage (R) and heart (Ht) projecting anteriorly.
B: Bowed femur with better modelling than in Figure 9C.

dactyly). Saldino-Noonan (SRPS type I) typically has
shortened long bones with pointed metaphyses. Majewski
(SRPS type II) may be distinguished from SRPS Type I
by finding median cleft lip or palate and disproportionately
short and ovoid tibiae. Ambiguous external genitalia may
also occur in Type II. There are reports of prenatal diagnosis using ultrasound for both types.[40-42]

Conditions characterised by rhizomelic shortening
Chondrodysplasia punctata (rhizomelic type) is a condition
characterised by rhizomelic shortening (particularly of the
humerus) and joint contractures. There is also stippling of
the epiphyses which can be detected in utero during the
second trimester. This rhizomelic form of chondrodysplasia
punctata is inherited in an autosomal recessive pattern and

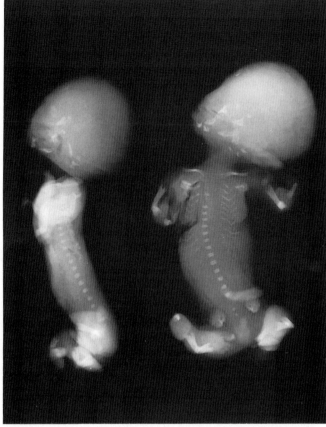

B

Fig. 11   Hypophosphatasia. A: Scan from a fetus with
hypophosphatasia showing a severely bowed femur measuring 15 mm
at 19 weeks. **B:** Radiograph of fetus in A (after rib biopsy) showing
marked angulation of femora and humeri, short distal extremities,
undermineralised skull and neural arch and thin, fractured ribs.

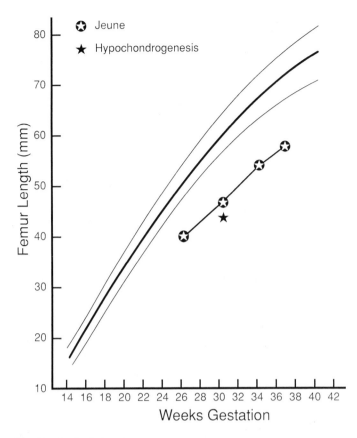

Fig. 12 **Asphyxiating thoracic dystrophy.** Nomogram of femur length showing femur growth in a case of asphyxiating thoracic dystrophy (adapted from O'Brien[3]).

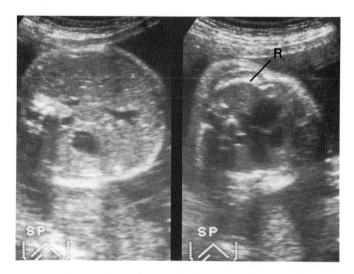

Fig. 13 **Asphyxiating thoracic dystrophy.** Axial scans of abdomen and thorax from a 32 week fetus with asphyxiating thoracic dystrophy. Note small thorax, short ribs (R) and protruding heart.

should not be confused with the non-rhizomelic form (Conradi-Hunermann syndrome) where both the genetics and prognosis are very different and prenatal diagnosis with ultrasound is probably not possible. The prognosis for the rhizomelic form is bad with death usually occurring within the first 2 years of life. All affected children have severe microcephaly and global developmental delay.

A recent case occurring de-novo in a primigravida mother showed short fetal humeri and femora at routine 18 week scan. More detailed examination revealed the typical splayed metaphyses and disorganised echoes around the epiphyses (stippled epiphyses) (Fig. 17). The limbs were flexed and showed severe limitation of movement. Fetal radiography performed in utero gave no useful additional information. The pregnancy was terminated and the diagnosis confirmed by fetal radiography (Fig. 17C) and biochemistry.[43]

Diastrophic dysplasia is characterised by rhizomelic micromelia, flexion deformities of the arms and legs, severe talipes equinovarus and proximal displacement of the thumbs ('hitch-hiker' thumbs). Micrognathia and cleft palate are sometimes associated. Reports of prenatal diagnosis are mainly in high-risk pregnancies and are based on short flexed limbs. 'Hitch-hiker' thumbs have been recognised on ultrasound in the first and second trimester.[44-47]

The spectrum of this disease is broad and prenatal diagnosis may not be possible before viability. There is an increased neonatal mortality, usually secondary to respiratory distress and pneumonia. The majority of affected infants who survive are intellectually unimpaired, but progressive kyphoscoliosis and arthropathy usually lead to severe physical handicap.

Non-lethal dysplasias Heterozygous achondroplasia has been diagnosed by ultrasound mensuration of the long bones in the second trimester of pregnancy. Considerable caution should be exercised making a definitive diagnosis before the twenty fourth week of pregnancy and clinicians should resist pressure from patients to do so. Limb measurements in this condition may not deviate from the normal range until 24 weeks or so (Fig. 3). This experience is confirmed by other reports of ultrasonic diagnosis.[21,32]

The condition is associated with good survival and normal intelligence although orthopaedic problems are common. Inheritance is dominant and more than half of the cases arise as the result of a new mutation.

Cleidocranial dysostosis is characterised by shortened or absent clavicles and skull undermineralisation. These and other features of the condition are variable in expression.

Conditions associated with spinal abnormalities Jarcho-Levin syndrome is a congenital skeletal disorder characterised by disorganisation of the spine with multiple fused and hemivertebrae and an abnormal rib cage. The long bones are unaffected. The vertebral anomalies cause a short neck and the spine is often shortened and has a kyphosis and/or scoliosis. As a result of the vertebral

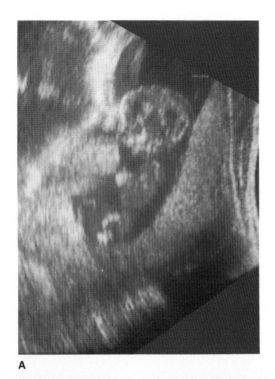

A

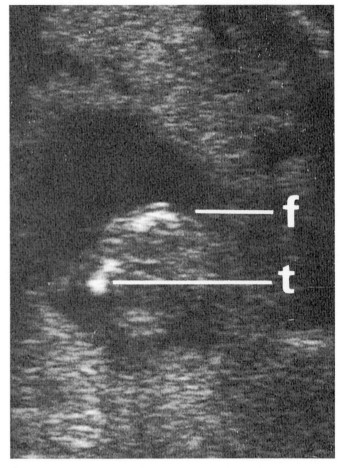

C

Fig. 14 Campomelic dysplasia. A: Fetus with campomelic dysplasia at 15+ weeks. **B:** Radiograph of the fetus at 17 weeks showing bowed femora and tibia and normal upper limbs. **C:** Lower limb shows short bowed femur (f), short tibia (t) and absent fibula. **D:** Upper limb shows humerus, radius and ulna with normal length and modelling.

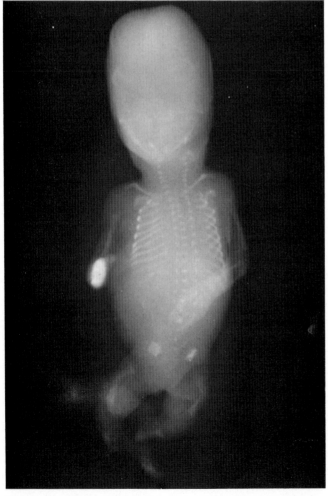

B

changes there is often posterior fusion of the ribs with anterior flaring resulting in a 'crab-chest' deformity. It is inherited in an autosomal recessive pattern and usually results in death from respiratory failure within the first year of life. Clinically there is some overlap with spondylocostal dysplasia where there are similar abnormalities but usually in a much milder form. Spondylocostal dysplasia is inherited in an autosomal dominant fashion.

Prenatal diagnosis of Jarcot-Levin syndrome based on the finding of disorganisation of the spine (particularly the thoracic region) in association with normal limb biometry has been made in both high- and low-risk cases.[48–52]

Dyssegmental dysplasia is a lethal syndrome characterised by marked shortening of the extremities and a deformed, undermineralised spine. It has been diagnosed

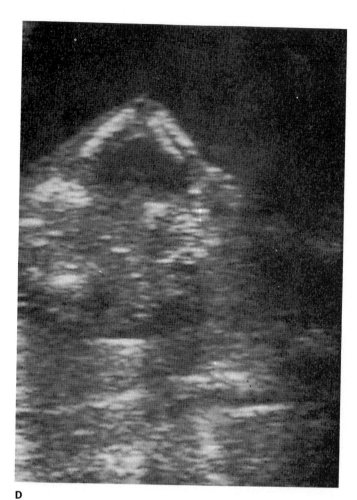

D

by antenatal ultrasonography at 18 weeks.[53] The inheritance is autosomal recessive.

Many other skeletal dysplasias may not show sufficient limb shortening or other features for second trimester diagnosis. Malformation of the spine because of hemivertebrae[54] may give a clue to diagnosis in high-risk pregnancies.

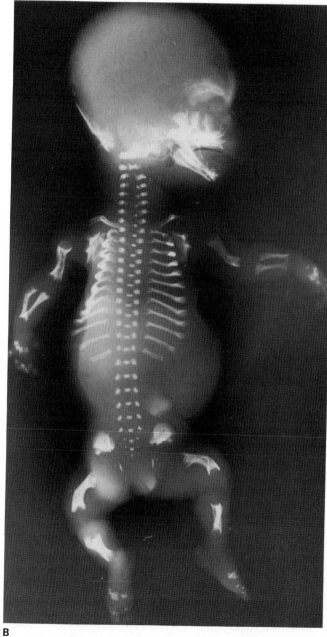

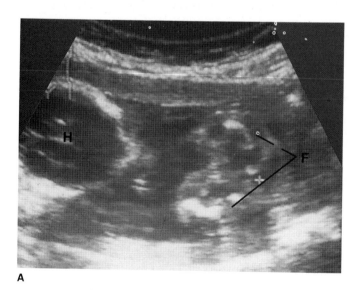

A

B

Fig. 15 **Thanatophoric dysplasia at 19 weeks. A:** Scan showing short, bowed femora (F) and large head (H). **B:** Radiograph of a similar fetus.

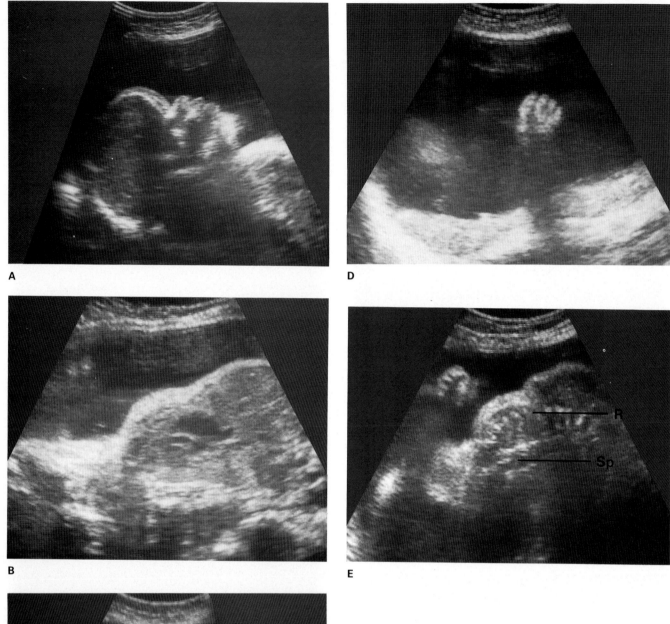

Fig. 16 Thanatophoric dysplasia at 31 weeks. A: Facial profile showing frontal bossing and depressed nasal bridge. **B:** Small thorax and normal liver giving 'champagne cork' appearance. **C:** Redundant folds of skin on the arm. **D:** Short, stubby fingers of 'trident hand' and polyhydramnios. **E:** Coronal scan of the thoracic spine (Sp) and short, thick ribs (R). **F:** Photograph of a term infant following neonatal death showing typical features of thanatophoric dysplasia.

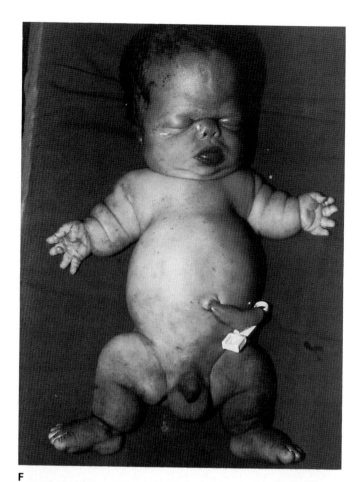

F

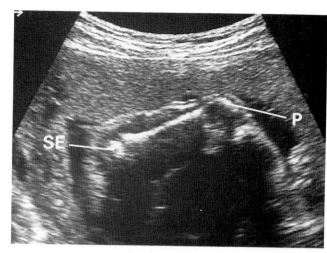

B

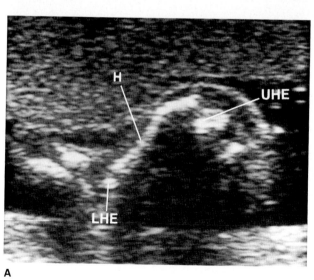

A

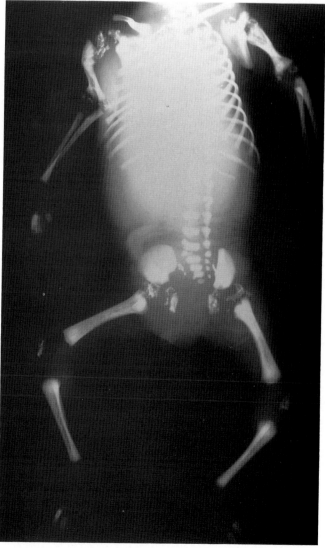

C

Fig. 17 Rhizomelic chondrodyplasia punctata. Scans from the upper arm and leg of a 19 week fetus with rhizomelic chondrodysplasia punctata. **A:** The humerus (H) is thick, short and bowed and shows disorganised upper humeral (UHE) and lower humeral (LHE) epiphyses. **B:** Mineralised stippled epiphysis at the upper femur (SE) and mineralised patella (P). **C:** Radiograph showing marked shortening of the humerus and disorganised, stippled epiphyses at upper and lower humerus, upper femur and patella. Note also fixed flexion deformity of the elbow.

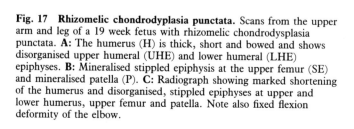

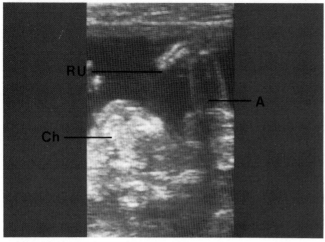

A

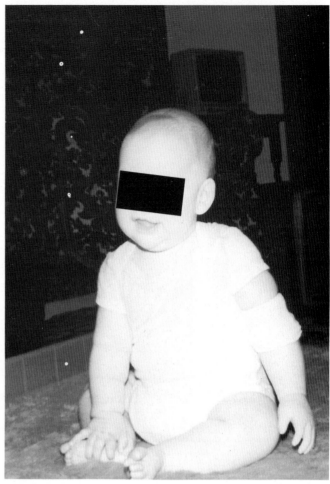

C

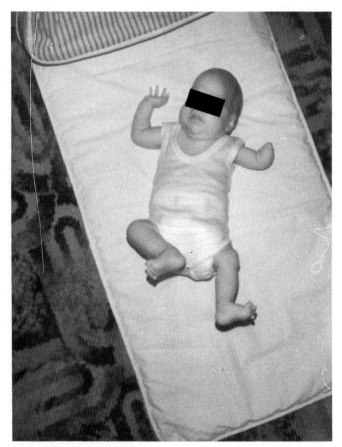

B

Fig. 18   Reduction defect. A: Scan of an isolated amputation-like reduction defect of the forearm showing shortened radius and ulna (RU) and absent hand. A – upper arm, Ch – chin. **B:** Photograph of infant at 8 weeks of age without prosthesis; **C:** with prosthesis at 6 months.

Limb reduction deformities

This group of deformities is characterised by absence or reduction of limbs or segments of limbs. In general this is a heterogeneous group of disorders many of which are not of genetic origin. The deformity may involve absence of all limbs (amelia) or reduction (phocomelia) of one, more or all limbs (tetraphocomelia). There may also be reduction of a longitudinal segment of a limb (hemimelia) such as the radius. In the absence of associated abnormalities prognosis is generally good as technological advances in limb prostheses are such that excellent functional and cosmetic results can be obtained, even in apparently severe reductions (Fig. 18). However a detailed general examination of the fetus is indicated as a limb reduction deformity may be part of a spectrum of abnormalities which will increase the risk of an underlying chromosomal defect (Fig. 19) or genetic syndrome.

Amniotic band syndrome (ABS) This group of disorders shows great variation in severity from minor digital constriction rings or amputations to major structural disruption of the head (encephalocele) and face, trunk (ventral wall defects) and limbs (deformity and amputations). The lesions are asymmetrical. Careful ultrasonic examination may reveal bands of amnion attached to and immobilising deformed fetal parts.[55]

If multiple asymmetrical abnormalities are found ABS should be considered and bands sought. A fetal karyotype should be obtained to exclude a chromosomal anomaly.

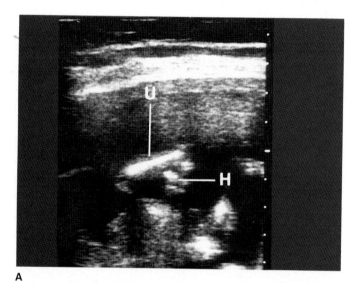

A

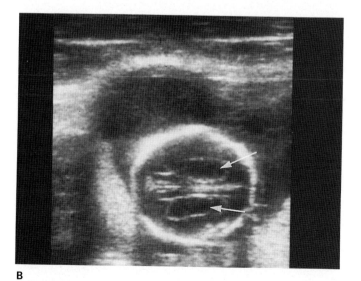

B

Fig. 19 Trisomy 18. Scan at 18 weeks showing: **A:** Radial aplasia and wrist deformity. U – ulna, H – hand. **B:** Large bilateral choroid plexus cysts (arrows).

Bands or ridges in the amnion may be seen in normal pregnancies. If these are not attached to the fetus and a careful search reveals no deformity they should be regarded as harmless.

The aetiology of the amniotic band syndrome is a source of continuing debate. It may be due to early amnion rupture, vascular occlusion during embryonic or fetal development or result from a gene mutation.

Genetic syndromes associated with limb reduction deformities Roberts syndrome is a recessive syndrome characterised by severe tetraphocomelia and median facial clefting associated with marked growth deficiency. Other features of the syndrome are syndactyly, talipes and microcephaly. Many are stillborn or die in infancy. Mental retardation is a common complication in the few survivors. An affected individual presents features similar to those associated with the teratogenic effects of the drug thalidomide. The syndrome has been diagnosed prenatally in a high-risk family.[13] The main differential diagnosis is hypoglossia-hypodactyly syndrome where there may be limb reduction defects in all limbs but a major distinguishing feature is the presence of micrognathia and a small tongue. Clefting does not usually occur. The other distinguishing feature is the presence of premature separation of the centromeres (chromosome puffing) which can be seen in most cases of Roberts syndrome on cytogenetic examination.[56] This may be of use prenatally if it is necessary to distinguish the two syndromes. The prognosis for intellectual development in hypoglossia-hypodactyly syndrome is good and most cases are sporadic, arising as new dominant mutations.

Thrombocytopaenia-absent radius (TAR) syndrome. The defects are usually bilateral radial aplasia or variable degrees of hypoplasia. The thumbs are always present. Ulnar or humeral reductions are seen in some cases. These deformities are diagnostic markers for the underlying haemopoietic defect of hypomegakaryocytic thrombocytopaenia which may be recognised on fetal blood sampling. In one third of cases there is coexistent congenital heart disease (Fallot's tetralogy, VSD). Successful ultrasonographic diagnosis in the second trimester has been reported.[13,57,58]

The prognosis depends on the severity of the cardiac lesion rather than the bleeding diathesis. The majority survive infancy and the thrombocytopaenia improves with age and, in badly affected cases, support with platelet transfusions.[59,60] Inheritance is autosomal recessive.

Fanconi pancytopaenia syndrome is an autosomal recessive syndrome associated with bone marrow failure and severe anaemia. Nearly 80% of affected individuals have aplasia or hypoplasia of the thumb and radius which may be unilateral. The anaemia tends to be progressive, usually presenting in the later part of the first decade of life. Prenatal diagnosis of this syndrome has not been reported but there is potential for diagnosis in high-risk families.

Other congenital anaemias (Aase and Blackfan Diamond) are also associated with radial defects in a significant proportion of cases.[59]

Holt-Oram syndrome is an autosomal dominant syndrome of upper limb/girdle deformity and congenital heart disease of very variable degree. The limb reductions vary in severity. They may involve any part of the upper limb and shoulder girdle. Thumbs may be absent, hypoplastic or triphalangeal (finger-like) or associated with syndactyly. ASD and VSD are the commoner cardiac abnormalities. Successful diagnosis in the second and third trimesters of high-risk pregnancies has been based on the ultrasonographic demonstration of both limb and cardiac deformities.[61,62] The expression of this disorder within a family is extremely variable and a gene carrier may have only the minimum of signs (e.g. difficulty in pronation of the forearm or minor abnormalities of the thumb).[62]

Polysyndactyly

Abnormalities of the fingers are best seen in a fully fanned hand (see Ch. 10, Fig. 56). The fetus is not always obliging enough to give this view and a section across the clenched hand in the axial plane will suffice to detect extra (or a deficiency of) bones. A full plantar view of the foot should display polydactyly (Fig. 20D).

Polydactyly may be pre-axial (Fig. 20) (duplicate or bifid thumbs or big toes) or post-axial (on the ulnar side of the index finger or lateral aspect of the foot). Syndactyly de-

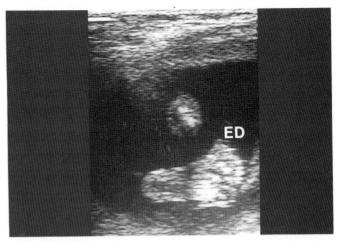

B

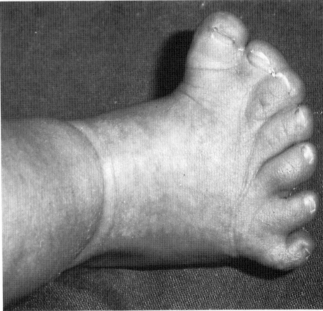

C

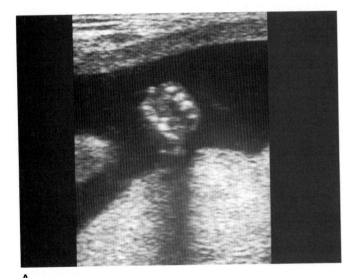

A

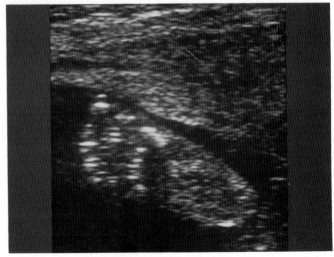

D

Fig. 20 Cephalopolysyndactyly syndrome. Scan and photograph from a fetus and infant with Greig cephalopolysyndactyly syndrome with dominant inheritance. **A:** Clenched hand showing post-axial extra digit. **B:** Plantar view of foot showing pre-axial polysyndactyly. ED – extra digit. **C:** Photograph of foot after birth. **D:** Scan of normal foot for comparison.

Table 5 Some syndromes associated with polysyndactyly

Polydactyly	Syndactyly
Meckel Gruber	Apert (acrocephalosyndactyly)
Ellis-van-Creveld	Oral facial digital
Greig cephalopolysyndactyly	Roberts (pseudothalidomide)
Grebe	Carpenter
SRP	
Oral facial digital	
Carpenter (acrocephalopolysyndactyly)	
Jeune (asphyxiating thoracic dystrophy)	
Jouberts	
Trisomy 13	

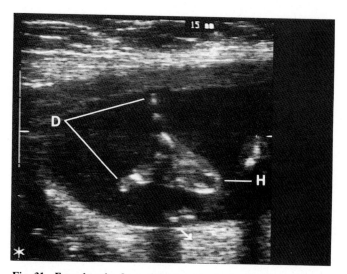

Fig. 21 Ectrodactyly. Scan of the foot of a fetus with bilateral ectrodactyly of the feet ('lobster claw' deformity). The hands appeared normal. H – heel, D – two digits. (Figure courtesy of Professor S. Campbell).

notes fusion of either the bones (osseous syndactyly) or soft tissues (cutaneous syndactyly) of the fingers or toes.

There are many syndromes with these abnormalities as a feature (Fig. 20). The commoner ones are listed in Table 5. For a more detailed list and description of the syndromes the reader is referred to Smith[59] and Winter et al.[2] As the syndromes have differing prognostic significance it behoves the ultrasonologist to make a detailed search for other fetal abnormalities before coming to a diagnosis. Fetal karyotyping should also be considered. Isolated polysyndactyly occurs as an autosomal dominant condition in some families.

Ectrodactyly

Ectrodactyly, or split hands or feet (Fig. 21), can occur as part of the ectrodactyly ectodermal dysplasia clefting syndrome (EEC) or as an isolated abnormality. Both conditions are inherited as autosomal dominant traits, but ectrodactyly may be associated with other syndromes with variable inheritance. EEC is associated with difficulty in sweating, sparse hair, abnormal teeth and facial clefts. The degree of penetrance within families can be very variable. Isolated ectrodactyly can affect one or more limbs to variable degrees. Isolated cases are new dominant mutations but before counselling low occurrences to apparently normal parents careful examination is mandatory as they may have very minimal signs (e.g. extra longitudinal skin creases on feet or hands).[63] A case of ectrodactyly diagnosed in a low-risk pregnancy is shown in Figure 21. Both feet had complete ectrodactyly. The diagnosis in severe cases such as this should not be a problem. However, more minor degrees may not be amenable to prenatal detection with ultrasound.

Positional deformities

Talipes (club foot)   In this condition the foot is plantar flexed and internally rotated. The condition may be detected on ultrasound examination by observing the relationship between the shaft of the tibia and the axis of the toes or plantar surface of the foot. The views of the leg employed to detect abnormalities are shown in Chapter 10, Figures 50 to 52. Talipes may occur as an isolated malformation in about one in 1200 births, as a result of asymmetrical intra-uterine environmental pressures (oligohydramnios, amniotic bands or intra-uterine tumours), as a marker of chromosomal abnormality or as an integral part of a multitude of genetic syndromes (Fig. 22).[59] Fetal karyotyping should be considered if talipes is present with another structural abnormality.

Rocker bottom feet are a feature of trisomy 18 (Edwards' syndrome), 18q syndrome, trisomy 13 (Patau syndrome) and Pena-Shokeir type II syndrome. The deformity is characterised by a prominent heel, and replacement of the normal concavity of the plantar arch by convexity. The finding of this deformity should be a stimulus to detailed fetal examination for other defects (Fig. 23) and fetal karyotyping.

Multiple congenital contractures (arthrogryposis multiplex congenita)   This is a heterogeneous group of disorders all of which have multiple joint contractures present at birth. These are a result of limitation of fetal joint mobility and may be secondary to neurological (central or peripheral), muscular, connective tissue or skeletal abnormalities. Intra-uterine crowding as with oligohydramnios may also cause multiple joint contractures. Hageman et al reviewed 75 newborns with

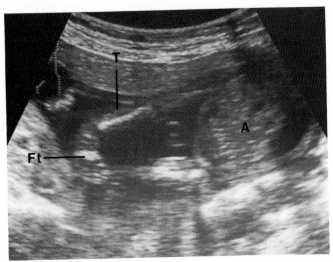

Fig. 22 Congenital muscular dystrophy. Scan of the leg of a fetus with congenital muscular dystrophy showing severe talipes. Note that the plantar view of the foot (Ft) is seen in the same plane as the tibia (T). A – abdomen.

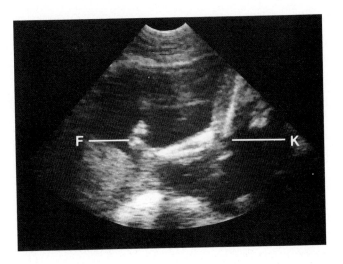

Fig. 24 Arthrogryposis. Scan of a fetal leg in a case of arthrogryposis multiplex congenita. The hips were adducted and the knee (K) hyperextended so that the foot (F) pointed directly at the face. There were also marked fixed positional deformities of the upper limb.

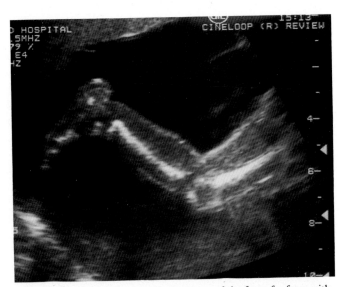

Fig. 23 Rocker bottom foot. Sagittal scan of the foot of a fetus with trisomy 18 showing prominent heel (H) suggestive of 'rocker bottom' feet. This deformity was found in association with omphalocele and cleft lip and palate.

multiple congenital contractures and found abnormalities in the central nervous system in 55%, the peripheral neuromuscular system in 8% and connective tissues and skin in 11%.[64] Oligohydramnios was associated in 7%.

These conditions should be recognised on ultrasound examination in the second trimester when fixed, immobile limbs are found in bizarre positions (Figs 22 to 25). Polyhydramnios and hydrops are frequent accompanying features. Specific syndromes such as Pena-Shokeir syndrome type I,[65,66] lethal multiple pterygium syndrome[67] and congenital muscular dystrophy have been described.

These syndromes are mainly autosomal recessive. Kirkinen et al describe ultrasonic observation of six high-risk pregnancies from the first trimester.[68] Although apparently normal at between 8 and 12 weeks, all six fetuses showed severe generalised subcutaneous oedema with restricted fetal movement by the sixteenth week. In two there was ascites or hydrothorax which are common accompaniments to these syndromes.[69–75] The prognosis in these cases is usually poor with a high incidence of stillbirth and neonatal deaths secondary to pulmonary hypoplasia.

The distal arthrogryposes are a group of milder conditions affecting peripheral joints such as hands, feet and the jaw.[76] The deformities may be corrected with surgery and life expectancy and neurological function are normal. These conditions are autosomal dominant. Prenatal ultrasound diagnosis in an affected family has been described on the detection of flexed fingers and extended wrists.[77,78]

Counselling and follow up

Some of the characteristic features of a wide spectrum of skeletal and postural deformities have been described. Diagnostic accuracy will be improved if time is spent examining the fetus in detail. A reference textbook may be very helpful in coming to an accurate diagnosis of many of the lethal dysplasias. In cases where the diagnosis or prognosis are in doubt it may be prudent to consult a geneticist or paediatrician before finally counselling a couple who may themselves wish a further specialist consultation before they come to a final decision on management.

On delivery of the affected fetus anteroposterior and lateral photographs and detailed X-rays should be taken. If the fetus is dead but fresh ask that fetal blood or skin be

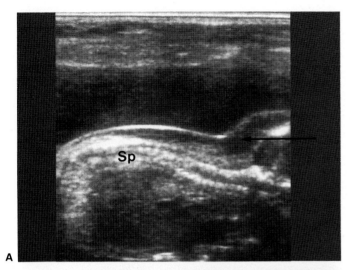

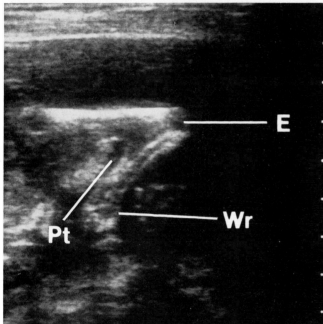

Fig. 25 Multiple pterygium syndrome. Scans from a fetus with lethal multiple pterygium syndrome. **A:** Posterior sagittal section of the spine (Sp) and occipital region showing nuchal oedema (arrow). **B:** The arm is in fixed flexion at the elbow (E). There is a skin web or pterygium (Pt) in the antecubital fossa. The wrist (Wr) shows a flexion deformity. Similar pterygia were apparent in the popliteal fossae.

sent for cytogenetic studies. In many cases consultation with a geneticist may be appropriate to discuss storage of DNA which may be useful for future early diagnosis. It is also important, where appropriate, that post-mortem examination is performed by a pathologist interested in skeletal dysplasias. Only when all this information has been gathered should the definitive diagnosis be made and the couple finally counselled by a geneticist as to risks of recurrence in future pregnancies and the implications for other family members.

REFERENCE

1 Koren G, Edwards M B, Miskin M. Antenatal sonography of fetal malformations associated with drugs and chemicals: a guide. Am J Obstet Gynecol 1987; 176: 79

2 Winter R M, Knowles S A S, Bieber F R, Baraitser M. The malformed fetus and stillbirth; a diagnostic approach. Chichester: John Wiley. 1988: p 166–201

3 O'Brien G D, Queenan J T, Campbell S. Assessment of gestational age in the second trimester by real-time ultrasound measurement of the femur length. Am J Obstet Gynecol 1981; 139: 540–545

4 Orioli I M, Castilla E E, Barbosa-Neto J G. The birth prevalence rates for the skeletal dysplasias. J Med Genet 1986; 23: 328–332

5 Glenn L W, Teng S S K. In utero sonographic diagnosis of achondrogenesis. JCU 1985; 13: 195–198

6 Golbus M S, Hall B D, Filly R A, Poskanzer L B. Prenatal diagnosis of achondrogenesis. J Paediatr 1977; 91: 464

7 Donnenfeld A E, Mennuti M T. Second trimester diagnosis of fetal skeletal dysplasias. Obstet Gynecol Surv 1987; 42: 199–217

8 Muller L M, Cremin B J. Ultrasonic demonstration of fetal skeletal dysplasia. S Afr Med J 1985; 65: 222–226

9 Griffin D, Campbell S, Allan L, Roberts A, Little D. Fetal anomalies. In: Barnet E, Morley P. eds. Clinical diagnostic ultrasound. Oxford: Blackwell Scientific Publications. 1985: p 559–580

10 Borochowitz Z, Ornoy A, Lachman R, Rimoin D L. Achondrogenesis II – hypochondrogenesis: variability versus heterogeneity. Am J Med Genet 1986; 24: 273–288

11 Stoll C, Manini P, Bloch J, Roth M-P. Prenatal diagnosis of hypochondroplasia. Prenat Diagn 1985; 5: 423–426

12 van der Harten J J, Brons J T J, Dijkstra P F, et al. Paediatr Pathol 1988; 8: 233–252

13 Hobbins J C, Bracken M B, Mahoney M J. Diagnosis of fetal dysplasias with ultrasound. Am J Obstet Gynecol 1982; 142: 306–312

14 Milsom I, Mattsson L-A, Dahlen-Nilsson I. Antenatal diagnosis of osteogenesis imperfecta by real-time ultrasound: two case reports. Br J Radiol 1982; 55: 310–312

15 Shapiro J E, Phillips J A, Byers P H, et al. Prenatal diagnosis of lethal osteogenesis imperfecta (OI type II). J Pediatr 1982; 100: 127–133

16 Dinno N D, Yacuob U S, Kadlec J F, Garver K L. Midtrimester diagnosis of osteogenesis imperfecta, type II. Birth Defects 1982; 18: 125–132

17 Elejalde B R, de Elejalde M M. Prenatal diagnosis of perinatally lethal osteogenesis imperfecta. Am J Med Genet 1983; 14: 353–359

18 Brons J T J, van der Harten J J, Wladimiroff J W, van Geijn H P. Prenatal ultrasonographic diagnosis of osteogenesis imperfecta. Am J Obstet Gynecol 1988; 159: 176–181

19 Young I D, Thompson E M, Hall C M, Pembrey M E. Osteogenesis imperfecta type IIA: evidence for dominant inheritance. J Med Genet 1987; 24: 386–389

20 Thompson E M, Young I D, Hall C M, Pembrey M E. Recurrence risks and prognosis in severe sporadic osteogenesis imperfecta. J Med Genet 1987; 24: 390–405

21 Kurtz A B, Wapner R J. Ultrasonographic diagnosis of second trimester skeletal dysplasias: a prospective analysis in a high risk population. J Ultrasound Med 1983; 2: 99–106

22 Wladimiroff J W, Niermeijer M F, Van der Harten J J, Stewart F G A, Bloms W, Huijmans J G M. Early prenatal diagnosis of congenital hypophosphatasia: case report. Prenat Diagn 1985; 5: 47–52

23 Mulivor R A, Mennuti M, Zackai E H, Harris H. Prenatal diagnosis of hypophosphatasia: genetic, biochemical and clinical studies. Am J Hum Genet 1978; 30: 271–282

24 Warren R C, McKenzie C F, Rodeck C H, Moscoso G, Brock D J, Barron L. First trimester diagnosis of hypophosphatasia with a monoclonal antibody to the liver/bone/kidney isoenzyme of alkaline phosphatase. Lancet 1985; 2: 856

25 Little D. Prenatal diagnosis of skeletal dysplasias. In: Rodeck C H, Nicolaides K H. eds. Prenatal Diagnosis. London: Royal College of Obstetricians and Gynaecologists. 1984: p 301–306

26 Elejalde B R, de Elejalde M M, Pansch D. Prenatal diagnosis of Jeune Syndrome. Am J Med Genet 1985; 21: 433–438

27 Donaldson M D C, Warner A A, Trompeter R S, Haycock G B, Chantler C. Familial juvenile nephronophthisis, Jeune's syndrome and associated disorders. Arch Dis Child 1985; 60: 426–434

28 Fryns J P, van den Berghe K, van Assche A, van den Berghe H. Prenatal diagnosis of campomelic dwarfism. Clin Genet 1981; 19: 199–201

29 Redon J Y, Le Grevellec J Y, Marie F, Le Coq E, Le Guern H. Un diagnostic antenatal de dysplasie campomelique. J Gynecol Obstet Biol Reprod 1984; 13: 437–441

30 Winter R, Rosenkranz W, Hofmann H, Zierler H, Becker H, Borkenstein M. Prenatal diagnosis of campomelic dysplasia by ultrasonography. Prenat Diagn 1985; 5: 1–8

31 Mahoney M J, Hobbins J C. Prenatal diagnosis of chondroectodermal cysplasia (Ellis-van-Creveld syndrome) with fetoscopy and ultrasound. N Engl J Med 1977; 297: 258–260

32 Filly R A, Golbus M S, Cary J C, Hall J G. Short limbed dwarfism: ultrasonographic diagnosis by mensuration of fetal femoral length. Radiology 1981; 138: 653–656

33 Filly R A, Golbus M S. Ultrasonography of the normal and pathologic fetal skeleton. Radiol Clin North Am 1982; 20: 311–323

34 Elejalde B R, de Elejalde M M. Thanatophoric dysplasia: fetal manifestations and prenatal diagnosis. Am J Med Genet 1985; 22: 669–683

35 Weiner C P, Williamson R A, Bonsib S M. Sonographic diagnosis of cloverleaf skull and thanatophoric dysplasia in the second trimester. JCU 1986; 14: 463–465

36 Chervenak F A, Blakemore K J, Isaacson G, Mayden K, Hobbins J C. Antenatal sonographic findings of thanatophoric dysplasia with cloverleaf skull. Am J Obstet Gynecol 1983; 146: 984–985

37 Beetham F G T, Reeves J S. Early ultrasound diagnosis of thanatophoric dwarfism. JCU 1984; 12: 43–44

38 Burrows P E, Stannard M W, Pearrow J, Sutterfield S, Baker M L. Early antenatal sonographic recognition of thanatophoric dysplasia with cloverleaf skull deformity. AJR 1984; 143: 841–843

39 Camera G, Dodero D, De Pascale S. Prenatal diagnosis of thanatophoric dysplasia at 24 weeks. Am J Med Genet 1984; 18: 39–43

40 Wladimiroff J W, Niermeijer M F, Laar J, Jahoda M, Stewart P A. Prenatal diagnosis of skeletal dysplasia by real-time ultrasound. Obstet Gynecol 1984; 63: 360–364

41 Meizner I, Bar-Ziv J. Prenatal ultrasonic diagnosis of short-rib polydactyly syndrome (SRPS) Type 3: a case report and a proposed approach to the diagnosis of SRPS and related conditions. JCU 1985; 13: 284–287

42 Gembruch U, Hansmann M, Frodisch H J. Early prenatal diagnosis of short rib-polydactyly (SRP) syndrome type 1 (Majewski) by ultrasound in a case at risk. Prenat Diagn 1985; 5: 357–362

43 Hoefler S, Hoefler G, Moser A B, Watkins P A, Chen W W, Moser H W. Prenatal diagnosis of rhizomelic chondrodysplasia punctata. Prenat Diagn 1988; 8: 571–576

44 Mantagos S, Weiss R W, Mahoney M, Hobbins J C. Prenatal diagnosis of diastrophic dwarfism. Am J Obstet Gynecol 1981; 139: 111–113

45 Gembruch U, Niesen M, Kehrberg H, Hansmann M. Diastrophic dysplasia: a specific prenatal diagnosis by ultrasound. Prenat Diagn 1988; 8: 539–545

46 O'Brien G D, Rodeck C, Queenan J T. Early prenatal diagnosis of diastrophic dwarfism by ultrasound. BMJ 1980; 280: 1300

47 Kaitila I, Ammala P, Karjalainen O, Liukkonen S, Rapola J. Early prenatal detection of diastrophic dysplasia. Prenat Diagn 1983; 3: 237–244

48 Campbell S, Griffin D, Roberts A, Little D. Early prenatal diagnosis of abnormalities of the fetal head, spine, limbs and abdominal organs. In: Orlandi P, Polani P, Bovicelli L. eds. Recent advances in prenatal diagnosis. Chichester: John Wiley. 1981: p 41–59

49 Tolmie J T, Whittle M J, McNay M B, Gibson A A M, Connor J M. Second trimester prenatal diagnosis of the Jarcho-Levin syndrome. Prenat Diagn 1987; 7: 129–134

50 Apuzzio J J, Diamond N, Ganesh M S, Despostio F. Difficulties in the prenatal diagnosis of Jarcho-Levin syndrome. Am J Obstet Gynecol 1987; 156: 916–918

51 Romero R, Ghidini A, Eswara M S, Seashore M R, Hobbins J C. Prenatal findings in a case of spondylocostal dysplasia type I (Jarco-Levin syndrome). Obstet Gynecol 1988; 71: 988–991

52 Marks M, Hernanz-Schulman M, Horii S, et al. Spondylothoracic dysplasia. Clinical and sonographic diagnosis. J Ultrasound Med 1989; 8: 1–5

53 Kim H J, Costales F, Bouzouki M, Wallach R C. Prenatal diagnosis of dysegmental dwarfism. Prenat Diagn 1986; 6: 143–150

54 Benacerraf B R, Greene M F, Barss V A. Prenatal sonographic diagnosis of congenital hemivertebra. J Ultrasound Med 1986; 5: 257–259

55 Mahony B S, Filly R A, Callen P W, Golbus M S. Amniotic band syndrome: antenatal sonographic diagnosis and potential pitfalls. Am J Obstet Gynecol 1985; 152: 63–68

56 Parry D M, Mulvihill J J, Tsai S, Kaiser-Kupfer M I, Cowan J M. SC phocomelia syndrome, premature centromere separation, and congenital nerve paralysis in two sisters, one with malignant melanoma. Am J Med Genet 1986; 24: 653–672

57 Luthy D A, Mack L, Hirsch J, Cheng E. Prenatal diagnosis of thrombocytopenia with absent radii. Am J Obstet Gynecol 1981; 141: 350–351

58 Filkins K, Russo J, Bilinki I. Prenatal diagnosis of thrombocytopaenia absent radius syndrome using ultrasound and fetoscopy. Prenat Diagn 1984; 4: 139

59 Smith D W. Recognizable patterns of human malformations: genetic, embryologic and clinical aspects. Philadelphia: W B Saunders, 1982

60 Hall J G. Thrombocytopenia and absent radius (TAR) syndrome. J Med Genet 1987; 24: 79–83

61 Muller L M, de Jong G, van Heerden K M M. The antenatal ultrasonographic detection of the Holt-Oram syndrome. S Afr Med J 1985; 68: 313–315

62 Brons J T J, Van Geijn H P, Wladimiroff J W, et al. Prenatal ultrasound diagnosis of the Holt-Oram syndrome. Prenat Diagn 1988; 8: 175–181

63 Penchaszadeh V B, Negrotti T C. Ectrodactyly-ectodermal dysplasia-clefting (EEC) syndrome: dominant inheritance and variable expression. J Med Genet 1976; 13: 281–284

64 Hageman G, Ippel E P F, Beemer F A, de Pater J M, Lindhout D, Willemse J. The diagnostic management of newborns with congenital contractures: a nosologic study of 75 cases. Am J Med Genet 1988; 30: 883–904

65 Pena S D J, Shokeir M H K. Syndrome of camptodactyly, multiple ankyloses, facial anomalies and pulmonary hypoplasia: a lethal condition. J Pediatr 1974; 85: 373–375

66 Hall J G. Invited editorial comment: analysis of Pena-Shokeir phenotype. Am J Med Genet 1986; 25: 99–117

67 Hall J G. The lethal multiple pterygium syndromes. Am J Med Genet 1984; 17: 803–807

68 Kirkinen P, Herva R, Leisti J. Early prenatal diagnosis of a lethal syndrome of multiple congenital contractures. Prenat Diagn 1987; 7: 189–196

69 Shenker L, Reed K, Anderson C, Hauck L, Spark R. Syndrome of camptodactyly, ankyloses, facial anomalies and pulmonary hypoplasia (Pena-Shokeir syndrome): obstetric and ultrasound aspects. Am J Obstet Gynecol 1985; 152: 303–307

70 Chen H, Immken L, Lachman R, et al. Syndrome of multiple pterygia, camptodactyly, facial anomalies, hypoplastic lungs and heart, cystic hygroma and skeletal anomalies: delineation of a new entity and review of lethal forms of multiple pterygium syndrome. Am J Med Genet 1984; 17: 809–823

71 Jeanty P, Romero R, D'Alton M, Venus I, Hobbins J. In utero sonographic detection of hand and foot deformities. J Ultrasound Med 1985; 4: 595–601

72 MacMillan R, Harbart G, Davis W, Kelly T. Prenatal diagnosis of Pena-Shokeir syndrome type I. Am J Med Genet 1985; 21: 279–284

73 Muller L M, de Jong G. Prenatal ultrasonic features of the Pena-Shokeir I syndrome and the trisomy 18 syndrome. Am J Med Genet 1986; 25: 119–129

74 Goldberg J D, Chervenak F A, Lipman R A, Berkowitz R L. Antenatal sonographic diagnosis of arthrogryposis multiplex congenita. Prenat Diagn 1986; 6: 45–49

75 Zeitune M, Fejgin M D, Abramowicz J, B-Aderet N, Goodman R. Prenatal diagnosis of the pterygium syndrome. Prenat Diagn 1988; 8: 145–149

76 Hall J G, Reed S D, Green G. The distal arthrogryposes: delineation of new entities – review and nosological discussion. Am

J Med Genet 1982; 11: 185–239

77 Baty B J, Cubberley D, Morris C, Cary J. Prenatal diagnosis of distal arthrogryposis. Am J Med Genet 1988; 29: 501–510

78 Griffin D R. Detection of congenital abnormalities of the limbs and face by ultrasound. In: Chamberlain G. ed. Modern antenatal care of the fetus. Oxford: Blackwell Scientific Publications. 1990: p 389–427

21

The thorax

Lyn S. Chitty, David R. Griffin and J. Malcolm Pearce

INTRODUCTION

Congenital abnormalities of the fetal lungs that can be recognised on ultrasound examination are rare. Attempts have been made to determine the maturity of the fetal lungs and the presence or absence of pulmonary hypoplasia by comparing the echo pattern with that from the liver, but the method is too inaccurate to be useful in patient management. Likewise nomograms for thoracic dimensions do not successfully predict pulmonary hypoplasia.[1]

Bronchogenic cyst

Definition and aetiology A bronchogenic cyst is a cystic structure which is lined with bronchial epithelium and may contain cartilage, muscle and mucous glands. The incidence is unknown since many are asymptomatic in early life.[1,2] These cysts arise from an abnormal budding of the foregut and they can remain attached to the tracheo-bronchial tree, in the mediastinum or within the pulmonary parenchyma. Bronchogenic cysts vary in size and location. They may become separated from their origin during development and migrate into the mediastinum, neck, pericardium and other sites.[3]

Associated abnormalities Bronchogenic cysts arise as a result of a bronchopulmonary foregut anomaly and are therefore associated with other abnormalities which have a common embryological origin. These include oesophageal duplications, diverticulum and cysts, tracheo-oesophageal fistula, neuro-enteric cysts and lung sequestration.[4,5] Vertebral anomalies are often associated with bronchogenic cysts.[6] There is one report of such a cyst occurring in a child with trisomy 21 and congenital heart disease.[3]

Diagnosis There are very few reports of prenatal diagnosis of bronchogenic cysts.[5,7–9] The earliest, at 17 weeks gestation, was a unilocular cystic lesion.[5] This infant also had extralobar pulmonary sequestration and duplication of the oesophagus. A bronchogenic cyst at 36 weeks gestation appeared highly reflective.[7]

The differential diagnosis of a bronchogenic cyst includes other mediastinal and pulmonary masses listed below.

Differential diagnosis of intrathoracic abnormalities
Solid lesions
    cystic adenomatoid malformation type III
    pulmonary sequestration
    mediastinal teratoma
    rhabdomyoma
Cystic lesions
    cystic adenomatoid malformation types I and II
    bronchogenic cyst
    mediastinal encephalocele
    congenital diaphragmatic hernia
    pericardial and pleural effusions

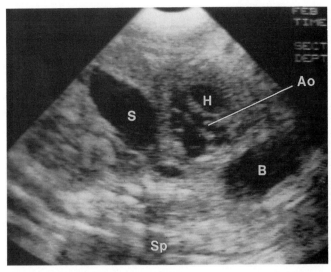

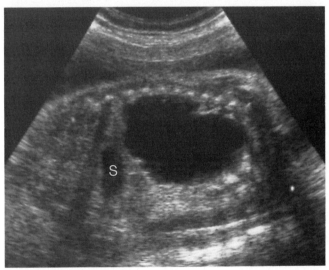

Fig. 1 Bronchogenic cyst. A: Longitudinal view through the fetal thorax and abdomen showing a bronchogenic cyst (B). **B:** A very large cyst filling the chest. Heart (H) with aortic root (Ao), S – stomach, Sp – spine.

A definitive diagnosis cannot usually be made prenatally and the final diagnosis depends on surgical and histological examination (Fig. 1).

Management and prognosis Many bronchogenic cysts are asymptomatic and are only discovered as an incidental finding on a chest radiograph[1] whilst others (particularly if located in the mediastinum) may cause airway compression sufficient to produce respiratory distress in the newborn period or recurrent respiratory tract infections in later life.[1–3] Delivery in a unit with intensive care facilities is recommended. Treatment is by surgical excision with lobectomy or pneumonectomy if the lesion is large. The

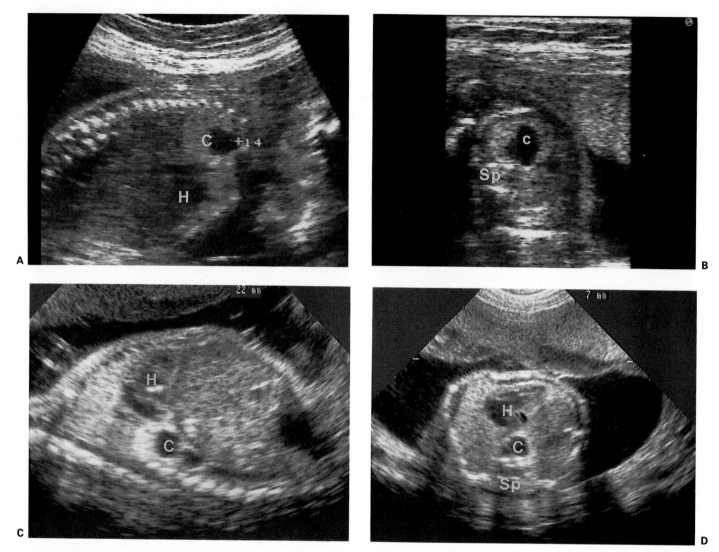

Fig. 2 Intrathoracic cystic lesions. A: Longitudinal and **B:** transverse views showing the cystic lesion (C) at the apex with the heart (H) and spine (Sp). **C:** The cyst (C) at the lung base is shown in longitudinal and **D:** transverse section.

long-term prognosis for those who survive surgery is good.[1,2]

Occasionally thoracic cysts may be demonstrated antenatally (Fig. 2) which are not substantiated post-natally. Both infants were well at birth and their chest radiographs showed minimal abnormalities and so further investigations were not thought to be justified. The first infant remains asymptomatic at $2\frac{1}{2}$ years.

Lung sequestration

Definition and aetiology Lung sequestration is a rare congenital abnormality of bronchopulmonary foregut origin in which some pulmonary parenchyma is separated from normal lung. The sequestrated lobe does not usually communicate with an airway and it has an independent blood supply directly from the systemic circulation.[10–12]

Two types of lung sequestration are recognised: intra- and extralobar. In the intralobar type the sequestrated and normal lung share a common pleura, whereas in the commoner extralobar variety the sequestrated lobe is covered by its own layer of visceral pleura. A male preponderance of 3:1 has been noted and they are usually unilateral and only include a part of the lung[13] although cases with bilateral lesions have been reported.[14] The most common location is between the lower lobe and the diaphragm. Other locations include paracardiac, mediastinal and abdominal sites. The sequestrated lobe is of variable size and has arterial and venous communication with systemic vessels.

In the majority of cases of intralobar sequestration the lower lobes are affected. The arterial supply arises most commonly from the thoracic or abdominal aorta with venous drainage into the pulmonary veins.

Associated anomalies As lung sequestration is one of the bronchopulmonary foregut malformations it has similar associations as bronchogenic cysts.[4,15-17] It is often found in association with cystic adenomatoid malformation.[1,18] Extrapulmonary abnormalities occur in 10% of patients with intralobar sequestration.[13] These include skeletal deformities, diaphragmatic hernia, congenital heart disease, renal and intracranial anomalies.[13,19,20] The incidence of extrapulmonary abnormalities in extralobar pulmonary sequestration is much higher (59%), diaphragmatic hernia being the most common.[1,10,13,18]

Lung sequestration may be associated with fetal hydrops and pleural effusions.

Diagnosis In the fetus this condition is most often discovered as a tumour of uncertain origin in the chest and a definitive diagnosis is not possible without histology.[7,21-25] The sequestrated lobe appears as a highly reflective, intrathoracic or intra-abdominal mass. Three of the cases reported had hydrops and polyhydramnios.[21,23,24] The differential diagnosis includes other intra-abdominal solid masses such as a mesonephroma, and other masses occurring in the lower part of the thorax, such as cystic adenomatoid malformation. Extralobar sequestration may simulate the pyramidal shape of the lower lobe of lung.

Prenatal diagnosis of intralobar pulmonary sequestration has been reported twice.[5,26] Both cases were detected at routine ultrasound examinations at 21 or 22 weeks gestation. In one case a highly reflective, well-defined mass in the right hemithorax suggestive of pulmonary sequestration or adenomatoid malformation was seen. The neonate had mild tachypnoea and surgical exploration at 5 days of age revealed intralobar pulmonary sequestration.[26] In the perinatal period a pre-operative diagnosis is only made in 39% of cases[13] and so accurate prenatal diagnosis may well be very difficult (Fig. 3).

Management and prognosis If the diagnosis is made before viability, particularly if there is associated hydrops, then the option of termination of pregnancy should be considered. In cases detected later in pregnancy, or where the decision to continue the pregnancy has been made, standard obstetric management should be followed. Delivery in a centre with neonatal intensive care and surgical facilities is advised as respiratory support and early surgery may be required.

The spectrum of these conditions is wide. Some cases may be discovered as an incidental finding on a routine chest radiograph. Many infants are asymptomatic until later in life when recurrent pulmonary infections or haemorrhage, gastrointestinal symptoms or heart failure from a left-to-right shunt occur.[10,16,18,20,26,27] However, the anomalous blood supply to the sequestrated lung can cause a sufficiently severe left-to-right shunt to cause cardiac failure soon after birth.[27,28] The prognosis for extralobar sequestration presenting in infancy is poor, the majority of cases having associated abnormalities and dying shortly

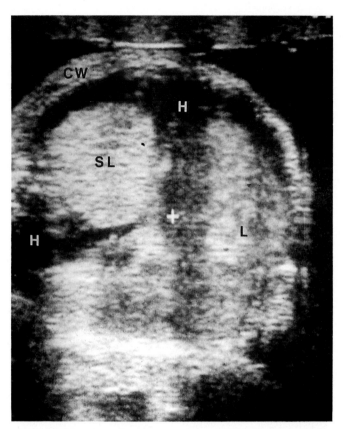

Fig. 3 Sequestrated lobe. Transverse view through the fetal chest demonstrating a sequestrated lobe (SL). Note the hydrothorax (H), chest wall (CW) and liver (L) which is visible in this section due to depression of the liver by the intrathoracic mass.

after diagnosis.[13] Of the cases detected antenatally only one of the four reported survived. The three who died had extralobar sequestration and hydrops. The survivor had intra-abdominal sequestration with no hydrops.[22] When the condition presents later in life the prognosis after surgery is good.

Cystic adenomatoid malformation

Definition and aetiology Cystic adenomatoid malformation (CAM) of the lung is a rare congenital cystic malformation characterised by excessive overgrowth of the terminal respiratory structures (hence adenomatoid) resulting in the formation of various sized intercommunicating cysts. CAM has been classified into three subgroups according to the size of the cysts.[29] The type I lesion is composed of single or multiple large cysts of greater than 2 cm in diameter. CAM type II is composed of multiple small cysts of less than 1 cm in diameter while type III is a large, bulky, microcystic lesion which often produces mediastinal shift. The lesion is usually unilateral.[30]

Associated anomalies The most common associations with CAM are polyhydramnios and fetal hydrops which

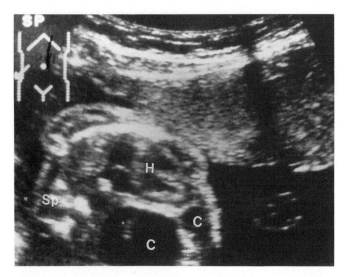

Fig. 4 Cystic adenomatoid malformation. Transverse view through the fetal chest demonstrating the large cystic areas (C) associated with CAM I. Note the mediastinal shift with the displacement of the heart (H). Sp – spine.

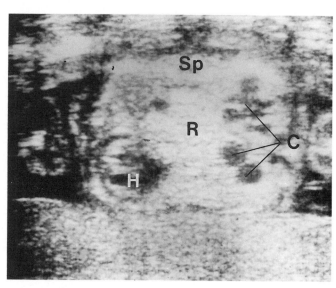

Fig. 5 CAM type II. Transverse view through the fetal chest showing the spine (Sp) and combination of highly reflective (R) and cystic (C) areas in CAM II. Note the displacement of the heart (H).

may occur in up to 80%, most commonly in type III.[31,32] Many of the cases detected prenatally are associated with these changes[32–34] although they may not be present when the initial diagnosis is made.[34] There are cases reported in the literature where the abnormality was not detected at an early routine scan but gross changes were seen later in pregnancy when the mother was scanned for another obstetric indication, usually polyhydramnios.[32,34] It has been suggested that the hydrops results from venous obstruction by the expanding mass which compresses the inferior vena cava and the hydrops may decrease after surgical decompression.[33]

Associated bronchial abnormalities have been reported in a number of cases,[1,18,35] mostly with CAM type II.[29] They include renal anomalies (in particular agenesis), diaphragmatic hernia, bowel atresia, hydrocephaly, spinal anomalies, sirenomelia and cardiac abnormalities.[36]

CAM type III has been reported in association with grossly elevated amniotic fluid alpha-fetoprotein.[37]

Diagnosis The diagnosis of CAM depends on the demonstration of an intrathoracic mass which may contain large cysts (CAM I, Fig. 4), a combination of smaller cysts with solid areas (CAM II, Fig. 5) or which may have the appearance of a uniformly reflective area (CAM III, Fig. 6). Mediastinal shift can occur in all types and this is manifested as displacement of the heart within the chest. The differential diagnosis includes other intrathoracic lesions such as congenital diaphragmatic hernia, pulmonary cysts and sequestration (see p. 408). Congenital diaphragmatic hernia can usually be distinguished by observation of peristalsis of the bowel in the chest or paradoxical visceral movement with fetal breathing.

There are several reports of prenatal diagnosis in the literature[7,30,32–34,37–42] the earliest being at 20 weeks gestation.[33,42] The majority are diagnosed later in pregnancy when an ultrasound scan is performed for another reason, often because the uterus is large for dates.

Management and prognosis The diagnosis of CAM should stimulate a careful search for other anomalies, particularly in type II. In type I decompression of the cyst(s) has been reported with good result[32,38,42] even in the presence of hydrops fetalis.[33] Spontaneous improvement in utero has been observed in three cases (one CAM I and

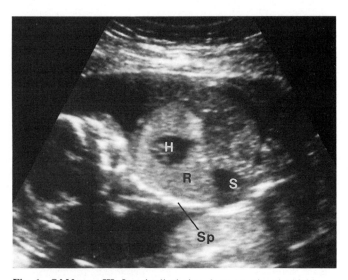

Fig. 6 CAM type III. Longitudinal view demonstrating the highly reflective appearance of CAM III (R) which is involving the entire lung. The heart (H), spine (Sp) and stomach (S) can be seen.

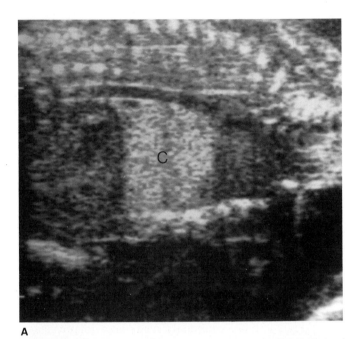

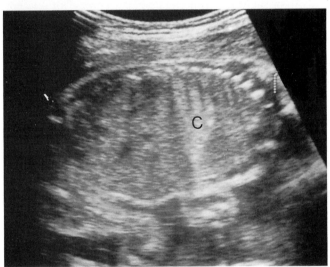

Fig. 7   Resolving CAM type III. Apparent CAM III (C) confined to the right lower lobe. **A:** Shows the early appearances. **B:** Note the apparent diminution.

two CAM II).[43,44] We have seen an apparently typical CAM type III case involving the right lower lobe, apparently showing partial resolution in utero (Fig. 7). These observations make it difficult to predict the outcome of CAM diagnosed prenatally. However, in general, the prognosis and survival of fetuses with CAM seem to vary with histological type and the presence of other abnormalities.[29,32] In the neonate CAM can be asymptomatic or may be fatal.[29,32,45] In one series five of the seven fetuses with CAM II diagnosed prenatally survived compared with only one of five with CAM III.[32] In another series all cases of CAM types II and III were either stillborn or died in

the neonatal period, whereas 11 of 19 cases with CAM I survived.[29] When hydrops, polyhydramnios or mediastinal shift occur the prognosis is usually poor, nearly 50% of cases with these associations resulting in stillbirth.[32] These signs occur more often in CAM III. In a series of 17 cases without polyhydramnios or hydrops presenting from a few hours of age to $3\frac{1}{2}$ years, only three infants died.[36] Prematurity is a common feature of cases diagnosed prenatally or in the newborn period and this can further complicate the already compromised respiratory state.[29,32] Cases undetected prenatally may present in the neonatal period with acute progressive respiratory distress because of mediastinal displacement and pulmonary compression by the expanding cystic lesion. Others develop recurrent respiratory infections in infancy and childhood.[36,45]

The management of CAM in the newborn is surgical removal, usually by lobectomy or pneumonectomy rather than segmentectomy. The prognosis for those infants who survive surgery is good.[32] Obstetric management should include delivery in a centre with neonatal intensive care and surgical facilities.

Congenital diaphragmatic hernia

Incidence and aetiology Congenital diaphragmatic hernia has an incidence of approximately one in 2000 births.[46] It occurs when a defective fusion or formation of the pleuroperitoneal membrane allows herniation of abdominal contents into the thoracic cavity. Congenital diaphragmatic hernias are classified according to the location of the defect and occur most commonly in the posterior part of the diaphragm through the foramen of Bochdalek. The majority (75%) are left sided with only 3% being bilateral.[46]

Associated anomalies Congenital diaphragmatic hernia is associated with a wide variety of abnormalities, the most common of which are malrotation of the gut and pulmonary hypoplasia, occurring as secondary phenomena. Normal lung development begins at about 5 weeks gestation. The full adult number of bronchioles is developed by the sixteenth week of gestation but alveoli continue to develop up to and beyond birth. Abdominal contents within the chest inhibit normal lung development, reducing the number of conducting airways and alveoli and resulting in pulmonary hypoplasia.[47] The severity of the hypoplasia depends on the stage of pulmonary development when herniation takes place and the volume of viscera herniated into the chest. Other structural abnormalities occur in 24% to 57% of all cases.[46,48–51] However, the incidence of associated anomalies is much lower in infants who survive the perinatal period.[51] Neural tube defects and other central nervous system abnormalities are the most frequent extrathoracic findings. Congenital heart lesions may occur in up to 23% of cases.[52] Renal and skeletal abnormalities are also major associations. Congenital diaphragmatic

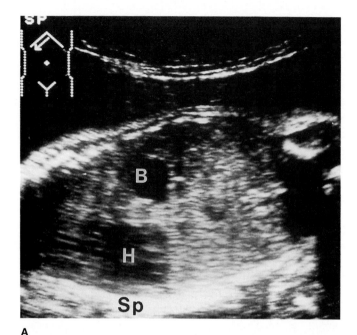

A

B

Fig. 8 **Congenital diaphragmatic hernia. A:** Longitudinal and **B:** transverse views through the chest in a fetus with a congenital diaphragmatic hernia. Note the bowel (B) in the chest, the absence of the normally situated stomach, spine (Sp) and heart (H).

hernia may also be found as a component of a number of syndromes.[53]

Chromosomal abnormalities, including trisomy 13, 18 and 21, and tetraploidy have been reported in cases of diaphragmatic hernia.[46,48,51-53] The precise risk of an associated karyotypic abnormality in the presence of a diaphragmatic hernia is difficult to assess and reports of the incidence vary from 5% to 21%.[48,54]

Diagnosis The diagnosis of a diaphragmatic hernia can be made if abdominal organs are visualised in the thorax (Fig. 8). However, bowel loops may be difficult to distinguish from other cystic lesions.[54] The differential diagnosis includes all other causes of cystic lesions in the chest (see p. 407). Paradoxical movement of the viscera with fetal respiration may be a useful discriminatory sign and, in later pregnancy, peristalsis of the bowel may be seen.[55] Other features include mediastinal shift (Fig. 9) and polyhydramnios.[54] Although prenatal diagnosis of a right sided hernia has been reported[45,55] it may be extremely difficult as in these cases the stomach maintains its normal position within the abdomen and it is the liver which herniates into the chest. The reflectivity of liver and lung are similar in mid-pregnancy, making diagnosis difficult. In two reported cases pleural effusions were present and in a third the gallbladder was identified within the chest.

The diagnosis of congenital diaphragmatic hernia has been made at the time of a routine second trimester scan[54,56] but is more commonly made later in pregnancy (usually in the third trimester) when scanning for another indication.[54,56,57] In a retrospective review of 94 cases of diaphragmatic hernia, 88 were diagnosed prenatally.[54] 76% had associated polyhydramnios and this was the indication for the scan in 66% and was associated with a poor prognosis. However, Crawford et al report a 33% incidence of associated polyhydramnios and they did not find it a poor prognostic sign.[56]

Not all cases of diaphragmatic hernia can be detected in utero because, whilst the defect may be present at an early stage, herniation of abdominal contents need not necessarily occur in utero. Approximately 5% of all cases present

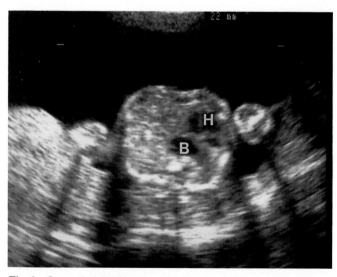

Fig. 9 **Congenital diaphragmatic hernia.** Transverse view through the chest of a fetus with a congenital diaphragmatic hernia demonstrating the mediastinal shift as indicated by the displacement of the heart (H). Note the bowel (B) in the chest.

after the neonatal period, even in adulthood.[58,59] Harrison et al report a case where a diaphragmatic hernia was clearly visible at 26 weeks but had not been detected at a routine 20 week scan.[54] They also refer to three other cases where the diagnosis had not been made at an earlier scan. They suggest that either small defects are not amenable to early detection or late herniation of the viscera occurs. All four of these cases survived. They postulate that the non-survivors have large defects and early visceral herniation resulting in more severe pulmonary hypoplasia and, incidentally, easier prenatal detection. This hypothesis is supported by the data from Crawford et al.[56] They report only two survivors from seven fetuses with isolated diaphragmatic hernia scanned prior to 24 weeks whereas seven of nine cases seen later in pregnancy survived. They make no comment on whether those cases diagnosed later in pregnancy had had a normal routine scan earlier.

Management and prognosis The prognosis for neonates with a diaphragmatic hernia is poor, the major causes of death being pulmonary hypoplasia and/or the associated anomalies. Many fetuses with major extrathoracic anomalies are stillborn or die in the neonatal period.[50,51,54] Those with cardiac malformations often die in the neonatal period.[52,54,56] Many who have an isolated diaphragmatic hernia die from respiratory insufficiency prior to surgery. In cases diagnosed in utero overall survival rates for those with an isolated diaphragmatic hernia range from 20% to 66%.[48,56] In those neonates who survive to undergo surgical repair, survival rates may be as high as 82%.[51] In a recent review of the outcome of surgery in 92 cases at the Hospitals for Sick Children, Great Ormond Street, 56 babies survived. The majority of deaths occur in the immediate post-operative period due to pulmonary hypoplasia.

There is much debate as to which prenatal features are useful prognostic indicators. The presence of associated anomalies is a bad sign. Some authors report that in isolated cases polyhydramnios predicts a poor outcome[54] whereas others do not find this association.[56] The site of the fetal stomach in left sided hernias may have prognostic importance, an abdominal site being favourable.[56] Evidence of cardiac ventricular disproportion before 24 weeks gestation is a poor prognostic sign. All four infants reported by Crawford et al showing this sign prior to 24 weeks died. When detected in the third trimester this sign appeared to be associated with a longer duration as an inpatient but not necessarily with death.[56]

The management of cases diagnosed prenatally should include fetal karyotyping and a detailed careful search for other structural abnormalities which may influence the prognosis. In particular women should be referred for expert fetal echocardiography as cardiac lesions may be very difficult to detect and classify in the presence of a distorted mediastinum.[56] As the prognosis is so variable, even when the lesion is isolated, termination of pregnancy should be discussed.

Family studies have shown that the recurrence risk for an isolated diaphragmatic hernia is about 2%.[46,60] When it occurs as part of a syndrome, the risk is that of the syndrome.

The prospects of open fetal surgery

Harrison[47,61-63] has developed an animal model of diaphragmatic hernia by inserting a balloon into the thorax of both the fetal lamb and Rhesus monkey. His group initially demonstrated that inflation of the balloon caused fatal pulmonary hypoplasia. Deflating the thoracic balloon but inflating an intra-abdominal balloon allowed sufficient lung development to allow survival after birth.

After devising an appropriate surgical technique which avoids impeding umbilical blood flow, Harrison[64] has now reported the outcome of the first six pregnancies. These women all had poor prognostic indicators and therefore underwent hysterotomy between 21 and 30 weeks with the fetus being externalised whilst the umbilical circulation was maintained. The diaphragmatic defect was repaired and an abdominoplasty was performed to prevent the returned bowel from impairing umbilical blood flow. There were three fetal deaths at the time of surgery, one immediate neonatal death while the two remaining infants died after birth from non-pulmonary causes. Post-mortem appeared to demonstrate that relative normal lung growth was possible after such a repair. None of the mothers suffered significant morbidity and four of the six have had further pregnancies without complication. The group have recently reported a further nine cases resulting in four living children.[65]

Pleural effusion

Incidence and aetiology Pleural effusions often occur as part of generalised fetal hydrops, but may be isolated. Only isolated pleural effusions are considered here: they are either idiopathic or due to chylothorax.[11] The incidence is not known.

Associated abnormalities Pleural effusions may be found in association with other bronchopulmonary abnormalities including sequestrated lobes, bronchogenic cysts, CAM and tracheo-oesophageal fistula. Chylothorax has been found in association with pulmonary lymphangiectasia and with trisomy 21[66] and Noonan's syndrome. Polyhydramnios is a frequent association.[8,66]

Diagnosis The diagnosis of a pleural effusion is easily made when the mediastinal contents and lungs are found displaced towards the centre of the thorax surrounded by an anechoic area (Fig. 10). The lesion may be uni- or bilateral, but chylothorax is usually unilateral. A specific diagnosis of the nature of the fluid cannot be made by ultrasound as the lymph appears serous and therefore echo-free until after commencement of oral feeds.

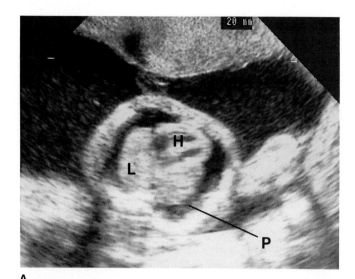

A

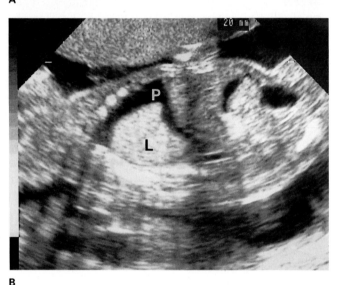

B

Fig. 10 Pleural effusions. A: Transverse and **B:** longitudinal views in a fetus with pleural effusions. Note the hydrothorax (P), compressed lungs (L) and the heart (H).

Management and prognosis When a pleural effusion is detected the rest of the fetus should be carefully examined to exclude other abnormalities. Skilled fetal echocardiography should be performed as pleural effusions may be the first manifestation of hydropic changes secondary to a congenital cardiac lesion.[67] Other causes of fetal hydrops should be excluded as far as possible and fetal karyotyping and virology studies performed.

In the absence of any other abnormality the prognosis for a fetus with pleural effusions is difficult to assess. There is the theoretical risk of pulmonary hypoplasia secondary to compression, as with all other intrathoracic space occupying lesions, and death due to pulmonary hypoplasia has been reported in cases diagnosed prenatally.[8] In addition, if left untreated, the fetus may develop generalised hydrops.[68] In an attempt to prevent these problems in utero thoracocentesis has been performed with reports of varying success rates.[68] Pijpers et al report a series of eight cases of isolated bilateral hydrothorax diagnosed prenatally at between 25 and 33 weeks gestation. No attempts at thoracocentesis were made and all infants were alive and well at the age of 1 month.[69] However it may be that diagnosis in later pregnancy is associated with a more favourable outcome. These authors conclude that a prospective study should be carried out to compare survival with and without pleuro-amniotic shunting. This may well be relevant as there are reports of spontaneous resolution of hydrothorax in utero.

The recurrence risk for hydrothorax in future pregnancies depends on the aetiology. There are some families where x-linked inheritance of idiopathic hydrothorax seems possible.

REFERENCES

1 Bailey P V, Tracy T, Connors R H, deMello D, Lewis J E, Weber T R. Congenital bronchopulmonary malformations. Diagnostic and therapeutic considerations. J Thorac Cardiovasc Surg 1990; 99: 597–603

2 Eraklis A J, Griscom N T, McGovern J B. Bronchogenic cysts of the mediastinum in infancy. N Engl J Med 1969; 281: 1150–1155

3 Ramenofsky M L, Leape L L, McCauley R G K. Bronchogenic cyst. J Paed Surg 1979; 14: 219–224

4 O'Connell D J, Kelleher J. Congenital intrathoracic bronchopulmonary foregut malformations in childhood. Can Assoc Radiol J 1979; 30: 103–108

5 Vergnes P, Chateil J F, Boissinot F, et al. Malformations pulmoaires de diagnostic antenatal. Chir Pediatr 1989; 30: 185–192

6 Fallon M, Gordon A R G, Lendrum A C. Mediastinal cysts of foregut origin associated with vertebral anomalies. Br J Surg 1954; 41: 520–533

7 Mayden K L, Tortora M, Chervenak F A, Hobbins J C. The antenatal sonographic detection of lung masses. Am J Obstet Gynecol 1984; 148: 349–351

8 Reece E A, Lockwood C J, Rizzo N, Pilu G, Bovicelli L, Hobbins J C. Intrinsic intrathoracic malformations of the fetus: sonographic detection and clinical presentation. Obstet Gynecol 1987; 70: 627–632

9 Young G, L'Heureux P R, Krueckeberg S T, Swanson D A. Mediastinal bronchogenic cyst: prenatal sonographic diagnosis. AJR 1989; 152: 127

10 Buntain W L, Woolley M M, Mahour G H, et al. Pulmonary sequestration in children: a twenty-five year experience. Surgery 1977; 81: 413–420

11 Ryckman F C, Rosenkrantz J G. Thoracic surgical problems in infancy and childhood. Surg Clin North Am 1985; 65: 1423–1454

12 Carter R. Pulmonary sequestration. Ann Thorac Surg 1969; 7: 68–89

13 Savic B, Birtel F J, Tholen W, et al. Lung sequestration: report of seven cases and review of 540 published cases. Thorax 1979; 34: 96–101

14 Wimbish K J, Agha F P, Brady T M. Bilateral pulmonary sequestration: computerised tomographic appearance. AJR 1983; 140: 689–690

15 Demos N J, Teresi A. Congenital lung malformations: a unified concept and case report. J Thorac Cardiovasc Surg 1975; 70: 260–264

16 Gerle R D, Jaretzki A, Ashley C A, Berne A S. Congenital bronchopulmonary-foregut malformation: pulmonary sequestration communicating with the gastrointestinal tract. N Engl J Med 1968; 278: 1413–1419

17 Heithoff K B, Sane S M, Williams H J, et al. Bronchopulmonary foregut malformations. A unifying etiological concept. AJR 1976; 126: 46–55

18 Stocker J T, Kagan-Hallet K. Extralobar pulmonary sequestration. Analysis of 15 cases. Am J Clin Pathol 1979; 72: 917–925

19 Iwa T, Watanabe Y. Unusual combination of pulmonary sequestration and funnel chest. Chest 1979; 76: 314–316

20 White J J, Donahoo J S, Ostrow P T, et al. Cardiovascular and respiratory manifestations of pulmonary sequestration in childhood. Ann Thorac Surg 1974; 18: 286–294

21 Jouppila P, Kirkinen P, Herva R, et al. Prenatal diagnosis of pleural effusions by ultrasound. JCU 1983; 11: 516–519

22 Mariona F, McAlpin G, Zador I, et al. Sonographic detection of fetal extrathoracic pulmonary sequestration. J Ultrasound Med 1986; 5: 283–285

23 Romero R, Chervenak F A, Kotzen J, et al. Antenatal sonographic findings of extralobar pulmonary sequestration. J Ultrasound Med 1982; 1: 131–132

24 Weiner C, Varner M, Pringle K, et al. Antenatal diagnosis and palliative treatment of non-immune hydrops secondary to pulmonary extralobar sequestration. Obstet Gynecol 1986; 68: 275–280

25 Choplin R H, Siegel M J. Pulmonary sequestration: six unusual presentations. AJR 1980; 134: 695–700

26 Maulik D, Robinson L, Dailey D K, et al. Prenatal sonographic depiction of intralobar pulmonary sequestration. J Ultrasound Med 1987; 6: 703–706

27 Goldblatt E, Vimpani G, Brown L H, et al. Extralobar pulmonary sequestration. Presentation as an arteriovenous aneurysm with cardiac failure in infancy. Am J Cardiol 1971; 29: 100

28 Ransom J M, Norton J B, Williams G D. Pulmonary sequestration presenting as congestive heart failure. J Thorac Cardiovasc Surg 1978; 76: 378–380

29 Stocker J T, Madewell J E, Drake R M. Congenital adenomatoid malformation of the lung. Classification and morphologic spectrum. Hum Pathol 1977; 8: 155–171

30 Rempen A, Feige A, Wunsch P. Prenatal diagnosis of bilateral cystic adenomatoid malformation of the lung. JCU 1987; 15: 3–8

31 Oster A G, Fortune D W. Congenital cystic adenomatoid malformation of the lung. Am J Clin Pathol 1978; 70: 595–604

32 Adzick N S, Harrison M R, Glick P L, et al. Fetal cystic adenomatoid malformation: prenatal diagnosis and natural history. J Pediatr Surg 1985; 20: 483–488

33 Clark S L, Vitale D J, Minton S D, Stoddard R A, Sabey P L. Successful fetal therapy for cystic adenomatoid malformation associated with second trimester hydrops. Am J Obstet Gynecol 1987; 157: 294–295

34 Fitzgerald E J, Toi A. Antenatal ultrasound diagnosis of cystic adenomatoid malformation of the lung. Can Assoc Radiol J 1986; 37: 48–49

35 Cachia R, Sobonya R E. Congenital cystic adenomatoid malformation of the lung with bronchial atresia. Hum Pathol 1981; 12: 947–950

36 Miller R K, Sieber W K, Yunis E J. Congenital adenomatoid malformation of the lung. Ann Pathol 1980; 15: 387–407

37 Petit P, Bossens M, Thomas D, Moerman P, Fryns J P, Van den Berghe H. Type III congenital cystic adenomatoid malformation of the lung: another cause of elevated alpha fetoprotein? Clin Genet 1987; 32: 172–174

38 Nugent C E, Hayashi R H, Rubin J. Prenatal treatment of type I congenital cystic adenomatoid malformation by intrauterine fetal thoracocentesis. JCU 1989; 17: 675–677

39 Pezzuti R T, Isler R J. Antenatal ultrasound detection of cystic adenomatoid malformation of the lung: report of a case and review of the recent literature. JCU 1983; 11: 342–346

40 Carles D, Serville F, Mainguene M, Glycos E, Herfaut G, Naya L. Prenatal diagnosis of type III congenital cystic adenomatoid malformation of the lung. J Genet Hum 1986; 34: 339–341

41 Vesce F, Garutti P, Grandi E, Perri G, Altavilla G. Prenatal diagnosis of cystic adenomatoid malformation of the lung. Clin Exp Obstet Gynecol 1989; 16: 121–125

42 Nicolaides K H, Blott M, Greenough A. Chronic drainage of fetal pulmonary cyst. Lancet 1987; I: 618

43 Fine C, Adzick N S, Doubilet P M. Decreasing size of a congenital cystic adenomatoid malformation in utero. J Ultrasound Med 1988; 7: 405–408

44 Saltzmann D H, Adzick N S, Benacerraf B R. Fetal cystic adenomatoid malformation of the lung: apparent improvement in utero. Obstet Gynecol 1988; 71: 1000–1002

45 Wolf S A, Hertzler J H, Philippart A I. Cystic adenomatoid malformation of the lung. J Pediatr Surg 1980; 15: 925–930

46 David T J, Illingworth C A. Diaphragmatic hernia in the southwest of England. J Med Genet 1976; 13: 253–262

47 Harrison M R, Jester J A, Ross N A. Correction of congenital diaphragmatic hernia in utero. I. The model: intrathoracic balloon produces fetal pulmonary hypoplasia. Surgery 1980; 88: 174–182

48 Benacerraf B R, Adzick N S. Fetal diaphragmatic hernia: ultrasound diagnosis and clinical outcome in 19 cases. Am J Obstet Gynecol 1987; 156: 573–576

49 Nakayama D K, Harrison M R, Chinn D H, et al. Prenatal diagnosis and natural history of the fetus with a congenital diaphragmatic hernia: initial clinical experience. J Pediatr Surg 1985; 20: 118–124

50 Butler N, Claireaux A E. Congenital diaphragmatic hernia as a cause of perinatal mortality. Lancet 1962; 1: 659–663

51 Hansen J, James S, Burrington, et al. The decreasing incidence of pneumothorax and improving survival of infants with congenital diaphragmatic hernia. J Pediatr Surg 1984; 19: 385–388

52 Greenwood R D, Rosenthal A, Nadas A S. Cardiovascular abnormalities associated with congenital diaphragmatic hernia. Pediatrics 1976; 57: 92–97

53 Winter R M, Knowles S A S, Bieber F R, Baraitser M. Respiratory tract anomalies. In: The malformed fetus and stillbirth – a diagnostic approach. Chichester: John Wiley. 1988: p 121–129

54 Harrison R H, Adzick N S, Nakayama D K, deLorimier A A. Fetal diaphragmatic hernia: fatal but fixable. Semin Perinatol 1985; 9: 103–112

55 Chinn D H, Filly R A, Callen P W, Nakayama D K, Harrison M R. Congenital diaphragmatic hernia diagnosed prenatally by ultrasound. Radiology 1983; 148: 119–123

56 Crawford D C, Wright V M, Drake D P, Allan L D. Fetal diaphragmatic hernia: the value of fetal echocardiography in the prediction of postnatal outcome. Br J Obstet Gynaecol 1989; 96: 705–710

57 Comstock C H. The antenatal diagnosis of diaphragmatic anomalies. J Ultrasound Med 1986; 5: 391–396

58 Ruff S J, Campbell J R, Harrison M W, et al. Pediatric diaphragmatic hernia: an 11 year experience. Am J Surg 1980; 139: 641–645

59 Osebold W R, Soper R T. Congenital diaphragmatic hernia past infancy. Am J Surg 1976; 131: 748–754

60 Norio R, Kaariainen H, Rapola J, Herva R, Kekomaki M. Familial congenital diaphragmatic defects: aspects of aetiology, prenatal diagnosis and treatment. Am J Med Genet 1984; 17: 471–483

61 Harrison M R, Ross N A, deLorimier A A. Correction for congenital diaphragmatic hernia in utero. III. Development of a successful surgical technique using abdominoplasty to avoid compromise of umbilical blood flow. J Paediatr Surg 1981; 16: 934

62 Harrison M J, Golbus M S, Filly R A. The unborn patient. In: Orlando F. ed. Prenatal diagnosis and treatment. Grune and Stratton. 1984: p 257–275

63 Harrison M R, Bressack M A, Churg A M, et al. Correction of congenital diaphragmatic hernia in utero. II. Simulated correction permits fetal lung growth with survival at birth. Surgery 1980; 88: 260

64 Harrison M R, Langer J C, Adzick N S, et al. Correction of congenital diaphragmatic hernia in utero. V. Initial clinical experience. J Pediatr Surg 1990; 25: 47–55

65 Harrison M R, Adzick N S, Longaker M T, et al. Successful repair in utero of a fetal diaphragmatic hernia after removal of herniated viscera from the left hemithorax. N Engl J Med 1990; 322: 1582–1584

66 Alonso C R P, Lozano G B, Andres M C B, Puerto M J M, Lopez M C, Posadas A S. Quilotorax espontaneo: Siete casos de diagnostico prenatal. An Esp Pediatr 1989; 30: 19–22

67 Allan L D, Crawford D C, Sheridan R, Chapman M G. Aetiology of non-immune hydrops: the value of echocardiography. Br J Obstet Gynaecol 1986; 93: 223–225

68 Benacerraf B R, Frigoletto F D, Wilson M. Successful midtrimester thoracocentesis with analysis of the lymphocyte population in the pleural effusion. Am J Obstet Gynecol 1986; 155: 396–399

69 Pijpers L, Reuss A, Stewart P A, Wladimiroff J W. Noninvasive management of isolated bilateral fetal hydrothorax. Am J Obstet Gynecol 1989; 161: 330–332

22

Miscellaneous abnormalities

Umbilical cord
Single umbilical artery
Umbilical hernia
Allantoic and omphalomesenteric cysts
Umbilical cord haematoma
The face
Normal anatomy
Abnormalities of the orbit
   Hypertelorism
   Hypotelorism
   Microphthalmia
Abnormalities of the nose
Cleft lip and palate
The Pierre-Robin syndrome
Abnormalities of the tongue

Unusual abdominal cysts
Choledochal cyst
Ovarian cyst
Mesenteric, omental and retroperitoneal cysts
Fetal tumours
Cystic hygroma
Isolated neck cysts
Fetal goitre
Cervical teratoma
Haemangiomata
Sacro-coccygeal teratoma

J. Malcolm Pearce

Umbilical cord (see also Ch. 23)

In the normal umbilical cord two umbilical arteries and a single, larger umbilical vein are visible (Fig. 1A). Abnormalities of the cord are rare but should not be overlooked as they may be markers of more serious pathology.

Single umbilical artery

A single umbilical artery may arise from agenesis of one umbilical artery (or persistence of the original allantoid artery of the body stalk) or atrophy of an artery (Fig. 1B). The condition is three to four times more common in dizygotic but not monozygotic twins[1] and has a male to female incidence of 0.85:1.[2] Approximately 20% of fetuses with a single umbilical artery have an associated abnormality; Table 1 lists those that are detectable on ultrasound examination. The incidence of associated chromosome abnormalities is unknown but may be as high as 60% (six out of nine),[3] so serious consideration should be given to karyotyping.

The overall perinatal mortality for fetuses with a single umbilical artery is 20%,[1] 60% of the deaths being stillbirths. Although most deaths are due to associated abnormalities, the perinatal mortality is increased even in normally formed fetuses with a single umbilical artery[3] mostly because of prematurity and intra-uterine growth retardation, and serial growth measurements are therefore indicated. Long-term follow up studies on survivors that were structurally normal do not show any evidence of intellectual impairment.[4]

Umbilical hernia

The prevalence of this condition is not known and it is an abnormality that is easily overlooked as the contents of the sac may not be within the cord at the time of examination (Fig. 2).[5] The differential diagnosis is with a small omphalocele, in which the intrahepatic portion of the umbilical vein is visible within the hernia; and with gastroschisis, which can usually be visualised as being separate to the umbilical cord (see Ch. 18). Approximately 1% of such fetuses demonstrate a chromosome abnormality and therefore karyotyping should be performed; if normal, the child is usually completely normal.

Allantoic and omphalomesenteric cysts

An allantoic cyst appears as a cystic mass within the umbilical cord close to the fetus and is a cyst of a remnant of the allantois. The solitary example that has been detected prenatally and reported was not associated with any perinatal problems.[6]

Omphalomesenteric cysts form in remnants of the duct that joins the yolk sac to the fetal gut. Remnants are not uncommon, the most well-known of which is Meckel's

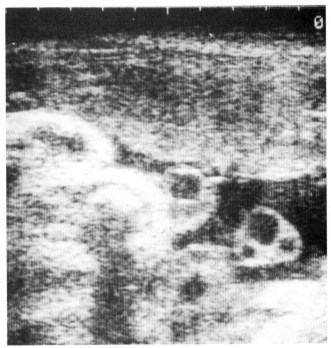

A

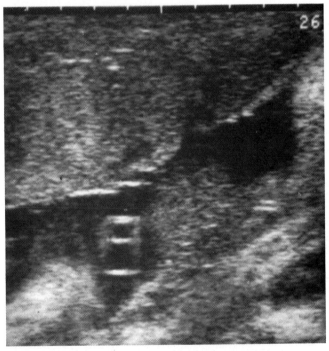

B

Fig. 1 Umbilical cord. A: Normal umbilical cord in transverse section demonstrating two arteries and a vein. **B:** An umbilical cord in transverse section demonstrating a single artery.

diverticulum. Remnants in the umbilical cord may become cystic and have been identified antenatally. They do not appear to grow antenatally and, although there is an isolated case report of a fetal death due to erosion of the

Table 1 Ultrasound detectable abnormalities associated with a single umbilical artery. (Modified from Heifetz[1].)

Abnormality	Approximate incidence (%)
Urinary tract	
Renal dysplasia	19
Renal agenesis	11
Hydronephrosis/hydroureter	11
Cardiac	
Ventricular septal defect	21
Atrial septal defect	9
Hypoplastic left heart	3
Truncus arteriosis	7
Fallot's tetralogy	3
Coarctation of the aorta	3
Skeleton	
Cleft lip and palate	13
Talipes	12
Polydactyly	8
Long bone abnormalities	8
Sacral agenesis	1
Gastrointestinal tract	
Omphalocele	13
Gastroschisis	3
Tracheo-oesophageal fistula	8
Gut atresia	4
Imperforate anus	16
Craniospinal defects	
Anencephaly	11
Spina bifida	8
Hydrocephaly	3
Holoprosencephaly	4
Microcephaly	2
Cerebellar abnormalities	2
Miscellaneous	
Diaphragmatic hernia	8
Cystic hygroma	9
Sacro-coccygeal teratoma	3

Overall 158 fetuses demonstrated 753 abnormalities at post-mortem. Editor's note: These figures are not representative of the incidence of associated anomalies in all cases of single umbilical artery since the above were detected as they died of their abnormalities and came to post-mortem.

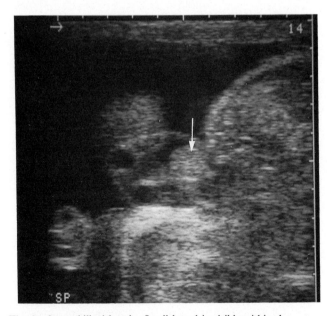

Fig. 2 An umbilical hernia. Small bowel is visible within the umbilical cord (arrow). This lesion was only apparent on two out of five ultrasound examinations.

umbilical vein by the gastric mucosa that lined the cyst,[7] most are harmless. The paediatricians should be alerted to their presence because the majority of cases are associated with a Meckel's diverticulum.

Umbilical cord haematoma

Although these may occur spontaneously[8–10] they are now increasingly being seen following cordocentesis or fetoscopic blood sampling.[11] They may be fatal if they burst into the amniotic cavity and cause fetal exsanguination or they may cause compression of the umbilical vessels. Iatrogenic haematomata may be extremely large (Fig. 3) if they result from needle tears of the umbilical vein, though size does not seem to correlate well with outcome. They may be associated with bradycardia and asystole.

Spontaneous haematomata are usually diagnosed long after the initial haemorrhage and, if the Doppler waveforms from the umbilical artery and vein are normal, no special action is needed. Management of iatrogenic haematomata depends upon the gestational age and the presence or absence of fetal distress.

The face

Normal anatomy

The bony features of the face can be visualised from 14 weeks gestation but detailed study of soft tissue structures is only feasible from 16 to 18 weeks gestation. A sagittal view of the fetal face (see Fig. 16A) demonstrates the normal relationships of the forehead, nose and chin and, with experience, variations can be recognised. Sliding the transducer caudally from the axial section on which

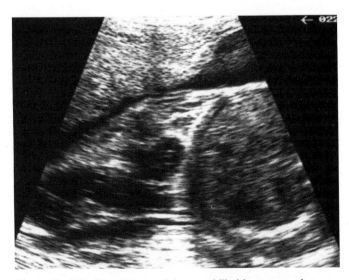

Fig. 3 Umbilical haematoma. A large umbilical haematoma that arose following fetal movement at cordocentesis at 24 weeks gestation. The haematoma stopped enlarging after 10 minutes and Doppler waveforms from the umbilical circulation remained normal.

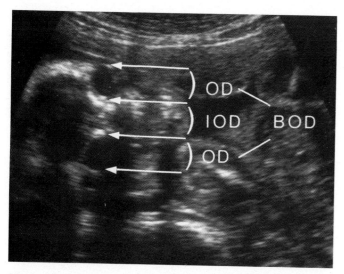

Fig. 4 Measurement of ocular distances. (OD – ocular diameter, IOD – interocular diameter, BOD – binocular diameter.)

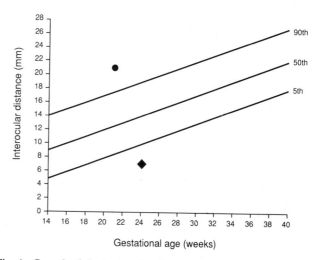

Fig. 6 Growth of the interocular distance (from Jeanty et al 1982). The dot is the measurement from the fetus illustrated in Figure 11B, whilst the diamond is the measurement from the fetus in Figure 12B.

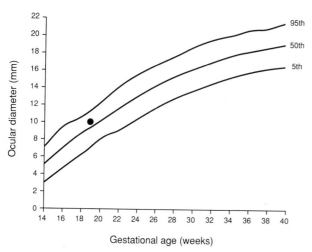

Fig. 5 Growth of the ocular diameter (from Jeanty et al 1982). The dot represents the diameters from the fetus illustrated in Figure 13.

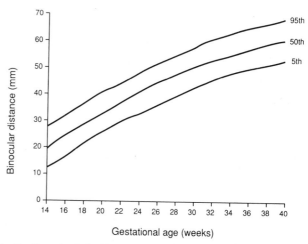

Fig. 7 Growth of the binocular diameter (from Jeanty et al 1982).

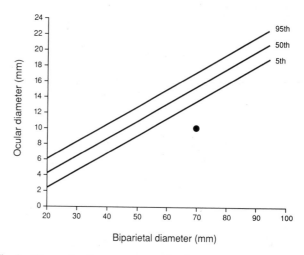

Fig. 8 The ocular diameter versus biparietal diameter (from Jeanty et al 1982). The dot is the measurement from the fetus illustrated in Figure 13 at 19 weeks gestation. BPD = 70 mm and OD = 10 mm. (Macrocephalic fetus.)

the biparietal diameter (BPD) is measured, demonstrates the orbits and then the palate. The intra-orbital distance and orbital diameters can be measured (Fig. 4). Figures 5 to 7 illustrate the growth of the ocular diameters with gestation whilst Figure 8 compares ocular diameters with the BPD.

In order to visualise the palate, the transducer is then slid caudally until the tongue can be seen fasciculating in the fetal mouth. A slight cephalad movement then demonstrates the palate (Fig. 9). Rotating the transducer through 90° and making a slight forward sliding movement then demonstrates the face in coronal view (Fig. 10). This view allows the lips and the nose to be examined in detail.

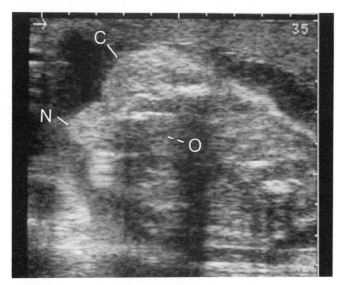

Fig. 9 Fetal palate. A transverse section through the fetal head showing a normal fetal palate. C – cheek, N – nose, O – oropharynx.

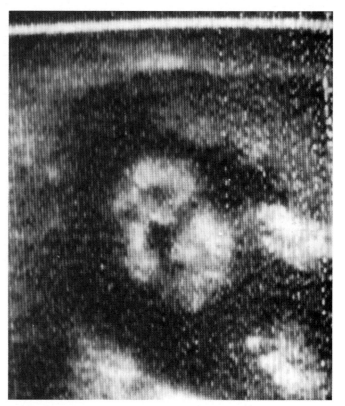

A

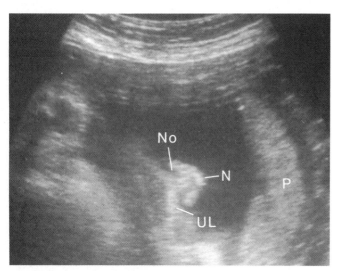

Fig. 10 Fetal lips and nose. A coronal view of the face demonstrating the normal lips and nose (N). No – nostril, UL – upper lip, P – placenta.

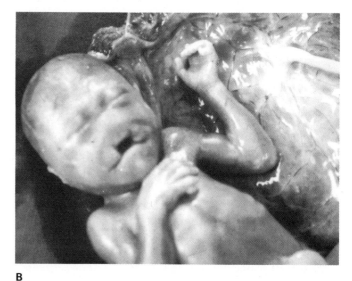

B

Fig. 11 Midline cleft. A: A coronal view of a fetal face demonstrating a midline cleft. **B:** The post-mortem specimen. The fetus also demonstrated hypertelorism (see Fig. 6, dot), holoprosencephaly and was an example of trisomy 13 (Patau's syndrome).

Abnormalities of the orbits

Hypertelorism Hypertelorism is an increase in interocular distance and, although it may be an isolated finding, when obvious antenatally, it is usually associated with other severe anomalies. Many of these form part of the median facial cleft syndrome of hypertelorism, median cleft lip and palate, agenesis of the corpus callosum and a defect in the midline of the frontal bone (cranium bifidum occultum). The syndrome can be diagnosed antenatally (Fig. 11).[12] Figure 6 illustrates the interorbital distance plotted against the data reference range. The median cleft face syndrome

is usually a sporadic mutation, although there are a few families that seem to be at risk from an autosomal dominant form.

Hypertelorism is also seen with some of the craniosynostoses, particularly Apert's and Crouzon's syndromes (see Ch. 20). It is also associated with some of the rarer chromosomal anomalies, particularly trisomy 9, Turner's syndrome (XO) and the syndromes of multiple extra sex chromosomes, so consideration should be given to karyotyping the fetus.

The sensitivity of the diagnosis of hypertelorism has not been systematically tested so that, in the absence of other abnormalities, prognosis should be guarded.

Hypotelorism Hypotelorism is a decrease in inter-orbital distance. It is rare and all the cases that have been described prenatally[13–15] have been associated with the holoprosencephaly malformation sequence (see Ch. 16) (Fig. 12).

Microphthalmia Strictly the term microphthalmia refers to decreased size of the eyeball but the prenatal diagnosis is suggested by a decreased size of one or both orbits. Figure 5 illustrates the growth of the orbits (ocular diameter) with gestational age. Care should be taken with the diagnosis unless it is unilateral as these charts are derived from a normal population so that 10% of normal infants will be below the tenth percentile. When the condition is suspected and is bilateral, the ocular diameters should be plotted against both the gestational age (Fig. 5) and the biparietal diameter (Fig. 8). Figure 13 illustrates a potential trap for the unwary. The ocular diameters both look small and when plotted against the BPD fell below the fifth centile (Fig. 8) but when plotted against the gestational age they were normal. Careful measurement showed that the trunk was appropriate for gestational age

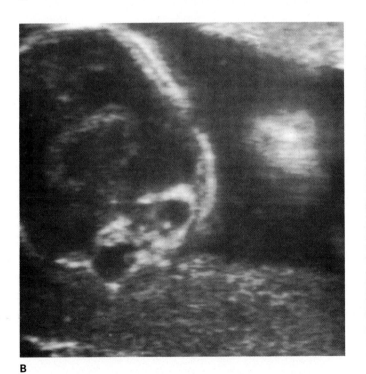

A

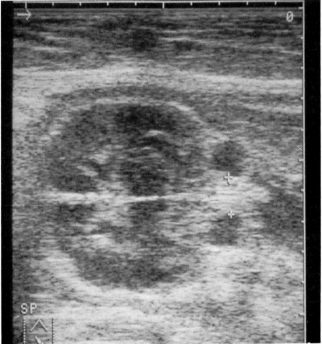

B

Fig. 12 Hypotelorism. A: A coronal view of the fetal face demonstrating severe hypotelorism with a midline facial cleft. **B:** An oblique view of the fetus demonstrating the hypotelorism. (Courtesy of Dr. Peter Rose, Queen Elizabeth Hospital, Gateshead.)

Fig. 13 Apparent microphthalmia. A fetus with apparent microphthalmia in that the orbital diameters are reduced compared to the BPD (Fig. 8). Detailed measurements, however, showed them to be normal when compared to the gestational age (Fig. 5) and the diagnosis of camptomelic dwarf with macrocephaly was made.

but that the limbs were short. The correct diagnosis of camptomelic dwarfism with macrocephaly and normal orbital distances was made.

Microphthalmia is usually seen in association with other severe abnormalities, particularly triploidy and trisomies 13 and 18, and karyotyping is therefore indicated. It may also arise following intra-uterine infection, particularly with rubella or toxoplasmosis, and is a part of the fetal alcohol syndrome. It is also part of several syndromes which involve congenital heart defects, ear abnormalities, renal agenesis and skeletal deformities, all of which should be carefully sought.

Abnormalities of the nose

Absence of the fetal nose (arhinia) is extremely rare and is usually associated with other severe deformities such as the holoprosencephaly sequence.

A proboscis is a trunk-like appendage that is almost inevitably part of the holoprosencephaly sequence which includes cyclops, cebocephaly, ethmocephaly and a median cleft (Fig. 14) (see also Ch. 16). The sequence is extremely rare but is more often found in abortuses, suggesting a high natural wastage rate. Its primary associations are trisomies 13 and 18, teratogenic agents such as irradiation and possibly maternal diabetes mellitus. Alobar holoprosencephaly is usually present, such that most die in utero or within the first year of life. With such an appalling prognosis most parents will opt for termination of pregnancy. The fetus should be karyotyped as the risk of recurrence of a trisomy is empirically quoted as 1% as opposed to a 6% risk of recurrent holoprosencephaly sequence.

Cleft lip and palate

Facial clefts occur in approximately one in 700 live births[16] and account for just over 10% of all congenital anomalies. Most clefts are lateral defects involving the upper lip and/or the palate but, in 0.5% of cases, there is a median cleft.

The fetal palate is best seen in the transverse view (Fig. 9) whereas the lips are best visualised in the coronal view (Fig. 10). The development of the midline structures of the face is closely linked with the differentiation of the forebrain so that the presence of a midline cleft (Figs 11 and 12A) should lead to a search for cerebral abnormalities, particularly the holoprosencephaly sequence. The median cleft syndrome (see above) is recognised by the presence of hypertelorism.

Lateral clefting of the lips and/or palate has been diagnosed prenatally[15,17,18] although the diagnosis of isolated cleft palate is difficult[15] and there has not been a systematic study evaluating the accuracy (Fig. 15). Over 60% of fetuses have associated abnormalities[19] although these are rarely syndromic. Isolated clefts of the lips or palate are most commonly associated with club foot whereas polydactyly is the most frequent anomaly associated with cleft lip and palate. Syndromic associations occur in 3% of cases and chromosome abnormalities occur in only 0.7% of liveborn children with clefts.[20,21] Common associations that are amenable to detection by ultrasound or karyotyping are listed in Table 2. Karyotyping is only indicated if there is a median cleft or other structural markers to suggest a chromosomal anomaly.

Lateral facial clefts largely have a multifactorial pattern of inheritance and the risks of recurrence are related to the severity of the lesion. Table 3 indicates the risk for future children.

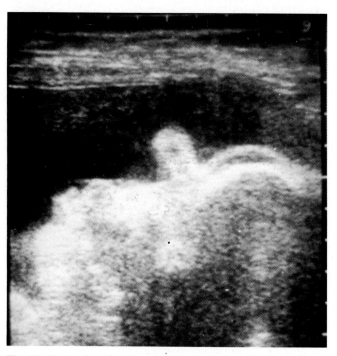

Fig. 14 Proboscis. A midline sagittal view of the fetal face demonstrating a proboscis.

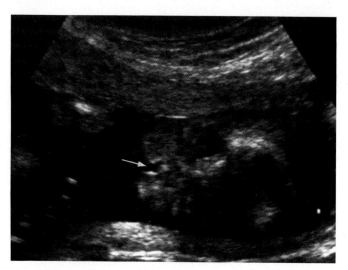

Fig. 15 Facial cleft. Unilateral cleft lip.

Table 2 Common associations with lateral facial clefts that are amenable to detection by ultrasound or karyotyping. (Modified from Gorlin et al.[16])

Syndromes		
Limbs		
Ectrodactyly	EEC syndrome	S, AD(p)
Hypomelia, absent thumb, radial aplasia, severe IUGR	Roberts'	AR
Popliteal pterygia Syndactyly	Popliteal web	AD
Hypertelorism Multiple dislocations	Larsen syndrome	?AD
Multiple pterygia	Escobar's	AR
Micromelia (after 20 weeks) Symmetrical IUGR	Diastrophic dwarfism	AR
Femoral hypoplasia Micrognathia	Femoral hypoplasia-unusual facies	?
Cerebral malformations		
Craniosynostosis, hypertelorism syndactyly	Apert's	S, AD
Microcephaly, micrognathia polydactyly, cardiac anomalies	Smith-Lemli Opitz	AR
Encephalocoele, microcephaly, polydactyly, polycystic kidneys	Meckel's	AR
Chromosomal syndromes		
Trisomy 13, 18 and 21 Triploidy XXXXY syndrome		
Non-syndromic associations		
Congenital heart disease Amniotic bands		

Key:
  S   – sporadic
  AD(p) – autosomal dominant with partial penetrance
  AD   – autosomal dominant
  AR   – autosomal recessive

Table 3 Risks of cleft lip (from Smith[16])

Defect/affected individual	Risk to subsequent children
Unilateral cleft	3%
Bilateral cleft	5%
Affected father	3%
Affected mother	14%
One affected sibling	4%
Two affected siblings	10%

The Pierre-Robin syndrome

This is a syndrome of micrognathia and a cleft in the soft palate. The primary defect is believed to be the under-development of the mandible which allows the tongue to occupy a posterior position thus interfering with the closure of the soft palate. In most cases this is an isolated deformity with an excellent long-term prognosis but in 25% the Robin sequence is part of a syndrome.[22] Associated syndromes that have ultrasonically recognisable features are diastrophic dwarfism (late onset micromelia), camptomelic dwarfism (micromelia with bowed tibia, macrocephaly, polyhydramnios) and the Beckwith-Wiedemann syndrome (omphalocele). Chromosomal abnormalities are extremely rare.

The syndrome has been described prenatally[23] (Figs 16 and 17). The diagnosis relies upon the demonstration of micrognathia on a mid-sagittal section of the fetal face. The cleft is in the soft palate in the Robin sequence and is probably not detectable on ultrasound. If there are no features of an associated syndrome spontaneous onset of labour can be awaited but an experienced paediatrician should be present at the delivery because the tongue may obstruct the neonatal airway and intubation may be difficult.

Abnormalities of the tongue

Macroglossia is a large tongue which may be so large as to cause severe respiratory obstruction at birth. In a mid-sagittal profile view of the face the tongue is not normally visualised outside of the mouth. The Beckwith-Wiedemann syndrome has been diagnosed in an at-risk mother at 30 weeks gestation,[24] allowing surgical reduction of the tongue soon after birth. The Beckwith-Wiedemann syndrome is an autosomal dominant condition but most of the reported cases are new mutations. Pettenati et al[25] reviewed 200 cases and described macroglossia in 98% whilst an omphalocele occurred in only 60%. Affected infants usually have a birthweight well over the ninetieth centile for gestational age.

Unusual abdominal cysts (see also Ch. 18)

Choledochal cyst

These are rare, sporadic cystic dilations of the common bile duct. They have been correctly diagnosed prenatally[26–29] and appear as a cystic space in the fetal abdomen (Fig. 18). The major differential diagnosis is from duodenal atresia, a distinction that is important as the latter condition has a 30% association with chromosomal anomalies whereas choledochal cysts have no association. The diagnosis can be made prenatally if dilated hepatic ducts can be seen adjacent to the cyst[27,29] but in most cases peristalsis and/or a connection to the stomach allows the diagnosis of duodenal atresia to be made, as does associated polyhydramnios.

No change is needed in antenatal management as the cysts are isolated lesions that do not reach sufficient size to cause dystocia. Surgery is recommended in the neonatal

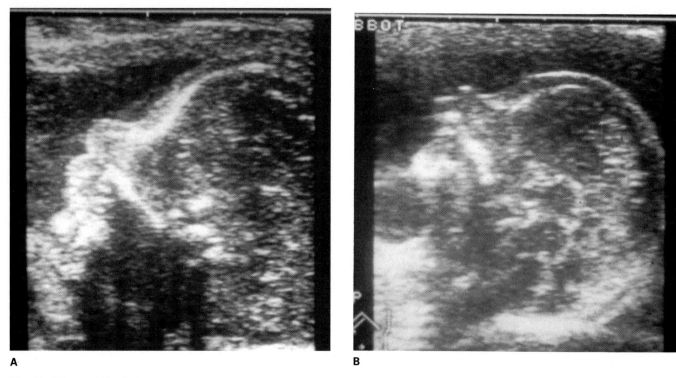

A

B

Fig. 16 Micrognathia. A: A mid-sagittal section of a normal fetal face demonstrating the relationship and size of the chin to the nose and forehead. **B:** A case of micrognathia showing the obvious receding chin. (Courtesy of Prof. Stuart Campbell, King's College Hospital, London.)

period because of the risk of biliary obstruction, progressive biliary cirrhosis and portal hypertension.

Ovarian cysts

An ovarian cyst produces an obvious echo-free mass within the abdomen (Fig. 19) which should be differentiated from a hydronephrosis, distended bladder or mesenteric cyst. It is important to remember that the fetus has almost no true pelvic cavity and that ovarian cysts may lie in the mid or even upper abdomen (see *Abdominal and General Ultrasound*, Vol. 2, Ch. 56). Differentiation may not always be possible but demonstrating that the fetus is male excludes this diagnosis.[30,31] Conservative management is advised for cysts less than 2 cm but there is debate as to whether this is appropriate for larger cysts[32] or whether they should be punctured under ultrasound guidance.[33] Installation of tetracycline to cause sclerosis has been successfully carried out.[34]

To date none of the antenatally diagnosed cysts have been malignant and those managed conservatively appear to resolve within 6 months. After delivery the child's thyroid function should be checked as hypothyroidism has been described in association with ovarian cysts.[30]

Mesenteric, omental and retroperitoneal cysts

All these cysts are extremely rare with only a few hundred case reports in the world literature. Figure 20 illustrates a mesenteric cyst detected on routine ultrasound examination at 34 weeks gestation. The precise diagnosis was not clear antenatally but other cystic masses in the abdomen were excluded. The cyst did not change in size over the next 6 week period and the child was delivered vaginally following spontaneous labour at term. The diagnosis was firmly established after surgical resection at 3 months of age.

Fetal tumours

Cystic hygroma

This is the most common fetal tumour, occurring in up to one in 200 pregnancies.[35] A cystic hygroma is a pathological dilatation of the jugular lymphatic sac, a primitive structure which drains the embryological lymphatic system and usually becomes connected to the jugular vein at about 9 weeks menstrual age. Complete failure of this link causes progressive peripheral oedema that eventually results in heart failure and non-immune hydrops fetalis. If the connection forms after the cystic hygroma has arisen, the fluid is resorbed and the child is born with a webbed neck.

Virtually all cases of cystic hygromata and non-immune hydrops fetalis are associated with Turner's syndrome[36–40] and most suffer intra-uterine death. Trisomies 18, 21,[41] 13,[42] 47 XXY and mosaics[39] have also been described in association with cystic hygromata. The incidence of a normal karyotype in a fetus with an isolated cystic hygroma is difficult to determine but is probably no greater than 10%.

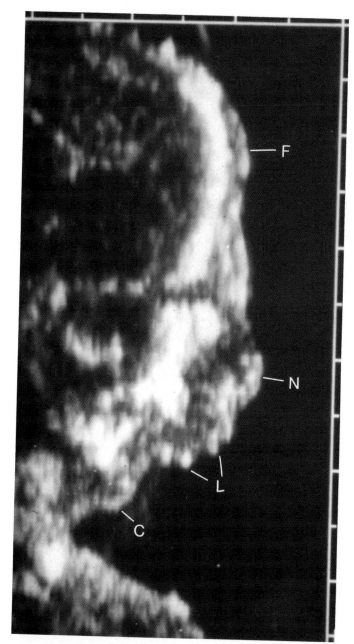

Fig. 17 **Robin sequence.** A mid-sagittal view of the fetal face demonstrating micrognathia as part of the Robin sequence F – forehead, N – nose, L – lips, C – chin. (Courtesy of Dr. Twining, Consultant Radiologist, Queens Medical Centre, Nottingham.)

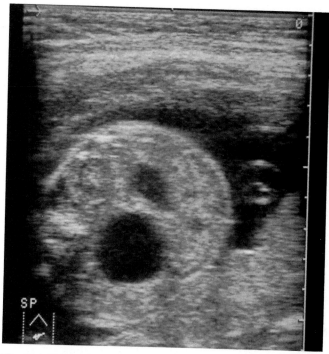

Fig. 18 **Choledochal cyst.** A transverse section of the fetal abdomen demonstrating an apparent 'double bubble'. The upper echo-free space is the stomach and the lower proved to be a choledochal cyst.

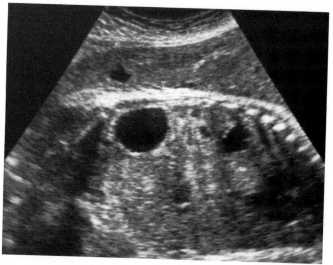

Fig. 19 **Ovarian cyst.** An oblique section of a fetal abdomen demonstrating an ovarian cyst. This cyst did not increase in size antenatally and disappeared over a 3 month period.

Prenatal diagnosis is usually straightforward with the appearance of a cystic lesion that contains septa in the region of the fetal neck (Fig. 21). The lesion may extend up onto the occiput and has been mistaken for an encephalocele; Table 4 lists the differences. Careful scanning should reveal the skull defect in the case of the encephalocele.[38] The diagnosis is feasible in the first trimester with the aid of trans-vaginal scanning.

The fetus should be karyotyped even if hydrops fetalis is present as this is more likely to succeed from a live fetus than an abortus. The precise diagnosis is important for genetic counselling; recurrence of Turner's syndrome is thought to be no greater than the background risk of one in 200 whereas the risk of recurrence of trisomy is empirically one in 100 but may be higher with advanced maternal age or if the parents carry a translocation. Isolated cystic hygromata are usually sporadic but there has been a suggestion that they may occasionally be inherited in an autosomal recessive manner.[43]

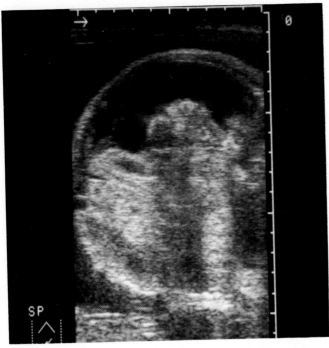

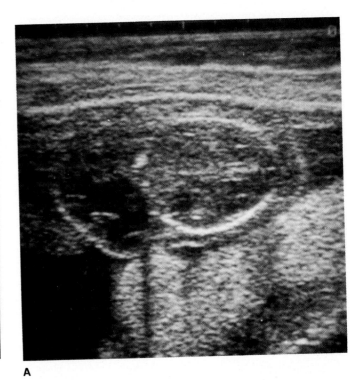

Fig. 20 Mesenteric cyst. A transverse section of the fetal abdomen. The echo-free space did not demonstrate peristalsis and was separate from other abdominal organs. This is a mesenteric cyst.

A

The prognosis depends largely upon whether there is non-immune hydrops fetalis; if present 99% die in utero with the survivors dying in the early neonatal period. Isolated cystic hygromata carry an excellent prognosis with a relatively normal outlook. Fetuses with Turner's syndrome who do not have hydrops fetalis should have detailed scanning of the fetal heart looking for coarctation of the aorta. Prognosis should be guarded as hydrops may develop late in pregnancy. The long-term outlook is of the classical Turner's phenotype but some of these patients may achieve fertility by ovum donation.[44]

Very rarely in cases of Turner's syndrome cystic hygromata may resolve in utero.[45] Cystic hygromata (lymphangiomata) may rarely occur in the fetal abdomen (Fig. 22) or in the limbs.[46] Such cases are usually unassociated with chromosome abnormalities but the tumour may be of such a size as to warrant delivery by caesarean section. Post-natal surgical removal can often be achieved and there are only cosmetic long-term sequelae.

Isolated neck cysts

Figure 23 illustrates an isolated cyst of the fetal neck. This was detected on routine ultrasound at 22 weeks gestation. A precise diagnosis was not determined but there were no other abnormalities seen. At delivery it measured only 1.5 cm in diameter and proved to be arising from the submandibular gland.

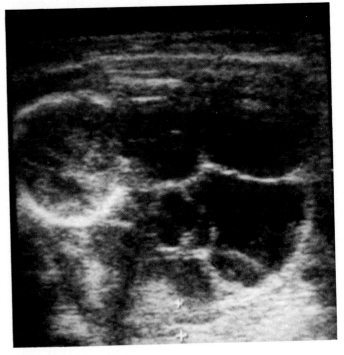

B

Fig. 21 Cystic hygroma. A: A transverse section of the fetal head at the level of the cavum septum pellucidum at 22 weeks gestation. There is marked scalp oedema and an echo-free mass over the occiput which is a cystic hygroma. The karyotype was XO. **B:** An oblique section of a fetal head at 18 weeks gestation demonstrating the usual septate appearances of a cystic hygroma.

Table 4 Cystic hygromata versus encephalocele (from Pearce et al[38])

Ultrasound findings	Cystic hygromata	Encephalocele
1. Bone defect in skull	Never	Always
2. Septa	Obvious multiple	Only as midline echo
3. Contents	Fluid	Variable, but often brain
4. Origin	Postero-lateral neck	Skull occiput (70%)
5. Extent	Nuchal but it may extend to face, vertex and trunk	Always arise from skull, never seen below neck
6. Microcephaly	Rare	Common
7. Other	Short limbs Hydrops fetalis Cardiac anomalies Turner's syndrome	Multicystic kidneys Polydactyly
8. Oligohydramnios	Common	Rare
9. Amniotic AFP	High if hygroma is punctured	Normal

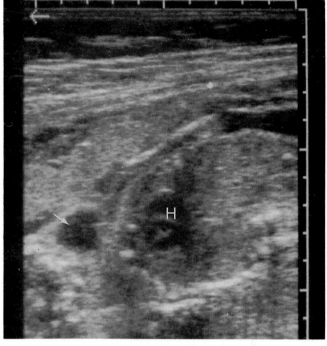

Fig. 23 Isolated neck cyst. An isolated neck cyst (arrow) that proved to be arising from the submandibular gland. H – heart. (Courtesy of Dr. Pat Hill, St. Helier Hospital, Carshalton, London.)

Fetal goitre

Fetal goitre can be diagnosed.[47–49] It is seen as a highly reflective mass anterior to the fetal cervical spine almost exclusively associated with maternal hypothyroidism or antithyroid medication.

Cervical teratoma

These are extremely rare tumours with just over 100 cases being reported in the paediatric literature.[50] The tumour is predominantly of nervous tissue and over half of the cases are calcified.

A complex mass is found in the region of the fetal neck (Figs 24 and 25). They are usually predominantly solid with some cystic areas. The main differential diagnosis is from haemangiomata of the neck (see below) which rarely demonstrate calcification.

The prognosis depends upon determining the upper limit of the lesion. Lesions that extend above the maxilla

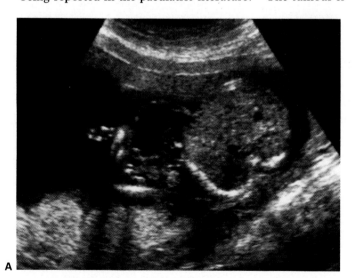
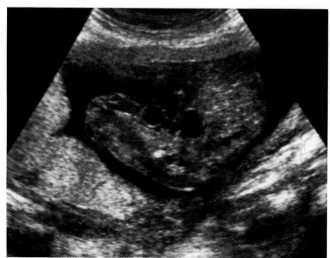

Fig. 22 Abdominal lymphangioma. A: A transverse section of the fetal abdomen demonstrating an abdominal lymphangioma. **B:** The tumour extends down to the level of the fetal pelvis and upper thigh.

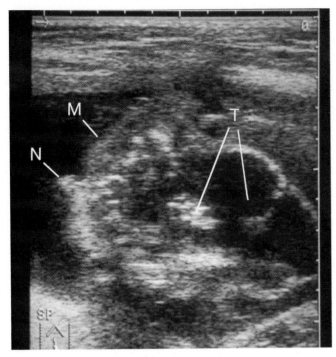

Fig. 24 Teratoma. A coronal section demonstrating a teratoma arising from the fetal face and neck. This patient was referred because of the finding of a trisomy 20 following amniocentesis for a maternal age of 36 years. This was thought to be a culture artefact and the teratoma was an incidental finding. The pregnancy was terminated.

are not surgically resectable and usually end in neonatal death due to respiratory obstruction; lesions that do not reach the maxilla carry approximately a 50% survival rate following surgery.[51] Unlike sacro-coccygeal teratomas the tumours are all benign (see below and *Abdominal and General Ultrasound*, Vol. 2, Ch. 53).

Haemangiomata

Figure 26 illustrates the ultrasound findings of a case of multiple haemangiomata. The patient presented with a persistent breech presentation at 32 weeks gestation and was thought to have a cervical teratoma by the referring hospital. On detailed ultrasound examination there was a separate tumour visible in the fetus' left humerus (Fig. 26C) and the fetal heart was massively dilated with a high time averaged mean velocity in the fetal descending aorta. The cervical tumour was thought to be involving the oropharynx and the fetal tongue. Multiple haemangiomata were diagnosed and a poor prognosis was given. A differential diagnosis of Klippel-Trenaunay-Weber syndrome was considered but the tumours were seen to be bilateral. A rapid increase in the size of the cervical tumour led to the induction of labour at 33 weeks gestation in order to avoid a caesarean section for dystocia. The baby died from respiratory obstruction within a few minutes of birth and post-mortem confirmed multiple haemangiomata (tongue,

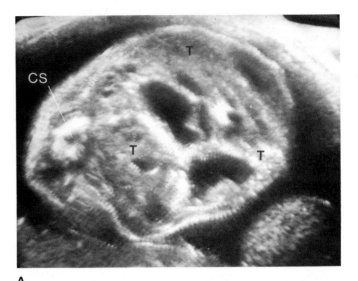

A

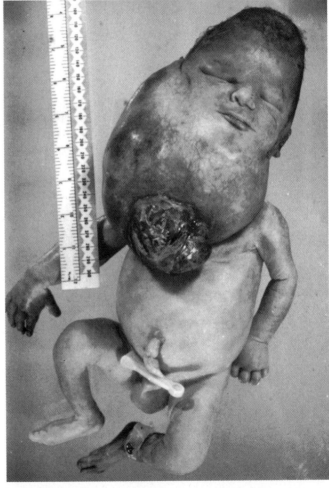

B

Fig. 25 Teratoma. A: A transverse section of the fetal neck demonstrating a massive teratoma (T). CS – cervical spine.
B: The infant. Death occurred almost immediately after delivery because of respiratory obstruction.

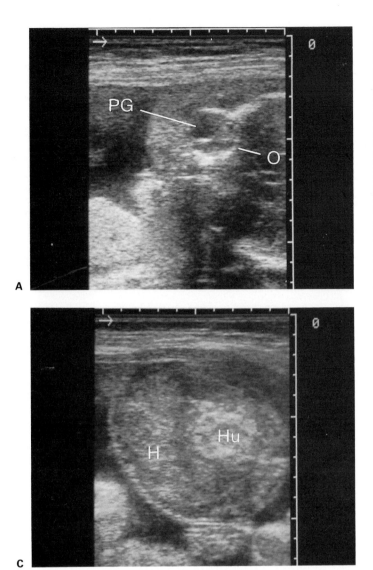

A

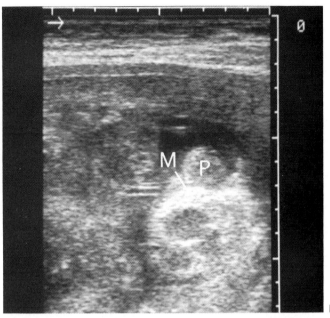

B

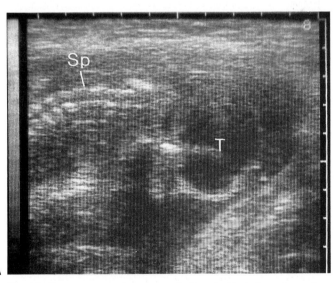

C

Fig. 26 Haemangioma. A: A coronal section of the fetal face demonstrating a prolapsed globe (PG) due to multiple haemangiomata. O – orbit. **B:** A parasagittal view. M – maxilla, P – prolapsed globe. **C:** The left arm of the fetus demonstrating a separate haemangioma (H). Hu – humerus.

neck, left humerus, right kidney and both feet). This appears to be the first prenatal diagnosis of an exceedingly rare tumour.

Sacro-coccygeal teratoma

This tumour is estimated to occur in about one in 40 000 births, with a male to female ratio of 1:4.[52] The tumour

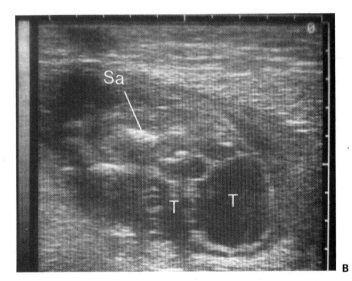

A   B

Fig. 27 Sacro-coccygeal teratoma. A: Longitudinal view of a cystic sacro-coccygeal teratoma (T) Sp – spine. **B:** Transverse section demonstrating that the tumour (T) is entirely post-sacral. Sa – sacrum.

is thought to arise from an embryonic rest of pluripotential cells known as Hensen's node. This node is thought to be remnant of a tail and usually migrates to finally lie anterior to the coccyx.

Over 30 cases have now been reported prenatally with the first 20 cases being reviewed in 1985.[53] All the described cases have been either largely or completely external to the sacrum, there being no prenatal reports of an entirely presacral tumour. In 15% the tumour is entirely cystic (Fig. 27) whilst the remainder are either completely solid or mixed (Fig. 28). The ultrasonic diagnosis is reasonably straightforward although they may be mistaken for a meningomyelocele. Careful examination of the spine, however, shows it to be intact.

The long-term prognosis depends upon the risk of malignancy and the size of the tumour. Tumours that have no presacral component are rarely if ever malignant[54] as are purely cystic tumours. As the presacral component increases the malignancy rate increases from 5% for a small presacral component, 20% for a largely presacral tumour with some external extension and 75% for entirely presacral tumours. Large teratomas have significant operative mortality (3%) usually due to bleeding. Malignant tumours are usually derived from the endodermal sinus or yolk sac components and therefore secrete alpha-fetoprotein, which allows their early detection in infancy. The median time of survival after diagnosis is 9 months[55] but this may be improved with recent advances in chemotherapy.

As the resolution of ultrasound equipment increases the degree of presacral involvement should become more

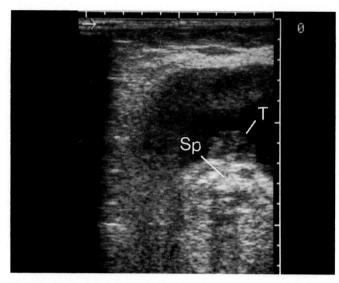

Fig. 28 Sacro-coccygeal teratoma. A transverse section at the level of the sacral vertebrae (Sp) demonstrating a solid and cystic sacro-coccygeal tumour (T). The patient was referred with a diagnosis of spina bifida but the neural arch is intact.

amenable to antenatal assessment such that a reasonable prognosis may be given. Until then most authors have given a guarded but favourable prognosis but this has still resulted in an elective termination rate of about 25%. In the series from Valdiserri[55] the perinatal mortality of the remainder was some 40%.

REFERENCES

1 Heifetz S A. Single umbilical artery. A statistical analysis of 237 autopsy cases and a review of the literature. Perspect Paediatr Pathol 1984; 8: 345–349
2 Bryan E M, Kohler H G. The missing umbilical artery. I. Prospective study based on a maternity unit. Arch Dis Child 1974; 49: 844
3 Bryan E M, Blanc W A. Malformations and chromosome anomalies in spontaneously aborted fetuses with a single umbilical artery. Am J Obstet Gynecol 1985; 151: 340
4 Froehlich L A, Fujikura T. Follow up of infants with a single umbilical artery. Paediatrics 1973; 52: 6
5 Colley N, Knott P D, Gould S J. Misdiagnosis of omphalocele associated with Edward's syndrome and congenital heart disease. Prenat Diagn 1987; 7: 377–380
6 Sachs L, Fourcroy J L, Wenzel D J, et al. The prenatal detection of an umbilical cord allantoic cyst. Radiology 1982; 145: 445
7 Blanc W A, Allan G W. Intrafunicular ulceration of a persistent omphalomesenteric duct with intra-amniotic hemorrhage and fetal death. Am J Obstet Gynecol 1961; 82: 1392
8 Breen J L, Riva H L, Hatch R P. Hematoma of the umbilical cord: case report. Am J Obstet Gynecol 1958; 76: 1288
9 Ruvinsky E D, Wiley T L, Morrison J C, et al. In utero diagnosis of umbilical cord hematoma by ultrasonography. Am J Obstet Gynecol 1981; 140: 833
10 Sutro W H, Tuck S M, Loesevits A, et al. Prenatal observation of umbilical cord hematoma. AJR 1984; 142: 801

11 Romero R, Chervenek F A, Coustan D, et al. Antenatal diagnosis of umbilical cord laceration. Am J Obstet Gynecol 1982; 143: 719
12 Chervenak F A, Tortora M, Mayden K, et al. Antenatal diagnosis of median cleft face syndrome: sonographic demonstration of cleft lip and hypertelorism. Am J Obstet Gynecol 1984; 149: 94
13 Chervenak F A, Isaacson G, Mahoney M J, et al. The obstetric significance of holoprosencephaly. Obstet Gynecol 1984; 63: 115
14 Mayden K L, Tortora M, Berkowitz R L, et al. Orbital diameters: a new parameter for prenatal diagnosis and dating. Am J Obstet Gynecol 1982; 144: 289
15 Pilu G, Romero R, Jeanty P, et al. Prenatal diagnosis of craniofacial malformations with ultrasonography. Am J Obstet Gynecol 1986; 155: 45
16 Gorlin R J, Cervenka J, Pruzansky S. Facial clefting and its syndromes. Birth Defects 1971; 7: 3
17 Benacerraf B R, Frigoletto F D, Bieber F R. The fetal face: ultrasound examination. Radiology 1984; 153: 495
18 Savoldelli G, Schmid W, Schinzel A. Prenatal diagnosis of cleft lip and palate by ultrasound. Prenat Diagn 1982; 2: 313
19 Kraus B S, Kitamura H, Ooe T. Malformations associated with cleft lip and palate in human embryos and fetuses. Am J Obstet Gynecol 1963; 86: 321
20 Pashayan H M. What else to look for in the child born with a cleft of the lip and palate. Cleft Palate J 1983; 20: 54–82
21 Smith D W. Recognisable patterns of human malformation. Philadelphia: Saunders and Co. 3rd edition. 1982

22 Cohen M M. The Robin anomalad – its nonspecific and associated syndromes. J Oral Surg 1976; 34: 587

23 Pilu G, Romero R, Reece E A, et al. The prenatal diagnosis of the Robin anomalad. Am J Obstet Gynecol 1986; 154: 630

24 Cobellis G, Iannoto P, Stabile F, et al. Prenatal ultrasound diagnosis of macroglossia in the Wiedemann-Beckwith syndrome. Prenat Diagn 1988; 8: 79–82

25 Pettenati M J, Haines J L, Higgins R R, et al. Wiedemann-Beckwith syndrome: presentation of clinical and cytogenetic data on 22 new cases and review of the literature. Hum Genet 1986; 74: 143

26 Dewbury K C, Aluwihare A P R, Birch S J, Freeman N V. Antenatal ultrasound demonstration of a choledochal cyst. Br J Radiol 1980; 53: 906–907

27 Elrad H, Mayden K L, Ahart S, et al. Prenatal ultrasound diagnosis of a choledochal cyst. J Ultrasound Med 1985; 4: 553

28 Frank J L, Hill M C, Chirathivat S, et al. Antenatal observation of a choledochal cyst by ultrasound. AJR 1981; 137: 166

29 Howell C G, Templeton J M, Wiener S, et al. Antenatal diagnosis and early surgery for choledochal cyst. J Pediatr Surg 1983; 18: 387

30 Alvear D T, Rayfield M M. Bilateral ovarian cysts in early infancy. J Pediatr Surg 1976; 11: 993

31 Rizzo A, Gabrielli S, Perolo A, et al. Prenatal diagnosis and management of fetal ovarian cysts. Prenat Diagn 1989; 9: 97

32 Ikeda K, Suita S, Nakano H. Management of ovarian cyst detected antenatally. J Pediatr Surg 1988; 5: 432

33 Eggermont E, Lecoutere D, de Vlieger H, et al. Ovarian cysts in newborn infants. Am J Dis Child 1988; 142: 702

34 Giorlandino C, Rivosecchi M, Bilancioni E, et al. Successful intrauterine therapy of a large ovarian cyst. Prenat Diagn 1990; 10: 473

35 Byrne J, Blanc W A, Warburton D, et al. The significance of cystic hygromas in the fetus. Hum Pathol 1984; 15: 61

36 Chervanek F A, Isaacson G, Blakemore K J, et al. Fetal cystic hygroma. Cause and natural history. N Engl J Med 1983; 309: 822

37 Garden A S, Benzie R J, Miskin M, Gardner H A. Fetal cystic hygroma colli. Am J Obstet Gynecol 1986; 24; 389

38 Pearce J M F, Griffin D, Campbell S. The differential prenatal diagnosis of cystic hygromata and encephalocele by ultrasound examination. JCU 1984; 13: 317

39 Redford D H A, McNay M B, Ferguson-Smith M E, et al. Aneuploidy and cystic hygroma detectable by ultrasound. Prenat Diagn 1984; 4: 377

40 Chervanek F A, Isaacson G, Tortora M. A sonographic study of fetal cystic hygromas. JCU 1985; 13: :311

41 Pearce J M F, Griffin D, Campbell S. Cystic hygromata in trisomy 18 and 21. Prenat Diagn 1984; 4: 371

42 Greenberg F, Carpenter R J, Ledbetter D H. Cystic hygromata and hydrops fetalis in a fetus with trisomy 13. Clin Genet 1983; 24: 389

43 Dallapiccola B, Zelante L, Perla G, et al. Prenatal diagnosis of recurrence of cystic hygroma with normal chromosomes. Prenat Diagn 1984; 4: 383

44 Connor J M. Prenatal diagnosis of Turner's syndrome; what to tell the patients. BMJ 1988; 293: 711–712

45 Chodirker B N, Harman C R, Greenberg C R. Spontaneous resolution of a cystic hygroma in a fetus with Turner's syndrome. Prenat Diagn 1988; 4: 291–296

46 Kozlowski K J, Frazier C N, Quirk J G. Prenatal diagnosis of an abdominal cystic hygroma. Prenat Diagn 1988; 8: 405–410

47 Weiner S, Scharf J I, Bolognese R J, et al. Antenatal diagnosis and treatment of fetal goiter. J Reprod Med 1980; 24: 39

48 Kourides I A, Berkowitz R L, Pang S, et al. Antenatal diagnosis of goitrous hypothyroidism by fetal ultrasonography and amniotic fluid thyrotropin concentration. J Clin Endocrinol Metab 1984; 59: 1016

49 Barone C M, Van Natta F C, Kourides I A, et al. Sonographic detection of fetal goiter, an unusual cause of hydramnios. J Ultrasound Med 1985; 4: 625

50 Gundry S R, Wesley J R, Klein M D, et al. Cervical teratomas in the newborn. J Paediatr Surg 1983; 18: 382

51 Spitz L. Personal communication. 1990

52 Donnellan W A, Swenson O. Benign and malignant sacro-coccygeal teratomas. Surgery 1968; 64: 834

53 Holzgreve W, Mahoney B S, Glick P L, et al. Sonographic demonstration of fetal sacrococcygeal teratoma. Prenat Diagn 1985; 134: 228

54 Altman R P, Randolph J G, Lilly J R. Hereditary presacral teratoma. J Paediatr Surg 1974; 9: 691

55 Valdiserri R O, Yunis E J. Sacrococcygeal teratomas. A review of 68 cases. Obstet Gynecol 1981; 53: 660

Placenta and cord

Eric Jauniaux and Stuart Campbell

INTRODUCTION

Before the development of prenatal investigation techniques, morphological examination of the placenta and the cord was limited to retrospective information and therefore was of little value in pregnancy management. With the improvement of ultrasound equipment it is possible to examine the placenta and the cord in detail before delivery.

The sonographic differential diagnoses of the principal placental abnormalities are reviewed in this chapter as well as their pathophysiological significance. The ultrasound features have been correlated with pathological findings.

Placental development and maturation

The developing placenta (chorion frondosum) can be observed by transabdominal ultrasound between 6 and 8 weeks of gestation.[1] At this time it appears as a thickening of a portion of the gestational sac (Fig. 1). At the end of the twelfth week of gestation the enlarging gestational sac fills the entire uterine cavity and fusion of the decidua capsularis surrounding the amniotic sac and the decidua parietalis completely obliterates the uterine cavity.[2] From this moment the components of the definitive placenta can be clearly discerned in vivo (Fig. 2).

The three basic placental structures are the chorionic or fetal plate, the placental villous tissue or substance and the basal or maternal plate. The placental mass is divided into 20 to 40 cotyledons or functional units determined by the branching pattern of the villous tree and includes the primary villous trunk with its derivatives.[3] The maternal surface is also divided in lobes, of no physiological signifi-

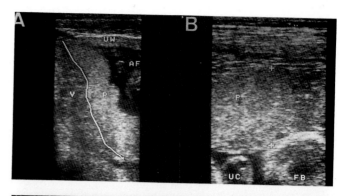

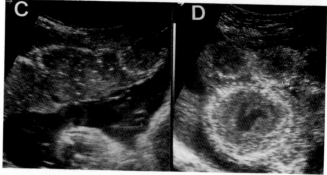

Fig. 2 **Placental grading.** Composite scans of the four placental grades. **A:** Grade 0 at 14 weeks of gestation. **B:** Grade I at 30 weeks of gestation. **C:** Grade II, partially grade III at 38 weeks of gestation. **D:** Premature grade III at 32 weeks in a pregnancy complicated by chronic hypertension.

cance, by septa extending from the basal plate towards the chorionic plate.[2]

The circulation of maternal blood through the intervillous chamber is a dynamic process that requires a continuous adaptation of the individual cotyledon to the blood flow offered to it by the corresponding uteroplacental artery. During the first trimester of pregnancy the growing embryo and its placenta are separated from the maternal circulation.[4] Trans-vaginal sonography, hysteroscopy and examination of chorionic villous sampling material are unable to detect a real continuous blood flow in the intervillous spaces before 12 weeks of gestation.[4] The early placenta is bathed by a fluid possibly composed of maternal plasma and uterine gland secretions.[4] After 12 weeks the trophoblastic plugs in the spiral arteries, still remaining from the first extravillous trophoblastic wave, no longer obliterate the uteroplacental arteries and a real intervillous circulation is then established.[4] A second wave of endovascular trophoblast migration now invades the myometrial segments of the spiral arteries allowing the progressive dilatation of these vessels.[5–7] By the end of pregnancy the placental blood supply is estimated to be around 600 ml/min.[7]

A sonographic classification system for grading placentae in utero according to maturational changes was developed by Grannum and associates.[8]

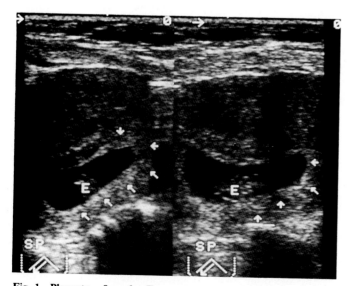

Fig. 1 **Placenta – 8 weeks.** Transverse and longitudinal sonograms of a gestational sac at 8 weeks of pregnancy. The developing placenta appears as a thick echogenic line at the posterior pole of the sac (arrows) (E – embryo).

Placental grading system (modified from Grannum et al. Am J Obstet Gynecol 1979).

Grade 0:   The placental tissue and the basal plate are homogeneous without the presence of linear highly reflective foci. The chorionic plate is smooth and well-defined.

Grade I: The placental tissue contains a few linear highly reflective areas parallel to the basal plate which remains unchanged. The chorionic plate presents subtle undulations.

Grade II: The placental tissue contains randomly dispersed echoes and is divided by comma-like reflective structures continuous with the chorionic plate. The marked indentations of the chorionic plate do not reach the basal plate which is well-defined by small linear highly reflective areas.

Grade III: The placental tissue is divided in compartments containing central echo-free areas. The chorionic plate indentations reach the basal plate which contains almost confluent very highly reflective areas.

The placentae were graded from 0 to III on the basis of static B-scan changes in the placental structures and the results were correlated with fetal pulmonary maturity evaluated by amniotic fluid lecithin-sphingomyelin (L/S) ratios. Mature L/S ratios were found in 68% of grade I, 88% of grade II and 100% of grade III placentae suggesting that invasive amniocentesis could be replaced by ultrasound placental grading as a standard test to assess fetal pulmonary maturity.[8] However, subsequent reports did not support these findings and showed that a grade III placenta was associated with an immature L/S ratio in 8% to 42% of cases and was therefore not accurate enough to replace amniocentesis in predicting fetal pulmonary maturity.[9–12]

Factors such as chronic hypertension (Fig. 2), pre-eclampsia, intra-uterine growth retardation and maternal smoking are associated with accelerated placental maturation[13,14] whereas diabetes and fetomaternal immunisation are associated with delayed placental maturation.[13] Earlier maturational changes were also described in twin fetuses compared with singleton fetuses.[15] Recently a randomised controlled trial has demonstrated that pregnant women with mature placental appearance (grade III) on ultrasonography between 34 and 36 weeks gestation have an increased risk of problems during labour and their babies have an increased risk of low birth weight, intrapartum distress and perinatal death.[14]

Therefore, though the placental sonographic grading system is not accurate enough to replace amniocentesis in the assessment of fetal pulmonary maturity, it may be useful as a predictive indicator of potential perinatal problems.

Placental localisation

The importance of accurate localisation of the placenta in patients with antepartum haemorrhage and in those requiring invasive procedures (amniocentesis, cordocentesis or placental biopsy) is well-established. Placental localisation by ultrasound was introduced by Donald in 1965, shortly after his first recording of an early gestation sac.[16,17] Placental visualisation by sonography rapidly became standard practice[18,19] replacing ancient methods such as soft tissue radiography[20] and radio-isotope scanning.[21]

Respiratory distress syndrome associated with premature delivery and severe fetal anaemia related to antepartum maternal haemorrhage are the major causes of neonatal morbidity and mortality associated with placenta praevia.[22] Placenta praevia also causes maternal morbidity due to massive intra- or post-partum haemorrhage sometimes requiring therapeutic hysterectomy.[22,23]

The pathogenesis of placenta praevia is still obscure but predisposing factors include advancing maternal age, multiparity and prior caesarean sections.[23] A uterine scar in the lower segment not only predisposes to placenta praevia but also to placenta accreta, increasing the overall rate of maternal complications such as uterine rupture or heavy post-partum haemorrhage.[23]

The incidence of placenta praevia varies from 0.3% to 0.5% of third trimester pregnancies, the range probably reflecting differences in definition.[23] The majority of cases of 'low placentae' in early pregnancy have been shown not to be praevia at delivery, 90% of such placentae appear subsequently to move into the upper portion of the uterus.[24–26] Placental 'migration' or 'ascension' due to progressive development of the lower uterine segment is put forward as the explanation for the difference in the incidence of placenta praevia encountered in the second and third trimesters.[25]

If a low-lying placenta is diagnosed in the second trimester the patient should be examined between 32 weeks and term to exclude placenta praevia. Placenta praevia can be divided into four categories:

I – low-lying placenta positioned close to the os (within 5 cm);

II – marginal placenta praevia located at the margin of the os;

III – partial placenta praevia partially covering the internal os;

IV – total placenta praevia completely covering the internal cervical os.

The prenatal ultrasound diagnosis of total placenta praevia is usually easy because of the large amount of placental tissue overlying the internal os (Fig. 3). However, low-lying placentae may not be distinguishable by sonography from marginal or partial placenta praevia (Fig. 4). Several conditions such as maternal obesity, posterior localisation of the placenta, overdistended bladder, local myometrial thickening or acoustic shadows from the fetal head can make accurate transabdominal ultrasound diagnosis of the different grades of placenta praevia difficult.[27] Asymptom-

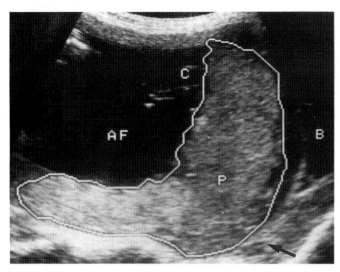

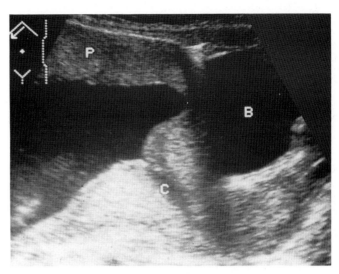

Fig. 3 Placenta praevia. Longitudinal sonogram of a total placenta praevia at 28 weeks of gestation. The placenta (P) completely covers the os (arrow) and separates the amniotic fluid (AF) from the bladder (B). Note the marginal insertion of the cord (C).

Fig. 5 Placental 'migration'. Longitudinal sonogram at 32 weeks of gestation of a placenta shown to be low-lying at 20 weeks. The placenta (P) appears clearly located above the internal cervical os (C). (B – bladder).

atic low placentae which do not completely cover the internal os in the mid-trimester are not associated with significant increase of maternal or neonatal complications.[26] Furthermore, a conversion to normal position (Fig. 5) of these cases has been demonstrated by serial ultrasound examinations.[26] These problems have lead to the introduction of trans-vaginal sonography as a more accurate method of diagnosis of placenta praevia.[27] In comparative series this new technique appears to be safe and diagnostically superior to transabdominal sonography.[27]

Placental size

Determination of the placental size is part of the overall assessment of the intra-uterine environment. Placental growth can be estimated by measuring the placental thickness or by estimation of the placental volume.

The placental thickness is measured at the thickest portion of the placenta or beneath the cord insertion.[8] There is a gradual decrease of the placental thickness from 32 weeks of gestation until term.[8] Placental thickness is not diagnostic of any particular condition but can contribute to

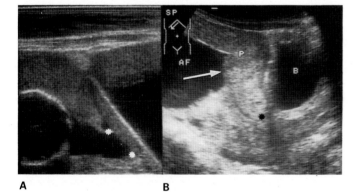

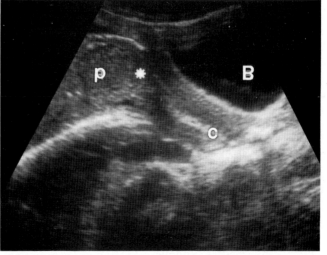

Fig. 4 Low-lying placentae. A: Low-lying placenta at 20 weeks of gestation. The distance between the placental edge (*) and the margin edge of the internal cervical os (*) can be estimated by ultrasound. **B:** Spurious placenta praevia at 32 weeks. The placental edge (P) is situated at a distance from the internal os (*). The false impression of placenta praevia is due to focal thickening of the posterior myometrium (arrow). **C:** Posterior placenta praevia (P) at term, partially covering the os (*). The bladder (B) distension can modify the relative position of the placental edge (*).

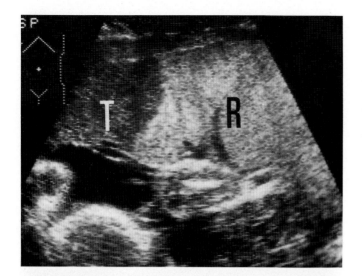

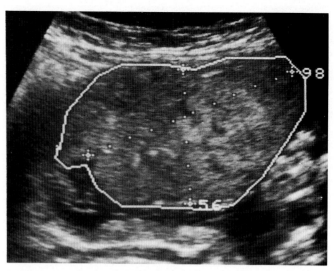

Fig. 7   **Large placenta in diabetes**. Transverse sonogram at 24 weeks showing a thick, heterogeneous placenta in a pregnancy complicated by uncontrolled class A diabetes mellitus.

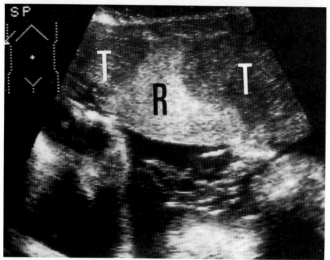

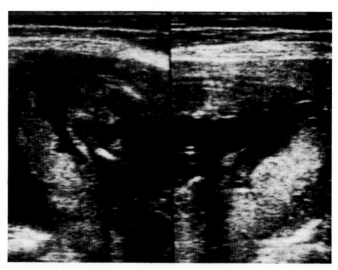

Fig. 6   **Twinning**. Transverse and longitudinal scans of the placenta in a monochorionic-diamniotic twin pregnancy at 30 weeks complicated by a twin-transfusion syndrome. The hemi-placenta corresponding to the recipient (R) or perfused twin is thicker and highly reflective (oedematous) compared with the placental area corresponding to the transfuser (T) or donor.

Fig. 8   **Placental atrophy in dead twin**. Sonograms of a monochorionic-diamniotic twin pregnancy at 21 weeks complicated by the death of one of the twins. The hemi-placenta corresponding to the dead fetus (left) is thinner compared to the placental area of the living twin (right).

the management of a fetus at risk.[28] Thick placentae (> 4 cm) can be an early sign of developing fetal hydrops of various causes (Fig. 6) or of uncontrolled maternal diabetes mellitus (Fig. 7). Placentae measuring up to 6 cm can also be found in pregnancies with elevated mid-trimester maternal serum alpha-fetoprotein (AFP) and an anatomically normal fetus.[29] Thin placentae (< 2.5 cm) are often seen in patients with intra-uterine growth retardation or fetal death (Fig. 8).

Sonographic methods for determination of the placental volume are usually complex and time consuming. However, these studies have highlighted important pathophysiological information. Longitudinal sonographic studies of the placental volume have shown a wide varia-

tion at each stage of gestation from approximately 110 to 425 ml at 23 weeks to 340 to 1000 ml at term.[30] As with the placental thickness, the growth rate of the placental volume decreased after 30 weeks and even falls towards term.[31] There is some evidence that fetal growth retardation is preceded by reduced placental volume growth in the first half of pregnancy.[32] Small placental volumes clearly denote fetal complications.[33] These preliminary results need to be confirmed by larger studies.

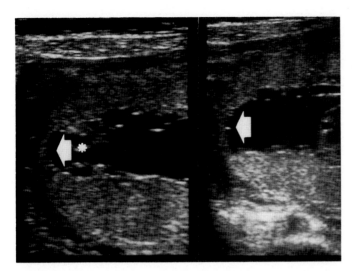

Fig. 9 **Bilobate placenta**. Longitudinal sonograms showing a bilobate fundal placenta at 26 weeks of gestation. The placental lobes are connected by a thin bridge of placental tissue (arrow) where the cord is inserted (*).

Major structural abnormalities of the placenta

Abnormalities of placentation

The placenta is normally a circular discoid organ but there is wide variation in its shape which is usually of no clinical significance.[2] However, some unusual placental shapes are associated with perinatal complications and their diagnosis in utero can influence the pregnancy management.[3] For most of these cases there is good evidence that the abnormality develops during implantation of the fertilised ovum or during the early stage of placental development.[3]

Placenta multilobata and accessory lobes Bilobate placentae consisting of two lobes of approximately equal size are found in less than 4% of pregnancies.[3] Macroscopically and sonographically the placental lobes appear as two well-defined masses connected by a thin bridge of chorionic tissue where the cord is usually inserted (Fig. 9). The bilobate placenta is in general of no direct clinical significance but is often associated with velamentous insertion[3] of the cord which should be excluded before the onset of labour (see p. 457).

Multilobate placentae consisting of three or more lobes are extremely rare and their clinical significance is not well-established.[3]

Fig. 10 **Circumvallate placenta. A:** Macroscopic view of a complete circumvallate placenta showing the abnormal membrane insertion away from the placental margin. **B:** Transverse and **C:** longitudinal scan at 20 weeks of the marginal zone of the placenta demonstrating multiple subamniotic echo-poor areas of various size and shape (*).
(Reproduced with permission of the publisher from Jauniaux et al. JCU 1989; 16: 126–131.)

An accessory lobe adjacent to the main placental mass is reported in about 3% of pregnancies.[3] The lobe is often linked to the main placental mass by a thin bridge of cho-

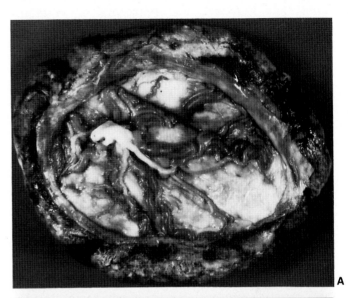

A

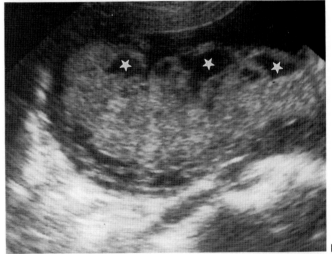

B

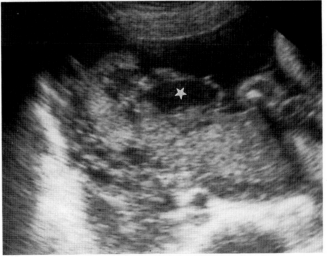

C

rionic vessels (succenturiata) but it can be entirely separate (spuria) and connected only by the membranes alone.[2] Their clinical significance lies in the risk of vessel rupture during labour, with severe fetal haemorrhage when the accessory lobe is located near the cervical os, or in the retention of the lobe in utero after delivery.[2,3] Accessory lobes are usually small and difficult to diagnose antenatally.

Placenta extrachorialis The placenta extrachorialis is a common abnormality found in about 25% of all placentae and characterised by a transition of membranous to villous chorion at a distance from the placental edge.[2,3] Insertion of the membranes within the placental margin results in placental tissue not covered by the chorionic plate (extrachorialis) and in a smaller than normal amniotic cavity.[2] Two forms can be distinguished.

a) circummarginate placenta presents with a flat ring of membranes comprising only amnion and chorion with fibrin and is practically asymptomatic.[2,3]

b) circumvallate placenta has a raised, often rolled ring of membranes (Fig. 10A), which contains amnion, chorion and decidual tissue.[2] As the uterine wall stretches in the second half of gestation the placenta cannot adapt and there is tearing of membranes and bleeding from the edge of the chorionic plate. Circumvallate placentation is, therefore, accompanied by a relatively high rate of premature rupture of the membrane, antepartum bleeding and preterm onset of labour.[2,3,34] This form of placentation is also associated with an increased incidence of low birth weight infants.[3]

Two cases of circumvallate placentae diagnosed in utero by sonography were recently reported.[34] The 'mammelonnated' appearance of the marginal chorionic plate was the main feature (Fig. 10B). The ultrasound images are made of multiple empty subamniotic echo-free areas of various sizes and shapes (Fig. 10C). These sonographic features are strictly limited to the marginal zone of the placenta and persist throughout pregnancy.[34] In contrast, the 'mammelonnated' appearance of the marginal chorionic plate is less pronounced in circummarginate placentae (Fig. 11). In the only case we have observed in utero the abnormal placental sonographic features disappeared during the second half of gestation, probably because the placenta in these cases can adapt to stretching of the myometrium.

Rare abnormalities of placentation Fenestrate placentae are extremely rare and are characterised by the absence of the central portion of a discoid placenta; there are no prenatal complications.[3]

Placentae membranacea or placentae diffusa are characterised by persistence of the villous growth over the whole surface of the placental membrane covering the entire uterine cavity.[2,3,35] This abnormality is extremely rare and is associated in nearly all cases by early antepartum bleeding and either abortion or premature labour due to the fact that a part of the placenta is necessarily praevia.[3,35]

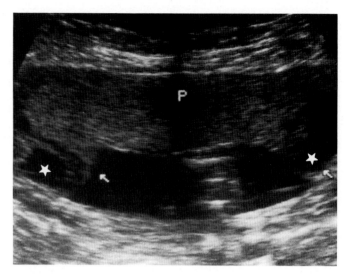

Fig. 11 Circummarginate placenta. Transverse sonogram of the upper part of the amniotic cavity at 17 weeks showing bilateral subamniotic (⋆) echo-poor areas (arrows). These features could not be identified on the scans from 22 weeks of gestation. Pathological examination demonstrated a circummarginate placenta. (P – placenta).

When the placenta is uniformly distributed over the membranes and of reasonable thickness, the prenatal diagnosis can be made by ultrasound.[35,36]

Placenta accreta has been defined as a placenta with abnormal adherence, either in whole or in part to the uterine wall.[3,37] This abnormality is characterised by myometrial invasion by the villi and occurs when the decidua basalis is partially or completely absent.[3] According to the degree of myometrial invasion this condition is subdivided into placenta accreta vera, when the villi are simply attached to the myometrium; placenta increta, when the villi invade deeply the myometrium; and placenta percreta when the villi penetrate the entire thickness of the uterine wall.[3,37] Placenta accreta is a rare but very serious abnormality. All conditions or procedures which affect the integrity of the internal uterine walls, such as caesarean section and other uterine surgery, curettage, sepsis or fibroids, are predisposing factors for abnormal villous penetration.[3] In many patients there is a combination of aetiological factors[3] and the association of a prior uterine scar and a low placental insertion is a particular risk.[23] Placenta accreta has both an overall maternal and fetal mortality of around 10% due to antepartum or post-partum bleeding, uterine rupture and uterine inversion.[3] Placenta percreta is clearly the most dangerous condition with a perinatal mortality rate of 96%.[37] On ultrasound the decidual interface between placenta and myometrium is absent at the level of the abnormal villous penetration.[37] Prenatal diagnosis of this condition may allow the obstetrician to demarcate the areas of the placenta that require resection prior to undertaking surgery.[37]

Placental vascular lesions

Many inaccurate and misleading expressions have been used by ultrasonographers to describe placental vascular lesions. This is probably due to the fact that little attempt has been made to compare ultrasound and pathological findings. The terms most currently used in the literature are placental cyst, thrombotic cyst and intraplacental haemorrhage. Until a better terminology can be proposed we will refer to the classical pathological terminology to categorise these placental lesions.

Avillous spaces or placental caverns Echo-free spaces within the placental tissue vary from small poorly reflective areas to large echo-free spaces also called 'maternal lakes'. Large echo-free spaces are found in 67% of placentae examined at any stage of gestation from the first half of pregnancy to term.[38] To some extent careful sonographic examination reveals maternal lakes of different sizes and shapes in virtually all placentae, mainly under the chorionic plate near the umbilical cord insertion or in the marginal zone (Fig. 12).

Small spaces in the centre of the cotyledon have been described in mature placentae (Fig. 2D). These cavities within the cotyledons are secondary to the dispersion of the free floating terminal villi by maternal arterial jets of blood entering the intervillous space.[2,7] These modifications observed in utero by ultrasound correspond anatomically to avillous zones and can be demonstrated in vitro by perfusion of the placenta after delivery.[39]

Large echo-free spaces (maternal lakes) can be found by ultrasound within the placental tissue from the second trimester until the end of pregnancy.[40,41] They contain turbulent blood flow on real time imaging and their shape can be modified by maternal position or by uterine contractions. Two categories must be distinguished.

a) Stable maternal lakes characterised sonographically by the constancy of their appearance on repeated examinations (Fig. 13A). The large lesions are almost unaffected by placental collapse during delivery (Fig. 13B). Microscopically they correspond to large avillous areas (caverns) surrounded by normal villous tissue (Fig. 13B) and are a non-pathological persistence of the placental anatomical structure from early in pregnancy.[41]

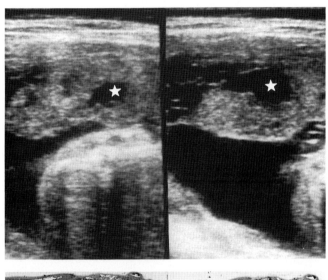

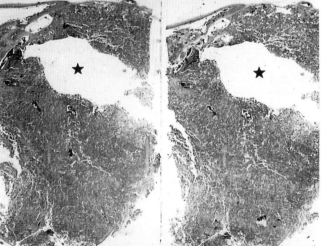

Fig. 13 Avillous placental space. A: Transverse sonograms at 37 weeks of gestation of a large echo-free space (★), identified at the end of the second trimester. The shape of the lesion and the reflectivity of the surrounding placental tissue remained unchanged until delivery. **B:** Histological sections of the lesion showing a large avillous space (★) surrounded by normal placental tissue.

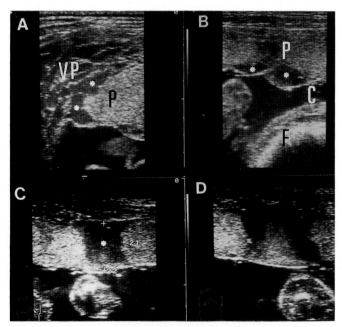

Fig. 12 Vascular spaces in the placenta. Sonograms of intraplacental echo-free spaces (★). **A:** Marginal between the placental mass (P) and the uterine draining venous plexus (VP). **B:** Under the cord insertion (C) (P – placenta, F – fetus). **C:** Transverse and **D:** longitudinal views of a large echo-free space containing turbulent blood flow.

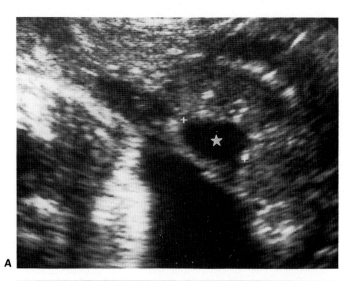

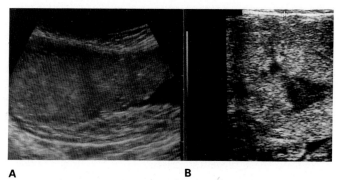

Fig. 15 **Vascular space in the placenta**. Sonograms at 20 weeks of gestation showing a large placenta (thickness > 4 cm) with **A**: patchy decreased reflectivity and **B**: large echo-free spaces containing turbulent blood flow. These placental sonographic features (jelly-like placenta) were associated with elevated maternal serum alpha-fetoprotein.

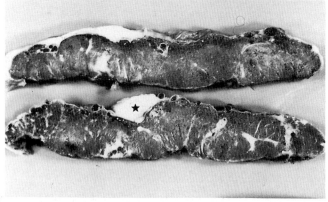

Fig. 14 **Subchorionic thrombosis. A**: Sonogram at 32 weeks showing a large echo-free space (*) beneath the chorionic plate. **B**: Macroscopic examination of the placenta at term demonstrating a subchorionic thrombosis (*).

b) Variable maternal lakes which correspond to the first stage of the development of a placental thrombosis. Their size is extremely variable and their reflectivity may change from one examination to another as blood coagulation and fibrin deposition lead to intervillous, subchorionic or marginal thrombosis (Fig. 14) classically described by the pathologists.[2,3,41]

These two categories can only be differentiated by serial ultrasound examinations. Large echo-free spaces may be found in pregnancies with elevated maternal serum alpha-fetoprotein (MSAFP) if they develop at the time of AFP screening.[29,42] Large spaces can also be observed in placentae of excessive thickness (Fig. 15) and may be associated with fetal growth retardation and premature delivery.[29,43]

Thrombosis Placental thromboses are the result of focal coagulation of blood in the intervillous spaces.[2,3] Intervillous thromboses are found in about 40% of placentae[2,3] and contain an admixture of fetal and maternal blood.[44]

Large echo-free spaces containing turbulent flow on real time imaging are the early stages of the development of intervillous, subchorionic or marginal placental thromboses.[38,41] Turbulence of maternal blood, with low flow laterally and relatively high flow in the central part, may result from the failure of the cotyledon to expand in response to the increasing jet of blood from the corresponding uteroplacental artery. Due to focal overpressure the surrounding villi are pushed away, compressed (Fig. 16) and gradually atrophy as fibrin is progressively laid down in the periphery. Finally the maternal blood coagulates in the placental tissue causing focal obliteration of the intervillous circulation (Fig. 17A). This failure to accommodate may be secondary to an inadequate venous drainage from the cotyledon, to alteration of the villous trophoblast with release of thromboplastic substances,[2] or to villous oedema as has been described in maternofetal incompatibility.[45,46]

Placental thrombosis may be detected by ultrasound early in the second trimester,[41,46] while serial ultrasound examinations can demonstrate the evolution of a simple maternal lake to an intervillous thrombosis. A progressive laying down of fibrin and degeneration of the surrounding villi will result in increased reflectivity of the lesion (Fig. 17A). Old thrombosis (Fig. 17B) may be difficult to differentiate from infarcts if repeated ultrasound examinations are not performed. The sonographic identification of intervillous thrombosis is of clinical importance as an indicator of abnormal placental function or of isoimmunisation.[45,46]

Single subchorionic and marginal thromboses are not associated with increased fetal and/or maternal risk.[2,3] However, massive subchorionic thrombosis, also known as 'Breus mole', separating the chorionic plate from the underlying villous tissue is associated with perinatal complications.[3,47] The development of this lesion predis-

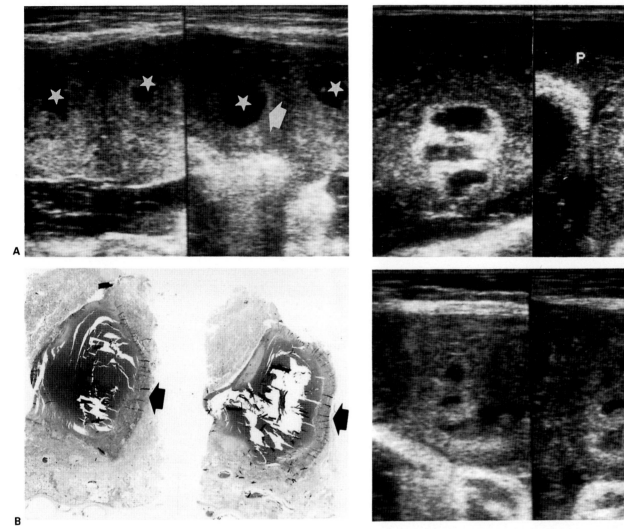

Fig. 16 Placental space. A: Sonograms at 35 weeks showing large placental echo-free spaces (*), which contained turbulent blood flow. Note the increased reflectivity of the surrounding villi (arrow). **B:** Histological section of the largest lesion. The surrounding villi opposite to the entrance of the maternal blood are compressed and degenerated (arrows).

Fig. 17 Intervillous thrombosis. A: Sonograms at 39 weeks showing abnormal placental features corresponding to an organised intervillous thrombosis with extensive fibrin deposition in the periphery. **B:** Sonograms of a placenta at 35 weeks showing small echo-free spaces surrounded by large areas of reflective tissue corresponding to an old intervillous thrombosis.

poses to premature onset of labour and can compromise the placental circulation with fetal distress or death. Sonographically the placenta appears enlarged with multiple echo-free spaces elevating the fetal plate.[47]

Infarcts Placental infarcts are similar to infarcts observed in any other organs and are the result of obstruction of the uteroplacental circulation. The relationship between placental infarcts and maternofetal complications has been well-documented in pathological studies.[2,3] Small infarcts are found in about 25% of placentae from uncomplicated pregnancies.[3]

The incidence of placental infarction is significantly increased in pregnancies complicated by pre-eclampsia or essential hypertension and is directly related to the severity of the disease.[3] In these maternal hypertensive disorders infarction is usually extensive and involves more than 10% of the placental tissue. These large placental infarcts are associated with an excess of perinatal mortality and intra-uterine growth retardation.[2,3]

Recent or acute infarcts appear macroscopically as red lesions which on histology consist of congested villi with widely dilated vessels and narrowed intervillous spaces. Old or chronic infarcts are yellow-white on macroscopic examination and are composed microscopically of necrotic ghost-like villi often with fibrin deposition in the periphery of the lesion.[2,3]

The sonographic features of placental infarcts have only recently been reported.[41,48] They appear as large irregular intraplacental areas, with reduced reflectivity in the acute stage and of similar reflectivity to adjacent normal placenta

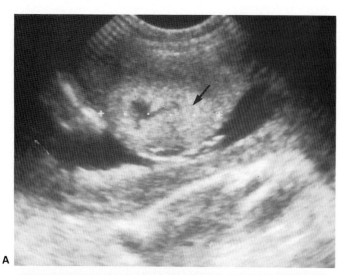

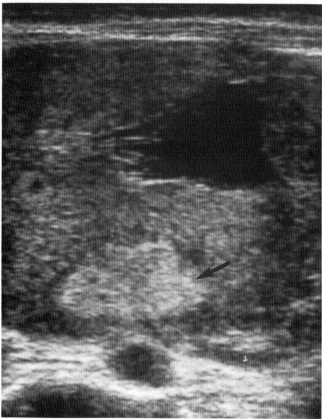

Fig. 18 Placental infarct. A: Large highly reflective lesion (arrow) of the placenta at 35 weeks of gestation in a pregnancy complicated by pre-eclampsia, corresponding to an acute infarct. **B:** Large placental area of high reflectivity (arrow) located near the basal plate at 32 weeks in an uncomplicated pregnancy corresponding to a chronic infarct. (Reproduced with permission of the publisher from Jauniaux et al. JCU 1990; in press.)

in more advanced stages (Fig. 18). They are usually located near the basal plate.

Fibrin deposition Perivillous fibrin deposition is more often a diffuse and microscopic phenomenon.[2,3] However,

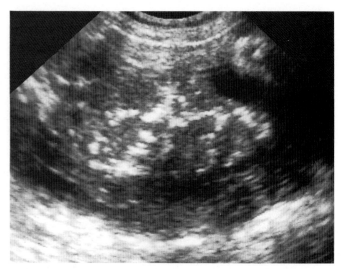

Fig. 19 Placental calcification. Sonogram of a third trimester placenta showing diffuse intensely reflective foci corresponding histologically to perivillous fibrin and calcium deposits.

large plaques of fibrin are found in 20% of the placentae examined at birth.[1] They are secondary to turbulence of maternal blood in the intervillous space. Perivillous fibrin deposition usually occurs during the second half of pregnancy and large lesions are often found in contact with the fetal plate of the placenta. Subchorionic fibrin deposition is similar sonographically and macroscopically to subchorionic thrombosis. Small diffuse fibrin deposits can be detected by ultrasonography and are frequently mixed with calcium deposits (Fig. 19). Extensive fibrin deposition involving more than 30% to 40% of the placental tissue is associated with fetal growth retardation.[2,3]

Haematomas Placental haematomas are localised masses of blood resulting from extravasation of maternal or fetal blood.

Haematomas from fetal origin are secondary to rupture of a chorionic vessel before or during delivery and are localised under the amniotic layer (subamniotic) covering the fetal plate. Their incidence is unknown but most of them are found in third trimester placentae and are thought to occur during delivery due to excessive traction on the umbilical cord.[11] However, when haematomas develop earlier in pregnancy they are associated with elevated maternal serum AFP and the lesion can be diagnosed by ultrasound.[29] Early subamniotic haematomas are sometimes complicated by fetal growth retardation and abnormal Doppler traces.[29,49] Sonographically they appear as a single mass protruding from the fetal plate and surrounded by a thin membrane. While the newly formed clot is moderately reflective (Fig. 20), the lesion becomes less so as the clot resolves (Fig. 21).

Haematomas of maternal origin are the pathological basis of placental abruption which is recognised as one of the most serious complications of pregnancy.[2,3,50] Vaginal

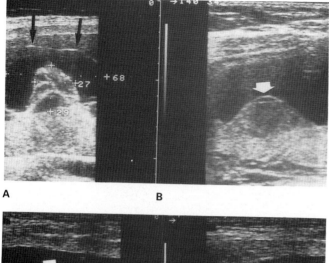

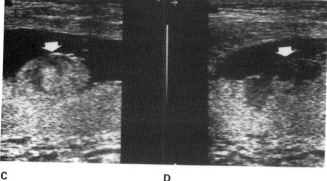

Fig. 20 Subamniotic haematoma. A: Subamniotic haematoma containing a newly formed clot on top of the fetal plate and surrounded by a thin membrane (arrow) corresponding to the amnion. **B,C** and **D:** (for comparison). Large echo-free subchorionic spaces (arrows) or maternal lakes elevating the fetal plate. These lesions are secondary to pooling and stasis of maternal blood under the fetal plate.

bleeding affects 25% of pregnancies before 20 weeks of gestation[51] and 4% during the third trimester.[50] In this context sonographic examination is important during the first half of gestation. Significant correlation is reported between the size of the haematoma and subsequent pregnancy complications.[52-55] The development of a haematoma is also associated with elevated maternal serum AFP and positive Kleihauer test suggesting fetomaternal admixture of blood in some of these cases.[42,55] By contrast the value of ultrasound in this condition is limited during the second half of pregnancy. The diagnosis of placental abruption in preterm or term pregnancies is based on the clinical triad (pain, uterine rigidity and vaginal bleeding) and sonographic investigations can only be used in non-acute cases to confirm the clinical diagnosis and to exclude placenta praevia.[50] Placental haematomas produce a wide spectrum of sonographic features depending on the location of the lesion and the degree of organisation of the blood clot. Acute haemorrhage may be of greater or similar reflectivity to the placenta, while resolving haematomas are poorly reflective after 1 week and echo-free after 2 weeks.[53] From a pathological point of view placental haematomas are separated into two categories which can be distinguished on ultrasound findings.

a) Marginal haematomas are found in 1% of all placentae and occur more often[2] in placentae partly implanted in the lower segment of the uterus (Fig. 22) or in placenta extrachorialis (Fig. 23). Retrospectively, at term, these lesions seem to be of no clinical importance.[2,3] However, sonography can detect subchorionic lesions often associated with marginal detachment of the placenta in patients with vaginal bleeding during the first half of pregnancy.[52-55] These subchorionic haematomas probably result from early marginal placental abruption with collection of blood be-

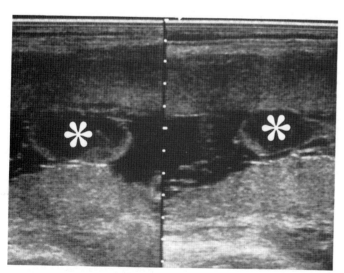

Fig. 21 Subamniotic haematoma. Poorly reflective mass protruding from the fetal plate of the placenta (*) corresponding to a subamniotic haematoma due to the rupture of fetal vessels.

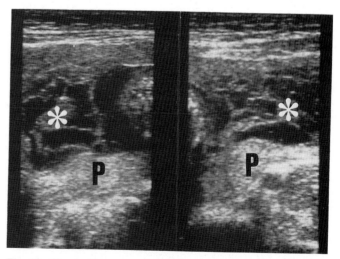

Fig. 22 Marginal haematoma. Transverse sonograms at 18 weeks of a heterogeneous mass (*) at the margin of a low inserted placenta (P), corresponding to a marginal placental haematoma.

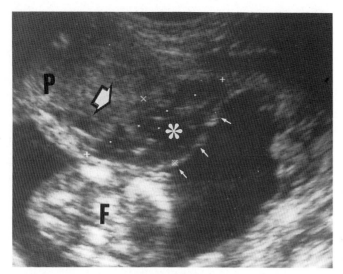

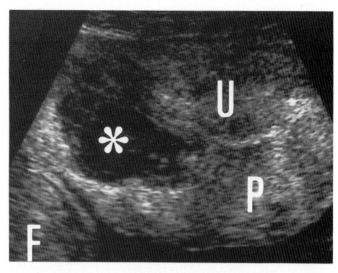

Fig. 23 Placental haematoma. Sonogram at 15 weeks showing a poorly reflective lesion (*) between the placental margin (large arrow) and fetus (F), displacing the chorionic membranes (small arrows). Pathological examination of the placenta demonstrated a marginal haematoma and extrachorialis insertion of the membranes (circumvallate placenta).

Fig. 24 Retroplacental haematoma. Sonogram at 32 weeks showing a poorly reflective mass (*) between the uterine wall (U), placenta (P) and fetus (F) 2 weeks after an umbilical cord puncture with passage of the needle through the placenta. Pathological examination demonstrated a large retroplacental haematoma.

neath the chorionic membrane, instead of collecting behind the placenta as happens during the third trimester.[52,53] The haematomas can also accumulate on the myometrial surface opposite the placenta.[53] Early intra-uterine haematomas are observed more frequently in patients with a history of spontaneous abortion, uterine malformation or myomas and are associated with an increased risk of subsequent fetal growth retardation (22%), a high rate of caesarean sections (26%) and manual removal of the placenta (7%) after delivery is often required.[55]

b) Retroplacental haematomas are found in 5% of all placentae and 15% of placentae from women with pregnancy induced hypertension.[3] Retroplacental bleeding with premature placental separation is thought to be due to rupture of a maternal uteroplacental artery.[2,3] Retroplacental haematomas are often accompanied by infarction of the overlying villous tissue and decidual necrosis.[2,3] Pathological evidence of a retroplacental haematoma is found in only 30% of placentae from women with clinical symptoms of placental abruption.[56] These lesions can develop in anteriorly located placentae during or after an invasive procedure such as amniocentesis or cordocentesis (Fig. 24). Acute haematomas are often of similar reflectivity to the surrounding placental tissue which may explain why they are difficult to diagnose antenatally. Thus negative sonographic examination of the placenta does not exclude the diagnosis of retroplacental haematoma, while other intra-uterine abnormalities such as leiomyomas or placental tumours can simulate placental haematomas on sonography.[53] Ultrasound visualisation of a retroplacental haematoma in both acute and non-acute clinical situations

is of little value in deciding when to undertake an emergency delivery.[50]

Placental tumours

Placental tumours include a wide range of placental abnormalities with different fetal and maternal implications. Prenatal differential diagnosis of both trophoblastic and non-trophoblastic tumours is based on symptoms, on specific ultrasound features and on biological investigations. The main characteristics of the different placental tumours are summarised below.

Differential diagnosis of placental tumours

a) Trophoblastic tumours
   – Classical hydatidiform mole
1. Complete mole: mainly diploid (46, XX in 90%; 46, XY in 10%):
   • Generalised swelling of the villous tissue (macroscopic).
   • Diffuse trophoblastic hyperplasia (microscopic).
   • No embryonic or fetal tissue (no gestational sac).
   • High levels of maternal serum human chorionic gonadotrophin (MShCG) and low levels of maternal serum alpha-fetoprotein (MSAFP) in all cases.
2. Twin pregnancy combining a complete diploid mole and a normal fetus with a normal placenta:
   • Molar mass associated with a normal fetus and placenta.
   • High levels of MShCG and normal levels of MSAFP.

3. Partial diploid mole:
- Focal swelling and trophoblastic hyperplasia.
- Normal embryo or fetus.
- High levels of MShCG and high levels of MSAFP.
  - Partial triploid mole (69,XXY in 70%; 69,XXX in 27%; 69,XYY in 3%)
- Focal swelling and trophoblastic hyperplasia (70%).
- Abnormal embryo or fetus (intra-uterine growth retardation (IUGR) (100%) + malformations (50%)).
- Elevated levels of MShCG and high levels of MSAFP with normal levels of amniotic fluid alpha-fetoprotein (AFAFP) in most of the cases.

b) Non-trophoblastic tumours
  - Chorioangiomas (0.5% to 1% of placentae)
- Well-circumscribed round mass, protruding from the fetal plate.
- Large tumours (> 5 cm diameter) associated with IUGR and non-immune hydrops fetalis.
- Elevated levels of MSAFP and AFAFP with normal levels of MShCG.
  - Teratomas
- Isolated mass developing over the chorion with no umbilical cord.
  - Metastasis
- From various maternal or fetal origin.
- Thick placenta.

Trophoblastic tumours The principal pathological finding of this category of placental abnormalities is the presence of microscopic trophoblastic hyperplasia often associated with enlargement of the placenta and macroscopic hydropic (molar) transformation (swelling) of the villous tissue. Molar changes of the placenta are not pathognomonic of trophoblastic disorders and can be found in other placental pathologies such as diffuse mesenchymal hyperplasia[29] or in prolonged placental retention in utero after fetal death. Hyperplasia of the trophoblast is associated with elevated levels of human chorionic gonadotrophin (hCG) in the maternal serum[57] and the rise of hCG levels is related to the extent of abnormal trophoblastic development.[57,58] The major prenatal features associated with placental trophoblastic disease are heavy vaginal bleeding, severe vomiting, pregnancy induced hypertension, a uterus enlarged above expected size and bilateral ovarian theca lutein cysts.[58] Pathological examination of the products of conception in these cases is of paramount importance as patients with trophoblastic tumours may develop persistent trophoblastic disease.[3,57] The placental trophoblastic disorders can be classified in two groups.

a) Classical hydatidiform moles. They are mainly represented by the complete hydatidiform mole characterised by generalised swelling of the villous tissue, diffuse trophoblastic hyperplasia and no embryonic or fetal tissue.[3,57]

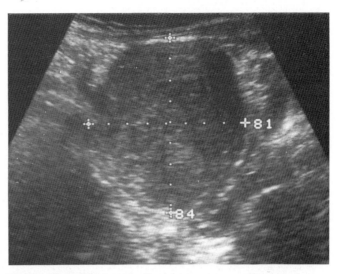

Fig. 25 Hydatidiform mole. Transverse sonogram at 8 weeks of gestation (calculated from the last menstrual period) showing an enlarged uterus with heterogeneous central echoes and no gestational sac. The patient presented with bleeding and had a positive pregnancy urine test. Pathological examination demonstrated a complete hydatidiform mole.

Complete moles are almost always diploid with 46,XX chromosomal constitution in 90% of the cases and a 46,XY karyotype in the remainder.[59] About 15% to 20% of complete moles can become invasive and metastasise.[57] Sonographically the uterus is filled with echo-free spaces of various shapes and sizes.[1] Although the vesicles are present in the first trimester hydatidiform mole they may be too small to be delineated on sonography and the tumour appears as homogeneous tissue (Fig. 25). Complete moles are associated with high levels of hCG and very low levels of AFP.[57,60] Classical moles may transform to choriocarcinoma (Ch. 3).

Molar transformation of one ovum in a dizygotic twin pregnancy is a rare entity comprising a classical hydatidiform mole with a normal pregnancy.[61,62] In these cases the hCG levels are raised, the AFP levels are within the normal range and sonographic or pathological examination shows a molar placental mass together with a normal placenta and fetus (Fig. 26). Colour flow imaging can be helpful in these cases by confirming the avascular nature of the mass.[62]

Diploid partial mole is a recently described entity characterised by a diffuse molar placenta associated with a normal fetus and elevated levels of hCG and AFP.[63] Pathologically, areas bearing characteristic molar transformation (diploid cytogenetic constitution) are interdigitated with unaffected placental areas.[63,64]

b) Triploid partial moles. Characterised by the presence of an extra set of chromosomes (69,XXY in 70%; 69,XXX in 27%; 69,XYY in 3%), this chromosomal disorder is associated with focal swelling of the villous tissue, focal trophoblastic hyperplasia and embryonic or fetal tissue.[58,65,66] Triploidy is a common chromosomal anomaly

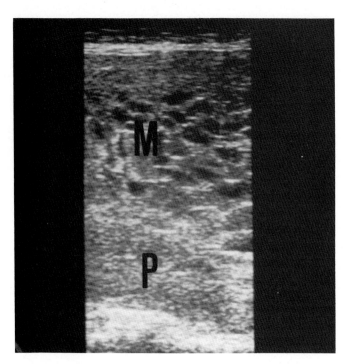

Fig. 26 Mole in a twin. Sonogram at 25 weeks of a molar mass (M) and a normal placenta (P) in a twin pregnancy combining a complete mole and a normal placenta and fetus. Note the vesicular nature of the well-developed hydatidiform mole. Colour flow mapping confirmed the avascular nature of the mass.

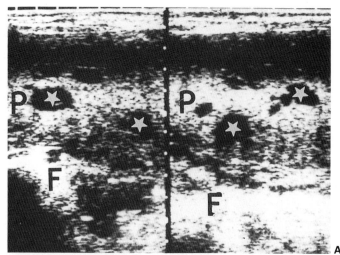

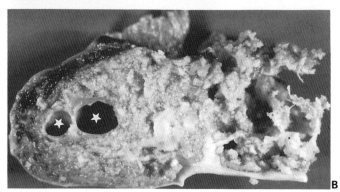

Fig. 27 Partial triploid mole. A: Transverse sonograms at 21 weeks of the placenta (P) and the fetus (F). The pregnancy was complicated by severe asymmetrical fetal growth retardation, oligohydramnios and early pregnancy induced hypertension. The placenta is enlarged and contains echo-free spaces of various sizes and shapes (*). **B:** Pathological and cytological investigations confirmed a partial triploid mole. The placenta was hydropic with focal villous swelling (*).

accounting for 1% to 2% of all clinically recognised human conceptions and for 20% of spontaneous abortions with chromosomal disorders.[65,66] The extra set of chromosomes is of paternal origin in 73% of the cases and of maternal origin in 27% of the cases.[66] There is a strong correlation between the origin of the extra set of chromosomes, the degree of the placental molar changes and the survival rate of the pregnancies.[66] All cases with an extra paternal set of chromosomes have significant molar changes (partial triploid mole) while few cases (14%) with an extra maternal set show these changes.[66] Placentae with non-molar changes are associated with better fetal survival and are more likely to be found near term.[66] These important findings suggest that the majority of placentae in triploidy should have molar changes detectable by sonography. However, absent placental molar changes on sonography does not exclude triploidy. In this disorder the fetus almost always presents with fetal growth retardation and/or major congenital defects (50%) including congenital heart disease, cystic renal dysplasia, hydrocephalus and neural tube defects.[66] After evacuation of a partial triploid mole 4% to 9% of the patients have been reported to develop a persistent trophoblastic tumour.[57]

The basis of the sonographic diagnosis of triploidy in the second and the third trimesters is severe asymmetrical growth retardation[67,68] associated with a relatively large placenta[69,70] containing sharply defined echo-free spaces of various sizes and shapes (Fig. 27). In the majority of triploidy cases, with or without associated fetal abnormalities, elevated levels of hCG and AFP are found in the maternal serum and normal levels of AFP are found in the amniotic fluid.[57,71] Sonographic criteria to differentiate triploid partial mole from other cases of first trimester missed abortion were recently proposed.[72] A ratio of transverse to anteroposterior dimension of the gestational sac > 1.5 with cystic changes, irregularity, or increased reflectivity in the decidual reaction, placenta or myometrium is in favour of a triploid partial mole.[72]

Non-trophoblastic tumours   This category of placental abnormalities includes tumours arising from any of the non-trophoblastic elements of the placenta.[3]

Chorioangiomas occur in 0.5% to 1% of the placentae examined at term.[2,3] The microscopic appearance may be that of a capillary angioma (vascular), mesenchymal hyperplasia (cellular) or usually a mixture of the two.[2] Most

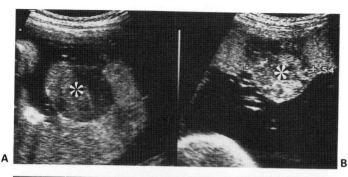

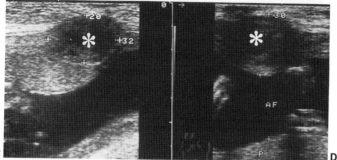

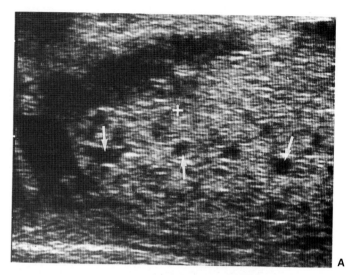

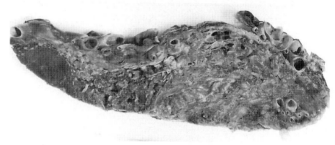

Fig. 28 Chorioangiomas. A and **B:** Composite compound sonograms of two placental chorioangiomas and **C** and **D:** two uterine leiomyomas. The chorioangiomas appear as heterogeneous and well-circumscribed masses (*), protruding from the fetal plate of the placenta. For comparison leiomyomas are poorly reflective and involve the uterine wall.

Fig. 29 False mole. A: Sonogram at 20 weeks of gestation showing a large placenta containing multiple echo-free spaces (arrows). **B:** Section showing the pseudomolar aspect of the placenta due to diffuse mesenchymal hyperplasia of the main villous trunks.

chorioangiomas are single, encapsulated, small, round and intraplacental.[2,3] Large tumours are of variable shape, divided by fibrous septa and often protrude from the fetal surface near the cord insertion.[2,3] Degenerative changes such as necrosis, calcification, hyalinisation or myxoid changes are frequently present in large tumours. A placental tumour combining a vascular chorioangioma and atypical trophoblastic proliferation (chorangiocarcinoma) was recently described suggesting that in rare cases chorioangiomas could be true neoplasms rather than hamartoma.[73]

Large chorioangiomas are well-circumscribed, have a different reflectivity from the rest of the placental tissue (Fig. 28) and are easily detectable early in pregnancy by sonography.[3,29,74–76] Chorioangiomas are associated with an increased incidence of polyhydramnios and fetal growth retardation.[3,29] Large tumours (< 5 cm in diameter) can also be complicated by fetal cardiac failure with hydrops due to the shunting of blood through the tumour.[3,29] Therefore, when a placental mass consistent with a chorioangioma is diagnosed antenatally, it is important to perform serial sonographic examinations. Increase in reflectivity of the tumour with gestation has been related to fibrotic degeneration of the lesion[29] which may reduce the risk of high output fetal cardiac failure. Placental chorioangiomas are associated with elevated levels of AFP in the maternal serum and in the amniotic fluid.[29,76] Associated fetal angi-

omas (cutaneous or hepatic) occur in 10% to 15% of cases of placental chorioangiomas and a detailed examination of the neonate is recommended in these cases.

Placentae containing multiple individual chorioangiomas or diffusely infiltrated by haemangiomatous tissue (chorioangiomatosis) or mesenchymal tissue (diffuse mesenchymal hyperplasia) have also been described.[3,29] Only the latter was observed prenatally on two occasions.[29] The placentae appeared massively enlarged containing multiple echo-free spaces on sonography (Fig. 29A). The maternal AFP levels were elevated in both cases. These prenatal findings were suggestive of a partial triploid or diploid mole.[29] However, the fetuses appeared anatomically normal and the hCG levels were within normal limits.[29] The pregnancies were otherwise uncomplicated and pathological investigations demonstrated in both cases diffuse mesenchymal hyperplasia of the main villous trunks (Fig. 29B).

Teratomas. These extremely rare benign tumours of the placenta lie between the amnion and the chorion.[3] They probably result from an abnormal migration of the primordial germ cells and can be distinguished from the fetus acardius amorphus by their lack of umbilical cord and polarity.[3] Teratomas have never been described sonographically.

Placental metastases. Placental malignant metastases are uncommon, may be of either maternal or fetal origin[3] and are often microscopic and multifocal. The only placental sonographic feature reported to date is increased thickness of the placenta in a case of fetal malignant melanoma.[77] Malignant metastases must be differentiated from septic 'metastases' observed in cases of infections in utero such as listerosis which may create a similar sonographic appearance.

Other placental abnormalities

Placental cysts   Placental cysts (cytotrophoblastic cysts) are found in 20% of the placentae examined at term.[2,3] Cytotrophoblastic cysts have a round or oval cavity, are isolated from the placental circulation and contain a gelatinous fluid (Fig. 30B). These cysts are located within the placental tissue (septal cyst) or under the fetal plate (subchorionic cyst) and they represent the only true placental cysts. Placental cysts occur more frequently in cases of di-

abetes mellitus or maternofetal rhesus incompatibility.[2,3] Sonographically they appear as single echo-free spaces (Fig. 30A) that persist unchanged on serial scans and contain no blood flow on real time imaging and give no Doppler signal.[41]

Amniotic band disruption complex   Early rupture of the amnion results in mesodermal bands emanating from the chorionic side of the amnion and which can tether parts of the developing embryo or fetus leading to a wide range of malformations.[78] Multiple anomalies such as limb deformities, craniofacial defects or ventral wall defects occur in 77% of the cases and the prognosis depends on the severity of the anomalies.[78] Sonographically amniotic bands appear as linear echoes floating in the amniotic fluid and anchored to the chorionic plate, but are not necessarily connected to the fetal body (Fig. 31).

Major structural abnormalities of the umbilical cord

The umbilical cord is derived from the stalk of the yolk sac and the allantois and normally contains two umbilical arteries and one vein surrounded by a clear gelatinous structure (Wharton's jelly) covered by amnion.[2,3] In transverse sonographic sections the arteries and umbilical vein appear as three separate rings while in longitudinal sections a portion of the cord will be seen as a series of parallel lines (Fig. 32) or as a central vein with the arteries looping around it. The mean umbilical cord circumference at term is 3.6 cm (1.2 cm diameter).[78]

Single umbilical artery (SUA) syndrome

The absence of one umbilical artery is amongst the most common congenital fetal malformations with an incidence

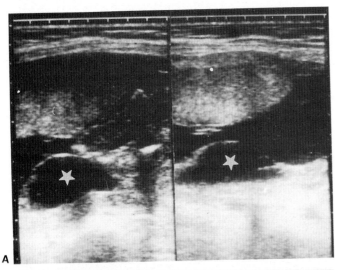

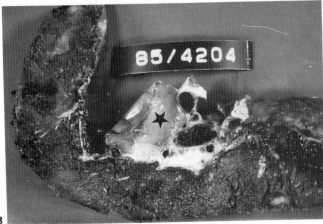

Fig. 30   Cytotrophoblastic cyst. A: Transverse scans at 32 weeks showing an echo-free cavity under the fetal plate (*) corresponding to **B:** a subchorionic cytotrophoblastic cyst (*).

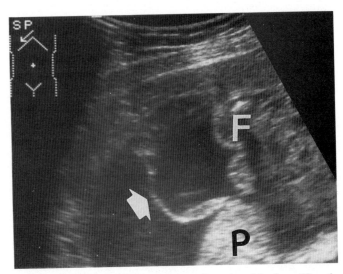

Fig. 31   Amniotic bands. Sonogram at 22 weeks of the fetus (F) and placenta (P) showing linear echoes floating in the amniotic fluid (arrow) not connected with the fetal body. The fetus was born with no abnormalities.

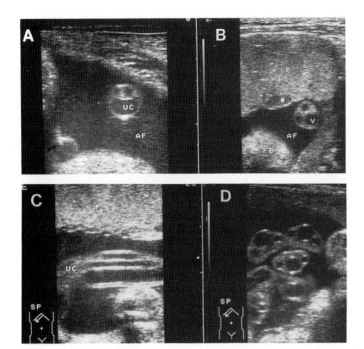

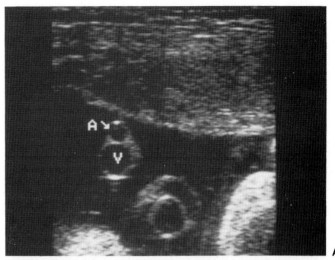

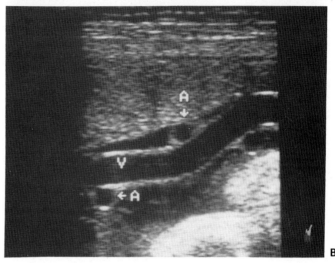

Fig. 32 Normal cord. Transverse and longitudinal scans at 28 to 32 weeks of gestation showing the normal anatomy of the umbilical cord (UC) with two arteries and one vein.

of approximately 1% of all deliveries.[79] Associated major fetal anatomical defects are largely responsible for the high fetal and neonatal loss from this pathology.[80] Fetal malformations are present in about 50% of the cases of SUA and can affect any organ system.[79,80] The incidence of intrauterine growth retardation is significantly elevated among fetuses with a SUA and are found without other congenital anomalies in 15% to 20% of the cases.[79,80] Table 1 summarises the retrospective results of a comparison of sonographic and post-natal findings in 80 cases of SUA

Fig. 33 Single umbilical artery. Transverse and longitudinal sonograms at 32 weeks demonstrating **A**: only one artery (A) and **B**: one vein (V). The fetus was growth retarded with no associated malformation.

Table 1 Comparison of the prenatal sonographic features and the post-natal findings in a series of 80 cases of single umbilical artery. (Modified from Jauniaux et al. J Gynecol Obstet Biol Reprod 1989).

Comparative data (N = 80)	Ultrasound findings		Neonatal findings	
Number of fetuses with associated malformation(s)	21	(26.6%)	34	(42.5%)
Incidence of total IUGR	28.3%		36.4%	
Incidence of isolated IUGR	15%		20%	
Distribution of the different associated fetal malformations:				
Musculoskeletal system	15	(28.8%)	32	(32%)
Urogenital system	11	(21.1%)	20	(20%)
Gastrointestinal system	3	(5.8%)	11	(11%)
Central nervous system	12	(23.1%)	11	(11%)
Integument	3	(5.8%)	9	(9%)
Cardiovascular system	4	(7.7%)	8	(8%)
Respiratory system	4	(7.7%)	6	(6%)
Miscellaneous	–	(0%)	3	(3%)
Total	52	(100%)	100	(100%)

IUGR = intrauterine growth retardation.

syndrome. In this context, minor malformations of the musculoskeletal system or of the genitourinary tract are often underdiagnosed by ultrasonography, especially if they are isolated.[79]

The prenatal diagnosis of the absence of one umbilical artery has been reported as early as 23 weeks of gestation.[81] The umbilical cord anatomy can often be visualised at that time but a precise diagnosis of a single umbilical artery is difficult and time consuming. At the end of the second trimester, or during the third trimester the umbilical cord anatomy can be examined in detail without difficulty (Fig. 33). However, various factors such as oligohydramnios or multiple loops in the cord can make accurate visualisation of the cord vessels impossible, even near term. High resolution colour Doppler imaging has an important role in early and accurate diagnosis of SUA

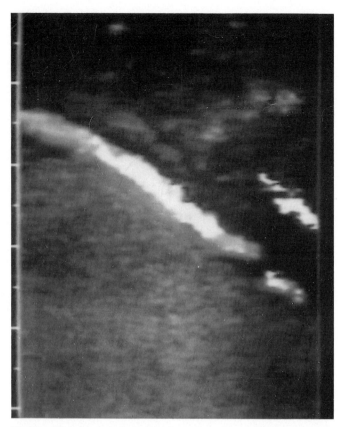
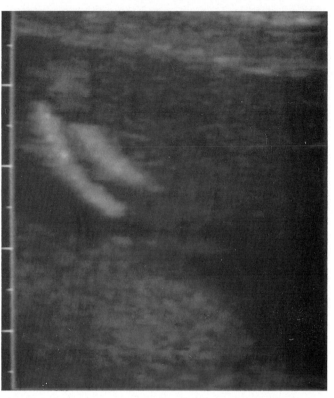

A   B

Plate 1   Normal cord. A: Colour flow image of a normal cord at 21 weeks of gestation for comparison with Plate 1B. **B:** Single umbilical artery. Colour flow image of single umbilical artery cord at 18 weeks associated with multiple fetal malformations and oligohydramnios. (Reproduced with permission of the publisher from Jauniaux et al. Am J Obstet Gynecol 1989; 161: 1195.) This figure is reproduced in colour in the colour plate section at the front of this volume.

(Plate 1) and is of clinical value in view of the possible association of a single umbilical artery and IUGR with no major fetal malformation.[82]

Tumours of the umbilical cord

Embryonic cysts   Umbilical cord remnants of the allantoic duct (urachus) and of the omphalomesenteric duct (vitelline duct) are common findings on microscopic examination of the cord.[2,3] Traces of the allantoic duct are found in 22.8% of cords examined histologically, located with a similar incidence on both ends of the cord.[83] Remnants of the vitelline duct are found in 2.4% of the cords examined, located mostly on the fetal end of the cord.[83] Cysts originating from these remnants have been reported very occasionally in the literature.

Although most of these cysts are small, some may exceed 5 cm in diameter and can be sonographically detected as a single fluid filled mass (Fig. 34). Allantoic cysts may co-exist with an omphalocele[84] or with a patent urachus secondary to a distal genitourinary tract obstruction.[85] Rarely structures arising from vitelline duct remnants differentiate to form gastric mucosa and if ulceration occurs it may cause serious damage to the umbilical vessels.[86] Al-

lantoic and omphalomesenteric cysts having a similar sonographic appearance cannot be distinguished in utero.

Angiomyxomas   The discovery of an umbilical cord angiomyxoma or haemangioma is a rare event. Although the condition was recognised early in the first half of this century, less than 30 cases have been recorded in the literature.[87–93] Cord angiomyxomas tend to be in intimate contact with one or more umbilical vessels from which they probably arise, at both fetal and placental extremities of the cord.[83,87] The majority consist of nodules clearly attached to the cord.[87,93]

Potential fetal complications of cord angiomyxomas include compression of the main vessels with retarded growth and possible intra-uterine death.[87] Angiomas of the cord may also be associated with non-immune hydrops fetalis.[89] While 16% to 33% of the placental chorioangiomas are accompanied by polyhydramnios[3] only rarely have cases of cord angiomyxomas been complicated in this way.[91] Ultrastructural studies of the umbilical cord amniotic epithelium reveal major differences from the placental amnion suggesting that passage of fluid occurs with far less ease through the cord amnion.[87] This explains the constant association of oedema and myxomatous degeneration of Wharton's jelly with angiomyxomas, a change that does not

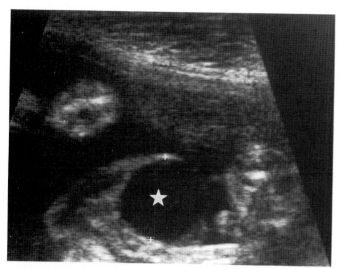

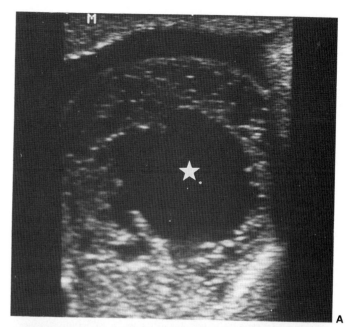

Fig. 34 Allantoic duct cyst. Sonogram of the cord near the fetal insertion at 32 weeks showing a poorly reflective round mass corresponding to an allantoic duct cyst (*). Blood flow within the mass was excluded by colour flow imaging.

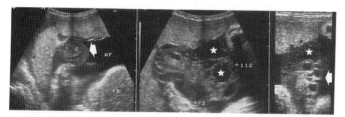

Fig. 35 Angiomyxoma of the cord. Heterogeneous multicystic mass involving the entire length of the cord at 36 weeks of gestation. The lesion is made of reflective zones (arrows) surrounded by echo-poor areas (*) and corresponds to an angiomyxoma of the cord (see also Plate 2).

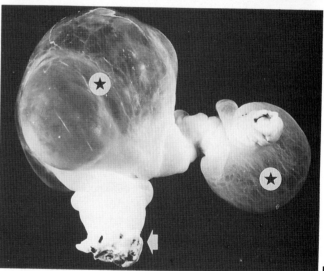

Fig. 36 False cyst of the cord. Same case as in Figure 35. **A:** Enlargement of an echo-free area (*) near the fetal insertion of the cord. **B:** View of the cord after delivery demonstrating two areas of oedema (*), corresponding to the echo-free areas (pseudocyst) described antenatally. The tumour starts near the placental insertion (arrow) and ends 2 cm from the umbilicus (see also Plate 2). (Reproduced with permission of the publisher from Jauniaux et al. J Ultrasound Med 1990; in press.)

occur with placental chorioangiomas.[87] Associated vascular neoplasms at other sites are known to occur in children born with a placental chorioangioma (see p. 450). Two cases of superficial skin angiomas and one case of hepatic angioma out of 30 cases of cord angiomyxomas have been reported.[89,93,94] Therefore, a careful post-natal examination of the neonate is recommended in case of a cord angiomyxoma.

These tumours appear sonographically as focal highly reflective areas corresponding to myxoid tissue and vascular proliferation (Fig. 35) with adjacent poorly reflective (pseudocystic) regions due to focal oedema (myxomatous degeneration) of the Wharton's jelly (Fig. 36). Angiomas involving the placental insertion of the cord sometimes extend on to the fetal plate and may be difficult to differentiate sonographically from a classical placental chorioangioma.[90,91] Complete infiltration of the cord by the angiomatous tissue and secondary progressive shortening of the cord have serious implications for vaginal delivery. When such a condition is discovered in the prenatal period

a caesarean section is recommended. Serial ultrasound examinations to monitor the enlargement of the lesion must be performed regularly and combined with Doppler measurements to detect the umbilical cord compression. Raised maternal serum AFP may be the earliest prenatal clue to the development of a cord angiomyxoma.[29,88,92] Colour flow Doppler imaging may also help the ultrasonographer (Plate 2) for early prenatal diagnosis of this cord abnormality.[82]

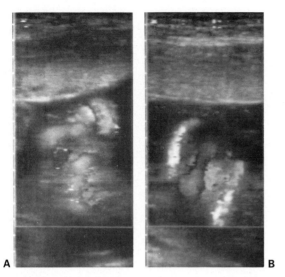

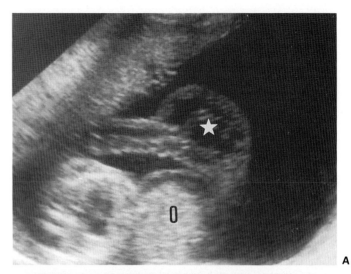

Plate 2 Angiomyxoma of the cord. A: Colour flow image of the cord tumour described in Figures 35 and 36 showing an abnormal vascular pattern at the placental insertion. **B:** Colour flow image showing the three vessels separated by a reflective structure partially compressing the umbilical vein. (Reproduced with permission of the publisher from Jauniaux et al. Am J Obstet Gynecol 1989; 161: 1195.) This figure is reproduced in colour in the colour plate section at the front of this volume.

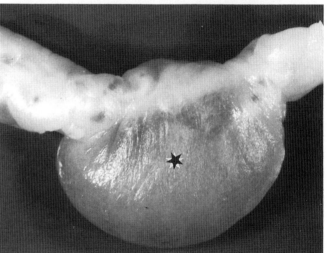

Fig. 37 False cyst of the cord. A: Transverse scan of the umbilical cord showing a large poorly reflective mass (★) juxtaposed with an omphalocele (O), corresponding to **B:** focal oedema (★) of the Wharton's jelly (pseudocyst). (Reproduced with permission of the publisher from Jauniaux et al. Prenat Diagn 1988; 8: 557.)

Pseudocysts Oedema of the Wharton's jelly has been associated with diabetes, maternofetal rhesus incompatibility and stillbirth.[95] Giant focal cord oedema is rare and gives an ultrasound appearance of an echo-free multicystic mass (Fig. 37). These pseudocysts are presumably due to the compression of umbilical cord vessels resulting from anterior fetal abdominal defects[96] or secondary to the development of a cord angioma (Fig. 36).

Teratomas The extremely rare teratoma of the cord is derived from primitive germ cells that aberrantly migrate from the primitive gut wall.[3] The tumour has not yet been documented by ultrasound.

Vascular lesions of the cord

Haematomas Spontaneous cord haematomas are occasional perinatal findings and are usually located near the fetal umbilicus.[3] Mechanical trauma of the cord such as prolapse, torsion, strangulation or dissecting aneurysm are all potential causes of cord haematoma. The vein appears to be affected more often than the arteries.[3] The implication of a cord haematoma may range from complete occlusion of the cord vessels with inevitable fetal death, to varying degrees of fetal distress, either acute or chronic.[97-101] Small haematomas will probably not affect fetal umbilical circulation because the blood may be reabsorbed before delivery. At ultrasound examination the cord appears markedly thickened, sausage shaped, and extremely highly reflective.[98-101]

Accidental laceration of umbilical cord vessels due to un-

controlled movements of the needle was reported during the early days of amniocentesis before ultrasound guidance was used when the estimated incidence was between 0.3% to 2.3%.[102] Most of the cases were reported after third trimester amniocentesis as the relatively small amount of liquor and the large size of the fetus at this stage reduced the possible movement of the cord away from the needle tip. Rare observations of haematoma leading to fetal death or cord laceration have been observed in utero by sonography during amniocentesis.[103]

Cases of fetal death have also been reported after cordocentesis.[104-106] However, compared to amniocentesis, uncontrolled movements of the needle in cordocentesis are reduced, presumably because in this new technique cord puncture is purposeful and precise and is performed under continuous ultrasound guidance. However, increased intra-vascular pressure which may be present in the recipient twin of a twin-twin syndrome[101] or following a top up fetal blood transfusion and direct blood injection in the Wharton's jelly during fetal transfusions[98] can result in haematoma (Fig. 38) and consequent tamponade of the umbilical cord vessels; the complication and mortality rates are higher following intravascular transfusion than after simple fetal blood sampling.[106] This accident should be suspected when fetal bradycardia develops during cordocentesis and ultrasound can readily detect the development of a potentially harmful haematoma at the site of puncture.

Thrombosis Thrombosis of one or more umbilical cord vessels is a rare complication with an incidence of approximately 0.08% among placentae examined prospectively at delivery.[107] Thrombosis of the umbilical vein occurs more frequently than thrombosis of one or both arteries and perinatal morbidity or mortality is more likely with umbilical artery thrombosis than with umbilical vein thrombosis.[107] The prevalence of antenatal and post-natal venous thrombosis is significantly higher in infants born to diabetic mothers.[107] Thrombosis of the umbilical vessels may also be secondary to localised increased resistance in the umbilical circulation in cases of torsion, compression and knotting of the cord.[3,107] It can affect the intra-abdominal portion of the umbilical vein and be associated with non-immune fetal hydrops.[108] Very highly reflective material within the lumen of the umbilical vessels is the main sonographic finding.[108]

Abnormalities of the cord insertion

The umbilical arteries branch off the hypogastric arteries, course lateral to the bladder, on to the anterior abdominal

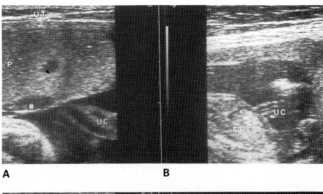
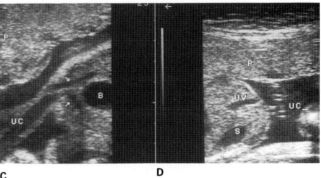

Fig. 39 Normal cord. Composite scans of the umbilical cord insertion (UC) showing: **A:** the placental (P) insertion of the cord, **B:** the fetal (FB) insertion of the cord, **C:** the two umbilical arteries (arrows) on both sides of the fetal bladder (B), **D:** the umbilical vein (UV) at the level of the fetal liver (S – stomach).

wall, and then through the umbilical cord to the placenta (Figs 3 and 39). The umbilical vein starts from the placenta, carrying the oxygenated blood and enters the fetal abdomen inferior to the level of the liver (Fig. 39). Both fetal and placental insertions of the cord should be evaluated during sonographic examination. The placental insertion is usually associated with a small echo-free space beneath the chorionic plate (Figs 12 and 39).

Marginal insertion of the cord Marginal and markedly eccentric insertions of the cord have not been clearly distinguished in the literature. This may explain the wide variation of their incidence in the general population.[3] By measuring the distance between the cord insertion and the closer placental margin one can avoid classification problems. With this method a significantly shorter distance was found in placentae from in vitro fertilisation and from the single umbilical artery syndrome compared to controls.[79,109] This form of cord insertion is not associated with an increase of pregnancy complications but may indicate a malrotation of the blastocyst at implantation.[3,109]

Velamentous insertion of the cord Placenta velamentosa (insertion of the umbilical cord into the membranes at the placental margins) is a well-defined pathological entity with a frequency around 1% of pregnancies.[2,3] The relation between this abnormal cord insertion and associated developmental defects is a matter

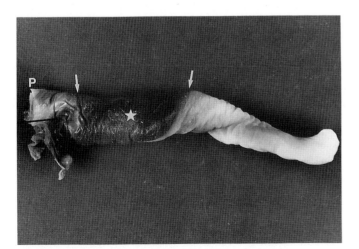

Fig. 38 Haematoma of the cord. Macroscopic appearance of the umbilical cord segment proximal to the placenta (P) 1 week after a fetal transfusion in utero. The arrows mark the extent of the haematoma (*).

of some debate. Some authors have observed a high incidence of fetal malformations associated with extraplacental cord insertions while others have only found an increased number of small for dates neonates but not of malformation.[3] From a clinical point of view, attachment of the cord to the extraplacental membranes is important because of the risk of severe fetal haemorrhage during labour.[110] Antenatal diagnosis of attachment of the cord to the membranes rather than the placental mass can be diagnosed before labour by ultrasonography.[78,110]

Other cord abnormalities

Abnormalities of the cord length   The umbilical cord has an average length of 54 cm at 34 weeks and 60 cm at term.[111] Male fetuses have significantly longer cords than females.[111] A cord less than 35 cm is defined as abnormally short. Short cords are found in fetuses with decreased in utero movements from a variety of causes or are due to a primary defect of umbilical cord and abdominal wall formation.[112,113] Excessive length of the cord may predispose to true knots or to cord prolapse during labour. It is almost impossible to determine umbilical cord length prior to delivery during routine sonographic examination. In cases of extended cord angiomyxoma the cord is highly reflective and rigid and its length can be estimated by ultrasound.[93]

Prolapse, looping and knots of the cord   Prolapse of the umbilical cord through the cervix into the vagina is an obstetric emergency,[114] with an incidence that varies between 0.5% and 0.6% of deliveries.[114–116] Cord prolapses are more likely to occur in premature deliveries, with a long umbilical cord, when the presenting part is unengaged and in pregnancies complicated by polyhydramnios.[78,114] Sonography can easily demonstrate fine parallel linear echoes corresponding to the cord, in the lower segment, below the presenting part.[78,116,117]

Looping of the cord may occur around the fetal neck, body or shoulder[114] and can be diagnosed by sonography (Fig. 40). Although in singletons looping of the cord around the neck is an uncommon cause of fetal death, a significant proportion of the high mortality of mono-amniotic twins can be attributed to umbilical cord problems.[114]

True knots of the cord are thought to be caused by excessive fetal movements early in pregnancy.[117] True knots must be distinguished from 'false knots' which are caused by focal aggregation of vessels.[3] True knots of the umbilical cord occur in 0.04% to 1% of pregnancies and are more frequent in mono-amniotic twins, in those with a long cord and in pregnancies complicated by polyhydramnios.[78] The umbilical vessels, protected by the Wharton's jelly, are rarely completely occluded. However, tight knots lead to vascular occlusion with fetal death in utero. Sonographically, a true umbilical knot appears as a complex homogeneous mass unmodified by fetal movements and unchanged on subsequent examinations (Fig. 41).

Stricture or coarctation of the cord   This rare abnormality is characterised by a localised narrowing of the cord with disappearance of Wharton's jelly, thickening of the vascular walls, and narrowing of their lumens.[78] The site of stricture or constriction is generally close to the fetus and this abnormality may result from a focal failure of the Wharton's jelly development.[78] Antenatal diagnosis has not as yet been achieved.

Conclusion

In the United Kingdom, the majority of pregnant women are scanned between 16 and 22 weeks of gestation for prenatal diagnosis of fetal malformation, confirmation of gestational age and the detection of multiple gestation. Detailed sonographic examination of the placenta at that time does offer clues as to the state of the fetus in its intra-uterine environment and can provide important information for pregnancy management.

Placental and cord lesions can occur at any time during gestation and may indicate the possibility of late fetal or

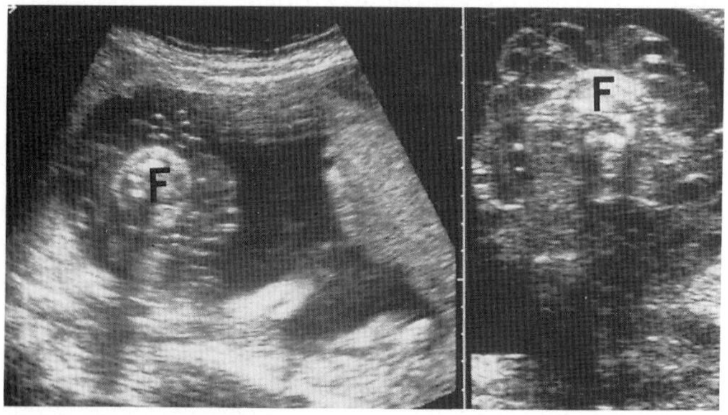

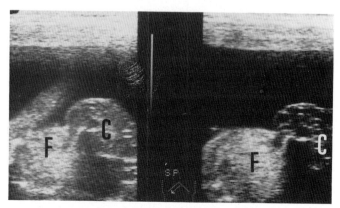

Fig. 40   Cord around the neck. Sonograms at 32 weeks showing cord loops surrounding the fetal neck (F).

Fig. 41   Knot of the cord. Sonograms at 28 weeks showing a homogeneous mass of the cord (C). The appearance of the mass was not modified by fetal (F) movements and persisted on subsequent examinations. A true knot of the umbilical cord was found after delivery.

maternal complications. Placental investigations require close collaboration between sonographers, clinicians and pathologists. Ultrasound/pathological correlation is necessary in cases where the nature of the lesion is not well-established in utero but can also help sonographers who are not familiar with placental pathology to improve the accuracy of their diagnoses.

The placenta is a dynamic organ. Depending on the delay between the development of a lesion in utero and delivery the ultrasound features and the pathological findings can be very different. Thus, serial ultrasound examination is recommended in cases where there may be an association between abnormal placental morphology and perinatal complications.

Advances in ultrasound equipment such as computerised sonography and colour Doppler imaging are likely to enhance the antenatal diagnosis of many placental and cord abnormalities described in this chapter.

Acknowledgements

This work was supported by the David & Alice Van Buuren Foundation (Hopital Universitaire Erasme, Free University of Brussels (ULB)). Eric Jauniaux is a recipient of the Sir Alexander Fleming Award (1989) from the British Council. The authors wish to acknowledge Dr G. Moscoso and Dr M. Driver (King's College Hospital, London University), Ms M. Florence and Mr Vanesse (ULB, Belgium) for invaluable technical assistance in pathological investigations of the specimens.

REFERENCES

1 Spirt B A, Gordon L P, Kagan E H. Sonography of the placenta. In: Sanders R C, James A E. The principles and practice of ultrasonography in obstetrics and gynecology. East Norwalk: Appleton-Century-Crofts. 1985: p 333–353

2 Wilkin P. Pathologie du placenta. Paris: Masson. 1965

3 Fox H. Pathology of placenta. Philadelphia: W B Saunders. 1978

4 Hustin J, Schaaps J P. Echographic and anatomic studies of the maternotrophoblastic border during the first trimester of pregnancy. Am J Obstet Gynecol 1987; 157: 162–168

5 Brossens I, Robertson W B, Dixon H G. The physiological response of the vessels of the placental bed to normal pregnancy. J Pathol Bacteriol 1967; 93: 569–579

6 Robertson W B, Khong M B, Brosens I, De Wolf F, Sheppard B L, Bonnar J. The placental bed biopsy: review from three European centers. Am J Obstet Gynecol 1986; 155: 401–412

7 Ramsey E M, Donner N W. Placental vasculature and circulation. Stuttgart: Georg Thieme. 1980

8 Grannum P A T, Berkowitz R L, Hobbins J C. The ultrasonic changes in the maturing placenta and their relation to fetal pulmonic maturity. Am J Obstet Gynecol 1979; 133: 915–922

9 Harman C R, Manning F A, Stearns E, Morrison I. The correlation of ultrasonic placental grading and fetal pulmonary maturation in five hundred sixty-three pregnancies. Am J Obstet Gynecol 1982; 143: 941–943

10 Quinlan R W, Cruz A M, Buhi W C, Martin M. Changes in placental ultrasonic appearance. I. Incidence of grade III changes in the placenta in correlation to fetal pulmonary maturity. Am J Obstet Gynecol 1982; 144: 468–470

11 Quinland R W, Cruz A M, Buhi W C, Martin M. Changes in placental ultrasonic appearance. II. Pathologic significance of Grade III placental changes. Am J Obstet Gynecol 1982; 142: 110–111

12 Gast M G, Ott W. Failure of ultrasonic placental grading to predict severe respiratory distress in a neonate. Am J Obstet Gynecol 1983; 146: 464–465

13 Hills D, Irwin G A L, Tuck S, Baim R. Distribution of placental grades in high-risk gravidas. AJR 1984; 143: 1011–1013

14 Proud J, Grant A M. Third trimester placental grading by ultrasonography as a test of fetal wellbeing. BMJ 1987; 294: 1641–1644

15 Ohel G, Granat M, Zeevi D, et al. Advanced ultrasonic placental maturation in twin pregnancies. Am J Obstet Gynecol 1987; 156: 76–78

16 Donald I. On launching a new diagnostic science. Am J Obstet Gynecol 1968; 103: 609–628

17 Campbell S, Kohorn E I. Placental localization by ultrasonic compound scanning. J Obstet Gynaecol Br Cwlth 1968; 75: 1007–1013

18 Gottesfeld K R, Thompson H E, Holmes J H, Taylor E S. Ultrasonic placentography: A new method for placental localization. Am J Obstet Gynecol 1966; 96: 539–547

19 Donald I, Abdulla U. Placentography by sonar. J Obstet Gynaecol Br Cwlth 1968; 75: 993–1006

20 Dippel A L, Brown W H. Roentgen visualization of the placenta by soft tissue technique. Am J Obstet Gynecol 1940; 40: 986–994

21 Kohorn E I, Walker R H S, Morrison J, Campbell S. Placental localization: a comparison between ultrasonic compound B scanning and radioisotope scanning. Am J Obstet Gynecol 1969; 103: 868–877

22 McShane P M, Heyl P S, Epstein M F. Maternal and perinatal morbidity resulting from placenta praevia. Obstet Gynecol 1985; 65: 176–182

23 Clark S T, Koonings P P, Phelan J P. Placenta previa/accreta and prior cesarean section. Obstet Gynecol 1985; 66: 89–92

24 Rizos N, Doran T A, Miskin M, Benzie B J, Ford J A. Natural history of placenta praevia ascertained by diagnostic ultrasound. Am J Obstet Gynecol 1979; 133: 287–291

25 Kurjak A, Borsic B. Changes of placental site diagnosed by repeat ultrasonic examination. Acta Obstet Gynecol Scand 1977; 56: 161–165

26 Andersen S, Steinke N M S. The clinical significance of asymptomatic mid-trimester low placentation diagnosed by ultrasound. Acta Obstet Gynecol Scand 1988; 67: 339–341

27 Farine D, Fox H E, Jakobson S, Timor-Tritsch I E. Is it really placenta previa? Eur J Obstet Gynecol Reprod Biol 1989; 31: 103–108

28 Grannum P A. Ultrasound examination of the placenta. Clin Obstet Gynecol 1983; 10: 459–473

29 Jauniaux E, Moscoso G, Campbell S, Gibb D, Driver M, Nicolaides K H. Correlation of ultrasound and pathologic findings of placental anomalies in pregnancies with elevated maternal serum alpha-fetoprotein. Eur J Obstet Gynecol Reprod Biol 1990: in press

30 Bleker O P, Kloosterman G J, Breur W, Mieras D J. The volumetric growth of the human placenta: a longitudinal ultrasonic study. Am J Obstet Gynecol 1977; 127: 657–661

31 Geirsson R T, Ogston S A, Patel N B, Christie A D. Growth of the total intra-uterine, intramniotic and placental volume in normal singleton pregnancy measured by ultrasound. Br J Obstet Gynaecol 1985; 92: 46–53

32 Wolf H, Oosting H, Treffers P E. Second-trimester placental volume measurements by ultrasound: prediction of fetal outcome. Am J Obstet Gynecol 1989; 160: 121–126

33 Wolf H, Oosting H, Treffers P E. A longitudinal study of the relationship between placental and fetal growth as measured by ultrasonography. Am J Obstet Gynecol 1989; 161: 1140–1145

34 Jauniaux E, Avni F E, Donner C, Rodesch F, Wilkin P. Ultrasonographic diagnosis and morphological study of placentas circumvallate. JCU 1989; 16: 126–131

35 Hurley V A, Beischer N A. Placenta membranacea. Case reports. Br J Obstet Gynaecol 1987; 94: 798–802

36 Molloy C E, McDowell W, Armour T, Crawford W, Bernstine R. Ultrasound diagnosis of placenta membranacea in utero. J Ultrasound Med 1983; 2: 377–379

37 Cox S M, Carpenter R J, Cotton D B. Placenta percreta: ultrasound diagnosis and conservative surgical management. Obstet Gynecol 1988; 71: 454–456

38 Hoogland H J. The ultrasound display of intervillous circulation. Placenta 1987; 8: 537–544

39 Vermeulen R C W, Lambalk N B, Exalto N, Arts N F T. An anatomic basis for ultrasound images of the human placenta. Am J Obstet Gynecol 1985; 153: 806–810

40 Cooperberg P L, Wright V J, Carpenter C W. Ultrasonographic demonstration of a placental maternal lake. JCU 1979; 7: 62–64

41 Jauniaux E, Avni F E, Elkazen N, Wilkin P, Hustin J. Etude morphologique des anomalies placentaires echographiques de la deuxieme moitie de la gestation. J Gynecol Obstet Biol Reprod 1989; 18: 601–613

42 Fleischer A C, Kurtz A B, Wapner R J, et al. Elevated alpha-fetoprotein and a normal fetal sonogram: association with placental abnormalities. AJR 1988; 150: 881–883

43 Haney A F, Trought W S. The sonolucent placenta in high-risk obstetrics. Obstet Gynecol 1980; 55: 38–41

44 Kaplan C, Blanc W A, Elias J. Identification of erythrocytes in intervillous thrombi: a study using Immunoperoxidase identification of hemoglobin. Hum Pathol 1982; 13: 554–557

45 Hoogland H J, De Haan J, Vooys J. Ultrasonographic diagnosis of intervillous thrombosis related to RH isoimmunization. Gynecol Obstet Invest 1979; 10: 237–245

46 Spirt B A, Gordon L P, Kagan E H. Intervillous thrombosis: sonographic and pathologic correlation. Radiology 1983; 147: 197–200

47 Olah K S, Gee H, Rushton I, Fowlie A. Massive subchorionic thrombohaematoma presenting as a placental tumour: case report. Br J Obstet Gynaecol 1987; 94: 995–997

48 Jauniaux E, Campbell S. Antenatal diagnosis of placental infarcts by ultrasound. JCU 1990; in press

49 Kirkinen P, Jouppila P. Intrauterine membranous cyst: a report of antenatal diagnosis and obstetrics aspects in two cases. Obstet Gynecol 1986; 67: 26–30

50 Sholl J S. Abruptio placentae: clinical management in nonacute cases. Am J Obstet Gynecol 1987; 156: 40–51

51 Fantel A G, Shepart T H. Basic aspects of early abortion. In: Iffy L, Kaminetzky H A. eds. Principles and practices of obstetrics and perinatology. Vol 1. New York: Wiley. 1981: p 533–563

52 Abu-Yousef M M, Bleicher J J, Williamson R A, Weiner C P. Subchorionic hemorrhage: sonographic diagnosis and clinical significance. AJR 1987; 149: 737–740

53 Nyberg D A, Cyr D R, Mack L A, Wilson D A, Shuman W P. Sonographic spectrum of placental abruption. AJR 1987; 148: 161–164

54 Sauerbrei E E, Pham D H. Placental abruption and subchorionic hemorrhage in the first half of pregnancy: US appearance and clinical outcome. Radiology 1986; 160: 190–195

55 Mandruzzato G P, D'Ottavio G, Rustico M A, Fonatana A, Bogatti P. The intrauterine hematoma: diagnostic and clinical aspects. JCU 1989; 17: 503–510

56 Howell R J G. Haemorrhage from the placental site. Clin Obstet Gynecol 1986; 13: 633–658

57 Berkowitz R, Ozturk M, Goldstein D, Bernstein M, Hill L, Wands J R. Human chorionic gonadotropin and free subunits' serum levels in patients with partial and complete hydatidiform moles. Obstet Gynecol 1989; 74: 212–215

58 Czernobilsky B, Barash A, Lancet M. Partial moles: a clinicopathologic study of 25 cases. Obstet Gynecol 1982; 59: 75–77

59 Kajii T, Ohama K. Androgenic origin of hydatidiform mole. Nature 1977; 268: 633–634

60 Grudzinkas J G, Kitau M J, Clarke P C. Extra-fetal origin of alphafetoprotein. Lancet 1977; II: 1088

61 Fisher R A, Sheppard D M, Lawler S D. Twin pregnancy with complete hydatidiform mole (46,XX) and fetus (46,XY): genetic origin proved by analysis of chromosome polymorphism. BMJ 1982; 284: 1218–1219

62 Jauniaux E, de Lannoy E, Moscoso G, Campbell S. Diagnostic prenatal des pathologies molaires associees a un fetus: revue de la litterature a propos d'un cas. J Gynecol Obstet Biol Reprod 1990; 19: in press

63 Crooij M J, Van Der Harten J J, Puyenbroek J I, Van Geijn H P, Arts N F T. A partial hydatidiform mole, dispersed throughout the placenta, coexisting with a normal living fetus: a case report. Br J Obstet Gynaecol 1985; 92: 104–106

64 Feinberg R F, Lockwood C J, Salafia C, Hobbins J C. Sonographic diagnosis of a pregnancy with a diffuse hydatidiform mole and coexistent 46,XX fetus: a case report. Obstet Gynecol 1988; 72: 485–488

65 Szulman A E, Philippe E, Boue J G, Boue A. Human triploidy: association with partial hydatidiform moles and nonmolar conceptuses. Hum Pathol 1981; 12: 1016–1021

66 Doshi N, Surti U, Szulman A E. Morphologic anomalies in triploid liveborn fetuses. Hum Pathol 1983; 14: 716–723

67 Lockwood C, Scioscia M, Stiller R, Hobbins J C. Sonographic features of the triploid fetus. Am J Obstet Gynecol 1987; 157: 285–287

68 Graham J M, Rawnsley E F, Millard Simmons G, et al. Triploidy: pregnancy complications and clinical findings in seven cases. Prenat Diagn 1989; 9: 409–419

69 Naumoff P, Szulman A E, Weinstein B, Mayer J, Surti U. Ultrasonography of partial hydatidiform mole. Radiology 1981; 140: 467–470

70 Rubenstein J B, Swayne L C, Dise C A, Gersen S L, Schwartz J R, Risk A. Placental changes in fetal triploidy syndrome. J Ultrasound Med 1986; 5: 545–550

71 Freeman S B, Priest J H, Macmahon W C, Fernhoff P M, Elsas L J. Prenatal ascertainment of triploidy by maternal serum alpha-fetoprotein screening. Prenat Diagn 1989; 9: 339–347

72 Fine C, Bundy A L, Berkowitz R S, Boswell S B, Berezin A F, Doubilet P M. Sonographic diagnosis of partial hydatidiform mole. Obstet Gynecol 1989; 73: 414–418

73 Jauniaux E, Zucker M, Meuris S, Verhest A, Wilkin P, Hustin J. Chorangiocarcinoma: an unusual tumour of the placenta. The missing link? Placenta 1988; 9: 607–614

74 Spirt B A, Gordon L, Cohen W N, Yambao T. Antenatal diagnosis of chorioangioma of the placenta. AJR 1980; 135: 1273–1275

75 O'Malley B P, Toi A, deSa D J, Williams G L. Ultrasound appearances of placental chorioangioma. Radiology 1981; 138: 159–160

76 Willard D A, Moeschler J B. Placenta chorioangioma: a rare cause of elevated amniotic fluid alpha-fetoprotein. J Ultrasound Med 1986; 5: 221–222

77 Campbell W A, Storlazzi E, Vintzileos A M, Wu A, Schneiderman H, Nochimson D J. Fetal malignant melanoma: ultrasound presentation and review of the literature. Obstet Gynecol 1987; 70: 434–439

78 Romero R, Pilu G, Jeanty P, Ghidini A, Hobbins J C. Prenatal diagnosis of congenital anomalies. Norwalk, Connecticut: Appleton and Lange. 1988: p 385–402

79 Jauniaux E, De Munter C, Pardou A, Elkhazen N, Rodesch F, Wilkin P. Evaluation echographique du sydrome de l'artere ombilicale unique: une serie de 80 cas. J Gynecol Obstet Biol Reprod 1989; 18: 341–348

80 Heifetz S A. Single umbilical artery: a statistical analysis of 37 autopsy cases and review of the literature. Perspect Pediatr Pathol 1984; 8: 345–378

81 Herrmann U J, Sidiropoulos D. Single umbilical artery: prenatal findings. Prenat Diagn 1988; 8: 275–280

82 Jauniaux E, Campbell S, Vyas S. The use of color Doppler imaging for prenatal diagnosis of umbilical cord anomalies: report of three cases. Am J Obstet Gynecol 1989; 161: 1195–1197

83 Jauniaux E, De Munter C, Vanesse M, Hustin J, Wilkin P. Embryonic remnants of the umbilical cord: morphological and clinical aspects. Hum Pathol 1989; 20: 458–462

84 Fink I J, Filly R A. Omphalocele associated with umbilical cord allantoic cyst: sonographic evaluation in utero. Radiology 1983; 149: 473–475

85 Renade R V, Nipladkar K B, Mtsorekar V R. Extraumbilical allantoic cyst: a case report. Indian J Pathol Bacteriol 1960; 9: 87–89

86 Heifetz S A, Rueda-Pedraza M E. Omphalomesenteric duct cysts of the umbilical cord. Pediatr Pathol 1983; 1: 325–335

87 Heifetz S A, Rueda-Pedraya M E. Hemangiomas of the umbilical cord. Pediatr Pathol 1983; 1: 385–393

88 Barson A J, Donnai P, Ferguson A, Donnai D, Read A P. Haemangioma of the cord: further cause of raised maternal serum and liquor alpha-fetoprotein. BMJ 1980; 281: 1252

89 Seifer D B, Ferguson J E, Behrens C M, Zemel S, Stevenson D K, Ross J C. Nonimmune hydrops fetalis in association with hemangioma of the umbilical cord. Obstet Gynecol 1985; 66: 283–286

90 Baylis M S, Jones R Y, Hughes M. Angiomyxoma of the umbilical cord detected antenatally by ultrasound. J Obstet Gynecol 1984; 4: 243–244

91 Mishriki Y Y, Vanyshelbaum Y, Epstein H, Blanc W. Hemangioma of the umbilical cord. Pediatr Pathol 1987; 7: 43–49

92 Resta R G, Luthy D A, Mahony B S. Umbilical cord hemangioma associated with extremely high alpha-fetoprotein levels. Obstet Gynecol 1988; 72: 488–490

93 Jauniaux E, Moscoso G, Chitty L, Gibb D, Driver M, Campbell S. An angiomyxoma involving the whole length of the umbilical cord: prenatal diagnosis by ultrasonography. J Ultrasound Med 1990; in press

94 Barry F L, McCoy, Callahan W P. Haemangioma of the umbilical cord. Am J Obstet Gynecol 1951; 62: 675–680

95 Coulter J B S, Scott J M, Jordan M M. Oedema of the umbilical cord and respiratory distress in the newborn. Br J Obstet Gynaecol 1975; 82: 453–459

96 Jauniaux E, Donner C, Thomas C, Francotte J, Rodesch F, Avni E. Umbilical cord pseudocyst in trisomy 18. Prenat Diagn 1988; 8: 557–563

97 Schreier R, Brown S. Hematoma of the umbilical cord. Obstet Gynecol 1962; 20: 798–800

98 Ruvinsky E D, Wiley T L, Morrison J C, Blake P G. In utero diagnosis of umbilical cord hematoma by ultrasonography. Am J Obstet Gynecol 1981; 140: 833–834

99 Moise K J, Carpenter R J, Huhta J C, Deter R L. Umbilical cord hematoma secondary to in utero intravascular transfusion for RH isoimmunisation. Fetal Ther 1987; 2: 65–70

100 Sutro W H, Tuck S M, Loesevitz A, Novotny P L, Archbald F, Irwin G L A. Prenatal observation of umbilical cord hematoma. AJR 1984; 142: 801–802

101 Jauniaux E, Donner C, Simon P, Vanesse M, Hustin J, Rodesch F. Pathologic aspects of the umbilical cord after percutaneous umbilical blood sampling. Obstet Gynecol 1989; 73: 215–218

102 Gassner C B, Paul R H. Laceration of umbilical cord vessels secondary to amniocentesis. Obstet Gynecol 1976; 48: 627–630

103 Romero R, Chervenak F A, Coustan D, Berkowitz R L, Hobbins J C. Antenatal sonographic diagnosis of umbilical cord laceration. Am J Obstet Gynecol 1982; 143: 719–720

104 Daffos F, Capella-Paviosky M, Forestier F. Fetal sampling during pregnancy with use of a needle guided by ultrasound: a study of 606 consecutive cases. Am J Obstet Gynecol 1985; 153: 655–660

105 Hogge W A, Thiagarajah S, Brenbridge A N, Harbert G M. Fetal evaluation by percutaneous blood sampling. Am J Obstet Gynecol 1988; 158: 132–136

106 Pielet B W, Socol M L, MacGregor S N, Ney J A, Dooley S L. Cordocentesis: an appraisal of risks. Am J Obstet Gynecol 1988; 159: 1497–1500

107 Heifetz S A. Thrombosis of the umbilical cord: analysis of 52 cases and literature review. Pediatr Pathol 1988; 8: 37–54

108 Abrams S L, Callen P W, Filly R A. Umbilical vein thrombosis: sonographic detection in utero. J Ultrasound Med 1985; 4: 283–285

109 Jauniaux E, Englert Y, Vanesse M, Hidden M, Wilkin P. Pathologic features of placentas from singleton pregnancies obtained by in vitro fertilization and embryo transfer. Obstet Gynecol 1990, in press

110 Gianopoulos J, Carver T, Tomich P G, Kalman R, Gadwood K. Diagnosis of vasa previa with ultrasonography. Obstet Gynecol 1987; 69: 488–491

111 Mills J L, Harley E E, Moessinger A C. Standards for measuring umbilical cord length. Placenta 1983; 4: 423–426

112 Grange D K, Arya S, Opitz J M, Laxova R, Herrmann J, Gilbert E F. The short umbilical cord. Birth defects 1987; 23: 191–214

113 Jauniaux E, Vyas S, Finlayson C, Moscoso G, Driver M, Campbell S. Early sonographic diagnosis of body stalk anomaly. Prenat Diagn 1990; 10: 127–132

114 Pritchard J A, MacDonald P C, Gant N F. Williams Obstetrics, 17th ed. New York: Appleton-Century-Crofts. 1985

115 Hales E D, Westney L S. Sonography of occult cord prolapse. JCU 1984; 12: 283–285

116 Johnson R L, Anderson J C, Irsik R D, Goodlin R C. Duplex ultrasound diagnosis of umbilical cord prolapse. JCU 1987; 15: 282–284

117 Chasnoff I J, Fletcher M A. True knot of the cord. Am J Obstet Gynecol 1977; 127: 425–427

Interventional procedures

Janet I. Vaughan and Charles H. Rodeck

INTRODUCTION

Reduction in perinatal mortality and long-term morbidity remains a challenge in modern obstetrics. Ultrasound imaging has enabled ready visualisation of the conceptus and has a unique potential for diagnosis of fetal problems so that management policies can be suitably altered. In addition, more subtle diagnoses may be achieved by an extensive range of invasive procedures, all ultrasound guided, which will be reviewed in this chapter. Although currently limited, the future use and scope of intra-uterine therapy is an exciting field of medicine which will be evaluated.

Counselling

All patients undergoing invasive antenatal procedures should have detailed counselling to inform them about the fetal disorder under consideration, the procedure involved for diagnosis or therapy, the risks and the management options. Ideally, this should be undertaken before pregnancy so that the parents can assess the facts objectively without threat to their current pregnancy. This is often not the case, particularly if the problem has only arisen in the pregnancy. Whatever the situation, counselling must still be optimal and should be given at a time and place separate to that of the procedure. More than one session may be required as the couple should have the opportunity to consider the issues before deciding on their management plan, which may be not to have any procedure at all. Obstetricians are responsible for ensuring that their patients are adequately informed and, if performing the counselling themselves, must be certain that the information given is accurate, current and non-directional. The skills of a geneticist or fetal medicine specialist will often be required as the diagnostic and therapeutic options are continually expanding.

Diagnostic procedures

Chorionic villus sampling

Background Chorionic villus sampling (CVS) has only been introduced clinically within the last decade. However, the concept of diagnostic placental biopsy for first trimester prenatal diagnosis was introduced in 1968 by Hahnemann and Mohr using trans-cervical endoscopy prior to termination of pregnancy.[1] Delayed termination revealed a high complication rate, mainly due to rupture of the amniotic sac and infection, but villi were obtained in 60% of the cases.[2] The success rate of chromosome analysis in these early attempts was low as difficulties were encountered with culturing the tissue.[3] The effect of these disappointing results combined with the information that early second trimester amniocentesis was safe and reliable, inhibited further progress in CVS.

Interest in the West was only rekindled after a report from the Tietung Hospital of the Anshan Iron and Steel Co; China in 1975 described the successful use of 'blind' trans-cervical needle aspiration of chorionic villi in 100 pregnancies.[4] The aim was to sex fetuses by chromatin analyses. This was achieved with a 94% success rate and of the pregnancies that were allowed to continue after CVS only 6% miscarried. There were no maternal, fetal or neonatal complications.

Additional motivation to develop a successful CVS technique followed advances in laboratory techniques for tissue analysis, in particular, the demonstration that villi could be used for gene analysis using recombinant DNA technology.[5] Williamson et al performed accurate globin gene hybridisation with DNA extracted from chorionic villi at termination of pregnancy in 1981. At the same time Niazi et al[6] described successful fetal karyotyping from pure mesenchymal trophoblast cell cultures also obtained at termination (Fig. 1). A year later control studies on enzyme activity in chorionic tissue confirmed the potential for first trimester detection of metabolic storage disorders.[7] An important advance was a direct cytogenetic analysis on spontaneous mitotic figures in the cytotrophoblast enabling rapid results in the first trimester (Fig. 1).[8]

Until 1980 the techniques that had been used for CVS included 'blind' aspiration,[4] endoscopic direct vision biopsy[1-3] and intra-uterine lavage.[9,10] In 1980, Kazy and Stigar from Moscow[11] reported 18 termination patients in whom flexible biopsy forceps were used in conjunction with continuous real time ultrasound guidance. This was

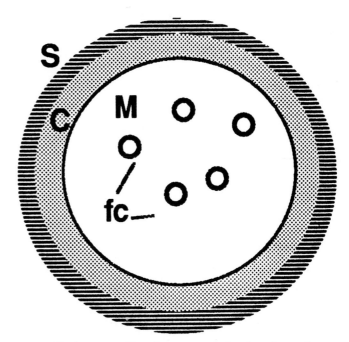

Fig. 1 Tertiary stem villus. A transverse section through a tertiary stem villus. M – mesenchymal core with fetal capillaries (fc), C – cytotrophoblast, S – syncytiotrophoblast.

the first reported series with a 100% success rate. In 1982, the same group used ultrasound guided trans-cervical methods to publish a larger series including the first diagnostic CVS series for genetic disease.[7] Subsequently diagnostic series were published for the haemoglobinopathies from England,[12] chromosomal and metabolic disorders from Italy[8] and sickle-cell disease from France.[13] All these groups used ultrasound guided trans-cervical methods which have become the most widely used.[13–15] Blind aspiration was shown to be unreliable[16,17] and endoscopy too complicated.[18]

Transabdominal sampling of the placenta was originally performed by Alvarez[19] to diagnose hydatidiform mole in 10 to 14 week pregnancies. Transabdominal CVS was introduced by the Scandinavians[20] in 1984 to reduce the risk of infection and avoid the relative technical contra-indications of trans-cervical CVS. It is becoming increasingly popular, both on its own and as a complimentary procedure to trans-cervical CVS.

A registry to collate data was initiated in 1983 under the auspices of Laird Jackson at Thomas Jefferson University in Philadelphia, USA. It is funded by the World Health Organisation and communicates through the 'Chorionic Villus Sampling Newsletter'. There are now over 57 000 cases recorded from 174 centres world-wide.[21] Criticism over the introduction of a new prenatal diagnostic technique prior to adequate assessment of risks, led to three multicentre randomised controlled trials being set up in the United Kingdom and North America.

Technique Ultrasonography is an integral part of the CVS technique. Real time sector scanners are the most useful because they give the best view of the pelvic organs. A preliminary scan should be performed to determine fetal viability, gestational age and the number of gestation sacs. Multiple pregnancy complicates CVS as there is an increased risk of abortion and a possibility that the chorion sampled does not represent each fetus. A routine scan for uterine, adnexal and pelvic pathology should be included.

Immediately prior to CVS a scan is performed to confirm the findings, to locate the placental site and assess the best route by which to perform the CVS. The chorion frondosum or definitive placenta is seen as the thickest region of endometrium surrounding the gestation sac and the insertion of the umbilical cord is usually visible after 9 weeks (Fig. 2). Early in the first trimester the placental site may be obscured by extraplacental villi which have not yet regressed to form the chorion laeve. The position of the uterus in the pelvis and in relation to the cervix has a profound effect on the success of CVS and can be manipulated to a certain extent by bladder filling and the use of a tenaculum. Fibroids may make CVS difficult and uterine contractions may alter the intra-uterine topography causing transient difficulties.

The trans-cervical procedure is guided throughout by real time ultrasound as 'blind' aspiration has an unaccept-

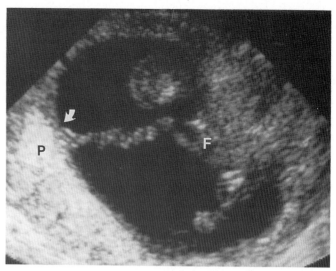

Fig. 2 Ultrasound scan of a 10 week pregnancy. The arrow shows the cord inserting into the definitive placenta (P). F – fetus.

able failure rate. This may be achieved by a single-operator technique[15] in which the sonographer guides the sampling instrument to the placenta; alternatively, an independent sonographer may assist. The biopsy instrument is identified in the cervical canal as a pair of bright lines and is guided from the internal os to the optimal placental site (Fig. 3). The position of the tip should be confirmed in both longitudinal and transverse planes prior to biopsy.

The transabdominal sampling is also performed under continual ultrasound surveillance. After locating the placenta the alignment is optimised by regulating the bladder volume. The sampling needle should be parallel to the chorionic plate once in the placental tissue (Fig. 4). Needle

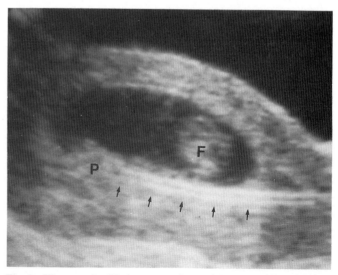

Fig. 3 Ultrasound guided trans-cervical CVS showing an aspiration cannula as a pair of bright lines (arrows). P – placenta, F – fetus.

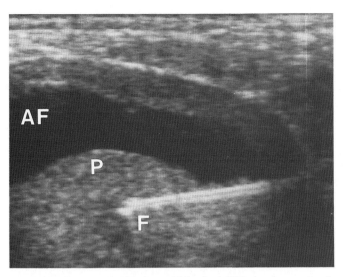

Fig. 4 **An ultrasound guided transabdominal CVS** showing a pair of biopsy forceps (F) as bright lines within the placenta (P). AF – amniotic fluid.

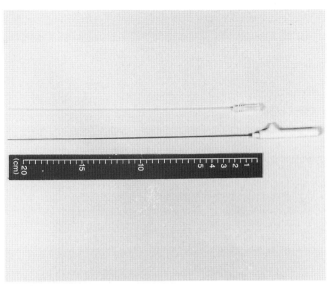

Fig. 5 'Trophocan' aspirating cannula, Portex Ltd.

guidance may be achieved either by a free-hand technique or by means of a needle guide system.

Following the CVS, real time ultrasound is used to check the fetal heart beat and to assess complications such as haematoma or amniotic sac rupture. A follow up scan is advisable to assess subsequent fetal development.

CVS is an outpatient technique, usually performed in the ultrasound department. Local anaesthetic or sedation are not usually required. Standard aseptic precautions are used and the patient is draped, but full gowning is not necessary. Prophylactic antibiotics are not needed. In the past, immediate microscopy was considered essential to distinguish villi from decidua and to assess its quantity and quality. With experience this is no longer found to be necessary. At present, it is not clear which method is optimal and much depends on operator preference and experience. Several of the most commonly used methods will be considered here; adequate samples can be obtained with any method in almost all cases.

Techniques of chorionic villous biopsy currently in use
Ultrasound guided trans-cervical
    a) aspirating cannula – plastic
                         – metal
    b) biopsy forceps

Ultrasound guided transabdominal
    c) aspirating cannula – double system
                          – single system
    d) biopsy forceps

a) Trans-cervical aspiration This method remains the most popular and is based on the 'blind' aspiration technique of the Chinese. It was originally described using the

Portex catheter (Fig. 5, Portex Ltd, England),[12] although a multitude of different catheters are now used.

The patient is positioned comfortably on a colposcopy chair, or if necessary in the lithotomy position on an operating table. Partners are encouraged to attend. The vulva and vagina are cleaned with an antiseptic solution and a speculum inserted to expose the cervix. An endocervical swab may be taken to exclude infection. CVS should be postponed until a florid infection has been treated. The cervical os is then meticulously cleaned. Prior to inserting the catheter it is not necessary to apply a tenaculum unless this is going to improve the access.

The majority of centres use a Portex catheter which is made of soft polyethylene and is disposable. It is 1.5 mm in external diameter with an overall length of 21 cm. An aluminium obturator enables it to be bent to the optimal shape depending on the relationship of the cervix, uterus and placental site. On correct placement, half way between the chorionic plate and decidua (Fig. 3) the obturator is removed and a 20 ml syringe containing some 3 to 5 ml heparinised culture medium attached. Suction is applied as the catheter is moved backwards and forwards ('hoovering') and slowly withdrawn. The contents of the catheter and syringe are then flushed into a Petrie dish for inspection. More than three catheter insertions at a single session increases the fetal miscarriage risk and the patient should be re-scheduled if this is necessary.

The most widely used metal catheter is that devised for single operator use (Fig. 6).[15] This is a 16 gauge malleable silver cannula which is 23 cm long and is reusable (Downs Surgical Ltd). It has an obturator to prevent decidual 'coring' and a suction control valve on the finger plate. After appropriate shaping the catheter is guided to the pla-

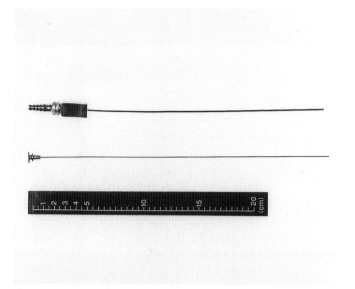

Fig. 6 **'KCH' CVS cannula**, Down's Surgical Ltd.

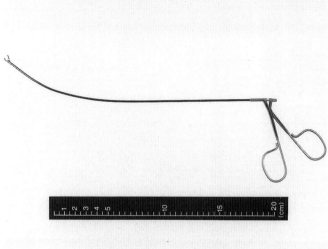

Fig. 7 **Transcervical biopsy forceps**, RM Surgical Developments.

centa with one hand whilst holding the transducer in the other. Once in position, the obturator is removed and villi are obtained by aspirating with a suction pump. Continuous ultrasound monitoring is maintained throughout.

b) Trans-cervical biopsy Kazy et al[7] in 1982 were the first to use biopsy forceps introduced through the cervix. They have been promoted by Dumez and his co-workers in France.[13] They use rigid straight metal forceps 2 mm in diameter, 20 cm in length with a cupped jaw (Storz Ref. 8591A). This system is simple to use, does not rely on aspiration and is suitable for a single operator. The tip is smooth when closed. Once in the placental substance, the jaws are opened, advanced, closed and the forceps withdrawn. Specimens largely uncontaminated with decidua or blood are reliably collected. Concerns about amniotic sac puncture have proved groundless. Other biopsy forceps have been introduced such as those used by Rodeck (Fig. 7). This has a curved shank and alligator jaws and does not require a tenaculum for use.

c) Transabdominal aspiration Original publications reported a double needle system[20,22] consisting of a co-axial 18 gauge guide cannula with a stylet and an inner 20 to 22 gauge aspirating cannula which is about 1.5 cm longer than the guide. It is important to use a very sharp pointed needle to penetrate the skin, rectus sheath and uterus with ease.

The patient is placed supine and her abdomen cleaned with an antiseptic solution. Using a sterile ultrasound technique, the needle guide with stylet is advanced so that the tip is just visible within the chorion frondosum. The stylet is then replaced with the aspirating needle and a 20 ml syringe attached to aspirate the villi in much the same way as is done trans-cervically. The inner needle is then with-

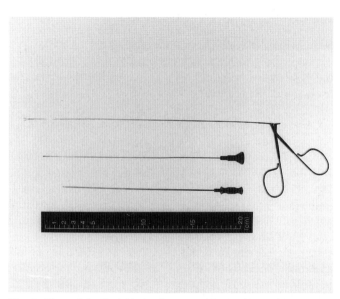

Fig. 8 **Transabdominal biopsy forceps** with the trocar and cannula used for insertion. (RM Surgical Developments).

drawn and the sample inspected after flushing into a Petrie dish. Additional tissue is collected if necessary. This is achieved simply by reinserting the inner needle and aspirating again. More recently, a simple 20 G spinal needle has been used.

d) Transabdominal biopsy A co-axial biopsy forceps system has also been devised[23] (Fig. 8). The technique is similar to that described, except that aspiration is avoided and clean samples are obtained.

Timing The optimal time to perform trans-cervical CVS is between 9 and 11 weeks' gestation. Before 9 weeks the definitive chorion frondosum may not be formed. In theory this may increase the chances of successful biopsy, but if degenerating villi are sampled no result may be obtained. At this stage there is a higher incidence of anembryonic pregnancies, which render CVS unnecessary, and spontaneous miscarriages which increase the apparent procedure-related miscarriage rate. Hogge et al describes an 11.8% fetal loss rate when CVS was performed prior to 9 weeks compared to a 3.5% loss rate at 9 to 11 weeks.[24] The percentage of unbalanced karyotypes found prior to 9 weeks is more than double that found at 9 to 11 weeks, which may account for some of this discrepancy.[25] After 12 weeks the increased uterine size may make the procedure difficult as the placenta may be out of reach.

One of the potential advantages of the transabdominal technique is that of a wider gestational age 'window'. The earliest practical time for sampling is 10 weeks but the method can be used until term, particularly for rapid fetal karyotyping.[26]

Experience Experience with CVS improves the success rate for obtaining samples and decreases the fetal loss rate. The learning curves for TC and TA are comparable,[27,28] with the maximum sampling success rate being achieved after 50 to 100 cases. Failure to obtain a satisfactory TC sample should then only occur in less than 2% of patients[29] and about 0.5% in TA CVS.[30] The ultrasonographer's experience seems most critical for success with TC CVS, whilst using a double needle guide system for TA enables multiple passes until an adequate sample is obtained. This basic difference in technique is probably the main reason for the faster learning curve for TA CVS suggested by Rosevear.[31] A flexible approach using the technique most appropriate to the clinical situation will achieve a 100% success rate[28] and performing at least 10 procedures a month will maintain the skill.[27]

Similarly, the fetal loss rate varies with experience. The average loss rate in 14 centres with less than 50 TC procedures is 7.3%, compared with a rate of 3.1% in the 8 centres with over 1000 cases (Table 1). The abortion rate after TC CVS is maintained at its lowest level only after 300 cases.[27] Fetal loss rate after TA CVS also declines with experience.[31]

Table 1 Fetal loss rates in centres with different experience[22]

	centres	cases	% fetal loss
> 1000 TC CVB	8	20 940	3.1
< 50 TC CVB	14	454	7.3

Indications The indications for CVS are:

— fetal karyotype
— inborn errors of metabolism
— DNA analysis
— fetal infection
— fetal blood group determination.

Chromosomes CVS is used for fetal karyotyping in the following situations:
investigation of aneuploidy in association with increasing maternal age;
the birth of a previous child with a non-disjunctional chromosomal abnormality;
a parental carrier for a balanced chromosomal translocation;
maternal carriers of X-linked disorders.

Of the cases reported to the collaborative cytogenetic study of CVS (Table 2), 75% were for advanced maternal age, 11.7% for a previous child with a non-inherited chromosome abnormality and 2.3% for parental rearrangements.[32] The high-risk group of X-linked disorders accounted for 5%, but in the future an increasing number of these conditions can be expected to be diagnosed specifically using DNA techniques. Structural abnormalities detected on ultrasound scanning have a high incidence of chromosomal abnormality and may be investigated by second and third trimester TA CVS in centres where fetal blood sampling is not available.[26]

Table 2 Results of chromosome analysis performed at chorionic villous biopsy[32]

Indication	% Total	(n)	% Abnormal	(n)
advanced maternal age	75.1	(5360)	4.3	(230)
prev. affected child	11.7	(835)	2.1	(18)
X-linked disease	5.0	(358)	33.8	(121)
parental rearrangement	2.3	(163)	30.7	(50)
other	5.9	(417)	1.6	(7)
	100		5.97	

Karyotyping can be performed on direct preparations or after tissue culture. For all methods it is essential that villi are meticulously cleaned of maternal cells.

a) The direct method depends on spontaneous mitoses in the Langerhans cells of cytotrophoblast layer of the tertiary stem villi (Fig. 1).[8] The advantages include rapid results (1 to 2 days), the avoidance of maternal cell overgrowth and bacterial infection. However, the accuracy of the results are jeopardised by too few good metaphase spreads and the poor quality of banding. It is ideal for determining fetal karyotype in X-linked disorders.

b) The short-term tissue culture is based on the same principles as the direct method except that the villi are cultured for 12 to 24 hours,[33] improving the quality of the G-banded metaphases.

c) High resolution banding for the detection of deletion breakpoints, small translocations and other subtle abnormalities requires long-term tissue culture as the banding is of better quality. It is the mesenchymal cells of the villi (Fig. 1) that are used for culture.[6]

Many laboratories have not had sufficient success with direct preparations and use either culture alone or both

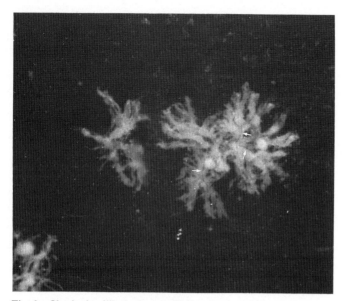

Fig. 9 Chorionic villi. Aspirated villi showing branching fronds with central fetal vessels (arrows).

methods in parallel. A minimum of 10 mg of villi is required for cytogenetic analysis. Villi with buds, sprouts and central vessels (Fig. 9) are said to contain more mitosis and are therefore most suitable for diagnosis.

The reliability of the cytogenetic results of CVS are crucial to its role as a first trimester diagnostic technique. Problems have arisen which are important in this regard and should be discussed when counselling patients.

a) Even in experienced laboratories failure to obtain a karyotype has been reported in 0.7% of direct preparations[34,35] and 1% to 3.2% of cultures.[24,35,36]

b) Maternal cell contamination is negligible in direct and short-term culture as there are no mitoses present in decidua. However, despite careful dissection, the risk of maternal cell contamination in long-term culture is about 12.5%.[35,37–41] This can be minimised by using Chang culture medium,[41] concurrent direct preparations and multiple cultures.

c) Discordance between chorionic villi and fetal karyotypes have been reported by several large studies[42–45] mostly using direct techniques. Pooling these results gives a frequency of discordance of 1.5% (n = 3812), which is 20-fold more than at amniocentesis.[46] The more common finding is that of a false positive result with a normal fetal karyotype and a mosaic placental karyotype. However, non-mosaic discordance has been reported with respect to trisomy 11, 16, 18, tetraploidy and monosomy X.[42,44,45,47] Mosaicism should be confirmed by amniocentesis before clinical decisions are made. Of more concern is the finding of a normal karyotype at CVS with an abnormal fetus (false negative), several cases of which have now been described with direct analysis,[35,45,48–52] the incidence being about one per 1000.[51]

d) Discordance between direct preparations and cultured villi are also reported. In the eight false negative cases above, all the long-term cultures correctly detected the fetal abnormality. This suggests that cultured cells more accurately represent the fetal karyotype. However, there have now been several reports of false negative long-term cultures which are discordant with both the direct preparation and the fetus.[35,53,54] The sensible approach to CVS for fetal karyotypes is to use both short- and long-term culture and to resort to amniocentesis if there is any discrepancy between them.

When advanced maternal age is the sole indication for performing first trimester CVS, the risk of detecting a chromosomal abnormality is significantly higher than at amniocentesis.[32,55] This would indicate the spontaneous loss of a number of chromosomally abnormal fetuses between weeks 9 to 11 and week 16.[56] Mosaicism comprises a quarter of these abnormalities and, although usually not present in the fetus, implies a much higher risk of spontaneous abortion.[24]

Inborn errors of metabolism (IEM) In 1986 there were 3900 human disorders known to be caused by a single gene defect.[57] The enzymal/protein defect has been identified in 44% of the recessive Mendelian conditions. This has important implications for first trimester prenatal diagnosis, as recessive conditions are usually severe with a one in four recurrence risk for parents with an affected child or known carrier status. Preconceptional screening for carrier detection is limited to populations in which there is a high incidence of a known enzyme or protein defect such as in Tay-Sachs disease amongst Ashkenazy Jews. The recurrence risk for dominant Mendelian conditions is one in two but there is usually variable expression and in only 4% has the defect been identified.

The first chorionic studies of enzymes known to be involved in inborn errors of metabolism were those of Kazy et al.[7] Subsequently, all enzyme deficiencies expressed in cultured amniotic fluid cells have been shown to be expressed in chorionic villi, but with the advantage that many results can be obtained without cell culture providing a result in 1 to 2 days. In most cases 5 to 10 mg of villi is adequate for diagnosis. It is imperative that the genetic and biochemical disorder, as well as the carrier status of the parents is confirmed before fetal diagnosis is undertaken.

Of 630 tested pregnancies 145 (23%) affected fetuses have been detected for over 40 conditions.[58] Misdiagnoses have been made in 1.6% but most would have been avoided with experience. For example, inadequate samples could have improved with cell culture and the presence of interfering isoenzymes could have been excluded.

DNA analysis DNA analysis was first used in the prenatal diagnosis of the haemoglobinopathies, with the diagnosis of sickle cell anaemia on amniotic cells.[59] Rapid advances in molecular genetics were a major stimulus to the development of CVS, but it was CVS in turn that really allowed DNA analysis for fetal diagnosis to evolve as more DNA can be extracted from villi than from amniotic fluid, 20 mg of villi yielding about 20 μg of DNA.

There are two basic approaches to DNA analysis. Firstly, if the genetic mutation causing the disease is known, fetal diagnosis may be made directly. Specific radioactive gene probes of cloned DNA search for the gene in the sampled DNA, once it has been cut up into small sequences by specific restriction endonucleases. Diseases caused by gene deletions, such as sickle cell anaemia,[13] can be diagnosed this way. Where a point mutation has been identified synthetic oligonucleotide probes may be used, as for α1-antitrypsin deficiency.[60]

Most diseases are heterogeneous and require linkage analysis using restriction fragment length polymorphisms (RFLPs). Even when the diagnostic gene is not known (for example, Duchenne muscular dystrophy), extra-genic probes can identify RFLPs in close proximity to the unknown gene. This involves extensive family studies, which unfortunately are not always informative. The risk of recombination during meiosis, which is higher the further away the RFLP is from the gene, can lead to misdiagnosis.[61]

The following conditions can currently be diagnosed by DNA analysis:

— α-thalassaemia
— β-thalassaemia
— sickle cell anaemia
— haemophilia A
— haemophilia B
— Huntington's disease
— myotonic dystrophy
— adult polycystic kidney disease
— cystic fibrosis
— α1-antitrypsin disease
— phenylketonuria
— congenital adrenal hyperplasia (21-hydroxylase deficiency)
— Duchenne muscular dystrophy.

Depending on the analytical method, 10 to 40 mg of villi are required. A result is usually available in 6 to 14 days. In 200 pregnancies investigated for haemoglobinopathies one misdiagnosis and one failed diagnosis occurred.[62] Misdiagnoses result from inadequate specimens, partial digestion, maternal tissue contamination, non-paternity, recombination and inadequate family studies.

Other Recently congenital rubella has been diagnosed in the first trimester by the detection of rubella antigen or ribonucleic acid sequences in chorionic villi. Monoclonal antibodies and a cloned complimentary DNA probe are used.[63]

Fetal blood grouping in the first trimester of pregnancy is now a diagnostic option in Rhesus and Kell alloimmunisation. Villi at 8 to 12 weeks' gestation contain enough fetal erythrocytes for red cell grouping either by micro-immunofluorescent or immunogold silver staining techniques.[64-66] Because fetomaternal haemorrhage resulting from the procedure can enhance the disease, this method of fetal grouping should be reserved for women with heterozygous partners and a history of severe disease, who would request termination of an antigenically positive fetus on the grounds that in utero treatment is likely to fail.[67]

Complications

Maternal Discomfort is minimal with TC CVS, although TA CVS may cause some pain. Abdominal cramping may occur up to 24 hours after either procedure. After TC CVS vaginal spotting occurs in 10% to 40% of cases, but rarely after TA CVS. Serious immediate post-CVS haemorrhage is rare and is not necessarily associated with fetal loss. Intra-uterine haematoma has been reported in 4.3% of patients, although with no serious consequences.[27]

Infection was a major deterrent to early TC CVS development.[3] Awareness of the problem has encouraged methodical aseptic techniques; subsequently infection has not been a major problem. Only two cases of serious maternal infection have been published.[68,69] In three published controlled trials comparing TC CVS with amniocentesis, there were no cases of maternal infection.[70-72] A potential advantage of the transabdominal technique is a reduction in infection.

Visceral trauma such as uterine perforation has not been reported with the trans-cervical route. Transabdominal uterine puncture should be atraumatic with the methods described but occasional bleeding and puncture of the bowel or bladder may occur with resultant peritonism in about 0.3%.[28]

Fetal The exact role of CVS in prenatal diagnosis has awaited the risks of fetal or neonatal complications derived from large multicentre randomised trials. The Canadian collaborative trial[70] is the only randomised study published to date and showed no significant difference in fetal loss rate between first trimester TC CVS and 16 week amniocentesis (Table 3). However, there was an unexplained trend towards fetal loss after 28 weeks in the CVS group.

The large United States (US) trial from the National Institute of Child Health and Human Development (NICHD)[71] was not randomised and had some difficulty recruiting amniocentesis controls of comparable maternal and gestational ages. However, they also reported no significant difference in fetal loss rates between the two procedures (Table 3). It must be remembered that amniocentesis itself has an inherent risk and in both the above trials the rate of fetal loss for CVS is above that for amniocentesis, so there is a suggestion that CVS does have an increased risk.

Table 3 Total fetal loss rate* (%) in chorionic villous sampling compared to amniocentesis

	CVS	amniocentesis
Canadian collaborative trial	7.6	7.0
NICHD	7.0	5.6

* includes termination of pregnancy

Recent data from 2058 late CVS cases indicate a 2% fetal loss in low-risk cases and 10% in those with ultrasound abnormalities.[73]

The fetal loss rate at CVS varies with several factors.

a) Operator experience (already discussed).

b) Sampling technique. Apart from direct vision biopsy, the type of instrument used has not been shown to alter significantly the fetal loss rate in TC CVS. Increasing the number of catheter insertions is dangerous and the NICHD[71] documented the loss of a chromosomally normal fetus in 10.8% with three to four attempts compared to 2.9% with one insertion. The transabdominal method is claimed to be a safer technique and preliminary results of a randomised trial of TA, TC and amniocentesis show respective loss rates of 3.4%, 6.4% and 0.7% but with small numbers.[74]

c) Background fetal loss for specific maternal age. It is now well-documented that the overall spontaneous fetal loss rate in ultrasonically viable pregnancies is about 2%.[75,76] However, the background fetal loss rate increases with increasing maternal age being 1.5% before 30 and 4.5% between 35 to 39 years.[75]

Infection and haemorrhage have been discussed in the context of the mother. Perforation of the membranes should be avoidable. Amniotic bands and abnormal embryogenesis have not been reported.

Feto-maternal haemorrhage after CVS has been documented by demonstrating a rise in maternal serum alpha-fetoprotein (msAFP) in the majority of patients.[29,77,78] Thus the potential for causing Rhesus isoimmunisation must be taken seriously and anti-D immunoglobulin prophylaxis is strongly recommended in Rhesus D negative women. Conversely, when anti-D antibodies are already present, CVS should be avoided as enhancement may accelerate the course of the disease. The post CVS rise in msAFP is transient so does not interfere with neural tube screening in the second trimester.[79]

Other fetal complications have not been shown to be increased with CVS. The Canadian trial showed no increase in either intra-uterine growth retardation (IUGR) or preterm labour, whilst the NICHD study could find no increase in placental abruption or preterm labour. The tendency towards late stillbirth in the CVS group in the Canadian trial has been mentioned.[70]

Neonatal There have been no reports of an increase in the neonatal death rate after CVS. Congenital defects were found in 2.6% of 615 completed pregnancies in one series.[27] The real risk of procedure related congenital abnormalities and later development of these children needs to be assessed in randomised trials.

Amniocentesis

Background Needles have been introduced into the human amniotic sac at least since 1877,[80] but the first clinical use of amniocentesis was reported in 1919 for a case of polyhydramnios.[81] Regular diagnostic amniocentesis began after Bevis reported its usefulness in the management of Rhesus isoimmunisation.[82] Diagnostic use remained limited to the third trimester, mainly for the management of Rhesus patients for the next decade. In 1960 fetal gender, established by sex chromatin analysis in amniotic fluid cells, enabled antenatal management of X-linked recessive disorders by termination of male fetuses.[83] This was the first use of amniocentesis in genetic disease. In 1965 Jeffcoate et al[84] used amniotic fluid to diagnose inborn errors of metabolism. They diagnosed the adrenogenital syndrome using amniotic fluid levels of 17-ketosteroid and pregnanetriol. Successful culture of amniocytes to yield a fetal karyotype was reported by Steele and Breg 1 year later.[85] The relationship of amniotic fluid AFP and open neural tube defects (NTD) was first described in 1972 by Brock and colleagues.[86,87]

Having established amniocentesis as useful in the antenatal diagnosis of common fetal disorders, investigators began to analyse the methodology to optimise its safety and accuracy. Trans-vaginal methods were tried and abandoned due to higher complication and failure rates.[88] Mid-trimester transabdominal amniocentesis remains the most established and widely used antenatal invasive procedure with 17 000 being performed annually in the United Kingdom. Even so this figure only represents about 30% of the high-risk pregnancies eligible for prenatal diagnosis,[89] reflecting such factors as ignorance of the procedure, religious or moral objections and the unacceptability of late therapeutic abortion.

Technique Ultrasound examination prior to amniocentesis allows confirmation of gestational age and fetal viability, evaluation of structural abnormalities, placental localisation and exclusion of multiple gestations. Although many early practitioners achieved a high degree of success with amniocentesis before ultrasound was available, few would want to proceed without it nowadays. Visualisation of a pool of amniotic fluid and localisation of the placenta enables more accurate and less frequent needle insertions to obtain fluid.[90–92] The report of the National Institute of Child Health and Development (NICHD) Amniocentesis Registry[91] showed a correlation between increasing the number of needle insertions and the rate of abortion. The scan must be performed at the time of the amniocentesis as the fetus and even the placenta may move.

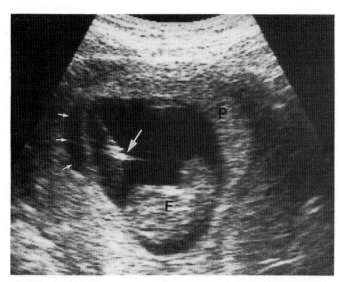

Fig. 10 Simultaneous monitoring during amniocentesis showing the needle passage avoiding the anterior placenta (P) and the extra-coelomic cavity (small arrows). Needle tip (large arrow). F – fetus.

Table 4 Comparison of chorionic villous sampling and amniocentesis

	CVS	amniocentesis
Advantages of CVS		
Gestation (weeks)	9–11	15–17
Result (days)	7–10	14–28
Termination	early	late
Disadvantages of CVS		
Procedure related loss	1–2%	1%
Additional procedure	1.5%	0.5%
Presentation	early	usual booking

Simultaneous ultrasound 'monitoring' is probably the best technique (Fig. 10). It has the advantage of allowing immediate adjustment of needle position as changes in the intra-uterine environment occur, and therefore a higher success rate with reduction in fetal, placental and cord trauma. Ch de Crespigny and Robinson[93] demonstrated a statistically significant reduction in technical difficulties, from 9.9% in those with prior ultrasound, to 3.7% in the monitored group. They also noted a fall in the number of spontaneous abortions from 2.4% to 0.8%. Similarly, in a series of 1300 patients undergoing genetic amniocentesis, Romero et al[94] compared 612 with prior ultrasound, to 688 with ultrasound monitoring and demonstrated a significant reduction in bloody or dry taps from 12.9% to 3.2% and in repeat taps from 8.2% to 2%.

Amniocentesis is performed as an outpatient procedure. Standard aseptic precautions are required, although full scrub, gowning and draping are not necessary provided a meticulous no touch technique is used. Prophylactic antibiotics and tocolytics are not necessary. Local anaesthetic is used by some operators. A 20 to 22 G spinal needle is used with a stylet to avoid maternal contamination. The Canadian MRC study associated needles greater than 19 G with increasing abortion risk.[95]

The initial collaborative studies did not report any increased risk with trans-placental amniocentesis.[90,95] More recently, a prospective randomised controlled trial of genetic amniocentesis in low-risk women reported a significantly increased risk of spontaneous abortion with placental perforation.[96] All the patients in this trial had ultrasound 'monitored' procedures and none had more than two needle insertions.

Timing For prenatal diagnosis the traditional timing of amniocentesis has been after 15 weeks. At this time the fundus is readily accessible transabdominally and the volume of amniotic fluid is approximately 150 to 200 ml, enabling aspiration of 15 to 20 ml without concern. Depending on the indication, a result may take 1 to 4 weeks, which precludes termination of an affected fetus much before 20 weeks. Obviously this increases the psychological and physical risks for the mother. In view of these disadvantages associated with mid-trimester amniocentesis and the complications associated with CVS (Table 4), there has been renewed interest in early amniocentesis (EA) as an alternative prenatal diagnostic procedure. The majority of EA reported have been between 12 to 15 weeks[97–101] and combined failure rates of only 2% have been reported using simultaneous ultrasound monitoring and 22 G needles.[98] However, technical problems, including bowel or bladder obstructing the path of the needle or no placenta free window, have dictated a variable rescheduling rate. Also, incomplete fusion of the chorion and amnion often found at EA (Fig. 10) may result in tenting of the membranes during the needling and necessitate more frequent needle passes.[97,101]

The success rate of cell culture after EA has been reported as 100% after 12 weeks,[102,103] but is lower prior to this gestation. Culture rates as short as 8 days have been reported,[104] but the more common experience is a delay of 1 to 2 days beyond that normal for mid-trimester samples. Successful diagnoses of some inborn errors of metabolism have also been performed by EA.[105] The accuracy of using amniotic fluid AFP for prenatal diagnosis in EA is also being investigated with preliminary reports showing a peak value at 13 weeks.[106,107] Simple extrapolation from existing regression line values in later pregnancy is therefore misleading and inappropriate for pregnancies of less than 13 weeks.

Despite this current interest in EA, there is only one report of a comparative trial with CVS; the pregnancy loss rates were 3.1% and 5% respectively.[100] However, selection was not randomised and the option of mid-trimester amniocentesis was included.

Of particular concern with EA is the respiratory function of the newborn, as the effects of removal of a relatively large proportion of amniotic fluid are unknown. In a series of 222 early amniocenteses performed between 9 and 14 weeks,[108] with a miscarriage rate of 1.4% and a 5% termination rate for fetal abnormality, there was one stillbirth and one congenital abnormality (bilateral talipes).[108] No infant had respiratory distress syndrome or pneumonia.

Experience Experience in performing amniocenteses has been shown to affect the success of the procedure. The United Kingdom MRC trial[90] reported that clinicians who had the experience of over 50 procedures had a failure rate of 1.1% compared with 9.9% for those with less than 50. Subsequent fetal loss is also related to the operator's experience, a spontaneous abortion rate of 0.3% with an experience of 50, increasing to 3.7% when this experience was limited to less than 10 in one series.[109]

Indications The indications for amniocentesis are shown below.

Before 20 weeks
Chromosome abnormalities (maternal age, previous affected child, translocation carrier, X-linked disorders)
Neural tube defects
Inborn errors of metabolism
DNA Analysis

After 20 weeks
Haemolytic disease of fetus (bilirubin via delta OD 450nm)
Fetal lung maturity (phospholipids)
Preterm premature ruptured membranes (microbiology)
Fetal maturity
Amniography or fetography

Chromosomes Fetal karyotyping is the most common indication for amniocentesis and the specific indications are the same as those for CVS. About two thirds are performed to investigate abnormalities associated with increasing maternal age. The age-specific risk figures are higher if amniocentesis data are quoted[55] rather than liveborn data.[110] This probably reflects the increased abortion and stillbirth rate associated with chromosomally abnormal fetuses, the incomplete reporting of chromosomal abnormalities amongst newborns and the fact that the liveborn data of Hook and Chambers[110] only include the risk for Down's syndrome, not all aneuploidy, as does the amniocentesis data.

The recurrence risk of non-disjunctional chromosomal abnormality is 0.5% to 1%[111] and prenatal diagnosis is most commonly utilised after a previous child with trisomy 21. In the case of a parent being a carrier for a balanced translocation, the risk of fetal abnormality varies with the specific aberration, but female carriers of an X-linked disorder risk 50% occurrence in male offspring.

Amniotic fluid contains cells desquamated from fetal skin, body tracts and amnion. Karyotyping is performed on cultured cells. Discordance between the karyotype obtained after amniotic cell culture and the actual fetal karyotype is possible, particularly in mosaicism. Failure to detect an abnormal karyotype at amniocentesis is very unlikely because of the variety of organs contributing to the cell culture. Mosaicism however, is not rare, with Level 2 (multiple cells with the same abnormality in a single flask) and Level 3 abnormalities (multiple cells with the same abnormality in multiple flasks) occurring with frequencies of 0.7% and 0.2% respectively.[46,112,113] However, only in 20% of Level 2 and 60% of Level 3 mosaicism will these karyotypes be confirmed in the fetus. Recently, fetal blood sampling (FBS) has been used to investigate this diagnostic dilemma.[114] Gosden et al reported 41 cases of amniotic cell mosaicism of which 31 fetuses had a normal karyotype on FBS, which was confirmed after delivery.

The issue of maternal cell contamination has been addressed by Thirkelsen who found a growth of mixed male and female cells in 0.229% of 40 000 cases with misdiagnosis resulting from maternal cell contamination in another 0.085%.[115] These figures should be doubled to include undetected maternal contamination with a female fetus.

Inborn errors of metabolism The principles of prenatal diagnosis are the same as for CVS. Over 100 different IEM have been diagnosed in utero by biochemical analysis of amniotic fluid or cultured cells.[58] For both fetal chromosome analysis and the diagnosis of IEM, the procedure is usually performed at 15 to 16 weeks and takes 3 to 4 weeks to obtain a result.

Neural tube defects Failure of closure of the neural tube results in a variety of abnormalities including anencephaly, encephalocele and spina bifida with or without associated meningomyelocele (see Ch. 16). Most isolated neural tube defects (NTD) are multifactorially inherited and the incidence varies with different populations. High-risk groups include parents with one or two previously affected children and women who themselves have spina bifida. The specific site of recurrence may vary amongst siblings.

For the diagnosis of NTD amniocentesis is more commonly performed at 18 to 20 weeks after suspicion has been raised by elevated msAFP at routine screening. Amniotic fluid AFP levels are more reliable with false positive and false negative rates of 0.03% and 10% respectively.[116] The amniotic AFP is normal in 'closed' skin-covered lesions.

Detailed ultrasound evaluation also has an important role in the evaluation of these high-risk pregnancies and is being used increasingly in the diagnosis of NTD, particularly anencephaly. Amniocentesis is now rarely indicated to confirm this diagnosis.[117]

DNA analysis DNA analysis is performed with the appropriate gene probe, but amniocytes are a poor source of DNA and culture delays diagnosis.[118] Villi are always preferable for this methodology and have the advantage of being obtainable in the first trimester.

Haemolytic disease of the fetus The severity of fetal red blood cell destruction in alloimmunisation has traditionally been measured indirectly by amniotic fluid bilirubin levels.[119,120] This is achieved by spectrophotometric measurement of the deviation in optical density of

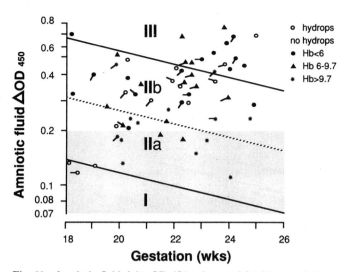

Fig. 11 Amniotic fluid delta OD 450 values and fetal haemoglobin concentration in 59 Rh alloimmunised pregnancies, plotted on the extrapolated Liley graph. In 25 patients who had a prior delta OD 450 measurement, a short line denotes the slope of change. (Reproduced from Nicolaides et al[122] with permission from CV Mosby Company.)

amniotic fluid at 450 nm (delta OD 450) and enables the definition of three zones which predict the severity of the anaemia. In the third trimester the accuracy of the prediction of Liley zone III is about 95% correct.[121]

However, extrapolation of these zones backwards into the second trimester gives inaccurate predictions of the severity of the disease, with a 68% false negative rate for severely affected fetuses[122] (Fig. 11).

Fetal lung maturity The amniotic fluid lecithin/sphingomyelin (L/S) ratio is an excellent predictor of fetal lung maturity,[123] and its introduction in 1971 revolutionised the obstetricians' ability to assess prenatally one of the functions vital to the infant's survival. In the current practise of obstetrics its use is declining. This is probably due to a combination of improvements in neonatal ventilatory support, frequent use of ultrasound dating, improved antenatal assessment of fetal wellbeing and the fact that maternal or fetal conditions necessitating preterm delivery are usually urgent and the use of the L/S ratio is inappropriate.[124] Despite the diminished use of the L/S ratio and the increased proportion of small babies, the incidence of respiratory distress syndrome has remained static and the perinatal mortality has continued to fall.

Other Amniocentesis for the investigation of preterm premature rupture of the membranes has not gained support, because low virulence micro-organisms that are not of any clinical significance are frequently identified.[125] The assessment of fetal maturity (gestational age) by amniotic fluid studies is inaccurate and now rarely used: neither is amniography nor fetography. All these procedures have been replaced by ultrasound.

Complications

Maternal There is minimal risk to the mother with amnionitis occurring in less than 0.1% of cases.[91] At the Montreal Workshop in 1979, only one maternal death was reported due to a direct complication out of 20 000 amniocenteses.[126] Psychological stress, however, is common, due to the indication for the procedure, the risk of fetal loss and the delay in obtaining the result.[127]

Fetal The risks to the fetus have been assessed in four major studies (Table 5). Of the three collaborative case controlled studies, only the UK MRC trial identified an increased risk (1.4%) of spontaneous abortion following amniocentesis.[90] The NICHD and the Canadian MRC studies found no complications attributable to the procedure, but had difficulty selecting matched controls.[91,95] In the only prospective randomised controlled study a 1% increment in the spontaneous abortion rate of the amniocentesis group was demonstrated.[96] Using a 20 G needle[128] under continuous ultrasound guidance, an increased risk of abortion was correlated with trans-placental sampling, the withdrawal of discoloured fluid and raised levels of msAFP prior to the procedure. An increase in the perinatal mortality rate was not demonstrated.

Table 5 Spontaneous abortion rate (%) in amniocentesis

	Subjects	Controls
Canadian MRC (1977)	0.9	1.6–1.9
NICHD (1978)	2.8	2.4
UK MRC (1978)	2.7	1.3
Tabor et al (1986)	1.7	0.7

Amniocentesis carries a risk of feto-maternal haemorrhage.[129] This is increased following trans-placental amniocentesis and if performed by less experienced operators. Unsensitised Rhesus negative patients having amniocentesis should be given prophlactic anti-D immunoglobulin (50 μg up to 20 weeks and 100 μg thereafter). A Kleihauer-Betke test may be performed to quantitate the fetomaternal haemorrhage and allow adjustment of the immunoglobulin dose as necessary.

Other less common risks include spontaneous rupture of membranes, fetal trauma and fetal exsanguination.

Neonatal The UK MRC study suggested that there was a higher incidence of postural deformities (talipes) and respiratory difficulties.[90] The former has not been confirmed, but the association of amniocentesis with respiratory distress and pneumonia was also reported by Tabor et al in the randomised trial.[96] Work in non-human primates supports this finding, but as yet the mechanism is unclear.[130] Fetal trauma is very rare. In the UK MRC study more skin marks and dimples were found in the control neonates than in the subjects.[90]

Fetal blood sampling

Background   Fetal blood sampling (FBS) was first performed experimentally in 1973 by Valenti, who aspirated the umbilical cord using a paediatric hysteroscope introduced into the amniotic cavity at hysterotomy.[131] Also in a series of patients prior to termination of pregnancy, Kan et al[132] described the technique of placentocentesis or 'blind' placental aspiration to obtain fetal blood suitable for the diagnosis of haemoglobinopathies. This was the first technique to be used clinically to obtain fetal blood for diagnosis.[133] After ultrasound localisation of the placenta, multiple needle punctures were made in the chorionic plate to induce fetal bleeding into the amniotic fluid. Blood-stained amniotic fluid samples were then aspirated to obtain fetal red cells. Samples were usually contaminated with maternal blood and often contained a very low proportion of fetal cells, with 10% or more of patients requiring a repeat procedure. Furthermore, a 10% fetal mortality rate, mainly due to fetal exsanguination, has ensured this procedure is now obsolete.[134]

Fetoscopy (Fig. 12) was the first satisfactory method for obtaining samples of fetal blood. Diagnostic application of fetoscopy was possible once the percutaneous transabdominal route was described by Hobbins and Mahoney in 1974.[135] Using local anaesthesia and an aseptic technique, they introduced a 1.7 mm rigid fibre-optic endoscope (Dyonics. Inc.) into the amniotic cavity to visualise the second trimester fetus. Fetal blood was obtained under direct vision by puncture of the vessels on the surface of the chorionic plate, but was often diluted with amniotic fluid and contaminated with maternal blood.

In 1978, using the same instrument, Rodeck and Campbell[136] sampled the umbilical cord vessels at the placental or fetal insertion and reliably obtained pure fetal blood. They also demonstrated that, despite the large diameter cannula (2.4 × 3.0 mm) which was used to house the fetoscope, the procedure could be performed on both anterior and posterior placentae as long as care was taken to avoid the placenta while introducing the trocar. An ultrasound scan was performed immediately before or during insertion to check placental localisation and cord insertion. Since that time, fetoscopy for FBS has become a precise ultrasound guided technique which can be performed from 18 weeks gestation into the third trimester and which enabled a variety of diagnostic and therapeutic procedures. However, it is a difficult technique to learn and in the most experienced centres had a fetal loss rate of about 2% to 5%.[137] There was also an increased risk of amniotic fluid leakage, preterm labour and amnionitis.

Improvements in ultrasound resolution enabled the introduction of ultrasound guided needling of fetal vessels. The most commonly used vessel is the umbilical vein. This was first reported by Daffos et al in 1983,[138] who successfully obtained fetal blood in 53 cases using a 20 G spinal needle under local anaesthetic. This procedure has become widely adopted and has now entirely displaced fetoscopy for fetal blood aspiration.

Technique   As with all invasive ultrasound procedures a preliminary real time scan should be performed prior to and independent of the procedure. In the case of FBS relevant features include the number of fetuses, viability, gestational age, amniotic fluid volume and the presence or absence of structural anomalies.

Just prior to the procedure the target organ is identified. This may be the placental or umbilical cord insertion, the intrahepatic vein,[139] the heart[140] or a free loop of cord. The most common site of sampling is the umbilical cord at its insertion into the placenta. It should be located in its long axis to allow optimal visualisation for sampling (Fig. 13). The optimal real time transducer to use is probably a curvilinear array. This transducer combines the advantages of sector and linear probes by allowing a large image field and visualisation of the whole course of the needle, whilst also being light and easy to manipulate. Use of colour flow imaging greatly facilitates location of the umbilical cord insertion.

Holding the transducer wrapped in a sterile plastic bag with the target organ visualised, the abdominal site of entry and direction of the needle is chosen. Using a free-hand technique the needle is then guided by simultaneous ultrasound to the chosen site and the needle tip identified as a clearly visible echo (Fig. 14). With the needle in situ, immediate complications may also be monitored ultrasonically. These include alterations in fetal heart rate, intra-amniotic bleeding seen as turbulent echoes in the am-

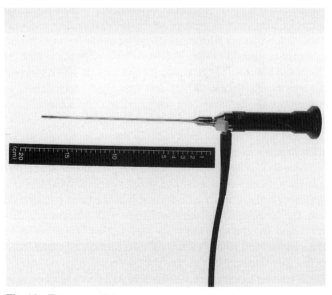

Fig. 12   Fetoscope, Olympus.

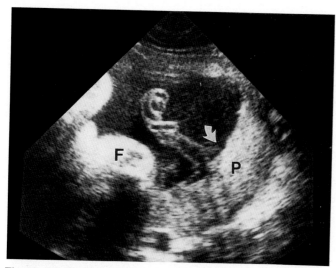

Fig. 13   Ultrasound scan of a posterior placental cord insertion (arrow). P – placenta, F – fetus.

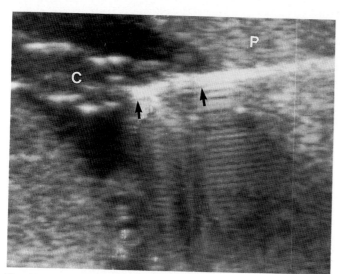

Fig. 14   Ultrasound guided fetal blood sampling from an anterior placental cord insertion showing the needle as a bright line (arrows). P – placenta, C – cord.

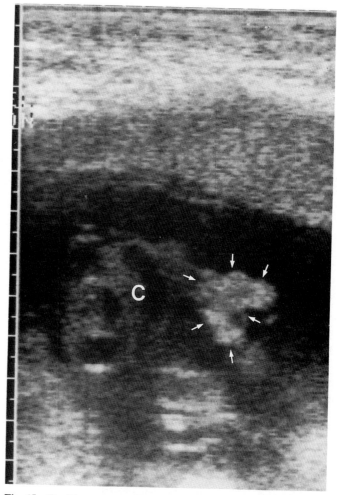

Fig. 15   Cord haematoma. Ultrasound image of a cord haematoma (arrows) after fetal blood sampling. C – cord.

niotic cavity and haematoma formation seen as reflective space-occupying lesions (Fig. 15).

Post-operatively potential complications can be monitored such as haematoma formation at the puncture site.

FBS is performed as an out-patient procedure. A partner or close relative is encouraged to attend for emotional support. Rarely is maternal or direct fetal sedation necessary. Standard aseptic conditions are maintained including a full scrub. With the patient wedged in a supine position with lateral tilt, the patient's abdomen is washed with antiseptic solution and 1% xylocaine infiltrated at the puncture site. A 20 G spinal needle is then advanced under continuous ultrasound guidance to the appropriate site and 2 to 5 ml of fetal blood aspirated, depending on the indication.

Confirmation that fetal blood has been aspirated is provided immediately by analysis on a Coulter Channelyzer, which detects the difference in mean cell volume (MCV) between maternal and fetal red blood cells (RBC). Other distinguishing haematological indices include a broad RBC distribution width and a single leukocyte peak in the fetus. Dilution by amniotic fluid occurs in about 1% of procedures, but maternal cell contamination is rare.[141] As either of these contaminants may alter the diagnostic results their presence should be checked. Maternal blood contamination is best detected by the presence of β-human chorionic gonadotrophin and amniotic fluid by coagulation factor assays.[141]

The different sites of sampling are:

a) placental cord insertion
b) fetal cord insertion (umbilicus)

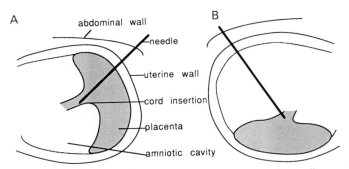

Fig. 16 **Fetal blood sampling**. The approach to fetal blood sampling in **A**: anterior placenta, **B**: posterior placenta.

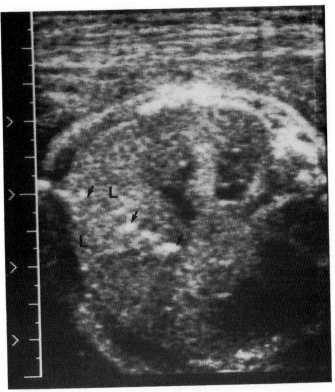

Fig. 17 **Fetal intra-abdominal blood sampling**. Transverse ultrasound section through a fetal abdomen showing the fetal blood sampling needle (small arrows) in the intrahepatic portion of the umbilical vein (large arrows). L – liver.

c) intrahepatic vein
d) fetal heart
e) free loop of cord.

a) Placental cord insertion. This is the original site described by Daffos et al[138] and is the most widely utilised. Both the artery and/or vein may be sampled and each is specifically identified by the direction of flow of the echoes seen when sterile saline (1 ml) is injected via the sampling needle. For anterior placentae the route to the umbilical cord is trans-placental and for posterior placentae the route is transamniotic (Fig. 16). The vessel is sampled about 1 cm from its placental insertion (Fig. 14). Failure to obtain fetal blood occurs in about 3% of cases and a second attempt may be necessary.[142]

Difficulties in sampling from the placental cord insertion may arise in cases of polyhydramnios, maternal obesity or when the fetus obscures a posterior placental cord insertion. This may be overcome by fetal manipulation, alteration of maternal position or postponing the procedure. Alternatively, another site may be chosen for the FBS.

b) Fetal cord insertion. Although possible, this site is not often used as passive mobility of the fetus makes successful sampling difficult.

c) Fetal intrahepatic umbilical vein. This method involves directing a needle through the fetal abdominal wall and liver substance into the intrahepatic portion of the umbilical vein (Fig. 17). In a transverse abdominal plane, the direction of approach is anterior, either midline or via either hypochondrium. Although this method was originally reported by Bang[143] and de Crespigny[144] as a route for intravascular transfusions in fetuses with Rhesus isoimmunisation, it was described by Koresawa[139] as the method of choice for second trimester diagnostic FBS. This approach is useful when difficulties arise, either with access or due to sampling failure at the placental cord insertion. Alternatively this site may be preferentially chosen when visualisation of the placental cord insertion is poor or to lessen the risks of fetomaternal haemorrhage.[145] Unlike

sampling at the placental cord insertion there is no need to confirm the fetal origin by mean corpuscular volume nor is infusion of saline needed to assess vessel origin. Nicolini et al[146] report success in obtaining a fetal blood sample in 92% of 214 cases. Analysis of changes in fetal liver enzymes following these procedures indicates there is no hepatic damage.[147]

d) Fetal heart. Prenatal diagnosis using blood obtained from the fetal heart is possible.[140] The technique described by Bang utilises a 1.2 mm diameter guide needle which is inserted into the fetal thorax. A 0.7 mm needle is then advanced into the fetal ventricle. Puncturing the atrium can be fatal and is best avoided. This method is commonly associated with the potentially severe complications of fetal bradycardia and asystole and is rarely used clinically except in emergencies.

e) Free loop of umbilical cord. The sampling needle is advanced within the amniotic cavity until it abutts an accessible loop of cord. The vessel is then penetrated with a quick thrust. Although a difficult technique in the presence of a normal amount of amniotic fluid because of cord mobility, this method is ideal in cases of oligohydramnios or anhydramnios as the cord becomes relatively fixed and the placental cord insertion is usually difficult to identify.

Timing Ultrasound guided FBS is usually performed from 16 to 42 weeks gestation depending on the indication. At the earlier gestations the procedure seems to be associated with a higher incidence of bradycardias and subsequent fetal deaths. This may be due to the relatively large size of the needle in relation to the vessel diameter for small fetuses. Also the relative paucity of Wharton's jelly may prolong traumatic haemorrhage. In a recent analysis of 500 early FBS (between 12 and 21 weeks gestation) 163 were performed at 16 weeks or earlier.[148] Using a 25 G needle and aspirating about 0.2 to 0.3 ml, a fetal loss rate of approximately 5% was reported; this figure dropped to 2.5% at 19 weeks gestation. Unfortunately the results in this study exclude 110 patients that underwent therapeutic abortion and a further 20 that were lost to follow up.

Experience It is important to realise that the excellent results reported are only achieved after a great deal of experience and training. After 606 procedures, Daffos et al report a 97% success rate at first attempt and failure rate of 0.5%.[142] In a smaller series of 96 procedures, however, rates of 63% and 5% respectively were reported.[149]

Indications Fetal blood sampling was introduced to diagnose genetic haemoglobinopathies, but is now used for a wide range of indications:

— haemoglobinopathies
— coagulopathies
— immunodeficiencies
— karyotyping
— isoimmunisation
— fetal infection
— non-immune hydrops
— metabolic disorders
— fetal blood gas and acid-base status.

Genetic blood disorders Prenatal diagnosis of haemoglobinopathies is made by measuring globin chain synthesis.[150] The major haemoglobin in the normal fetus is Hb F (alpha 2, gamma 2) and between 16 and 24 weeks gestation they have a beta/gamma ratio of 0.11 ± 0.005. Those affected with β-thalassaemia major have a ratio less than 0.02. Homozygous β-thalassaemia (gamma 4) causes fetal hydrops and intra-uterine death. The fetus with sickle cell anaemia has alpha, gamma, and $beta_s$ but no $beta_A$ chains.[151]

The diagnosis of fetal haemophilia A or B is made by quantification of factor VIIIC or factor IX respectively. Accurate diagnosis requires pure fetal blood free of clot initiation.[152] Many other coagulopathies and platelet disorders can be diagnosed prenatally as the relevant normal ranges are available.[152]

Increasingly first trimester diagnosis via DNA analysis of chorionic villi is replacing fetal blood analysis for these disorders, provided a family DNA marker has been identified and the pregnancy is sufficiently early.

Inherited severe combined immunodeficiencies can be diagnosed by monoclonal anti-T cell lymphocyte antibodies and a fluorescence-activated cell sorter.[153,154]

Karyotyping A karyotype can be obtained from cultured fetal lymphocytes within 3 days, which is far more rapid than from amniocytes. This is useful in the further investigation of fetal structural abnormalities identified by ultrasound in the second trimester, as they are associated with a higher incidence of chromosomal aberration than at term, particularly omphalocele, obstructive uropathy, cystic hygroma, duodenal atresia, non-immune hydrops and severe intra-uterine growth retardation.[155] Rapid karyotyping may also be useful for other markers of fetal chromosomal abnormality such as thickened nuchal skin fold, abnormal facies and abnormalities of hands and feet. Assessment of fetal structural anomalies now forms the largest group of patients having FBS.

Other indications for fetal blood karyotyping include: late booking or failed amniocentesis, fragile X-linked mental retardation[157] and the investigation of mosaicism or pseudomosaicism arising at amniocentesis.[114]

Alloimmunisation In pregnancies affected by red cell alloimmunisation (D, c, Kell), FBS is useful not only in the assessment of the severity of the disease, but also in the determination of the fetal blood group.

Determination of fetal blood group is justified in patients with a history of severe disease or with high circulating antibody levels, where the father is heterozygous.[158] A fetus that is found to be antigen negative needs no further investigation. There is a risk that the procedure itself will cause feto-maternal haemorrhage, resulting in a rise in maternal antibody levels and worsening the disease in an affected fetus.[159] This must be considered when offering the procedure and care must be taken to minimise the risk by avoiding a trans-placental needle passage.

Direct measurement of the fetal haemoglobin or haematocrit and a positive indirect Coombs test enables the most accurate assessment of the severity of red cell allo-immunisation. This is particularly useful in moderate to severe affliction and in the second trimester when Liley charts are unreliable.[122] The diagnostic FBS can be followed by an intra-uterine intravascular transfusion if necessary.[160,161]

Alloimmune thrombocytopenia is analogous to red cell alloimmunisation, except that fetal platelets are the target antigen for maternal IgG PLA1 antibodies. Because of the risk of antenatal intracranial haemorrhage and intra-uterine death,[162–165] second and third trimester determination of fetal platelet levels is appropriate in at risk pregnancies.[166] There is evidence that antenatal treatment by serial fetal intravenous platelet infusions may be more effective in preventing pathology than elective caesarean section after scalp puncture to assess fetal platelet count in early labour.[167]

Fetal infections As documented maternal rubella infection during early pregnancy does not always result in fetal infection, prenatal diagnosis by the detection of rubella-specific IgM antibody in fetal blood may be helpful.[168–170] No congenital abnormalities have been documented following maternal infection after the seventeenth week of pregnancy.[171] The assay should only be performed after 20 to 22 weeks when the fetus can reliably mount an immune response.

Fetal toxoplasmosis can be diagnosed with 92% accuracy using fetal blood to perform a specific IgM assay and mouse inoculation as well as white blood cell, platelet and eosinophil counts, measurement of total IgM and plasma gamma glutamyltransferase and lactic dehydrogenase. Serial ultrasound is useful to detect microcephaly, hydrocephaly, intracranial calcifications, ascites and hepatomegaly.[172] Successful prophylactic treatment has been achieved using a combination of spiramycin, pyrimethamine and sulphonamides.[172]

Other infections causing fetal teratogenesis include cytomegalovirus, varicella-zoster, human parvovirus and human immunodeficiency virus, all of which may be diagnosed antenatally with variable success.

Blood gas and acid-base status   In 1986 Soothill et al published reference ranges for blood gas and acid-base values in umbilical venous, umbilical arterial and intervillous blood from 16 weeks gestation until term.[173] They demonstrated that pO_2 decreases linearly with advancing gestation, but a constant oxygen content is maintained by a compensatory increase in fetal haemoglobin concentration (Fig. 18). The umbilical venous pCO_2, bicarbonate, base

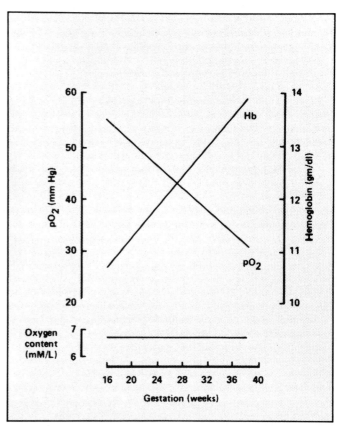

Fig. 18   Relationship between haemoglobin and pO_2. pO_2 decreases linearly with gestation as haemoglobin increases, maintaining a constant oxygen content (Reproduced from Soothill et al[173] with permission from S. Kager AG)

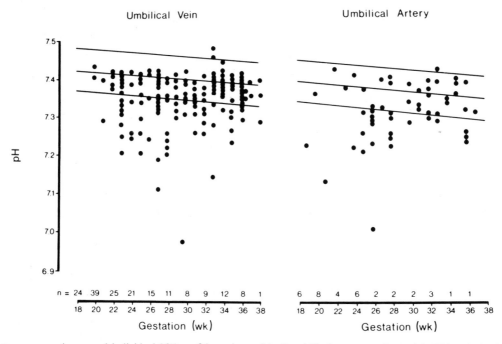

Fig. 19   Reference ranges (mean and individual 95% confidence intervals) **of umbilical venous and arterial pH** (vertical axis) with gestation. Individual values of small for gestational age fetuses are also shown (closed circles). (Reproduced from Nicolaides et al[174] with permission from CV Mosby Company.)

excess and plasma lactate rise with advancing gestation, but the pH remains the same (Fig. 19).[174]

Analysis of blood from small for gestational age (SGA) fetuses has shown that a substantial proportion are chronically hypoxic, the degree of which correlates with acidosis, hypercapnia, hyperlacticaemia, hypoglycaemia and erythroblastosis.[175] These changes seem to distinguish genetically small from growth retarded fetuses. However, the relevance of this information in planning the clinical management is controversial as fetuses may survive in utero for up to 5 weeks despite being small, hypoxaemic and/or acidaemic.[176] Also fetal hypoxaemia and acidaemia correlate well with an absence of end diastolic Doppler velocities, but not with perinatal outcome (Figs 20 and 21).[176]

Other In non-immune hydrops, FBS may be used to determine karyotype, viral infection or anaemia, when ultrasound has been unable to demonstrate a cause.

Although rapid diagnosis of many inborn errors of metabolism can be made on fetal blood, earlier diagnosis is possible on chorionic villi or amniotic fluid. FBS is therefore limited in use to late booking patients or failed amniocentesis.

Complications

Maternal Discomfort at the time of the procedure and for 1 to 2 days post-operatively is common, but no serious maternal complications have been reported.[138,142,149]

Fetal In the largest series reported spontaneous abortion or intra-uterine death occurred in 7 of 606 cases (1.9%), although only two were considered to be due to the procedure.[142] They also report no increase in preterm delivery or growth retardation. Such excellent results are only accomplished after considerable training and experi-

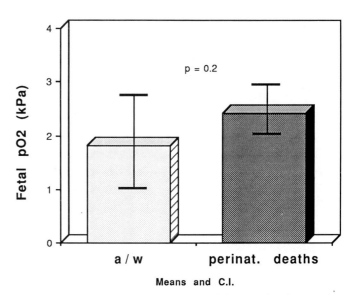

Fig. 21 Fetal pO₂ levels in growth retarded fetuses with absent end diastolic flow that survived (white) and died (grey) perinatally: means and confidence intervals.

ence. However, it is worthwhile to note that this series was based predominantly on normal fetuses greater than 21 weeks gestation undergoing prenatal diagnosis for congenital toxoplasmosis, and as such, may not represent the spectrum of patients seen in other centres. Loss rates are higher with compromised fetuses and at earlier gestational ages.[148]

Although intra-amniotic bleeding occurs in about 40% of cases it is transient.[142,149] Fetal bradycardia is observed more commonly with arterial samplings[149] and is usually transient. An uncommon but specific risk of fetal cord sampling is acute bleeding into the Wharton's jelly, producing cord haematoma and tamponade. In late pregnancy, emergency caesarean section should be performed to salvage these infants.

Neonatal No neonatal complications have been reported. Babies that have had intrahepatic vein FBS show no evidence of puncture marks or trauma.

Fetal skin biopsy

Unless characterised by a chromosomal abnormality or enzyme defect, prenatal diagnosis of hereditary skin disorders requires histology and ultrastructural studies on fetal skin biopsies[177] obtained either by fetoscopy or ultrasound guided techniques.[178,179]

Technique A biopsy assessment should be performed to confirm gestational age and fetal heart action, and to exclude structural anomalies and multiple pregnancy.

The preferential site for biopsy depends on the particular condition under investigation. Ultrasound is used to select the abdominal entry point which will allow access to the sampling site which depends on fetal position and placental

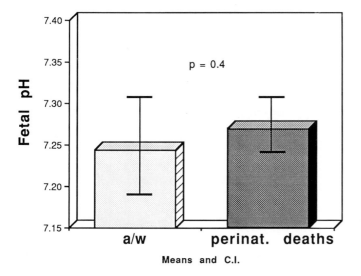

Fig. 20 Fetal pH levels in growth retarded fetuses with absent end diastolic flow that survived (white) and died (grey) perinatally: means and confidence intervals.

location. For example, fetuses at risk of epidermolysis bullosa are best sampled from the buttock or leg and those at risk of albinism should be biopsied from the eyebrow or scalp.

Method   Four techniques have been used:

a) Fetoscopy with direct vision. The fetoscope is inserted into the uterus under local anaesthesia. The fetus is examined, the area to be sampled identified, and several small biopsies of 1 to 2 mm are pinched out of the skin under direct vision using 20 gauge biopsy forceps (RM Surgical Developments) (Fig. 8) passed down the operating side arm of the fetoscope cannula.[178] This technique is still very useful in cases of oculocutaneous albinism, where skin specifically from the eyebrow region is required for correct diagnosis.

b) Fetoscopy with ultrasonically directed biopsy. Having chosen the biopsy site by inspection with fetoscopy the fetoscope is withdrawn and 18 gauge biopsy forceps are introduced down the centre of the cannula and guided by ultrasound to this site. This enables larger specimens to be taken, although samples of amnion are sometimes obtained.[180]

c) Fetoscopy with 'blind' biopsy. This technique is no longer practised as it is imprecise and has a high failure rate.[181]

d) Ultrasound guided biopsy is performed by introducing a 19 gauge cannula with trocar into the uterine cavity under ultrasound surveillance. After withdrawing the trocar fine 20 gauge cupped biopsy forceps (RM Surgical Developments) (Fig. 8) are directed to the appropriate site and multiple samples are pinched out.

Using direct vision fetoscopy or ultrasound guided biopsy in 52 patients at King's College Hospital and Queen Charlotte and Chelsea Hospitals between 1980 and 1988 there were no failed procedures.

The biopsy technique causes crush damage so the specimens are flushed from the forceps using sterile saline and fixed immediately without further handling. The samples can be processed in a matter of hours for analysis by light and electron microscopy.[182]

Timing   The majority of skin biopsies are performed at 18 to 22 weeks gestation, although differentiation of major fetal skin structures is not completed until 24 to 26 weeks.[183]

Indications   There are currently six conditions for which prenatal skin biopsy is indicated.

a) Epidermolysis bullosa lethalis is diagnosed by demonstrating separation of the epidermis from the dermis at the lamina lucida and a reduced number of malformed or rudimentary hemidesmosomes (Fig. 22).[178]

b) Epidermolysis bullosa dystrophica demonstrates a cleavage plane below the basal lamina and focal collagenolysis in the upper dermis below the dermo-epidermal junction in unseparated regions.[184]

c) Epidermolytic hyperkeratosis is distinguished by cy-

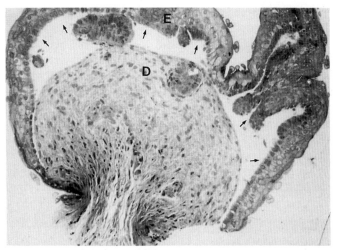

Fig. 22   Histological diagnosis of epidermolysis bullosa lethalis showing separation (arrows) of the epidermis (E) from the dermis (D).

tolysis of the suprabasal epidermal cells and clumping of the tonofilaments.[185]

d) Harlequin icthyosis shows premature hyperkeratosis, particularly around hair follicles and sweat gland ducts.[181]

e) Oculocutaneous albinism displays lack of active melanin synthesis in hair bulb melanocytes.[186]

f) Sjogren-Larsson syndrome is diagnosed by hyperkeratosis and increased keratohyaline.[187]

Complications   Review of the 52 skin biopsies performed at King's College Hospital and Queen Charlotte and Chelsea Hospitals between 1980 and 1988 revealed 13 affected fetuses. Of the 40 continuing pregnancies, there were no spontaneous abortions, four preterm deliveries and one neonatal death following premature delivery.

Liver biopsy

Prenatal diagnosis of inborn errors of metabolism is usually achieved through assay of chorion, fetal blood or cultured amniocytes for specific enzyme activity or metabolite detection. In a few rare disorders, diagnosis is only possible on liver tissue due to the localised protein expression.[188-192] In the future, it seems likely that the indications for liver biopsy will diminish as new gene probes enable first trimester diagnosis in at risk families.[193-195]

Technique   As usual a prebiopsy ultrasound is performed independently to the timing of the biopsy.

Initial experience of liver biopsy was with fetoscopy.[188] The site of entry is chosen by ultrasound to avoid damaging the placenta and to ensure access to the fetal liver.

More recently ultrasound guided transabdominal liver biopsies have been performed. The route to the fetal liver is selected on ultrasound and the needle is guided across the amniotic space to the right hypochondrium of the fetus. It is then introduced swiftly into the fetal trunk, as the fetus is likely to withdraw from the needle tip unless rapidly transfixed. This technique is more adaptable than fetoscopy as the needle tip is continuously visualised within the abdomen. It allows more oblique and lateral approaches to the fetal trunk and is particularly advantageous when the fetal spine is anterior. In this regard, the technique is similar to needling the intrahepatic portion of the umbilical vein (Fig. 17).

Following the procedure, the fetal heart rate is checked with ultrasound and the fetal peritoneal cavity scanned for evidence of bleeding.

Using fetoscopy, the umbilicus and right nipple of the fetus are identified by direct vision. After gentle palpation by the biopsy needle passed down the side channel, an entry is made just below the costal margin and away from the midline.[188] The aspiration needle is 19 gauge for its last 8 cm, the rest of the shaft being slightly narrower. A 10 ml syringe is attached to the hub and strong negative pressure is exerted after removal. The needle containing a core of liver tissue is flushed through with normal saline into a gallipot and the procedure repeated as necessary.

For ultrasound guided liver biopsies a double cannula (17 G/19 G) (Fig. 23) is used similar to that for transabdominal CVS. The back and forth aspirating motion is then confined to the inner cannula, which minimises maternal discomfort from peritoneal irritation and limits the movement of the needle within the fetal liver. The tissue is aspirated using negative pressure as for fetoscopy. Several insertions of the inner needle may be required to obtain the 10 to 25 mg of tissue required for analysis. A light microscope is useful to confirm that the correct tissue has been sampled.

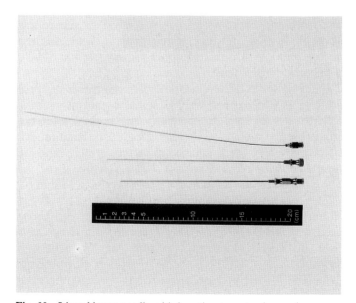

Fig. 23 Liver biopsy needle with inserting trocar and cannula.

Prior to undertaking liver biopsy for prenatal diagnosis the exact enzyme defect from a previous pregnancy or the maternal carrier status must be identified. For optimal results the procedure is best restricted to referral centres with operators skilled in invasive procedures. The laboratory must have established its own control ranges for enzyme activities in mid-trimester fetuses as these are lower than neonatal values.[188,192] Technical failures can be checked against other liver enzymes, which should be normal.[188–190] To date no failed procedures or incorrect diagnoses have been reported.

Timing Fetal liver biopsy for any current indication is delayed until 17 weeks gestation when the enzyme activity is first expressed. In the future sampling may be performed earlier as some enzyme activity has been demonstrated in fetal liver from first trimester terminations.[196,197]

Indications Fetal liver biopsy has been reported in the prenatal diagnosis of only four conditions: ornithine carbamyl transferase deficiency,[188,189] carbamyl phosphate synthetase deficiency,[190] glucose 6 phosphatase deficiency[191] and primary hyperoxaluria.[192]

a) Ornithine carbamyl transferase (OTC) deficiency is a rare X-linked condition where there is failure to convert ammonia into urea.[198,199] The affected males develop ammonia intoxication after birth and usually die in the first week.[200] Prenatal diagnosis is not possible from amniotic fluid or fetal blood as the placenta rapidly clears the metabolites,[188] but it is expressed in mitochondria of hepatocytes and intestinal tissue. Since carrier females have no clinical manifestations prenatal diagnosis has in the past been offered to at risk male fetuses, selected by high resolution ultrasound.[201] Many carriers can now be detected with gene probes and for them prenatal diagnosis is available by DNA analysis in the first trimester.[193]

b) Carbamyl phosphate synthetase (CPS) catalyses the first step of the urea cycle and is located in the mitochondria of the hepatocytes. Deficiency of this enzyme is rarer than OTC and the inheritance is autosomal recessive.[200] Most affected infants die from hyperammonaemia in the first weeks of life. Absence of CPS activity in a mid-trimester liver biopsy is diagnostic.[190]

c) Glucose 6 phosphatase deficiency (G6P) is also known as glycogen storage disease type I or Von Gierke's disease and prevents the liberation of hepatic glucose, resulting in hypoglycaemia, lactic acidaemia, hyperuricaemia and hyperlipidaemia.[202] This condition is autosomal recessive and mental impairment and death from the disease are common. As the enzyme is only expressed in hepatic, renal and intestinal tissue, liver biopsy is the best means of prenatal diagnosis.[191]

d) Primary hyperoxaluria type I (PHI) is an autosomal recessive condition involving a deficiency of the enzyme alanine glyoxalate aminotransferase (AGT). There is an excess synthesis of oxalate and glycolate resulting in neph-rolithiasis, nephrocalcinosis, systemic oxalosis and death in childhood unless a combined hepatic and renal transplant is performed.[203] The AGT enzyme is expressed exclusively in the liver and successful prenatal diagnosis using fetal liver biopsy has recently been reported.[192]

Complications The risk of fetal loss secondary to ul-trasound guided invasive intra-uterine procedures is 1% to 2%. General experience suggests that despite the small numbers, it is a safe procedure.[189,191] Of 13 procedures there were seven affected fetuses which were terminated. All six continuing pregnancies delivered livebirths with no complication. Occasional transient bradycardia was the most common complication. No evidence of intraperitoneal bleeding was found at autopsy following liver biopsy in 18 fetuses,[188,189] but a small skin puncture scar was noted in one neonate.[191]

Tumour biopsy

Altered pattern of fetal organs at ultrasound examination enables the identification of a wide variety of masses within the fetus. Definitive diagnosis is important to assess the fetal prognosis and plan the subsequent obstetric manage-ment. In some of these lesions definitive diagnosis is only possible by histopathology, for which biopsy is required. Lung biopsy under ultrasound control has been used to investigate strongly reflective fetal lungs and successfully diagnose type III congenital adenomatoid malformation by demonstrating elastin deposition on light microscopy.[204]

Fetal muscle biopsy

This has been employed using a Tru-cut needle to exclude Duchenne muscular dystrophy in a patient in whom gene probes were uninformative. The presence of dystrophia was demonstrated in the muscle fibres by an immunoflu-orescent technique.[205]

Fetal kidney biopsy

Kidney biopsy during the second trimester has enabled prenatal diagnosis in a case at risk of congenital nephrosis, by demonstrating podocyte fusion in the cortical nephrons on electron microscopy.[206]

Aspiration of fetal urine

Evaluation of fetal renal function by ultrasonic appearance is unreliable. Consequently aspiration of fetal urine to as-sess renal function has assumed an important role now that prenatal urethral bypass (vesico-amniotic) shunting is an available treatment for life-threatening lower urinary tract

obstruction associated with posterior urethral valves.[207] Success with shunting depends on the selection of appro-priate cases.

Technique Ultrasound prior to the procedure is essen-tial. Firstly the lesion must be definitively diagnosed and other causes for cystic structures in the fetal pelvis and ab-domen excluded. Secondly, the level and extent of the urinary tract obstruction must be established (Ch. 17). Lastly any other structural abnormalities must be excluded: these occur in about 30% of cases.[155]

The appearance of the renal tract and the amount of am-niotic fluid should be accurately documented. However, renal function does not correlate either with the degree of pelvi-calyceal dilatation, nor the degree of cortical thin-ning. Renal cortical cysts and increased parenchymal reflectivity (Ch. 17, Fig. 11), have been reported to pre-dict dysplasia with a sensitivity of 73% and a specificity of 80%.[208] Oligohydramnios carries a poor prognosis,[209,210] as it is associated with lung hypoplasia. However, oligohydramnios may be due to a treatable cause such as urethral obstruction as well as reduced urine production or renal function.[211]

Ultrasound is used to locate the sampling site for aspi-ration and guide the needle to this point using a free-hand technique. Although bladder sampling is more common (Fig. 24), aspiration of dilated renal pelves enables each kidney to be evaluated independently.[212] As with other procedures, the approach to the fetus should be anterior or lateral with the fetus imaged in transverse section. Once in the amniotic cavity the needle is thrust into the fetus with one movement as touching the body promotes a reflex withdrawal. Urine is aspirated until the bladder or pelvis is seen to be completely empty on ultrasound.

After the procedure the fetal heart rate and sampling site(s) are assessed for any complications. Documented bladder filling 24 hours later is suggestive of subsequent urine production, but may be unreliable if there has been passive filling from a dilated upper urinary tract or if there is polyuric renal failure.

Using a sterile technique and local anaesthesia the fetal urine is aspirated using a 20 G spinal needle. The urine biochemistry is then compared to the normal reference ranges for gestational age[211] (Figs. 25 and 26). Sodium, cal-cium, phosphate levels and the sodium/creatinine ratio are correlated with renal dysplasia. Urine calcium gives the best sensitivity and sodium the best specificity (Table 6). Values of urinary sodium < 100 mmol/l, chloride < 90 mmol/l and osmolality < 210 mosm/l have been corre-lated with good renal function,[213] but these findings have been challenged,[214] probably because they were derived retrospectively from the outcome of fetuses with obstruc-tive uropathy and because it was falsely assumed that fetal urine biochemistry did not alter with gestation or with the disease process.[211]

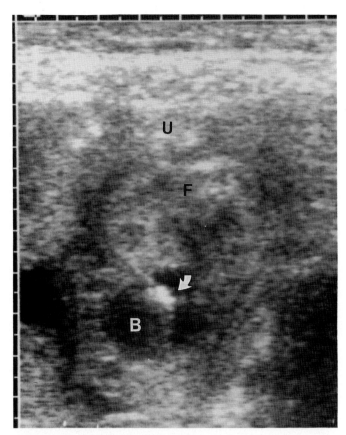

Fig. 24 Ultrasound guided fetal bladder aspiration showing needle tip (arrow) within the fetal bladder (B). F – fetus, U – uterus.

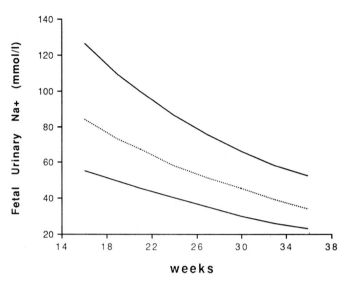

Fig. 25 Reference range for fetal urinary sodium (Na^+) throughout gestation: mean and 95% data intervals. (Reproduced from Nicolini et al[211] with permission.

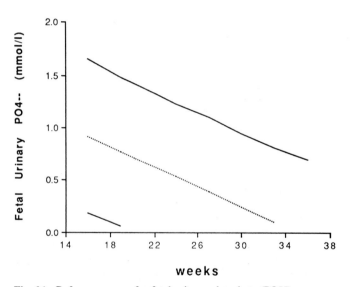

Fig. 26 Reference range for fetal urinary phosphate (PO^{--}) throughout gestation: mean and 95% data intervals. (Reproduced from Nicolini et al[211] with permission.

Timing The timing of fetal urinary aspiration to assess renal function in lower urinary tract obstruction depends on the time of onset and the extent of the lesion. The aim is to sample the urine prior to the onset of both renal dysplasia due to obstruction and pulmonary hypoplasia due to severe oligohydramnios. However, oligohydramnios is uncommon before the sixteenth to seventeenth week of gestation even in the complete absence of fetal micturition and it may be that in these early cases irreversible kidney damage has already occurred.[215] Alternatively, unless serial ultrasonic scans have proven a short duration of oligohydramnios this should be regarded as a poor prognostic sign.[209,210]

Indications The most frequent cause of lower urinary tract obstruction, and that with the best prognosis, is posterior urethral valves.[216] Urethral atresia and prune-belly syndrome are commonly associated.[207,210] Posterior urethral valves occur exclusively in males. The ultrasonic finding of bladder enlargement in females should therefore suggest urethral atresia which is unlikely to benefit from prenatal decompression.

Complications The risks of fetal urinary aspiration are similar to other fetal invasive procedures.

Table 6 Fetal urinary biochemical indices in the prediction of renal dysplasia

	Sensitivity	Specificity	K
Na^+	80%	80%	0.59
Ca^{++}	100%	60%	0.64
$PO4^{--}$	43%	62%	0.05
Na^+/Creatinine	64%	80%	0.42

K – Coehens Kappa value (statistical accuracy measurement)

Fetal thoracocentesis

This procedure has limited diagnostic use in utero as fluid obtained from cystic lesions within the lung does not have any distinguishing features. For example, the typical lymphocytosis or chylomicron content in a chylothorax is absent in the fetus because there is minimal gut absorption.[217]

Fetal diagnostic infusions

In severe oligohydramnios ultrasound visualisation of fetal anatomy is severely restricted due to lack of an acoustic window and abnormal fetal posture. Fluid instilled into either the amniotic[218] or the peritoneal[219] cavity can greatly improve the quality of the imaging.

Technique The finding of severe oligohydramnios necessitates a meticulous ultrasonic fetal examination to establish the aetiology, which is most commonly related to intra-uterine growth retardation or renal tract abnormalities, once preterm premature rupture of the membranes has been excluded. However, even with the improved resolution possible with trans-vaginal ultrasound, anatomical differentiation may still be difficult and false negative and false positive diagnoses of renal agenesis have been reported.[220]

For amnioinfusion ultrasound is used to identify a suitable entry point into the uterus. Care must be taken as echo-free areas suggestive of a small pocket of amniotic fluid may be umbilical cord: evaluation with Doppler (preferably colour) is a prerequisite. The needle is guided into the uterus under continuous ultrasound surveillance, and entry into the amniotic cavity is confirmed by observing injected saline dispersing around the fetus.

Following the procedure sonographic visibility is greatly improved and fetal movement facilitates the examination of fetal anatomy. Fetal breathing and swallowing are also commonly observed. As usual, the fetal heart rate should be checked.

This procedure should be performed under strict aseptic conditions and with antibiotic prophylaxis. A 20 G spinal needle is used and, before fluid instillation, aspiration with a 1 ml syringe will exclude the possibility of being in a vessel. Any fetal blood aspirated can be used to assess karyotype and blood gases. The amount of warm saline instilled depends on the amniotic fluid pressure, the resultant visibility and the gestational age of the fetus. Following the

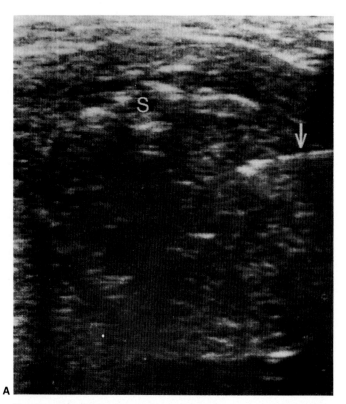
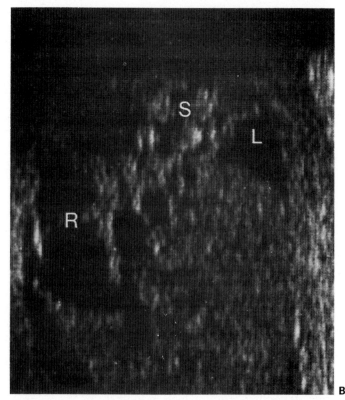

A   B

Fig. 27   Oligohydramnios and amnioinfusion. A: Ultrasound demonstrating oligohydramnios and the fetal abdomen in cross-section. No renal tissue is seen on either side of the fetal spine (S). The arrow indicates the needle inserted to instil saline. **B:** After the intraperitoneal infusion of saline, the right multicystic kidney (R), the liver and fluid in the position of the left kidney (L) are evident. (Reproduced from Nicolini et al[219] with permission from John Wiley and Sons.)

amnioinfusion leakage of fluid from the vagina confirms premature rupture of the membranes.

Occasionally ultrasound visualisation remains obscured despite amnioinfusion;[221] and another technique which may help clarify the fetal intra-abdominal and retroperitoneal anatomy is that of intraperitoneal saline infusion.[219] In particular renal agenesis may be diagnosed more accurately (Fig. 27).

Indications The current indication for performing amnioinfusion and/or peritoneal infusion is severe oligohydramnios or anhydramnios. Gembruch and Hansmann reported 50 such pregnancies in which the final diagnoses included Potter's syndrome, obstructive uropathy, cystic kidneys, Meckel syndrome, Cornelia de Lange syndrome, cytomegaly fetopathy, VATER association, triploidy, severe intra-uterine growth retardation and preterm premature rupture of the membranes.[218]

Complications The principal risks associated with amnioinfusion are rupture of the membranes and preterm labour, which have been reported in up to 10.5% of cases following a single procedure and in 28.9% overall.[218] Inadvertent fetal blood sampling at the time of amnioinfusion carries its own risks, such as arterial spasm and cord tamponade, and is of particular concern in these cases where poor visualisation inhibits the exact localisation of the needle tip. Other risks are similar to those for amniocentesis.

Intraperitoneal infusion will cause fetal heart rate changes if the intraperitoneal pressure is raised too high. Usually up to 100 ml can be infused safely.[219] Ultrasound guidance minimises fetal trauma from the procedure.

Intra-uterine pressure measurements

Intra-uterine pressure measurements during the antenatal period are technically simple to perform and are potentially useful in clinical practice. Accumulating evidence suggests that it is changes in intra-amniotic pressure rather than abnormalities of amniotic fluid volume that cause complications.[222–224] If this proves correct pressure measurements should be useful for both diagnosis and prognosis. Monitoring intravascular, intraperitoneal and intrapleural pressures during fetal therapy may improve the outcome.[222,225]

Technique Intra-amniotic pressure is measured using a saline filled catheter attached at one end to the needle in the amniotic cavity and at the other to a silicone strain gauge transducer (EM 750, Elcomatic Ltd, Glasgow, UK). The pressure scale is referenced to zero at the maternal skin surface. The output is then displayed on a chart recorder for 60 to 90 seconds to ensure stable readings which are free of artefact such as Braxton Hicks contractions and maternal respiratory movements. Normal amniotic fluid pressure increases slightly with advancing gestational age (Fig. 28).

Using a second needle and catheter fetal vascular or body

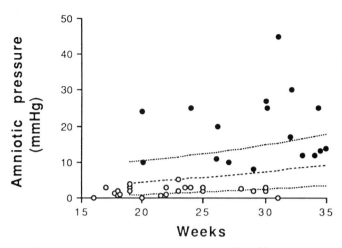

Fig. 28 Amniotic pressure in pregnancies complicated by polyhydramnios (closed circles) or oligohydramnios (open circles) shown against the normal range for gestation: mean and 95% data intervals. (Reproduced from Fisk et al[223] with permission from Elsevier Science Publishing Co.)

compartment pressures are obtained by measuring the differential from amniotic fluid by subtraction manometry.[222]

Indications Amniotic fluid aspiration in symptomatic polyhydramnios has traditionally focused on the volume seen and removed rather than the change in intra-amniotic pressure. The amniotic pressure is always above the normal mean for gestation in polyhydramnios (Fig. 28) and is correlated with the depth of the deepest pool and inversely with fetal pO_2.[223] Amniotic pressure is raised in all pregnancies with the deepest pool >15 cm and falls significantly with drainage. Pregnancies with raised pressures have a shorter interval to delivery.[223]

In oligohydramnios there is a reduction in intra-amniotic pressure (Fig. 28) and this is associated with pulmonary hypoplasia.[224] Amnioinfusion of normal saline in severe oligohydramnios will cause a significant rise in pressure.[222,223] From these data it seems that pressure monitoring is necessary during amnioinfusion and therapeutic amniocentesis.

Nicolini et al suggest a role for intraperitoneal pressure monitoring during intraperitoneal transfusion in patients with Rh alloimmunisation.[225] They report that basal intraperitoneal pressure is significantly lower than basal umbilical pressure and, during transfusions, is associated with fetal heart rate changes, the increment in intraperitoneal pressure in these cases being greater than in uncomplicated transfusions.

Raised intrapleural pressure has been found in association with fetal hydrothorax.[222] Further study is underway to determine whether intrapleural pressure is a useful predictor of the potential for lung re-expansion following pleuro-amniotic shunting[226] and the effect on pulmonary hypoplasia.

Fetal ECG waveform analysis

Clinical use of the fetal ECG in the assessment of wellbeing is limited to the analysis of changes in heart rate and heart rate variability. However, waveform changes such as ST segment elevation and increment in T wave amplitude reflect myocardial strain from hypoxia, anaemia, hypotension or fluid overload[227] and could provide useful information during FBS for growth retardation or transfusions for anaemia. Recent technological advances have made ECG waveform analysis possible during labour using a scalp electrode.[228] The same system has been adapted to record the fetal ECG directly at the time of FBS or intravascular transfusion performed through the intrahepatic umbilical vein.[145,229]

Contrast radiography

The use of radio-opaque contrast media is obsolete in amniography, fetography and intraperitoneal transfusion. However, occasionally, contrast X-rays help delineate structural abnormalities. In one case, ultrasound guided in-

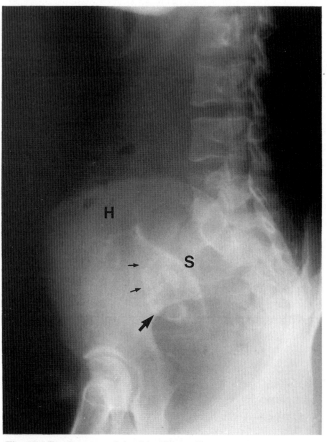

Fig. 29 Fetal contrast injection. X-ray of a maternal abdomen containing an 18 week fetus in whom dispersal of injected contrast throughout the pleural (small arrows) and peritoneal (large arrow) cavities confirmed congenital diaphragmatic hernia. H – head, S – spine.

jection of contrast medium into the fetal chest became dispersed throughout the peritoneal cavity (Fig. 29), proving that the lesion was a diaphragmatic hernia.

In the future, sonographic contrast media in the form of encapsulated microbubbles in suspension may help diagnose functional lesions such as ureteric reflux and cardiac abnormalities and further assist in our understanding of fetal pathophysiology.

Therapeutic procedures

Amniocentesis and amnioinfusion

Amniotic puncture can be used therapeutically to instil substances such as urea to induce second trimester abortion. Instillation of fetal nutrients or drugs has been practised. Therapeutic drainage of amniotic fluid in polyhydramnios was first described in 1919[81] but apart from reports documenting its use,[230,231] there is no controlled evidence as to its benefit. Fisk et al reported a series of patients with polyhydramnios in whom intra-amniotic pressure was measured.[223] Complications associated with the condition such as maternal discomfort and preterm labour only occurred in those with an elevated pressure, which in turn correlated with a deepest pool > 15 cm. Drainage is only indicated in this group of patients and only quite small volumes need to be removed to restore normal pressure. In this way complications of placental separation should be avoided. Recently medical treatment of polyhydramnios via maternal indomethacin has been used successfully,[232] but may lead to premature closure of the ductus arteriosus and/or cause fetal anuria.[233,234]

Therapeutic amnioinfusion to restore low intra-amniotic pressures to normal may have a role in the prevention of pulmonary hypoplasia in severe oligohydramnios and is under current investigation.[222–224]

Fetal transfusion

The first intra-uterine intravascular fetal blood transfusions were performed in the 1960s for severe Rhesus disease, and required hysterotomy and cannulation of the fetal femoral artery,[235] saphenous vein[236] or a chorionic plate vessel.[237] The high rates of fetal mortality and maternal morbidity associated with these techniques of open fetal transfusion prohibited their use. Instead, the more acceptable and less invasive technique of percutaneous intraperitoneal transfusion became the accepted method for performing transfusions in utero.

The procedure, first described by Liley in 1963,[238] requires an amniocentesis to inject urografin into the amniotic cavity with X-ray follow up to visualise the fetal bowel containing swallowed contrast medium. An epidural catheter was then inserted into the fetal peritoneal cavity via a 16 gauge Tuohy needle, and further X-ray films taken to ensure correct placement. Rhesus negative packed red cells were then transfused, and absorbed into the fetal circulation through the subdiaphragmatic lymphatics and the thoracic duct. Various modifications were introduced to improve the success of the technique, but it was only after the introduction of ultrasound that this was achieved. The risk of malignancy due to ionising radiation was also eliminated.

After two decades of intraperitoneal transfusion, the survival rates have improved dramatically from 24% to 56% in the decade to 1976 to 69% to 92% in the 1980s.[239-242] The principle factors which continued to limit the survival rates were an early gestational age at initial transfusion and the presence of hydrops fetalis. Thus the advent of fetoscopy fulfilled the continued interest in developing a direct intravascular route for transfusion.

In 1981, Rodeck et al reported on the first intravascular transfusion performed through an umbilical cord vessel using the fetoscope.[243] Three years later the same group published an overall survival rate of 72% in 25 severely affected Rhesus fetuses who underwent 77 fetoscopic intra-uterine transfusions.[244] In this series a survival rate of 84% was obtained amongst fetuses who had their first transfusion before 25 weeks, almost 50% of whom had hydrops at this early stage of gestation.

Subsequently the development of ultrasound guided percutaneous needling has simplified direct intravascular fetal transfusion and the technique most widely used now is modified from that described by Daffos et al[138] using the umbilical vein at the placental cord insertion.[245,160] Using this technique, Nicolaides et al[160] reported 21 fetuses, including 11 with hydrops, that had a total of 96 transfusions and a survival rate of 95%. Other sites which can be used for transfusion include the intrahepatic portion of the umbilical vein[143,144] and the fetal heart.[246] The advantages of transfusing intravascularly are summarised below:

— assess fetal blood group
— measure pre- and post-transfusion haematocrit
— time subsequent transfusions by % haematocrit fall/day
— perform before 20 weeks' gestation
— avoid lymphatic transport from peritoneal cavity
— reverse hydrops fetalis in utero
— continue treatment until pulmonary maturity confirmed.

Technique Weekly ultrasonic evaluation of the fetus remains an integral part of the management of Rh isoimmunisation and may detect fetal ascites, which is an early sign in the onset of hydrops (ascites, pericardial effusion, subcutaneous oedema, polyhydramnios and placentomegaly) thus prompting timely intervention. This applies both prior to the commencement of any intra-uterine therapy and after transfusions have begun. However, in the absence of hydrops, ultrasound measurements of abdominal circumference, head circumference, head/abdominal circumference ratio, intraperitoneal volume, extra- and intrahepatic vein diameters and placental thickness > 4 cm are not reliable in distinguishing mild from severe fetal haemolytic disease.[247,248]

The role of ultrasound in fetal procedures has already been described in this chapter.

a) Intravascular transfusion Fetal intravascular transfusion (IVT) is usually performed as an out patient procedure without maternal sedation. A fetal blood sample is taken in the usual manner using a 20 gauge spinal needle. If it is not appropriate to sample from the placental cord insertion, the needle is directed to the intrahepatic portion of the umbilical vein.[145] The fetal heart is rarely used due to the potentially dangerous complications such as asystole, haemopericardium and cardiac tamponade.[143] Prophylactic antibiotics are often given, but their benefit is unproven. Fetal movement during the IVT may cause needle displacement. Temporary paralysis may be achieved for about 2 hours using intramuscular or intravascular curare[144] or pancuronium bromide.[249]

Once a sample is obtained the fetal haematocrit is determined immediately using a Coulter counter. If this is 2 SD below the normal mean for gestation[160,161] (Fig. 30) the tip of the needle is kept in situ and a transfusion of fresh, concentrated (70% to 80%) Rh negative red cells, cross-matched with maternal blood, is given manually in 5 ml aliquots. Extension tubing connected to a three-way stopcock is attached to the needle (Fig. 31) to minimise movement of the needle after it is correctly placed. The fetal heart rate and the flow of the infused blood are monitored continually during the procedure by real time ultrasound.

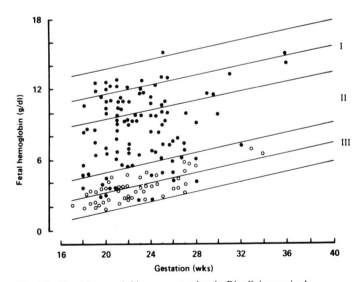

Fig. 30 Fetal haemoglobin concentration in Rh alloimmunised pregnancies with (open circles) and without (closed circles) fetal hydrops plotted on the normal range: mean and 95% data intervals. (Reproduced from Nicolaides et al[161] with permission from Lancet Ltd.)

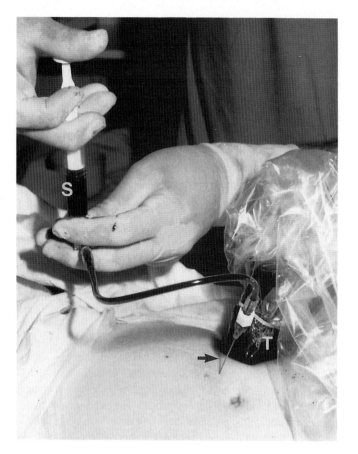

The amount of blood transfused depends on the initial haematocrit, the haematocrit of the donor blood and the gestational age. Nomograms have been calculated to provide an estimation of the volume of donor blood required to increase the fetal haematocrit to about 40%[160] (Fig. 32). Following the transfusion another fetal sample is aspirated to determine the actual haematocrit and further blood is given as necessary to bring the final value to 40% to 50%.

Two methods of IVT are in current use. A 'top up' or 'bolus' transfusion refers to the intravenous administration of blood into the fetus without removing any blood, and is the most commonly used technique. An 'exchange' transfusion consists of the administration and removal of approximately equal amounts of blood, the aim of which is to prevent hypervolaemia and further compromise of an already overburdened fetal myocardium, particularly in a severely hydropic fetus.[250,251] Clinically hypervolaemia has been of little concern, with reports of 'top up' transfusions of up to 100% to 150% of fetoplacental blood volume without any change in the fetal heart rate.[160,252] 'Top up' transfusions have the advantage of being simpler to per-

Fig. 31   Intravascular transfusion. Set-up for an ultrasound guided IVT in Rh disease showing needle (arrow) connected to an extension set and 3-way stop-cock for attaching syringe (S). The transducer is in a sterile plastic bag (T).

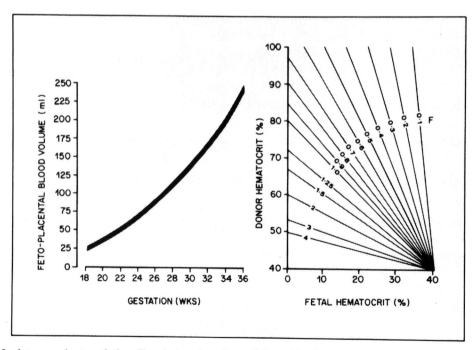

Fig. 32   Nomogram for intravascular transfusion. To calculate the volume of donor blood necessary to achieve a fetal haematocrit of 40%, the estimated fetoplacental blood volume (left, e.g. 100 ml at 27 weeks) is multiplied by F (right, e.g. 0.8 for a pre-transfusion haematocrit of 10% and a donor haematocrit of 80%). (Reproduced from Nicolaides et al[160] with permission from S Kager AG.)

form and of being completed in less than half the time it takes to do an 'exchange' transfusion, which decreases the probability of bacterial contamination, needle dislodgement and thrombosis in the umbilical vein. The fetus tolerates 'top up' transfusions given at a rate of 5 to 15 ml/min without obvious adverse effects[160] and only minor changes in acid-base and blood gas status.[253] Pressure increments in the umbilical vein of up to 12 mmHg have been recorded after transfusion without complication.[222,225]

b) Intraperitoneal transfusion Percutaneous ultrasound guided intraperitoneal transfusions are performed in the same way as the intravascular procedures, except that the needle is directed into the fetal abdominal cavity. Correct needle placement is verified in a hydropic fetus by aspirating ascitic fluid or by visualising sterile saline injected into the peritoneal cavity if there is no ascites. The amount of blood transfused is estimated by the empirical formula:

$$(\text{gestation in weeks} - 20) \times 10 \text{ ml}^{254}$$

and is transfused either at a rate of 5 to 15 ml/min with continual monitoring of the fetal heart rate or more slowly with a pump through an indwelling catheter.

Since the development of intravenous transfusions the intraperitoneal procedure has become second line therapy, mainly because of the inadequate absorption of erythrocytes from the peritoneal cavity in hydropic fetuses, so that in the moribund fetus IPT offers no hope.[255] However, it is very effective in the absence of hydrops, and may be used in combination with IVT to increase the total blood volume given to the fetus, thereby prolonging the interval between transfusions (up to 4 to 5 weeks) and reducing the total number of invasive procedures.[252,256]

Timing The first transfusion depends on the gestation at referral and the predicted severity of the disease. In general, for patients with a previous history of erythrocyte isoimmunisation, the first FBS and IVT are performed approximately 10 weeks prior to the earliest previous fetal or neonatal death, fetal transfusion, or birth of a severely affected baby, but not before 17 to 18 weeks' gestation.[160] It seems that neither fetal death nor hydrops occur before this gestation, presumably because the fetal reticuloendothelial system is too immature to destroy antibody-coated red cells. In patients without a previously affected pregnancy, the ideal time for the first procedure is after the fetus has become anaemic but before the onset of hydrops. Earlier sampling increases the risk of further maternal antibody production due to a fetomaternal bleed. Therefore FBS and IVT should be performed if the amniocentesis delta OD 450nm is worsening or if there is evidence of fetal hydrops.

The second transfusion is given within 2 weeks of the first because the rate of fall of haematocrit of each fetus is unpredictable.[256] This rate is on average 1% per day, but with a range from 0.2% to 3%.[160] The subsequent intervals can be planned depending on the rate of fall in the first interval and the degree of suppression of fetal erythropoiesis based on the Kleihauer-Betke test. Normally the subsequent transfusion is planned to prevent the development of hydrops by maintaining the fetal haematocrit above the critical level of one third of the normal mean for gestational age.[257]

Indications The conditions in which fetal transfusion may be required are:

a) red cell alloimmunisation (anti-D, c, Kell)
b) perinatal alloimmune thrombocytopenia
c) suppression of fetal erythropoiesis (parvovirus)
d) acute fetomaternal haemorrhage

a) Red cell alloimmunisation The most common cause of severe fetal haemolytic disease is Rhesus (Rh) anti-D antibodies developing in an Rh (D) negative mother with an Rh (D) positive fetus. Although the incidence of Rh alloimmunisation has been greatly reduced by the use of prophylactic Rh immunoglobulin, there are still 600 to 700 new Rh (D) immunisations per year in the United Kingdom.[258] The perinatal mortality for England and Wales due to Rh alloimmunisation is estimated at 5.0 per 100 000 births after 28 weeks[259] and is double if losses before 28 weeks are included. Once sensitisation has occurred and the fetus has developed severe anaemia and/or hydrops, prolonging life in utero is dependent on intra-uterine therapy until delivery is safe.

Although generally less serious than anti-D, anti-c antibodies can be associated with an anaemia severe enough to cause hydrops and the principles of management are similar to those in Rh (D) haemolytic disease. With anti-c confusion arises because this is an Rh antibody developing in a Rh-D positive woman. The incidence has been reported as 70 per 100 000 pregnant women.[260]

Anti-Kell antibodies can also cause severe anaemia and hydropic changes in the fetus; a recent survey showed the frequency of affected neonates to be 10 per 100 000.[261] Observation in a few cases of anti-Kell anaemia has shown that the percentage of reticulocytes in the fetal blood is much lower for a given haemoglobin level than that associated with anti-D.[262] In addition the amniotic fluid bilirubin concentration does not rise significantly despite the severity of the anaemia.[263] Though based on only a few patients, this suggests that the anti-Kell antibody causes suppression of effective erythroblastosis in the fetus rather than haemolysis,[67] and therefore the conventional criteria for management of fetal alloimmunisation should not be applied. Instead blood should be sampled early for Kell grouping and assessment of anaemia, followed by a combination of serial FBS and frequent ultrasound screening if immediate transfusion is not indicated.

b) Perinatal alloimmune thrombocytopenia Perinatal alloimmune thrombocytopenia mediated by PLA-1 antibody, causes a high rate of morbidity and mortality through intracranial haemorrhage. The insult may occur during intra-uterine life and in mothers at risk intra-uterine intravascular platelet transfusion may be used to prevent neonatal pathology.[167,264]

c) Suppression of fetal erythropoiesis   Parvovirus B19 infection during pregnancy causes fetal hydrops and subsequent pregnancy loss. 26% of fetuses developed hydrops following serologically documented maternal infection, which may be subclinical.[265] Fetal infection seems to cause inhibition of erythrocyte precursors leading to a severe aplastic crisis and subsequent hydrops.[266] Successful in utero therapy by serial intravascular blood transfusions has been reported in five cases with normal neonatal outcome.[265,267]

d) Acute fetomaternal haemorrhage   Life-threatening fetal anaemia subsequent to massive fetomaternal haemorrhage is uncommon. Recently two case reports of successful treatment by intra-uterine transfusion have been published[268,269] suggesting that Kleihauer-Betke stains on maternal blood are useful in the investigation of non-immune hydrops and fetal compromise. Intra-uterine death has also occurred following successful transfusion and suggests recurrent haemorrhage.[270]

Complications   At Queen Charlotte's Hospital, London from 1986 to 1990, 99 fetuses underwent 324 transfusions. The fetal loss rate was 5.6% per transfusion, the greatest risk occurring during the first transfusion. An initial transfusion before 20 weeks carries a risk of fetal loss of 14% whilst after 30 weeks this falls to 8% (Fig. 33). The survival rate of non-hydropic and hydropic fetuses is the same at 80%.

Chorio-amnionitis or ruptured membranes may result in spontaneous abortion or preterm labour. Fetomaternal haemorrhage complicates 50% to 75% of treated pregnancies, particularly after trans-placental passage of the needle,[159] and may further compromise this and future pregnancies.

Fetal shunting procedures

The concept of fetal therapy was established with the development of successful in utero transfusion. Improvements in ultrasound technology have enabled the identification of fetal structural anomalies that might be amenable to intra-uterine treatment. The aim of such therapy is to halt the progression in utero of a condition that is fatal or causes severe handicap at birth if left untreated. Obstructive uropathy, hydrocephalus, hydrothorax, diaphragmatic hernia, aortic stenosis and neural tube defects are all potentially correctable lesions. Prior to considering therapy the condition must be accurately diagnosed and there should be evidence, particularly from experimental animal studies, that intervention can improve the outcome.

In 1982 a group of early investigators in this field met at a conference sponsored by the Kroc Foundation to discuss the management of the fetus with a correctable congenital defect.[271] The participants set guidelines and selection criteria for the specific treatment of obstructive uropathy and hydrocephalus in utero:

Criteria for shunting fetal obstructive uropathy

— urethral obstruction
— oligohydramnios or reduction of amniotic fluid on serial scans
— adequate renal function
— normal karyotype

Criteria for ventriculo-amniotic shunting

— isolated ventriculomegaly with no other serious central nervous system abnormalities on ultrasound
— negative viral studies
— normal karyotype.

They suggested that any fetus being considered for therapy must be a singleton less than 32 weeks with a normal karyotype and without coexisting anomalies which might worsen the prognosis. The therapy should be provided by a multidisciplinary team and the patient must be prepared to return for follow up.

An International Fetal Surgery Registry (IFSR) was established to record the results of fetal surgery and to report on the outcome of all known cases treated.[271] In 1985 a natural history registry was added so that treated and untreated cases could be compared. The registry data were published in 1986[207] at which time 21 centres from seven countries had contributed 124 cases; 114 of those cases involved treatment of either obstructive uropathy (73 cases) or hydrocephalus (41 cases).

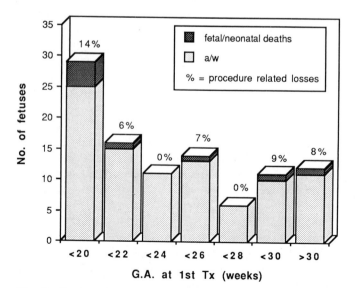

Fig. 33   Fetal survival rate following intravascular transfusion. Fetal survival rate (%) following first transfusion in relation to gestational age.

Obstructive uropathy   In 1982 Golbus et al reported the placement of a suprapubic catheter in a 32 week fetus with lower urinary tract obstruction.[272] In the period 1982 to 1985 73 vesico-amniotic shunts were placed in fetuses with lower urinary tract obstructive uropathy.[207] The mean age at the time of therapy was 24.2 weeks (range: 17 to 34). Chromosomal abnormalities were found in six (8.2%) of fetuses. All these fetuses were electively terminated subsequent to catheter placement, as were five others because of ultrasound evidence of renal dysplasia. The survival rate in the 62 continuing pregnancies was 48.4% and depended on the type of obstructive uropathy and in particular to pulmonary hypoplasia.

Posterior urethral valve syndrome was the most common diagnosis and had a 76.5% survival rate. This compares favourably with the 55% survival rate recently reported in neonates with untreated posterior urethral valves[209] and suggests that in utero therapy may be of benefit in this condition. All three fetuses with 'prune belly' syndrome survived but showed no anatomical evidence of urethral obstruction. Female fetuses with urethral atresia, both isolated and with a persistent cloaca, had the worst survival rate at 20%.

Selection for intra-uterine therapy depends initially on accurate ultrasound diagnosis of urethral obstruction and is covered in Chapter 17. Specific diagnosis of posterior urethral valves should be possible by determining male genitalia and visualising a dilated proximal urethra (Fig. 34). These signs may also be present in 'prune belly' syndrome which is uncommonly associated with urethral obstruction and is therefore unlikely to benefit from prenatal shunting.[215]

Diagnosis may be difficult in the presence of severe oligohydramnios and intra-amniotic[218] or fetal intra-abdominal[219] fluid instillation, as described in this chapter is recommended to improve ultrasound visualisation of fetal anatomy and exclude any associated structural anomalies. Chromosomal abnormalities are diagnosed by fetal blood sampling. To select those appropriate for shunting further fetal evaluation focuses on the assessment of renal function as prenatal recognition of pulmonary hypoplasia is difficult.[215]

Most intra-uterine fetal shunting procedures have used ultrasound guided percutaneous insertion of vesico-amniotic catheters. In cases of oligohydramnios catheter introduction is preceded by amnioinfusion to ensure that the fetal external abdominal wall is well-visualised. A trocar and cannula is then introduced through the maternal abdomen and uterus and directed into the fetal bladder through the anterior abdominal wall. Once the needle tip is seen inside the bladder the trocar is removed and the shunt is loaded into the cannula; the technique is illustrated in Figure 35. Following successful shunt insertion the catheter is seen as a pair of bright lines within the fetal pelvis and the bladder cannot be identified ultrasonically as it is continuously empty (Fig. 36). The distal end of the shunt is similarly seen protruding from the fetal anterior abdominal wall in the presence of amniotic fluid (Fig. 36). Reaccumulation of amniotic fluid is not a specific index of good renal function[215] as at Queen Charlotte's Hospital we have observed an adequate volume of amniotic fluid in three cases later found to have renal dysplasia. Thus the concept of a 'diagnostic catheter' is no longer supported by our experience.

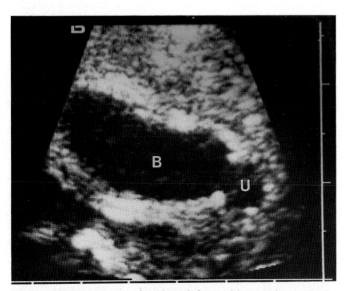

Fig. 34   Ultrasound scan of a 14 week fetus with posterior urethral valves, enlarged bladder (B) and dilated proximal urethra (U).

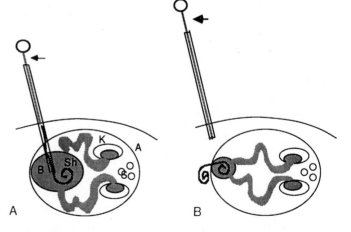

Fig. 35   Technique of bladder shunting. A: Cross-section of fetus in amniotic cavity (A), showing spine (S), kidneys (K) and dilated bladder (B). Insertion of proximal end of double pigtail catheter (Sh) is performed with the short introducer (thin arrow). **B:** The shunt insertion is completed by withdrawing the cannula into the amniotic cavity and discharging the distal end of the catheter with the long introducer (thick arrow).

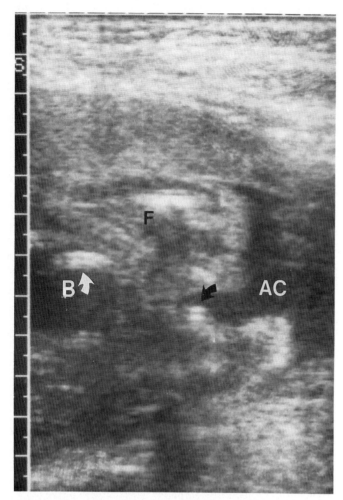

Fig. 36 Vesico-amniotic shunt in situ. Ultrasound scan of a 22 week fetus (F) with a vesico-amniotic shunt in situ. Proximal catheter (white arrow) within the fetal bladder (B), distal catheter (black arrow) in the amniotic cavity (AC).

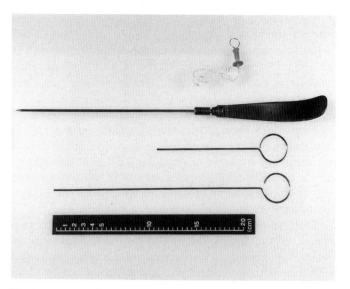

Fig. 37 Double pigtail catheter and insertion set, Rocket of London.

Weekly follow up to assess the volume of amniotic fluid, urinary tract dilatation and shunt location are recommended as the catheter may become blocked or dislodged, although this is not common with the instrument that we have designed (Fig. 37).

Fetal shunt placement is an outpatient technique performed under aseptic conditions with prophylactic antibiotic cover. Local anaesthesia is usually sufficient, although sedation is sometimes required.

Two different shunts have been used by most centres. The 'Harrison Fetal Bladder Stent' is made of polyethylene and manufactured by Cook Urological (Spencer, Indiana, USA). It has side holes in both ends, a curled end in the bladder and a flare in the amniotic cavity. Because it is introduced outside the needle placement may be difficult.[273] The Rocket catheter (London, UK), is a double pigtail with holes in both ends, and is introduced inside a cannula (Fig. 37). The amniotic coil is perpendicular to the rest of the catheter and lies flat against the anterior wall so as to minimise the risk of removal by the fetus.

Experience Although inadequate patient selection is probably the prime reason for the poor results reported by the International Fetal Surgery Registry, 7% of perinatal losses were attributable to the shunting procedure and in only 8.2% was the catheter correctly placed at the first attempt.[207] Elder et al reported a complication rate of 44% of attempted shunt placements or urine aspiration.[274] This high complication rate is probably related to the paucity of experience, as most centres reported only one case treated.

Complications The procedure related fetal loss rate in the 62 continuing pregnancies reported to the International Fetal Surgery Registry was 5% comprising two stillbirths due to fetal trauma and one neonatal death due to respiratory distress syndrome following premature labour induction.[207] Of the 29 neonatal deaths pulmonary hypoplasia was the cause in 27 while only one died from chronic renal failure. The quality of life in the survivors is good, with only two having a chronic illness. A controlled trial to test the efficacy of prenatal shunting for obstructive uropathy is needed.

Hydrocephalus In 1981 Birnholz and Frigoletto reported the first fetus treated in utero for hydrocephalus.[275] Ventriculocentesis was performed six times under ultrasound guidance and at birth the baby had multiple undiagnosed associated abnormalities and a poor outcome. Clewell et al developed an indwelling ventriculo-amniotic shunt which was first placed in a fetus with a family history of X-linked aqueductal stenosis.[276] Delivery at 34 weeks after shunt occlusion resulted in a child with severely delayed neurological development.

41 treated cases of hydrocephalus were reported to the International Fetal Surgery Registry from 1982 to 1985.[207]

Of these 39 were treated with long-term ventriculo-amniotic shunt placement and two with serial ventriculocentesis. The mean gestational age at the time of treatment was 27 weeks (range: 23 to 33). Although 83% survived, follow up between 2 and 14 months confirmed 65% to be abnormal. 18 treated fetuses (53%) have severe handicap with developmental quotients less than 60. Five of these infants have cortical blindness, three have a seizure disorder and two have spastic diplegia.

Aqueductal stenosis was the most common form of fetal hydrocephalus to be treated (77%), and was the diagnosis in the only neurologically normal fetuses in the series. Of the 32 cases with this diagnosis 37.5% are normal, 44% have a severe handicap and 12.5% died from complications due to the treatment. Other cases of hydrocephalus which were inappropriately shunted included Dandy-Walker syndrome, Arnold-Chiari malformation, porencephalic cyst, holoprosencephaly and three cases with associated lethal abnormalities.

Serial ultrasound evidence of a persistently elevated lateral ventricular width to hemisphere width ratio (LVW/HW) (Ch. 16) has been shown to be a reliable predictor of ventriculomegaly.[277] However, methods used to establish the cause of ventriculomegaly and exclude associated central nervous system and other structural anomalies are not so reliable.[278,279] In the series reported to the International Fetal Surgery Registry, 22% had undiagnosed associated abnormalities.[207]

The principles of ultrasound guided shunt placement are similar to those described for obstructive uropathy except that the needle and trocar are directed into the fetal lateral ventricle. Measurements of pressure within the amniotic cavity and fetal ventricle should be taken during placement of the needle, as shunting is only of benefit in cases with elevated intracranial pressure. Ultrasonic location of the catheter ends determines the correct placement and should be accompanied by a reduction in the LVW/HW ratio. Obstruction or dislodgement is diagnosed by a rapid increase in the LVW/HW ratio.

The most commonly used shunt was the 'Denver shunt', which contains a one way valve to prevent sudden decompression of the ventricles and back flow of amniotic fluid and was held in position by rubber flanges.[276] It has now been withdrawn from production so that there is no currently available shunt to treat prenatal hydrocephalus.

Risks The procedure related fetal loss rate reported to the International Fetal Surgery Registry was 10%: one stillbirth due to trauma and three neonatal deaths following prematurity due to chorio-amnionitis.[207] There were also considerable problems in keeping the shunts in position and in maintaining patency.

Manning et al compared the registry statistics for treated aqueductal stenosis with those managed expectantly in the literature.[207] In the registry's group 87.5% survived but only 37.5% were normal. In the untreated group only 40% survived but 75% were normal at follow up. Fetal intervention may improve survival at the expense of severe handicap, and as a consequence prenatal treatment of hydrocephalus has been abandoned. Challenges for the future include the prenatal assessment of neurological function and improvements in shunt design.

Hydrothorax Isolated fetal hydrothorax developing in the early mid-trimester has a high mortality from pulmonary hypoplasia (Fig. 38).[280] In addition, the raised intrathoracic pressure may compromise cardiac return and cause hydrops, which also causes high perinatal mortality. Decompression by thoracocentesis may be successful,[217]

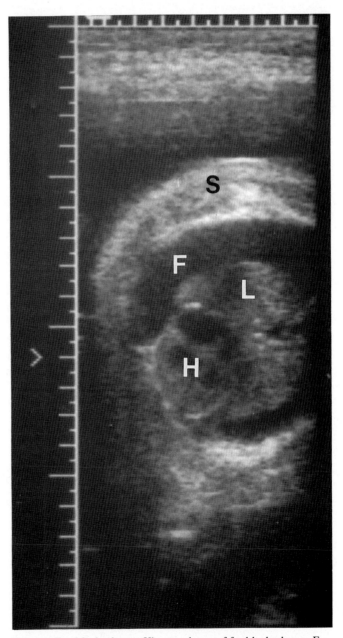

Fig. 38 Fetal hydrothorax. Ultrasound scan of fetal hydrothorax. F – fluid, L – lung, H – heart, S – subcutaneous oedema.

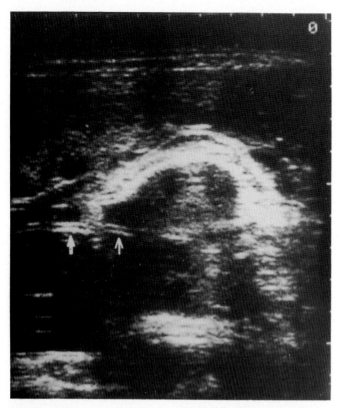

Fig. 39 Pleuro-amniotic shunt in situ. Ultrasound of a 32 week fetus with a pleuro-amniotic shunt in situ showing the intrapleural (thin arrow) and extrapleural (thick arrow) portions. The effusions have drained and the lungs re-expanded. (Reproduced from Rodeck et al[226] with permission from Massachusetts Medical Society.)

but rapid reaccumulation of fluid usually necessitates serial drainage. Pleuro-amniotic shunts have been inserted with successful neonatal outcome in isolated hydrothoraces[281,282] and Rodeck et al reported good neonatal outcome in three of five cases associated with hydrops.[226] The two that died had pulmonary hypoplasia and re-expansion of the lungs did not occur after insertion of the shunt.

Congenital chylothorax may be the primary cause but is difficult to diagnose prenatally. Prior to shunting chromosomal and structural abnormalities must be excluded and viral studies should also be performed. The shunt used is a double pigtail catheter (Rocket, London, UK) (Fig. 37), inserted under ultrasound guidance into the pleural cavity (Fig. 39). The risks are difficult to assess as only small numbers are available. However, fetal loss, trauma, premature labour, infection and repeat procedures due to dislodgement and obstruction are possible. Care must be taken post-delivery to clamp the shunt so as not to cause a pneumothorax.

Selective fetocide

Selective fetocide to reduce the number of fetuses in a multiple pregnancy is often the only option to achieve the birth of a healthy child. The ethics of fetocide are controversial, but as the intent is to promote the birth of the normal child, ethical approval should be justified as long as it is performed prior to the legal limit for termination and for medical, not social indications.[283] It may be performed via hysterotomy[284] or guided by fetoscopy.[285] Most selective terminations utilise ultrasound guided methods.[286–294]

Technique In multiple pregnancies where not all the fetuses are affected by a fetal genetic or structural abnormality ('discordant pregnancy') ultrasound has a major diagnostic role, either directly or by utilising ultrasound guided procedures. Prior to second trimester fetocide exclusion of monochorionicity is crucial, as death of the normal twin has occurred in all but one attempt.[295] Sonographic display of a thin septum suggests monochorionicity, whereas a thicker more easily seen membrane indicates dichorionicity. Fetal angiography has been used unsuccessfully in an attempt to determine vascular connections in monozygotic twins discordant for hydrocephalus.[291] A more successful alternative is to transfuse adult blood into the circulation of the affected fetus and then sample the unaffected one, using the Kleihauer-Betke test to check for adult red cells.[296]

Prior to fetocide the affected twin must be identified. This is not difficult where the fetuses are of different sexes or where there is a structural abnormality. However, in many cases it is the orientation of the fetal sacs within the uterus that distinguishes them, so this must be carefully documented at the time of initial diagnosis.

Fetal asystole is induced by cardiac puncture under continuous ultrasound guidance. A transabdominal approach is most common, but trans-vaginal aspiration has also been used in the first trimester.[297] Asystole is documented by ultrasound. The procedure is repeated if the first attempt is unsuccessful or if more than one fetus is to be terminated.

A scan is performed the next day to confirm the viability of the normal fetus. Serial scans are recommended throughout pregnancy to follow up the normal fetus and document the resorption of the affected one.

Selective fetocide is performed as an aseptic outpatient technique, with optional use of maternal and/or fetal sedation and antibiotics. The techniques which have successfully accomplished fetocide in the second trimester are exsanguination,[286,287] air embolisation,[285,288,289] pericardial tamponade[290] and intracardiac potassium chloride injection.[291,292] First trimester selective reduction has been achieved using a combination of sac aspiration and pericardial needling[293,294,297] or by pericardial injection of potassium chloride.[292,294]

Timing The recommended gestational age to begin performing first trimester reduction is 10 weeks, when the risk of background spontaneous loss is less than earlier in gestation.[292] Second trimester fetocide must be performed within the legal limits for fetal termination.

Indications In multiple pregnancies discordant for fetal abnormality selective fetocide offers the option of delivery of a normal infant without the birth of the affected one, and for some parents avoids the dilemma of terminating the entire pregnancy. Second trimester procedures have been successfully carried out in dizygotic pregnancies discordant for Down's syndrome, trisomy 18, Tay-Sachs disease, Hurler syndrome, San Fillipo A, haemophilia A, autosomal recessive microcephaly, isolated hydrocephalus and spina bifida.[285-288,290] More recently first trimester diagnosis via chorionic villus biopsy has enabled selective fetocide during the first trimester.

Multifetal pregnancy, in which there is an unacceptably high risk of spontaneous abortion or poor perinatal outcome, is another indication for first trimester selective termination.[292-294] The most common cause for this is the overzealous use of ovulation induction agents.[293]

Complications Selective reduction in monozygotic pregnancies almost uniformly leads to death in the normal twin[295] and theoretically could also risk embolic damage in the normal twin should it survive.[292] For these reasons selective reduction is contra-indicated in monozygotic gestations, unless performed by surgical removal or circulatory ablation. Although these complications could occur in dizygotic pregnancies they are very uncommon. Infection and maternal coagulopathy are potentially serious problems, but have not been reported following selective reduction. Abortion and preterm labour may be increased.

Fetomaternal haemorrhage does occur, so anti-D immunoglobulin must be given where appropriate. After first trimester procedures the sustained rise in maternal serum alpha-fetoprotein prohibits screening for neural tube defects.[293]

Conclusions

With the advent of high resolution ultrasound invasive intra-uterine procedures have become readily available. These relatively low-risk techniques allow extensive investigation and occasionally treatment of the fetus. In a society that is continually demanding improvements in perinatal outcome, these procedures will enable further understanding of fetal physiology and pathology. Specialised training is needed to acquire the necessary skills; however, it is the responsibility of every obstetrician to be aware of the scope of prenatal diagnosis and therapy, so that their patients benefit from appropriate referral.

Acknowledgements

JV is the recipient of a Fotheringham Research Fellowship from the Royal Australian College of Obstetricians and Gynaecologists and a RNSH Medical Board Centenary Fellowship from the Royal North Shore Hospital, Sydney, Australia.

REFERENCES

1 Hahnemann N, Mohr J. Genetic diagnosis in the embryo by means of biopsy from extra-embryonic membranes. Bull Eur Soc Human Genet 1968; 2: 23–29
2 Hahnemann N, Mohr J. Bull Eur Soc Hum Genet 1969; 3: 47–54
3 Kullander S, Sandahl B. Fetal chromosome analysis after transcervical placental biopsies during early pregnancy. Acta Obstet Gynecol Scand 1973; 52: 355–359
4 Tietung Hospital of Anshan Iron and Steel Co; Department of Obstetrics and Gynaecology. Fetal sex prediction by sex chromatin of chorionic villi cells during early pregnancy. Chin Med J 1975; 1: 117–126
5 Williamson R, Eskdale J, Coleman D V, Niazi N, Loeffler F E, Modell B. Direct gene analysis of chorionic villi, a possible technique for the first trimester diagnosis of haemoglobinopathies. Lancet 1981; ii: 1125–1127
6 Niazi M, Coleman D V, Loeffler F E. Trophoblast sampling in early pregnancy. Culture of rapidly dividing cells from immature placental villi. Br J Obstet Gynaecol 1981; 1: 1081–1085
7 Kazy Z, Rozovsky I S, Bakharev V A. Chorion biopsy in early pregnancy: a method of early prenatal diagnosis for inherited disorders. Prenat Diagn 1982; 2: 39–45
8 Simoni G, Brambati B, Danesino C, et al. Efficient direct chromosome analysis and enzyme determinations from chorionic villi samples in the first trimester of pregnancy. Hum Genet 1983; 63: 349–357
9 Rhine S A, Palmer C G, Thompson T. A simple first trimester alternative to amniocentesis for prenatal diagnosis. Birth Defects Orig Art 1977; Ser XII 3D: 231–247
10 Goldberg M F, Chen A T L, Young W A, Reidy J A. First trimester fetal chromosome diagnosis using endocervical lavage: a negative evaluation. Am J Obstet Gynecol 1980; 138: 435–440

11 Kazy Z, Stigar A M. Kozvetlin Real-time (ultrahang) kontroll melletti chorion biopsy. Orv Het 1980; 121: 2765–2766
12 Old J M, Ward R H T, Karagozlu F, Petrou M, Modell B, Weatherall D J. First trimester fetal diagnosis for haemoglobinopathies: three cases. Lancet 1982; ii: 1413–1416
13 Goosens M, Dumez Y, Kaplan Y, et al. Prenatal diagnosis of sickle cell anaemia in the first trimester of pregnancy. N Engl J Med 1983; 309: 831–833
14 Ward R H T, Modell B, Petriu M, Karagozlou F, Douratsos E. A method of chorionic villus sampling in the first trimester of pregnancy under real-time ultrasonic guidance. BMJ 1983; 286: 1542–1544
15 Rodeck C H, Nicolaides K H, McKenzie C M, Gosden C M, Gosden J R. A single-operator technique for first trimester chorion biopsy. Lancet 1983; ii: 1340–1341
16 Horwell D H, Loeffler F E, Coleman D V. Assessment of a transcervical technique for chorionic villus biopsy in the first trimester of pregnancy. Br J Obstet Gynaecol 1983; 90: 196–198
17 Lui D T Y, Mitchell J, Johnson J, Wass D M. Trophoblast sampling by blind transcervical aspiration. Br J Obstet Gynaecol 1983; 90: 1119–1123
18 Gosden J R, Mitchell A R, Gosden C M, Rodeck C H, Morsman J M. Direct vision chorion biopsy and chromosome-specific DNA probes for determination of fetal sex in first trimester prenatal diagnosis. Lancet 1982; ii: 1416–1419
19 Alvarez H. Diagnosis of hydatidiform mole by transabdominal placental biopsy. Am J Obstet Gynecol 1966; 95: 538–541
20 Smidt-Jensen S, Hahnemann N. Transabdominal fine needle biopsy from chorionic villi in the first trimester. Prenat Diagn 1984; 4: 163–169
21 Jackson L G. Chorion villus sampling. Newsletter 1989, 31

January, No 27, Thomas Jefferson University, Philadelphia, USA

22 Maxwell D, Lilford R, Czepulkowski B, Heaton D, Coleman D. Transabdominal chorionic villus sampling. Lancet 1986; i: 123–126

23 Rodeck C H. unpublished

24 Hogge W A, Schonberg S A, Golbus M S. Prenatal diagnosis by chorionic villus sampling: lessons of the first 600 cases. Prenat Diagn 1985; 5: 393–400

25 Mikkelsen M. Cytogenetic findings in first trimester chorionic villi biopsies: a collaborative study. In: Fraccaro M, Simoni G, Brambati B. eds. First trimester fetal diagnosis. Berlin: Springer-Verlag. 1985: p 109–120

26 Nicolaides K H, Soothill P W, Rodeck C H, Warren R C. Why confine chorionic villus (placental) biopsy to the first trimester? Lancet 1986; i: 543–544

27 Brambati B, Oldrini A, Ferrazzi E, Lanzani A. Chorionic villus sampling: an analysis of the obstetric experience of 1000 cases. Prenat Diagn 1987; 7: 157–169

28 Brambati B, Lanzani A, Oldrini A. Transabdominal chorionic villus sampling. Clinical experience of 1159 cases. Prenat Diagn 1988; 8: 609–617

29 Warren R C, Rodeck C H. Experience with a silver cannula for transcervical chorion villus sampling. Contr Gynae Obstet 1986; 15: 32–40

30 Smidt-Jensen S, Hahnemann N. Transabdominal chorionic villus sampling for fetal genetic diagnosis. Technical and obstetrical evaluation of 100 cases. Prenat Diagn 1988; 8: 7–17

31 Rosevear S K. Placental biopsy. Br J Hosp Med 1989; 41: 334–348

32 Mikkelsen M, Ayme I. Chromosomal findings in chorionic villi. A collaborative study. Proceedings of the 7th International Congress of Human Genetics. Berlin: Springer-Verlag. 1987

33 Gregson N, Seabright M. Handling chorionic villi for direct chromosome studies. Lancet 1983; ii: 1491

34 Simoni G, Terzoli G, Romitti L. Fetal karyotyping by direct chromosome preparation. In: Brambati B, Simoni G, Fabro S. eds. Chorionic villus sampling. New York: Marcel Dekker. p 99–117

35 Therkelsen A J, Jensen P K A, Hertz J M, Smidt-Jensen S, Hahnemann N. Prenatal cytogenetic diagnosis after transabdominal chorionic villus sampling in the first trimester. Prenat Diagn 1988; 8: 19–31

36 Czepulkowski B H, Heaton D E, Kearney L U, Rodeck C H, Coleman D V. Chorionic villus culture for first trimester diagnosis of chromosome defects: evaluation by two London centres. Prenat Diagn 1986; 6: 271–282

37 Cooke H M G, Penketh R J A, Delhanty J D A. An evaluation of maternal cell contamination in cultures of chorionic villi for the prenatal diagnosis of chromosome abnormalities. Clin Genet 1986; 30: 485–493

38 Olsen S, Buckmaster J, Bissonnette J, Magenis E. Comparison of maternal and fetal chromosome heteromorphisms to monitor maternal cell contamination in chorionic villus samples. Prenat Diagn 1987; 7: 413–417

39 Williams J, Medearis A L, Chu W H, Kovacs G D, Kaback M M. Maternal cell contamination in cultured chorionic villi: comparison of chromosome Q-polymorphisms derived from villi, fetal skin and maternal lymphocytes. Prenat Diagn 1987; 7: 315–322

40 Roberts E, Duckett D P, Lang G D. Maternal cell contamination in chorionic villus samples assessed by direct preparations and three different culture methods. Prenat Diagn 1988; 8: 635–640

41 Simoni G, Rossella F, Lalatta F, Fraccaro M. Maternal metaphases in direct preparation from chorionic villi and in cultures of villus cells. (letter) Hum Genet 1986; 72: 104

42 Hogge W A, Schonberg S A, Golbus M S. Chorionic villus sampling: Experience of the first 1000 cases. Am J Obstet Gynecol 1986; 154: 1249–1252

43 Simoni G, Gimelli G, Cuoco C, et al. First trimester fetal karyotyping: one thousand diagnoses. Hum Genet 1986; 72: 203–209

44 le Schot N J, Wolf H, Verjaal M, et al. Chorionic villi sampling: cytogenetic and clinical findings in 500 pregnancies. BMJ 1987; 295: 407–410

45 Callen D F, Korban G, Dawson G, et al. Extra-embryonic fetal karyotype discordance during diagnostic chorionic villus sampling. Prenat Diagn 1988; 8: 453–460

46 Worton R G, Stern R. A Canadian collaborative study of mosaicism in amniotic fluid cell cultures. Prenat Diagn 1987; 4: 131–144

47 Heim S, Kristofferson U, Mandahl N, et al. Chromosome analysis in 100 cases of first trimester trophoblast sampling. Clin Genet 1985; 27: 451–457

48 Eichenbaum S Z, Krumins E J, Fortune D W, Duke J. False-negative finding on chorionic sampling. Lancet 1986; ii: 391

49 Martin A O, Elias S, Rosinsky B, Bombard A T, Simpson J L. False-negative finding on chorionic villus sampling. Lancet 1986; ii: 391–392

50 Linton G, Lilford R J. False-negative finding on chorionic sampling. Lancet 1986; ii: 630

51 Simoni G, Fraccaro M, Gimelli G, Maggi F, Bricarelli F D. False-positive and false-negative findings on CVS (letter). Prenat Diagn 1987; 7: 671–672

52 Wirtz A, Seidel H, Brusis E, Murken J. Another false-negative finding on placental sampling (letter). Prenat Diagn 1988; 8: 321

53 Schulze B, Miller K. Chromosomal mosaicism and maternal cell contamination in chorionic villi cultures. Clin Genet 1986; 30: 239–240

54 Verjaal M, Leschot N J, Wolf H, Treffers P E. Karyotypic differences between cells from placenta and other fetal tissues. Prenat Diagn 1987; 7: 343–348

55 Ferguson-Smith M A, Yates J R W. Maternal age specific rates for chromosome aberrations and factors influencing them: report of a collaborative European study on 52965 amniocentesis. Prenat Diagn 1984; 4: 5–44 (special issue)

56 Mikkelson M. Chromosome analysis on chorionic villi. In: Rodeck C H. ed. Ballieres clinical obstetrics and gynaecology. Fetal diagnosis of genetic defects. London: Balliere Tindall. 1987: p 533

57 Galjaard H. Inborn errors of metabolism. In: Rodeck C H. ed. Ballieres clinical obstetrics and gynaecology. Fetal diagnosis of genetic defects. London: Balliere Tindall. 1987: p 547

58 Galjaard H. Worldwide experience with first trimester fetal diagnosis by molecular analysis. Proceedings of the 7th International Congress of Human Genetics. Berlin: Springer-Verlag. 1987: p 547

59 Kan Y W, Dozy A M. Antenatal diagnosis of sickle cell anaemia by DNA analysis of amniotic fluid cells. Lancet 1978; ii: 910

60 Kidd V J, Wallace R B, Hakura K, Woo S L C. α1-antitrypsin deficiency detection by direct analysis of the mutation in the gene. Nature 1983; 304: 230–234

61 Winter R M, Harper K, Goldman E, et al. First trimester prenatal diagnosis and carrier detection of haemophilia A using the linked DNA probe DX 13. BMJ 1985; 291: 765–769

62 Old J M, Fitches A, Heath C, et al. First trimester fetal diagnosis for haemoglobinopathies: report on 149 cases. Lancet 1986; ii: 763–767

63 Terry G M, Ho-terry L, Warren R C, Rodeck C H, Cohen A, Rees K R. First trimester prenatal diagnosis of congenital rubella: a laboratory investigation. BMJ 1986; 292: 930–933

64 Gemke R J B J, Kankai H H H, Overbeeke M A M, et al. ABO and Rhesus phenotyping of fetal erythrocytes in the first trimester of pregnancy. Br J Haemotology 1986; 64: 689–697

65 Furhman H C, Klink F, Grzejszczyk G, et al. First trimester diagnosis of RH(D) with an immunofluorescence technique after chorionic villus sampling. Prenat Diagn 1987; 7: 17–21

66 Rodesch F, Lambermont M, Donner C, et al. Chorionic biopsy in management of severe Kell alloimmunization. Am J Obstet Gynecol 1987; 156: 124–125

67 Rodeck C H, Letsky E. How the management of erythroblastosis fetalis has changed. Br J Obstet Gynaecol 1989; 96: 759–763

68 Blakemore K J, Mahoney M J, Hobbins J C. Infection and chorionic villus sampling. Lancet 1985; ii: 338

69 Barela A I, Kleinman G E, Golditch I M, Menke D J, Hogge W A, Golbus M S. Septic shock with renal failure after chorionic villus sampling. Am J Obstet Gynecol 1986; 154: 1100–1102

70 Canadian Collaborative CVS-Amniocentesis Clinical Trial Group. Multicentre randomized clinical trial of chorionic villus sampling and amniocentesis. Lancet 1989; i: 1–6

71 National Institute of Child Health and Human Development. The

safety and efficacy of CVS for early prenatal diagnosis of cytogenetic abnormalities. N Engl J Med 1989; 320: 609–617

72 Crane J P, Beaver H A, Cheung S W. First trimester chorionic villus sampling versus mid-trimester genetic amniocentesis – preliminary results of a controlled prospective trial. Prenat Diagn 1988; 8: 355–366

73 Holzgreve W, Miny P, Schloo R and participants of the 'late CVS' registry. 'Late CVS' international registry compilation of data from 24 centres. Prenat Diagn 1990; 10: 159–167

74 Smidt-Jensen S, Philip J. Transabdominal C V S versus transcervical versus amniocentesis: a randomized study. Am J Human Genet 1987; 41: 27 (abstract)

75 Wilson R D, Kendrick V, Whittman B K, McGillivray B C. Risk of spontaneous abortion in ultrasonically normal pregnancies. Lancet 1984; ii: 920–921

76 MacKenzie W E, Holmes D S, Newton J R. Spontaneous abortion rate in ultrasonically viable pregnancies. Obstet Gynecol 1988; 71: 81–83

77 Brambati G, Guercilina S, Bonacchi I, Oldrini A, Lanzani A, Piceni L. Feto-maternal transfusion after chorionic villus sampling: clinical implications. Human Reprod 1986; 1: 37

78 Blakemore K G, Baumgarten A, Schoenfeld-Dimaio M, Hobbins J C, Mason E A, Mahoney M J. Rise in maternal serum α-fetoprotein concentration after chorionic villus sampling and the possibility of isoimmunization. Am J Obstet Gynecol 1986; 155: 988–993

79 Sigler M E, Colyer C R, Rossiter J, Dorfmann A D, Jones S L, Schulman J D. Maternal serum alpha-fetoprotein screening after chorionic villus sampling. Obstet Gynecol 1987; 70: 875–877

80 Prochownick L. Beitrage zur leptre vom fruchtwasser und seiner entsehung. Archiv fur Gynaekologie 1877; 11: 304–345

81 Henkel M. Akutes hydramnion, leberkompression, enges becken. Punktion des hydramnion. Zentralblatt für Gynäkologie 1919; 43: 841

82 Bevis D C A. The antenatal prediction of haemolytic disease of the newborn. Lancet 1952; i: 395–398

83 Riis P, Fuchs F. Antenatal determination of foetal sex in prevention of hereditary diseases. Lancet 1960; ii: 180–182

84 Jeffcoate T N A., Fliegner J R N, Russel S N, Davis J C, Wade A P. Diagnosis of adrenogenital syndrome before birth. Lancet 1965; ii: 553–555

85 Steele M W, Breg W T. Chromosome analysis of human amniotic fluid cells. Lancet 1966; i: 383–385

86 Brock D J H, Scrimgeour J B. Early prenatal diagnosis of anencephaly. Lancet 1972; ii: 1252

87 Brock D J H, Sutcliffe R G. AFP in the antenatal diagnosis of anencephaly and spina bifida. Lancet 1972; ii: 197–199

88 Scrimgeour J B. Amniocentesis: technique and complications. In: Emery A E H. ed. Antenatal diagnosis of genetic disease. London: Churchill Livingstone. 1973: p 11

89 Turnbull A C, MacKenzie I Z. Second trimester amniocentesis and termination of pregnancy. Br Med Bull 1983; 39: 315–321

90 Medical Research Council. An assessment of the hazards of amniocentesis. Br J Obstet Gynaecol 1978; 85(suppl 2): 1–41

91 National Institute of Child Health and Development Amniocentesis Register. The safety and accuracy of midtrimester amniocentesis. US Department of Health, Education and Welfare. 1978: p 78–190

92 Crandon A J, Peel K R. Amniocentesis with and without ultrasound guidance. Br J Obstet Gynaecol 1979; 86: 1–3

93 Ch de Crespigny L, Robinson H P. Amniocentesis: a comparison of 'monitored' versus 'blind' needle insertion technique. Aust NZ J Obstet Gynaecol 1986; 26: 124–128

94 Romero R, Jeanty P, Reece A E, Grannum P, Bracken M, Berkowitz R, Hobbins J C. Sonographically monitored amniocentesis to decrease intraoperative complications. Obstet Gynecol 1985; 65: 426–430

95 Canadian Medical Research Council. Diagnosis of genetic disease by amniocentesis during the second trimester of pregnancy. A Canadian study. Report No.5 Supply Services. Canada. 1977

96 Tabor A, Philip J, Marsen M, Bang J, Obel E B, Norgaard-Pedersen B. Randomized controlled trial of genetic amniocentesis in 4606 low-risk women. Lancet 1986; i: 1287–1292

97 Hanson F W, Zorn E M, Tennant F R, Marianos M, Samuels S. Amniocentesis before 15 weeks gestation: outcome, risks and technical problems. Am J Obstet Gynecol 1987; 156: 1524–1531

98 Johnson J, Godmilow L. Genetic amniocentesis at 14 weeks or less. Clin Obstet Gynecol 1988; 31: 345–352

99 Benacerraf B R, Greene M F, Saltzman D H, et al. Early amniocentesis for prenatal cytogenetic evaluation. Radiology 1988; 169: 709–710

100 Godmilow L, Weiner S, Dunn L K. Early genetic amniocentesis: experience with 600 consecutive procedures and comparison with chorionic villus sampling. Am J Hum Genet 1988; 43: A232

101 Elejalde B R, de Elejalde M M. Early genetic amniocentesis, safety, complications, time to obtain results and contradictions. Am J Hum Genet 1988; 43: A234

102 MacLachlan N A, Rooney D E, Coleman D, Rodeck C H. Prenatal diagnosis: early amniocentesis or chorionic villus sampling. Contemp Rev Obstet Gynaecol 1989; 1: 173–179

103 Rooney D E, MacLachlan N, Smith J, et al. Early amniocentesis: a cytogenetic evaluation. BMJ 1989; 299: 25

104 Henry G, Peakman D C, Winkler W, O'Connor K. Amniocentesis before 15 weeks instead of CVS for earlier prenatal cytogenetic diagnosis. Am J Hum Genet 1985; 37(suppl): A835

105 Chadefaux B, Rabier D, Dumez Y, Oury J F, Kamoun P. Eleventh week amniocentesis for prenatal diagnosis of metabolic diseases. Lancet 1989; i: 849

106 Drugan A, Syner F N, Greb A, Evans M I. Amniotic fluid alpha-fetoprotein and acetylcholinesterase in early genetic amniocentesis. Obstet Gynecol 1988; 72: 35–38

107 Crandall B F, Hanson F W, Tennant F, Perdue S T. Alpha-fetoprotein levels in amniotic fluid between 11 and 15 weeks. Am J Obstet Gynecol 1989; 160: 1204–1206

108 Nevin J, Nevin N C, Dornan J C, Sim D, Armstrong M J. Early amniocentesis: experience of 222 consecutive patients, 1987–1988. Prenat Diagn 1990; 10: 79–83

109 Verjaal M, Leschot N J. Risk of amniocentesis and laboratory findings in a series of 1500 prenatal diagnoses. Prenat Diagn 1981; 1: 173–181

110 Hook E B, Chambers G M. Estimated rates of Down syndrome in live births by one year maternal age intervals for mothers aged 20–49 in a New York State study – implications of the risk figures for genetic counseling and cost-benefit analysis of prenatal diagnosis programs. Birth Defects 1977; 13: 124–141

111 Mikkelsen M, Stene J. Previous child with Down syndrome and other chromosome aberration. Proceedings of the 3rd European Conference on Prenatal Diagnosis of Genetic Disorders. Stuttgart: Ferdinand Enke Publishers. 1979: p 22

112 Bui T H, Iselius L, Lindsten J. European collaborative study on prenatal diagnosis: mosaicism, pseudomosaicism and single abnormal cells in amniotic fluid cell cultures. Prenat Diagn 1984; 4: 145–162

113 Hsu L Y F, Perlis T E. United States survey on chromosome mosaicism and pseudomosaicism in prenatal diagnosis. Prenat Diagn 1984; 4: 97–130

114 Gosden C, Nicolaides K H, Rodeck C H. Fetal blood sampling in investigation of chromosome mosaicism in amniotic fluid cell culture. Lancet 1988; i: 613–616

115 Thirkelsen A J. Cell culture and cell technique. Proceedings of the 3rd European Conference on Prenatal Diagnosis of Genetic Disorders. Stuttgart: Ferdinand Enke Publishers. 1979: p 258

116 Milunsky A, Sapirstein V S. Prenatal diagnosis of open neural tube defects using the amniotic fluid acetylcholinesterase assay. Obstet Gynecol 1982; 59: 1–5

117 Richards D S, Seeds J W, Katz V L, Lingley L H, Albright S G, Cefalo R C. Elevated maternal serum alpha-fetoprotein with normal ultrasound; is amniocentesis always appropriate? A review of 26069 screened patients. Obstet Gynecol 1988; 71: 203–207

118 Pembrey M E. The impact of DNA analysis on fetal diagnosis. In: Rodeck C H. ed. Ballieres Clinical Obstetrics and Gynaecology. London: Balliere Tindall. 1989: p 589

119 Liley A W. Liquor amnii analysis in the management of the pregnancy complicated by rhesus sensitization. Am J Obstet Gynecol 1961; 82: 1359–1370

120 Whitfield C R. A three-year assessment of an action line method

of timing intervention in rhesus isoimmunization. Am J Obstet Gynecol 1970; 108: 1239–1244

121 Bowman J M. The management of Rh-isoimmunization. Obstet Gynecol 1978; 52: 1–16

122 Nicolaides K H, Rodeck C H, Mishiban R S, Kemp J R. Have Liley charts outlived their usefulness? Am J Obstet Gynecol 1986; 155: 90–94

123 Gluck L, Kulovich M V. Lecithin/sphingomyelin ratios in amniotic fluid in normal and abnormal pregnancy. Am J Obstet Gynecol 1973; 115: 539–546

124 James D K, Tindall V R, Richardson T. Is the lecithin/sphingomyelin ratio outdated? Br J Obstet Gynecol 1983; 90: 995–1000

125 Fisk N M. Modifications to selective conservative management in preterm premature rupture of the membranes. Obstet Gynecol Surv 1988; 43: 328–334

126 Prenatal diagnosis – past, present and future. Report of the International Workshop held at Val David, Quebec, Canada. Nov 1979. London: John Wiley. 1980

127 Farrant W. Stress after amniocentesis for high serum alpha-fetoprotein concentrations. (letter) BMJ 1980; 281: 452

128 Tabor A, Philip J, Bang J, Madsen M, Obel E B, Norgaard-Pedersen B. Needle size and risk of miscarriage after amniocentesis. Lancet 1988; i: 183–184

129 Tabor A, Bang J, Norgaard-Pedersen B. Feto-maternal haemorrhage associated with genetic amniocentesis: results of a randomized trial. Br J Obstet Gynaecol 1987; 94: 528–534

130 Hislop A, Fairweather D V I, Blackwell R J, Howard S. The effect of amniocentesis and drainage of amniotic fluid on lung development in Macaca fascicularis. Am J Obstet Gynecol 1984; 91: 835–842

131 Valenti C. Antenatal detection of haemoglobinopathies. A preliminary report. Am J Obstet Gynecol 1973; 115: 851–853

132 Kan Y W, Valenti C, Guidotti R, Carnazza V, Rieder. Fetal blood sampling in utero. Lancet 1974; i: 79–80

133 Alter B, Modell B, Fairweather D, et al. Prenatal diagnosis of hemoglobinopathies: a review of 15 cases. N Engl J Med 1976; 295: 1437–1439

134 Fairweather D V I, Ward R H T, Modell B. Obstetric aspects of midtrimester fetal blood sampling by needling or fetoscopy. Br J Obstet Gynecol 1980; 87: 87–99

135 Hobbins J C, Mahoney M J. In utero diagnosis of hemoglobinopathies. Technique for obtaining fetal blood. N Engl J Med 1974; 290: 1065–1067

136 Rodeck C H, Campbell S. Sampling pure fetal blood by fetoscopy in second trimester of pregnancy. BMJ 1978; ii: 728–730

137 Rodeck C H, Nicolaides K H. Fetoscopy. Br Med Bull 1986; 42: 296–300

138 Daffos F, Capella-Pavlovsky M, Forestier F. A new procedure for fetal blood sampling in utero. Prenat Diagn 1983; 3: 271–274

139 Koresawa M, Inaba J, Iwasaki H. Fetal blood sampling by liver puncture. Acta Obstet Gynaecol Jpn 1987; 39: 395–399

140 Bang J. Ultrasound-guided fetal blood sampling. In: Albertini A, Crosignani P F. eds. Progress in perinatal medicine. Amsterdam: Excerpta Medica. 1983: p 223

141 Forestier F, Cox W L, Daffos F, Rainaut M. The assessment of fetal blood samples. Am J Obstet Gynecol 1988; 158: 1184–1188

142 Daffos F, Capella-Pavlovsky M, Forestier F. Fetal blood sampling during pregnancy with the use of a needle guided by ultrasound: a study of 606 consecutive cases. Am J Obstet Gynecol 1985; 153: 655–660

143 Bang J, Bock J E, Trolle D. Ultrasound-guided fetal intravenous transfusion for severe rhesus haemolytic disease. BMJ 1982; 284: 373–374

144 Ch de Crespigny L, Robinson H P, Quinn M, Doyle L, Ross A, Cauchi M. Ultrasound-guided fetal blood transfusion for severe rhesus isoimmunization. Obstet Gynecol 1985; 66: 529–532

145 Nicolini U, Santolaya J, Ojo O E, Fisk N M, Hubinot C, Tonge M, Rodeck C H. The fetal intrahepatic umbilical vein as an alternative to cord needling for prenatal diagnosis and therapy. Prenat Diagn 1988; 8: 665–671

146 Nicolini U, Nicolaidis P, Fisk N M, Tannirandorn Y, Rodeck C H. Fetal blood sampling from the intrahepatic vein: analysis of

safety and clinical experience with 214 procedures. Obstet Gynecol 1990; 76: 47–53

147 Nicolini U, Nicolaidis P, Tannirandorn Y, Fisk N M, Nasrat H, Rodeck C H. Fetal liver dysfunction in Rh alloimmunization. Br J Obstet Gynaecol; in press

148 Orlandi F, Damiani G, Jakil C, Lauricella S, Bertolino O, Maggio A. The risks of early cordocentesis (12–21 weeks): analysis of 500 procedures. Prenat Diagn 1990; 10: 425–428

149 Weiner C P. Cordocentesis for diagnostic indications: two years' experience. Obstet Gynaecol 1987; 70: 664–667

150 Weatherall D J, Clegg J B Naughton M A. Globin synthesis in thalassaemia: an in vitro study. Nature 1965; 208: 1061–1065

151 Nicolaides K, Rodeck C H. Fetal blood sampling. In: Rodeck C H. ed. Ballieres Clinical Obstetrics and Gynaecology. Fetal diagnosis of genetic defects. London: Balliere Tindall. 1987: p 623

152 Mibashan R S, Rodeck C H. Haemophilia and other genetic defects of haemostasis. In: Rodeck C H, Nicolaides K H. eds. Prenatal Diagnosis. Proceedings of the XIth Study Group of the Royal College of Obstetricians and Gynaecologists. Chichester: John Wiley. 1984: p 179

153 Linch D C, Beverly P C L, Levinsky R J, Rodeck C H. Phenotypic analysis of fetal blood leucocytes: potential for prenatal diagnosis of immunodeficiency disorders. Prenat Diagn 1982; 2: 211–218

154 Levinsky R J. Prenatal diagnosis of severe combined immunodeficiency. In: Rodeck C H, Nicolaides K H. eds. Prenatal Diagnosis. Proceedings of the XIth Study Group of the Royal College of Obstetricians and Gynaecologists. Chichester: John Wiley. 1984: p 137

155 Nicolaides K H, Rodeck C H, Gosden C M. Rapid karyotyping in non-lethal malformations. Lancet 1986; i: 283–286

156 Benacerraf B R, Frigoletto F D, Laboda L A. Sonographic diagnosis of Down Syndrome in the second trimester. Am J Obstet Gynecol 1985; 153: 49–52

157 Webb T P, Rodeck C H, Nicolaides K H, Gosden C M. Prenatal diagnosis of Fragile X syndrome using fetal blood and amniotic fluid. Prenat Diagn 1987; 7: 203–214

158 MacKenzie I Z, Bowell P J, Castle B M, Selinger M, Ferguson J F. Serial fetal blood sampling for the management of pregnancies complicated by severe rhesus (D) isoimmunization. Br J Obstet Gynaecol 1988; 95: 753–758

159 Nicolini U, Kochenour N K, Greco P, et al. Consequences of fetomaternal haemorrhage after intrauterine transfusion. BMJ 1988; 297: 1379–1381

160 Nicolaides K H, Soothill P W, Rodeck C H, Clewell W. Rhesus disease: intravascular fetal blood transfusion by cordocentesis. Fetal Ther 1986; 1: 185–192

161 Nicolaides K H, Soothill P W, Clewell W H, Rodeck C H, Mishaban R S, Campbell S. Fetal haemoglobin measurement in the assessment of red cell isoimmunisation. Lancet 1988; i: 1073–1075

162 Zalneraitis E L, Young R S K, Krishnamoorthy K S. Intracranial haemorrhage in utero as a complication of isoimmune thrombocytopenia. J Pediatr 1979; 95: 611–614

163 Jesurun C A, Levin G S, Sullivan W R, Stevens D. Intracranial haemorrhage in utero and thrombocytopenia. J Pediatr 1980; 97: 695–696

164 Kelton J G, Inwood M J, Barr R M, et al. The prenatal prediction of thrombocytopenia in infants of mothers with clinically diagnosed immune thrombocytopenia. Am J Obstet Gynecol 1982; 144: 449–454

165 De Vries L S, Connell J, Bydder G M, et al. Recurrent intracranial haemorrhages in utero in an infant with alloimmune thrombocytopenia. Case report. Br J Obstet Gynaecol 1988; 95: 299–302

166 Millar D S, Davis L R, Rodeck C H, Nicolaides K H, Mishiban R S. Normal blood cell values in the early midtrimester fetus. Prenat Diagn 1985; 5: 367–373

167 Daffos F, Forestier F, Muller J Y. Prenatal treatment of alloimmune thrombocytopenia (letter). Lancet 1984; ii: 623

168 Daffos F, Forestier F, Grangeot-Keros L, et al. Prenatal diagnosis of congenital rubella. Lancet 1984; ii: 1–3

169 Morgan-Capner P, Rodeck C H, Nicolaides K H, Cradock-Watson J E. Prenatal diagnosis of rubella. (letter) Lancet 1984; ii: 343

170 Morgan-Capner P, Rodeck C H, Nicolaides K H, Cradock-Watson J E. Prenatal detection of rubella-specific IgM in fetal sera. Prenat Diagn 1985; 5: 21–26

171 Munro N D, Sheppard S, Smithells R W, Holzel H, Jones G. Temporal relations between maternal rubella and congenital defects. Lancet 1987; ii: 201–204

172 Daffos F, Forestier F, Capella-Pavlovsky M, et al. Prenatal management of 746 pregnancies at risk for congenital toxoplasmosis. N Engl J Med 1988; 318: 271–275

173 Soothill P W, Nicolaides K H, Rodeck C H, Campbell S. The effect of gestational age on fetal and intervillous blood gas and acid-base values in human pregnancy. Fetal Ther 1986; 1: 166–173

174 Nicolaides K H, Economides D L, Soothill P W. Blood gases, pH and lactate in appropriate and small-for-gestational age fetuses. Am J Obstet Gynecol 1989; 161: 996–1001

175 Soothill P W, Nicolaides K H, Campbell S. Prenatal asphyxia, hyperlacticaemia, hypoglycaemia, and erythroblastosis in growth retarded fetuses. BMJ 1987; 1: 1051–1053

176 Nicolini U, Nicolaidis P, Fisk N M, et al. The limited role of fetal blood sampling in prediction of outcome in intrauterine growth retardation. Lancet 1990; 2: 768–772

177 Eady R A J, Rodeck C H. Prenatal diagnosis of disorders of the skin. In: Rodeck C H, Nicolaides K H. eds. Prenatal diagnosis. Proc. 11th study group of the Royal College of Obstetricians and Gynaecologists. Chichester: John Wiley. 1984: p 147

178 Rodeck C H, Eady R A J, Gosden C M. Prenatal diagnosis of epidermolysis bullosa letalis. Lancet 1980; i: 949–952

179 Bang J. Intrauterine needle diagnosis. In: Holm H H, Kristensen J K. eds. Interventional ultrasound. Copenhagen: Munksgaard. 1985: p 122–128

180 Hobbins J C, Mahoney M J, Goldstein L K. New method of intrauterine evaluation by the combined use of fetoscopy and ultrasound. Am J Obstet Gynecol 1974; 118: 1069

181 Elias J, Mazur M, Sabbagha R, Esterly J, Simpson J L. Prenatal diagnosis of harlequin ichthyosis. Clin Genet 1980; 17: 275–279

182 Eady R A J, Gunner D B, Tidman M J, Nicolaides K H, Rodeck C H. Rapid processing of fetal skin for prenatal diagnosis by light and electron microscopy. J Clin Pathol 1984; 37: 633–638

183 Bakharev V A, Aivazyan A A, Karetnikova N A, Mordovtsev V N, Yantovsky Y R. Fetal skin biopsy in prenatal diagnosis of some genodermatoses. Prenat Diagn 1990; 10: 1–12

184 Anton-Lamprecht I, Jovanovich V, Arnold M L, Rauskolb R, Kern B, Schenck W. Prenatal diagnosis of epidermolysis bullosa dystrophica Hallopeau Siemens with electron microscopy of fetal skin. Lancet 1981; ii: 1077–1079

185 Golbus M S, Sagebiel R W, Filly R A, Gindhart T D, Hall J G. Prenatal diagnosis of congenital bullous icthyosiform erythroderma (epidermolysis hyperkeratosis) by fetal skin biopsy. N Engl J Med 1980; 302: 93–95

186 Eady R A J, Gunner D B, Rodeck C H, Garner A. Prenatal diagnosis of oculocutaneous albinism by electron microscopy of fetal skin. J Invest Derm 1983; 80: 210–212

187 Kusseff B G, Matsouka L Y, Stenn K S, Hobbins J C, Mahoney M J, Hashimoto K. Prenatal diagnosis of Sjogren-Larsson syndrome. J Pediatr 1982; 101: 998–1001

188 Rodeck C H, Patrick A D, Pembrey M E, Tzannatos C, Whitfield A E. Fetal liver biopsy for prenatal diagnosis of ornithine carbamyl transferase deficiency. Lancet 1982; ii: 297

189 Holzgreve W, Golbus M S. Prenatal diagnosis of ornithine transcarbamylase deficiency utilizing fetal liver biopsy. Am J Hum Gen 1984; 36: 320

190 Piceni-Sereni L, Bachmann C, Pfister U, Buscaglia M, Nicolini U. Prenatal diagnosis of carbamoyl-phosphate synthetase deficiency by fetal liver biopsy. Prenat Diagn 1988; 8: 307

191 Golbus M S, Simpson T J, Koresawa M, Appelman Z, Alpers C E. The prenatal determination of glucose 6 phosphatase activity by fetal liver biopsy. Prenat Diagn 1988; 8: 401

192 Danpure C J, Jennings P J, Penketh R J, Wise P J, Rodeck C H. Fetal liver alanine: glyoxalate aminotransferase and the prenatal

193 Pembrey M E, Old J M, Leonard J V, Rodeck C H, Warren R, Davies K E. Prenatal diagnosis of ornithine carbamoyl transferase deficiency using a gene specific probe. J Med Gen 1985; 22: 462

194 Nussbaum R L, Boggs B A, Beaudet A L, Doyle S, Potter J L, O'Brien W E. New mutation and prenatal diagnosis in ornithine transcarbamylase deficiency. Am J Hum Genet 1986; 38: 149

195 Fox J, Hack A M, Fenton W A, et al. Prenatal diagnosis of ornithine transcarbamylase deficiency with the use of DNA polymorphisms. N Engl J Med 1986; 315: 1205

196 Meisel M, Amon I, Amon K, Huller H. Investigation of glucose-6-phosphatase in the liver of the human fetus. Biol Res Preg 1982; 3: 73

197 Raiha N C R & Suihkonen J. Development of urea-synthesising enzymes in human liver. Acta Pediatr Scand 1968; 57: 121

198 Scott C R, Teng C C, Goodman S I, Greensher A, Mace J W. X-linked transmission of ornithine carbamylase deficiency. Lancet 1972; ii: 1148

199 Short E M, Conn H O, Snodgrass P J, Campbell A G M, Rosenberg L E. Evidence for X-linked dominant inheritance of ornithine transcarbamylase deficiency. N Engl J Med 1973; 288: 7.

200 Walser M. Urea cycle disorders and other hereditary hyperammonemic syndromes. In: Stanbury J B, Wyngaarden J B, Fredrickson D S, Goldstein J L, Brown M S. eds. The metabolic basis of hereditary disease. New York: McGraw-Hill. 1983

201 Reece E A, Winn H N, Wan M, Burdine C, Green J, Hobbins J C. Can ultrasonography replace amniocentesis in fetal gender determination during the early second trimester? Am J Obstet Gynecol 1987; 156: 579–581

202 Howell R. The glycogen storage diseases. In: Stanbury J B, Wyngaarden J B, Fredrickson D S, Goldstein J L, Brown M S. eds. The metabolic basis of inherited disease. New York: McGraw-Hill. 1983

203 Danpure C J, Jennings P R. Perioxosomal alanine: glyoxalate aminotransferase deficiency in primary hyperoxaluria type I. FEBS Lett 1986; 201: 20

204 Rodeck C H, Nicolaides K H. Fetal tissue biopsy: techniques and indications. Fetal Ther 1986; 1: 46–58

205 Evans M. personal communication

206 Nicolini U, Rodeck C H, Gau G. unpublished

207 Manning F A, Harrison M R, Rodeck C H and members of the International Fetal Medicine and Surgery Society. Catheter shunts for fetal hydronephrosis and hydrocephalus. N Engl J Med 1986; 315: 336–340

208 Mahoney M S, Filly R A, Callen P W, Hricak H, Golbus M S, Harrison M R. Fetal renal dysplasia: sonographic evaluation. Radiology 1984; 152: 143–146

209 Nakayama D K, Harrison M R, de Lorimer A A. Prognosis of posterior urethral valves presenting at birth. J Pediatr Surg 1986; 21: 43–45

210 Reuss A, Wladimiroff J W, Stewart P A, Scholtmeijer R J. Non-invasive management of fetal obstructive uropathy. Lancet 1988; ii: 949–951

211 Nicolini U, Fisk N M, Beacham J, Rodeck C H. Fetal urine biochemistry: an index of renal maturation and dysfunction. Br J Obstet Gynaecol; in press

212 Nicolini U, Rodeck C H, Fisk N M. Shunt treatment for fetal obstructive uropathy. Lancet 1987; ii: 1338–1339

213 Glick P I, Harrison M R, Golbus M S, et al. Management of the fetus with congenital hydronephrosis II; prognostic criteria and selection for treatment. J Pediatr Surg 1985; 20: 376–387

214 Wilkins I A, Chitkara U, Lynch L, Golberg J D, Mehalek K E, Berkowitz R L. The non predictive value of fetal urinary electrolytes: preliminary report of outcomes and correlations with pathologic diagnosis. Am J Obstet Gynecol 1987; 157: 694–698

215 Nicolini U, Rodeck C H. Fetal urinary diversion. In: Chervenak F, Isaacson G, Campbell S. eds. Textbook of Ultrasound in Obstetrics and Gynecology. New York: Little Brown. 1990

216 Lebowitz R L, Griscom N T. Neonatal hydronephrosis: 146 cases. Radiol Clin North Am 1977; 15: 49–59

217 Schmidt W, Harms E, Wolf D. Successful prenatal treatment of

non-immune hydrops fetalis due to congenital chylothorax: case report. Br J Obstet Gynaecol 1985; 92: 685–687

218 Gembruch U, Hansmann M. Artificial instillation of amniotic fluid as a new technique for the diagnostic evaluation of cases of oligohydramnios. Prenat Diagn 1988; 8: 33–45

219 Nicolini U, Santolaya J, Hubinont C, Fisk N M, Maxwell D, Rodeck C H. Visualization of fetal intra-abdominal organs in second trimester severe oligohydramnios by intraperitoneal infusion. Prenat Diagn 1989; 9: 191–194

220 Romero R, Cullen M, Grannum P, et al. Antenatal diagnosis of renal anomalies with ultrasound. III. Bilateral renal agenesis. Am J Obstet Gynecol 1985; 151: 38–43

221 Hackelöer B J, Waldenfels H V, Martin K, Hamburg D. Treatment and results of oligohidramnios by instillation of artificial amniotic fluid (150 cases). Presented at the 5th Annual Meeting of the International Fetal Medicine and Surgery Society, Bonn 1988

222 Nicolini U, Fisk N M, Talbert D G, et al. Intrauterine manometry: technique and application to fetal pathology. Prenat Diagn 1989; 9: 243–254

223 Fisk N M, Tannirandorn Y, Nicolini U, Talbert D G, Rodeck C H. Amniotic pressure in disorders of amniotic fluid volume. Obstet Gynecol 1990; 76: 210–214

224 Nicolini U, Fisk N M, Rodeck C H, Talbert D G, Wigglesworth J S. Low amniotic pressure in oligohydramnios – is this the cause of pulmonary hypoplasia? Am J Obstet Gynecol 1989; 161: 1098–1101

225 Nicolini U, Talbert D G, Fisk N M, Rodeck C H. Pathophysiology of pressure changes during intrauterine transfusion. Am J Obstet Gynecol 1989; 160: 1139–1145

226 Rodeck C H, Fisk N M, Fraser D I, Nicolini U. Chronic in utero drainage of fetal hydrothorax. N Engl J Med 1989; 319: 1135–1138

227 Rosen K G. Alterations in the fetal electrocardiogram as a sign of fetal asphyxia: experimental data with a clinical implementation. J Perinat Med 1986; 14: 355–363

228 Lilja H, Arulkumaran S, Lindecrantz K, Ratnam S S, Rosen K. ECG during labour: a presentation of a microprocessor system. J Bio Med Eng 1988; 10: 348–350

229 Arulkumaran S, Nicolini U, Fisk N M, Tannirandorn Y, Rosen K, Rodeck C H. Antenatal ECG waveform analysis during intrahepatic vein fetal blood sampling. submitted for publication

230 Rivett L C. Hydramnios. J Obstet Gynaecol Br Cwlth 1933; 40: 522–525

231 Cabrera-Ramirez L, Harris R E. Controlled removal of amniotic fluid in hydramnios. South Med J 1976; 69: 239–240

232 Cabrol D, Landesman R, Muller J, Uzan M, Sureau C, Saxena B B. Treatment of polyhydramnios with prostaglandin synthetase inhibitor (indomethacin). Am J Obstet Gynecol 1987; 157: 422–426

233 Moise K J, Huhta J C, Sharif D S, et al. Indomethacin in the treatment of preterm labour: effects on the fetal ductus arteriosus. N Engl J Med 1988; 319: 307–313

234 Cantor B, Tyler T, Nelson R, Stein G H. Oligohydramnios and transient neonatal anuria. A possible complication of the maternal use of prostaglandin synthetase inhibitors. J Reprod Med 1980; 24: 220

235 Freda V J, Adamsons K J. Exchange transfusion in utero. Am J Obstet Gynecol 1964; 89: 817–821

236 Asensio S H, Figueroa-Longo J G, Pelegrina I A. Intrauterine exchange transfusion. Am J Obstet Gynecol 1966; 95: 1129–1133

237 Seelen J, van Kessel H, van Leusden H, et al. A new method of exchange transfusion in utero. Cannulation of vessels on the fetal side of the human placenta. Am J Obstet Gynecol 1966; 95: 872–876

238 Liley A W. Intrauterine transfusion of foetus in haemolytic disease. BMJ 1963; 2: 1107–1109

239 Bock J E. Intrauterine transfusion in the management of pregnant women with severe rhesus immunization. II Results and discussion. Acta Obstet Gynecol Scand (Suppl) 1976; 53: 29–36

240 Clewell W H, Dunne M G, Johnson M L, Bowes W A. Fetal transfusion with real-time ultrasound guidance. Obstet Gynecol 1981; 57: 516–520

241 Scott J R, Kochenour N K, Larkin R M. Changes in the management of severely Rh-immunized patients. Am J Obstet Gynecol 1984; 149: 3361

242 Harman C R, Manning F A, Bowman J M, Lange I R. Severe Rh disease: poor outcome is not inevitable. Am J Obstet Gynecol 1983; 145: 823–829

243 Rodeck C H, Holman C A, Karnicki J, Kemp J R, Whitmore D N, Austin M A. Direct intravascular blood transfusion by fetoscopy in severe rhesus isoimmunization. Lancet 1981; i: 625–628

244 Rodeck C H, Nicolaides K H, Warsof L S, Fysh W J, Gamsu H R, Kemp J R. The management of severe rhesus isoimmunization by fetoscopic intravascular tranfusions. Am J Obstet Gynecol 1984; 150: 769–774

245 Berkowitz R L, Chitkara U, Goldberg J D, Wilkins I, Chervenak F A. Intrauterine transfusion in utero: the percutaneous approach. Am J Obstet Gynecol 1986; 154: 622–627

246 Westgren M, Selbing A, Stragenberg M. Fetal intracardiac transfusion in patients with severe rhesus isoimmunization. BMJ 1988; 296: 885–886

247 Nicolaides K H, Fontanarosa M, Gabbe S G, Rodeck C H. Failure of ultrasonographic parameters to detect the severity of fetal anaemia in rhesus isoimmunization. Am J Obstet Gynecol 1988; 158: 920–926

248 Chitkara U, Wilkins I, Lynch L, Mehalek K, Berkowitz R L. The role of sonography in assessing severity of fetal anaemia in Rh- and Kell-isoimmunized pregnancies. Obstet Gynecol 1988; 71: 393–398

249 Grannum P A T, Copel J A. Prevention of Rh isoimmunization and treatment of the compromised fetus. Semin Perinatol 1988; 12: 324–335

250 Berkowitz R L, Chitkara U, Wilkins I A, Lynch L, Plosker H, Bernstein H H. Intravascular monitoring and management of erythroblastosis fetalis. Am J Obstet Gynecol 1988; 158: 783–795

251 Ronkin S, Chayen B, Wapner R J, et al. Intravascular exchange and bolus transfusion in the severely isoimmunized fetus. Am J Obstet Gynecol 1989; 160: 407–411

252 Nicolini U, Rodeck C H. A proposed scheme for planning intrauterine transfusion in patients with severe Rh-immunization. J Obstet Gynecol 1988; 9: 162–163

253 Nicolini U, Santolaya J, Fisk N M, et al. Changes in fetal acid-base status during intravascular transfusion. Arch Dis Child 1988; 63: 710–714

254 Bowman J M. Rh erythroblastosis. Semin Haematol 1975; 12: 189–207

255 Harman C R, Manning F A, Bowman J M, Lange I R, Menticoglou S M. Use of intravascular transfusion to treat hydrops fetalis in the moribund fetus. Can Med Assoc J 1988; 138: 827–830

256 Nicolini U, Kochenour N K, Greco P, Letsky E, Rodeck C H. When to perform the next intra-uterine transfusion in patients with Rh allo-immunization: combined intravascular and intraperitoneal transfusion allows longer intervals. Fetal Ther 1989; 4: 14–20

257 Nicolaides K H, Rodeck C H. Rhesus disease: the model for fetal therapy. Br J Hosp Med 1985; 34: 141–148

258 Urbaniak S J. Rh(D) haemolytic disease of the newborn: the changing scene. BMJ 1985; 291: 4–6

259 Clarke C A, Whitfield A G W, Mollison P L. Death from Rh haemolytic disease in England and Wales in 1984 and 1985. BMJ 1987; 294: 1001

260 Tovey L A D. Haemolytic disease of the newborn – the changing scene. Br J Obstet Gynaecol 1986; 93: 960–966

261 Caine M E, Mueller-Heubach M D. Kell sensitisation in pregnancy. Am J Obstet Gynecol 1986; 154: 85–90

262 Mollison P L, Engelfreit C P, Contreras M. Haemolytic disease of the newborn. In: Blood Transfusion in Clinical Medicine. 8th edn. Oxford: Blackwell Scientific Publications 1987: p 637–687

263 Berkowitz R L, Beyta Y, Sadovsky E. Death in utero due to Kell sensitization without excessive elevation of the delta OD 450 value in amniotic fluid. Obstet Gynecol 1982; 60: 746–749

264 Nicolini U, Rodeck C H, Kochenour N K, et al. In-utero platelet transfusion for alloimmune thrombocytopenia. Lancet 1988; ii: 506

265 Schwarz T F, Roggendorf M, Hottentrager B, et al. Human parvovirus B19 infection in pregnancy. Lancet 1988; ii: 566–567

266 Gray E S, Davidson R J L, Anand A. Human parvovirus and fetal anaemia. Lancet 1987; ii: 1144

267 Peters M T, Nicolaides K H. Cordocentesis for the diagnosis and treatment of human fetal parvovirus infection. Obstet Gynecol 1990; 75: 501–504

268 Cardwell M S. Successful treatment of hydrops fetalis by feto-maternal haemorrhage: a case report. Am J Obstet Gynecol 1988; 158: 131–132

269 Fischer R L, Kuhlman K, Grover J, Montgomery O, Wapner R J. Chronic, massive fetomaternal haemorrhage treated with repeated fetal intravascular transfusions. Am J Obstet Gynecol 1990; 162: 203–204

270 Tannirandorn Y, Nicolini U, Nicolaidis P, Nasrat H, Letsky E, Rodeck C H. Intrauterine death due to fetomaternal haemorrhage despite successful treatment of fetal anaemia. J Perinat Med 1990; 18: 233–235

271 Harrison M R, Filly R A, Golbus M S, et al. Fetal treatment 1982. N Engl J Med 1982; 306: 1651–1652

272 Golbus M S, Harrison M R, Filly R A, Callen P W, Katz M. In utero treatment of urinary tract obstruction. Am J Obstet Gynecol 1982; 142: 383–388

273 Glick P L, Harrison M R, Adzick N S, Noall R A, Villa R L. Correction of congenital hydronephrosis in utero IV: in utero decompression prevents renal dysplasia. J Pediatr Surg 1984; 19: 649–657

274 Elder J S, Duckett J W Jnr, Snyder H M. Intervention for fetal obstructive uropathy: has it been effective? Lancet 1987; ii: 1007–1010

275 Birnholz J C, Frigoletto F D. Antenatal treatment of hydrocephalus. N Engl J Med 1981; 303: 1021–1023

276 Clewell W H, Johnson M L, Meier P R, et al. A surgical approach to the treatment of fetal hydrocephalus. N Engl J Med 1982; 306: 1320–1325

277 Chervenak F A, Berkowitz R L, Tortora M, Chitkara U, Hobbins J C. Diagnosis of ventriculomegaly before fetal viability. Obstet Gynecol 1984; 64: 652–656

278 Chervenak F A, Berkowitz R L, Tortora M, Hobbins J C. The management of fetal hydrocephalus. Am J Obstet Gynecol 1985; 151: 933–942

279 Clewell W H, Meier P R, Manchester D K, Manco-Johnson M L, Pretorius D H, Hendee R W. Ventriculomegaly: evaluation and management. Semin Perinatol 1985; 9: 98–102

280 Roberts A B, Clarkson N S, Pattison M G, Mok P M. Fetal hydrothorax in the second trimester of pregnancy: successful intrauterine treatment at 24 weeks gestation. Fetal Ther 1986; 1: 203–209

281 Petres R E, Redwine F O, Cruickshank D P. Congenital bilateral chylothorax: antepartum diagnosis and successful intrauterine surgical management. JAMA 1982; 248: 1360–1361

282 Booth P, Nicolaides K H, Greenough A, Gamsu H R. Pleuro-amniotic shunting for fetal chylothorax. Early Hum Dev 1987; 15: 365–367

283 Evans M I, Fletcher J C, Rodeck C H. Ethical problems in multiple gestations: selective termination. In: Evans M I, Dixler A O, Fletcher J C, Schulman J D. eds. Fetal Diagnosis and Therapy. Philadelphia: JB Lippincott. 1989: p 266

284 Beck L, Terinde R, Dolff M. Zwillingsschwangerschaft mit freier Trisomie 21 eines Kindes; sectio parva mit Entfernung des kranken und spatere Geburt des gesunden Kindes. Geburtsh Frauenheilk 1980; 40: 397–400

285 Rodeck C H, Mibashan R S, Abramowicz J, Campbell S. Selective feticide of the affected twin by fetoscopic air embolism. Prenat Diagn 1982; 2: 189–194

286 Aberg A, Mitelman F, Cantz M, Gehler J. Cardiac puncture of fetus with Hurler's disease avoiding abortion of unaffected co-twin. Lancet 1978; ii: 990–991

287 Kerenyi T D, Chitkara U. Selective birth in twin pregnancy with discordancy for Down's syndrome. N Engl J Med 1981; 304: 1525–1527

288 Petres R, Redwine F. Selective birth in twin pregnancy. N Engl J Med 1981; 305: 1218–1219

289 Wittmann B K, Farquharson D F, Thomas W D, Baldwin V J, Wadsworth L D. The role of fetocide in the management of severe twin transfusion syndrome. Am J Obstet Gynecol 1986; 155: 1023–1026

290 Shalev E, Issacov D, Weiner E, Feldman E, Zuckerman H. Ultrasound-guided selective fetocide of hydrocephalic fetus in triplet pregnancy. JCU 1988; 16: 41–43

291 Donnenfeld A E, Glazerman L R, Cutillo D M, Librizzi R J, Weiner S. Fetal exsanguination following intrauterine angiographic assessment and selective termination of a hydrocephalic, monozygotic co-twin. Prenat Diagn 1989; 9: 301–308

292 Wapner R J, Davis G H, Johnson A, et al. Selective reduction of multifetal pregnancies. Lancet 1990; i: 90–93

293 Kanhai H H H, van Rijssel E J C, Meerman R J, Bennebroek Gravenhorst J. Selective termination in quintuplet pregnancy during first trimester. Lancet 1986; i: 1447

294 Berkowitz R L, Lynch L, Chitkara U, Wilkins I A, Mehalek K E, Alvarez E. Selective reduction of multifetal pregnancies in the first trimester. N Engl J Med 1988; 318: 1043–1047

295 Golbus M S, Cunningham N, Goldberg J, et al. Selective termination of multiple gestations. Am J Med Genet 1988; 31: 339–348

296 Fisk N M, Borrell A, Hubinot C, Tannirandorn Y, Nicolini U, Rodeck C H. Fetofetal transfusion syndrome: do the neonatal criteria apply in utero? Arch Dis Child 1990; 65: 657–661

297 Itskovitz J, Boldes R, Thaler I, Bronstein M, Erlik Y, Brandes J M. Transvaginal ultrasonography-guided aspiration of gestational sacs for selective abortion in multiple pregnancy. Am J Obstet Gynecol 1989; 160: 215–217

The post-partum uterus

Heather S. Andrews

Normal post-partum uterus

The puerperium is the post-partum period during which the body returns to its pre-pregnant state. This is usually completed within 6 weeks and in the vast majority of patients is uneventful.

Immediately after delivery the uterus weighs approximately 900 grams and the fundus is palpable some 12 cm above the symphysis pubis. There is a subsequent rapid reduction in uterine tissue mass, by 50% at the end of the first week post-delivery. By 6 weeks the uterus weighs less than 100 grams and is only very slightly bigger than it was in its pre-pregnancy state. Within 3 days of parturition the superficial layer of decidua becomes necrotic and is shed in the lochia. The restoration of the endometrial covering takes approximately 3 weeks by which time the uterine blood loss has been curtailed.[1]

Ultrasound appearance The uterus is significantly enlarged with a smooth and globular outline. Immediately post-partum the longitudinal dimension is approximately 20 cm. The myometrial echo pattern is homogeneous (Fig. 1). A small amount of fluid within the uterine cavity may be considered normal and the shedding endometrium and membranes may be visualised as thin sheets of reflective material. It is not uncommon for small amounts of air to be seen in the uterine cavity immediately post-partum. This air will have been incidentally introduced at delivery and is of no clinical significance. There is a steady reduction in uterine size over the next 6 weeks. When uterine fibroids are present, they may shrink post-partum and any areas of necrosis that have developed slowly resolve.

Post-partum complications

Retained products of conception

Incomplete evacuation of the uterus following either vaginal delivery or caesarean section generally presents with excessive bleeding within a few days of delivery, although in some cases presentation is delayed by some weeks. The uterus does not involute as fast as might normally be expected. This complication is associated with an increased risk of endometritis. Ultrasound shows the uterus to be of an inappropriate size with distension of the endometrial cavity. The contents of the cavity are of mixed reflectivity with varying amounts of fluid and blood clot, membranes and placental tissue (Fig. 2). Similar appearances may be seen following spontaneous or induced abortion. Where a significant amount of retained products of conception is present curettage will normally be performed. When only small amounts of abnormal tissue and fluid are present spontaneous resolution may occur and can be monitored with follow up ultrasound examinations.

Endometritis

Nowadays serious post-partum endometritis and myometritis is rarely encountered due to prompt treatment with antibiotics. The patient presents with uterine tenderness, pyrexia, abnormal bleeding and offensive lochia. This complication is commoner following caesarean section and secondary to serious lacerations resulting from vaginal delivery. Uterine infection following childbirth initially involves the endometrium and rapidly spreads to involve the myometrium and adnexae. Septicaemia may occur if prompt antibiotic treatment is not given.

The ultrasound appearances may be indistinguishable from those of retained products of conception and thus the diagnosis is generally made on clinical grounds. There may be inappropriate enlargement of the uterus and the myometrium may appear relatively echo-poor in severe infection. Varying amounts of tissue, fluid and occasionally gas may be present in the uterine cavity (Fig. 3).

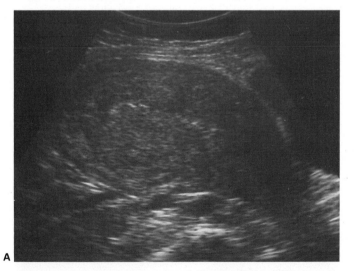
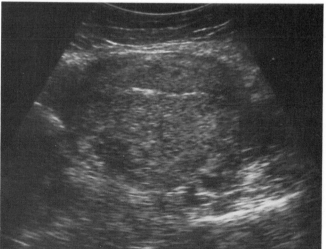

A B

Fig. 1 Normal post-partum uterus. A: Longitudinal and **B:** transverse scans show normal uterine appearances 5 days post-partum.

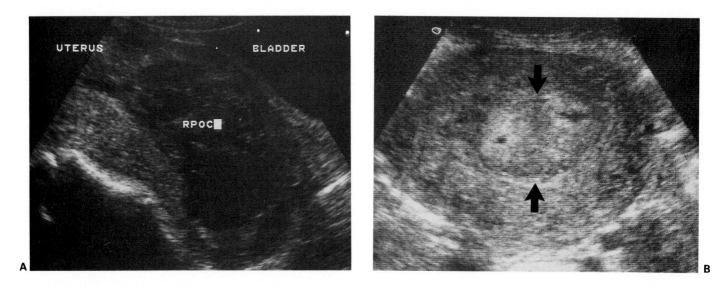

Fig. 2 Retained products of conception. A: Longitudinal scan 3 days post-partum shows uterine cavity markedly distended with retained products of conception (RPOC). **B:** Transverse scan 6 days post-partum shows retained products of conception (arrows) of a more moderate nature.

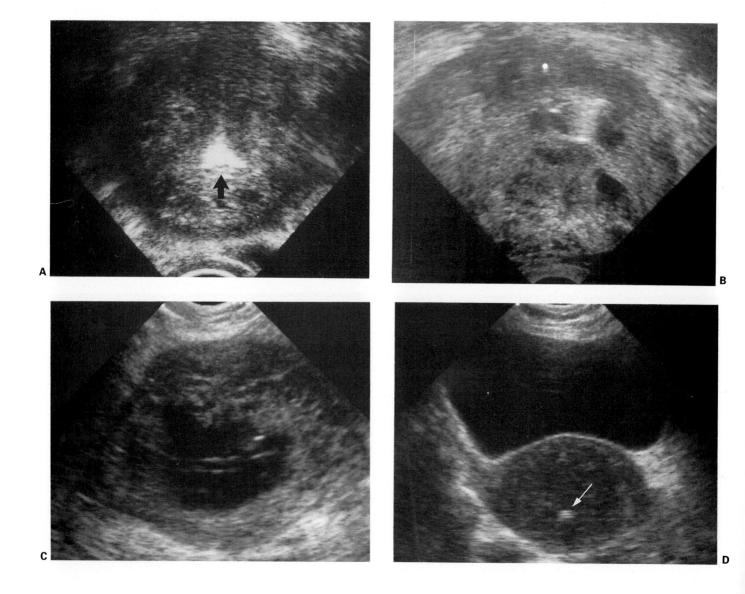

Post-partum haemorrhage

Ultrasound is rarely of value unless the haemorrhage is associated with retained products of conception.

Paravaginal haematoma

Following complicated vaginal delivery, with or without cervical or vaginal lacerations, damage to the paravaginal venous plexus may cause bleeding and may produce a paravaginal haematoma. This is visualised as a fluid collection lying lateral to the vagina. Of varying size, the haematoma may compress or deviate the vagina.

Uterine inversion

This is an unusual post-partum complication with an incidence of 1:30 000 deliveries. Complete uterine inversion is diagnosed clinically and is a devastating process which may result in severe shock and death. Partial uterine inversion is a less serious complication presenting with pelvic pain and abnormal bleeding. On ultrasound the uterine fundus is poorly visualised due to inversion of the uterus upon itself. The normal midline echo assumes a 'Y' shape. In transverse sections a ring is seen corresponding to the inverted endometrial cavity. The ultrasound appearance in some ways mimics that seen with an intussusception of the bowel. Treatment involves manual decompression of the uterus or, where that fails, emergency hysterectomy.[2]

Caesarean section

The incidence of caesarean section is steadily increasing and is performed in up to 20% of pregnancies depending on local practice. The uterine incision is either the classical vertical incision or, more commonly, a horizontal lower segment incision. Immediately post-operatively the incision site is clearly visible on ultrasound as a well-defined oval area interposed between the lower uterine segment and the posterior wall of the urinary bladder (Fig. 4). This produces a slight indentation of the bladder. Suture material appears as small punctate, regularly spaced highly reflective foci and may be clearly visualised.[3]

Within a few weeks, however, the wound heals, the suture material disappears and the scar is no longer visualised.[4] In some patients a small step-like deformity of

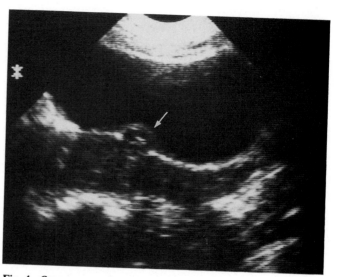

Fig. 4 Caesarean section scar. Longitudinal scan of uterus showing caesarean section scar (arrow) 10 days post-operatively.

the anterior uterine wall persists and may give rise to an acoustic shadow at the site of the scar. This may cause the erroneous impression of a small fibroid but the history and the classical site of the scar at the junction of the middle and lower thirds of the uterus allows a confident diagnosis. Vertical uterine scars however cannot be identified.[4] Post-operatively it is not uncommon for small, rapidly resolving fluid collections to develop adjacent to the uterine wound. Infection and haemorrhage are the commonest post-operative complications and may involve the uterine wound, the anterior abdominal wall or may develop in the peritoneal, extraperitoneal or paravesical spaces.[3] The so-called 'bladder flap' haematoma develops in relationship to the uterine wound. This occurs when haemostasis is not obtained after closure of the uterine wound and a retroperitoneal haematoma may form between the anterior uterine wall and posterior bladder wall.[5] Fluid collections in the abdominal wound may be localised or may track cephalad in the fascial planes of the anterior abdominal wall. Other complications associated with caesarean section include an increased incidence of endometritis and retained products of conception. In the long-term, there is said to be an increased risk of uterine adenomyosis developing as a result of caesarean section. Bleeding may occur at the site of a uterine scar during subsequent deliveries (Fig. 5).

Pelvimetry

The clinical value of pelvimetry is controversial and the use of conventional X-ray techniques has declined, principally due to a concern as to the effects of ionising radiation on the fetus. Prepartum pelvimetry is generally requested in order to assess the dimensions of the bony pelvis when vaginal delivery is contemplated in a breech presentation.

Fig. 3 Endometritis. A: Trans-vaginal scan 3 weeks post-partum in a patient with endometritis. Gas is seen in the uterine cavity (arrow). **B:** Trans-vaginal post-partum scan after caesarean section. The endometritis has progressed to involve the entire uterus. **C:** Severe endometritis after a procured abortion. **D:** Same case as C 2 weeks later following dilatation and curettage and antibiotic treatment. Retained products of conception are still present within the cavity (arrow) but the infection is largely resolved.

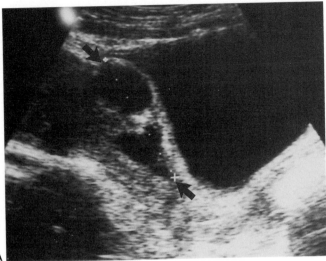

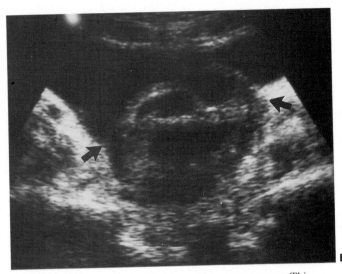

A

B

Fig. 5 Uterine haematoma. A: Longitudinal and **B:** transverse scans of a large haematoma (arrows) involving a previous caesarean scar. This occurred following a normal vaginal delivery.

Vaginal breech delivery is associated with an increased perinatal morbidity and mortality which has led to the considerable increase in the number of caesarean sections. However, favourable assessment of the pelvis by clinical imaging methods will provide confidence for a trial of labour in the breech presentation. Maternal short stature and pelvic deformity are other indications for prepartum pelvimetry. Post-partum pelvimetry is usually requested for pelvic assessment after unplanned caesarean section or where there has been previous dystocia.

X-ray pelvimetry has been the method of choice for many years but the arrival of modern cross-sectional imaging techniques has allowed the development of new methods. Ultrasound pelvimetry has proved unreliable and in particular does not allow proper visualisation of the pelvic configuration and thus this method has been abandoned. However, prior to pelvimetry by whatever method, an ultrasound examination of the fetus should be performed in order to confirm breech presentation, assess gestational age and to make a fetal weight estimation.

In recent years CT pelvimetry has become the method of choice and, with the advent of MRI, another satisfactory method of pelvic assessment has evolved. CT and MRI not only allow the pelvic dimensions to be measured but also allow assessment of the sacral curvature and bony ring of the pelvis. Fetal presentation is noted, particular reference being made to the attitude of the fetal head in the breech fetus.

Only dimensions of the true pelvis, i.e. below the pelvic brim, are of interest to the obstetrician. The axis of the pelvis rotates through 50° between the inlet and the outlet. The cross-sectional shape of the pelvis also changes, the inlet being wider in transverse diameter than the antero-posterior (AP) diameter – with the opposite situation ob-

tained at the outlet where the AP diameter is the greater. The absolute anterior dimensions of the inlet are of the greatest importance as the outlet can expand in all direc-

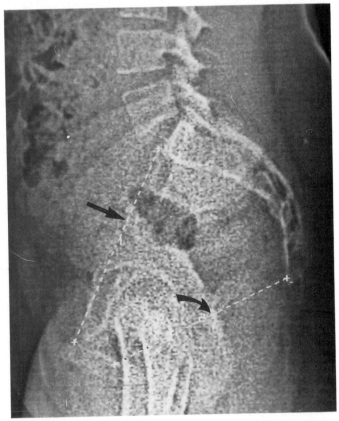

Fig. 6 CT pelvimetry. Lateral scanogram shows AP inlet measurement (straight arrow) and AP outlet measurement (curved arrow).

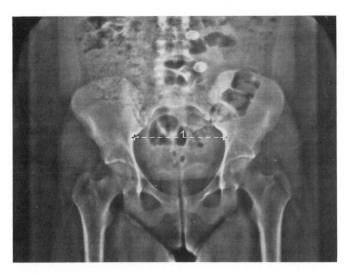

Fig. 7 CT pelvimetry. AP scanogram shows maximum transverse diameter of the pelvic inlet.

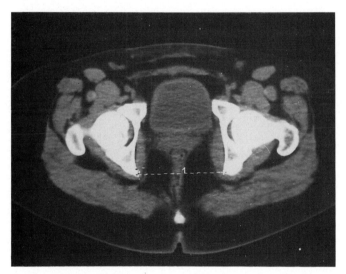

Fig. 8 CT pelvimetry. Axial scan at level of fovea of femoral head shows inter-spinous distance.

tions by relaxation of the sacro-iliac joints and symphysis pubis.

Various methods of CT pelvimetry have been described but in essence two digital radiographs are obtained together with one tomographic cross-section.[6] The examination is rapid with the patient lying in the dorsal supine position throughout. The lateral radiograph allows measurement of the AP dimensions of the pelvis. Using electronic calipers the pelvic inlet is measured from the anterior aspect of the sacral promontory to the posterior cephalad aspect of the symphysis pubis. The outlet is assessed by measuring from the last fixed sacral segment to the posterior caudal aspect of the symphysis pubis (Fig. 6). This view also allows assessment of the contour of the sacral body. The AP radiograph allows measurement of the maximum transverse diameter of the pelvic inlet (Fig. 7) and additionally a fetogram is obtained. Using this view as a guide an axial tomographic section is taken at the level of the fovea capitalis of the femur. This axial scan allows measurement of the inter-spinous diameter thus allowing assessment of the transverse diameter of the mid-pelvic cavity (Fig. 8).

Pelvic dimensions are said to be adequate when the AP diameter of the inlet is greater than 10 cm, the transverse diameter of the inlet is greater than 11.5 cm, the transverse inter-spinous diameter of the mid-pelvis is greater than 9.5 cm and the AP dimension of the pelvic outlet is greater than 11.5 cm.

When compared with conventional X-ray pelvimetry there is a very considerable reduction in radiation dose. Routine X-ray pelvimetry exposes the fetus to 1.3 rads but CT pelvimetry reduces the dose to 0.23 rads.[7]

MRI pelvimetry allows imaging in multiple planes and has the advantage over radiographic and CT methods that no ionising radiation is used. Similar views to those used for CT pelvimetry are obtained using sagittal and anterior/posterior coronal views. In a study of 10 patients at or near term MRI pelvimetry was compared with post-partum MRI pelvimetry and X-ray pelvimetry and all measurements were comparable.[8]

REFERENCES

1 Turnbull A, Chamberlain G. Obstetrics. Edinburgh: Churchill Livingstone. 1989: p 891
2 Gross R C, McGahan J P. Sonographic detection of partial uterine inversion. AJR 1985; 144: 761–762
3 Baker M E, Kay H, Mahony B S D, Cooper C J, Bowie J D. Sonography of the low transverse incision caesarean section: a prospective study. J Ultrasound Med 1988; 7: 389–393
4 Lonky N M, Worthen N, Ross M G. Prediction of caesarean section scars with ultrasound imaging during pregnancy. J Ultrasound Med 1989; 8: 15–19
5 Baker M E, Bowie J D, Killam A P. Sonography of post-caesarean section bladder-flap hematoma. AJR 1985; 144: 757–759
6 Christian S S, Brady K, Read J A, Kopleman J N. Vaginal breech delivery: a five-year prospective evaluation of a protocol using computed tomographic pelvimetry. Am J Obstet Gynecol 1990; 163: 848–855
7 Moore M M, Shearer D R. Fetal dose estimates for CT pelvimetry. Radiology 1989; 171: 265–267
8 van Loon A J, Mantingh A, Thijn C J P, Mooyaart E L. Pelvimetry by magnetic resonance imaging in breech presentation. Am J Obstet Gynecol 1990; 163: 1256–1260

Appendix

Charts of fetal size

Lyn S. Chitty and Douglas G. Altman

INTRODUCTION

There are hundreds of published papers presenting charts (standards) of fetal size (references and review[1,2]). Unfortunately, most of these have serious weaknesses in design or statistical analysis (or both). The working group of the British Medical Ultrasound Society (BMUS) had difficulty identifying even one appropriate study for some fetal measurements.[3]

In this Appendix we consider the appropriate design and analysis of studies to derive reference centiles for fetal size. We describe a study that meets these requirements and present centile charts for various fetal measurements and dating charts. We also compare these new charts with those recommended in the BMUS Report.[3]

Study design

Selection of the sample

As with any research the choice of an appropriate sample is of great importance. A serious weakness of many published studies is that they use routinely collected data, so that multiple observations on the same fetus are included. It is likely that many such fetuses are atypical, as multiple measurements are not taken unless there is some clinical concern. The best approach is to collect data expressly for the purpose of developing a reference range. The date of measurement for each woman can be chosen at random, to give about the same number at each week of gestation. Data can be collected at the time of a routine second trimester scan provided there is no selection for this examination, but each woman should be included only once. Later in pregnancy data should be collected only when examinations are performed specifically for the purpose of the study. Data collected from examinations performed later in pregnan for some other clinical indication (e.g. ? small for dates) should not be included as they may bias the results. Some further sampling is necessary to include sufficient numbers around term, because some women will deliver before the appointed ultrasound date.

A second problem relates to exclusions. Reference data should relate to normal fetuses. It is sensible to exclude data from fetuses subsequently shown to have had a serious congenital abnormality. The exclusion of neonatal deaths is questionable, except for this reason. It may also be appropriate to exclude those with a condition that affects growth, such as maternal diabetes. With these exceptions, it is wrong to make use of information not available at the time of the ultrasound measurement, most notably birth weight. It is reasonable, though, to exclude on the basis of data that are available when the measurement is taken, but we favour as unselected a group as possible. We cannot see the justification for excluding smokers, for example.

Size of sample

It is not as easy to specify the appropriate sample size as, say, for a controlled trial. It should be remembered that attention is concentrated on the tails of the distribution – i.e. the extreme values – and so a large sample is necessary to get a good fix on the placing of say the 5th and 95th centiles. It seems clear that several hundred observations are required; Royston discusses this issue further.[4]

The reference centiles should be calculated from single observations, if that is the usual clinical practice. It is wrong to use the average of two or more measurements.

Analysis

There are two basic approaches to the calculation of reference centiles that can be illustrated by considering the 5th and 95th centiles. The non-parametric approach involves calculating the observed 5th and 95th centiles at each week of gestation and joining these values. The resulting lines are not smooth, although smooth curves can be fitted. The problem with this approach is that a lot of data is needed at each week of gestation for a reasonable estimate of extreme centiles: at least 100 observations and preferably more. The total sample size would thus need to be several thousand. For this reason we do not think that this is a practicable method.

In the parametric approach the 5th and 95th centiles are derived as mean $\pm$ 1.645 SD, the value of 1.645 deriving from the theoretical Normal distribution. The method is based on the strong assumption that at each gestational age the data have a Normal distribution. Most published centiles are constructed in this way, but most studies have deficiencies in the analysis.

Reference centiles should have the following properties:

a) they should change smoothly with gestation;
b) they should be a good fit to the data;
c) the statistical model should be as simple as is compatible with a) and b).

The most common problems with published reference centiles are:

1) there is no explanation of the statistical method used;
2) the centiles do not change smoothly across gestation;
3) there is no assessment of whether the data have a (nearly) Normal distribution;
4) there is no verification that the centiles are a good fit to the data;
5) the authors have failed to take account of change in variability with gestation.

The last is an extremely common error. It has major consequences, because it leads to centiles that are too far apart early in pregnancy and too close later on. Most reports do not include a scatter diagram of the data with the centiles superimposed and therefore the deficiencies may not be readily apparent.

When these aspects are considered in conjunction with design weaknesses it is clear that very few published studies can be considered statistically acceptable. This includes studies whose data are included in the recent BMUS report.[3]

Recommended approach to analysis

The suggested approach to the derivation of centiles can be illustrated by the analysis of 450 measurements of foot length (Fig. 1). This analysis follows the recommendations of Royston[4] and Altman,[5] who give detailed explanations and discussion.

Step 1 – model the mean

A polynomial regression model is fitted to the data – a quadratic or cubic curve usually gives a reasonable fit. The 'linear-cubic' model seems to work well for fetal size data; this is given by

$$Y = b_0 + b_1X + b_2X^3$$

where X is gestational age and Y is the measurement. The model chosen is the simplest that gives a good fit to the data (see below). Figure 1 shows the linear-cubic model fitted to the foot measurements.

Step 2 – obtain residuals

Calculate the differences between the observed values and the fitted line (known as residuals). A plot of these values against gestational age shows how the variability changes with gestation.

Step 3 – check the distribution

Assess these for Normality using a Normal plot and perhaps also a formal test. If not Normal, the data may require transformation.

Step 4 – model the variability

The standard deviation (SD) of the residuals is modelled as a function of gestation. For fetal size, linear or quadratic regression is usually adequate. We have used the method described by Altman.[5] The values ± 1.645 SD can be superimposed on the residual plot to see how well the SD has been modelled (Fig. 2). The numbers above and below the range should be close to the expected proportions. Here 10% of the observations lie above the 90th centile and 11% below the 10th centile.

Step 5 – calculate standard deviation scores

Calculate for each observation a standard deviation score (SDS) (also called a standardised residual) as SDS = (observed value − fitted mean)/fitted SD.

Step 6 – check the distribution

Assess the SDSs for Normality as in step 3. Normally distributed data should lie on a straight line. Figure 3 shows the Normal plot for the foot measurements, and the associated Shapiro-Francia W test gives F = 0.6. Together these show that the model is a good fit to the data. Non-Normality would indicate the need to transform the data.

Step 7 – derive the centiles

The required centiles are calculated and superimposed on

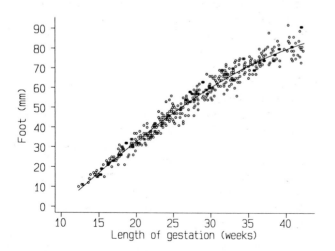

Fig. 1 450 measurements of foot length with fitted curve describing the mean.

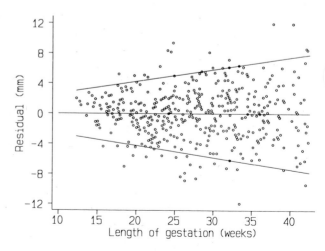

Fig. 2 Residuals from model describing mean with fitted 5th and 95th centiles.

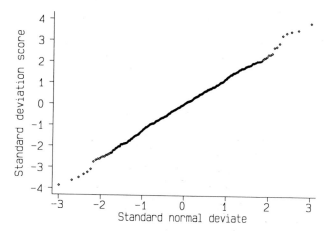

Fig. 3 Normal plot of standard deviation scores.

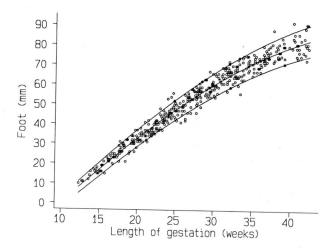

Fig. 4 Foot length measurements with fitted 5th, 50th and 95th centiles.

a scatter diagram of the observations as a final check of the fit. Figure 4 shows the 5th, 50th and 95th centiles for the foot measurements. The 5th and 95th centiles were obtained as mean ± 1.645 SD. If a transformation has been used, the mean and SD (and thus the centiles) are obtained in the transformed scale, and need to be back-transformed to the original scale.

The approach described above meets all the previously stated requirements. A major advantage is that any observation can be converted into a standard deviation score using the regression equations for the mean and SD. Thus a precise centile for any measurement can be obtained by reference to a table of the standard Normal distribution. Further, subgroups of fetuses can be compared, as can a new group with the reference group using simple t tests. For example, the European and Afrocarribean groups can be compared.

This method was used to produce the centile charts

shown on pages 523–555. The three kidney measurements were found to need a square root transformation to achieve a Normal distribution of SDSs. None of the other measurements needed transformation.

Dating charts

There are many reports of the value of ultrasound in the prediction of gestational age. The literature is comprehensibly reviewed by Geirsson.[6] The measurements which have been found to be of most value in the second trimester are the biparietal diameter (BPD), femur length and head circumference. In the first trimester, the crown-rump length is considered to be the most valuable measurement.[7] Charts for predicting gestational age from fetal size are produced in a similar fashion, except that they are based on regression of gestational age on fetal size.[3] Again, simple polynomial regression should suffice.

The dating charts shown on pages 557–567 were obtained using the same general approach as for the charts of fetal size. Only data up to approximately 30 weeks of gestation were included, i.e. BPD <76 mm, head circumference <281 mm and femur length <56 mm. In each case it was found necessary to apply a logarithmic transformation to gestational age.

Construction of new charts of fetal size

Patient selection and recruitment

All the patients included in this study were scanned by one of three operators using an Hitachi EUB-340 in the ultrasound department at King's College Hospital. As this was a cross-sectional study each fetus was measured once only between 12 and 42 weeks for the purposes of the study. Women were recruited in one of four ways.

1) Women scanned between 12 and 17 weeks were recruited prospectively at the time of booking for prenatal care and asked to attend for one extra examination before their routine second trimester scan.
2) Data were collected from women between 18 and 23 weeks at the time of a routine scan.
3) Women were recruited prospectively in the ultrasound clinic at the time of their routine examination and asked to return for an extra scan at a randomly allocated gestation from 23 weeks.
4) As the study progressed it became clear that many of the women asked to return at 37 weeks or later had delivered prior to the study scan. Women were therefore recruited and studied between 37 and 42 weeks at the time of their visit to the antenatal clinic.

Only western European and Afrocaribbean racial groups were included. All subjects had a known last menstrual period and the ultrasound and menstrual age at 18 to 20 weeks agreed to within 10 days. Exclusion criteria were:

1) maternal disease or medication which was likely to affect the growth of the fetus (diabetes mellitus, renal disease, hypertension requiring treatment etc.);
2) multiple pregnancies;
3) the presence of a fetal malformation;
4) cases where the neonate was found to have a significant congenital malformation, abnormal karyotype or other disease at birth.

A total of 669 fetuses were examined for the purpose of the study. There were two exclusions. One neonate who was scanned at 13 weeks gestation had trisomy 21. The other was scanned at 32 weeks, at which time marked asymmetrical intra-uterine growth retardation was noted. At birth the neonate had dysmorphic features compatible with trisomy 18, a diagnosis confirmed by karyotyping.

We aimed to obtain 20 measurements for each variable for each week of pregnancy from 12 until 42 weeks. It was not possible to obtain every measurement from each fetus due to fetal position and so this objective was not met in all cases. Only one measurement was taken of each variable.

Measurements

The BPD was measured in the axial plane at the level where the continuous midline echo is broken by the septum pellucidum cavum in the anterior third (see Ch. 11, Fig. 7 and Ch. 13, Fig. 2). The measurements were made from the proximal echo of the fetal skull to the distal side of the border deep to the ultrasound beam (outer–outer) or from the proximal edge to the proximal edge of the deep border (outer–inner). The head circumference was measured at the same level. The abdominal circumference was measured on a transverse section through the fetal abdomen which was as close as possible to a circle and at a level where the umbilical vein was seen in the anterior third and the stomach bubble was visualised in the same plane (see Ch. 13, Fig. 5). The head and abdominal circumferences were measured both directly by tracing around the perimeter and by derivation from the measurement of the diameters (OFD and BPD outer-outer for the head, and transverse and antero-posterior diameters for the abdomen).

All long bones (radius, ulna, humerus, tibia, fibula and femur) were measured in a plane such that the bone was as close as possible to a right angle to the ultrasound beam. Care was taken to ensure that the full length of the bone was visualised and the view was not obscured by shadowing from adjacent bony parts. The radius and ulna, tibia and fibula were measured independently. The foot was measured in the plantar view, the measurement being made from the heel to the end of the longest toe.

The kidneys were measured in three planes. The renal length was measured from the upper to the lower pole. The antero-posterior and transverse diameters were both measured in a transverse section through the fetal abdomen. The level taken was at the height of the renal pelvis if visible or, if not, in a plane where the kidney appeared largest. It was not always possible to visualise both kidneys well enough to obtain accurate measurements on both. We have included measurements of only one kidney per fetus in the construction of the kidney size charts.

The size charts derived from these measurements, shown on pages 523–555, refer to exact gestational age. Half a week should be added if age is recorded in completed weeks. We have also derived a head circumference/abdominal circumference (HC/AC) ratio chart for use in the assessment of fetal growth as described by Campbell and Thoms.[8]

These charts are based on cross-sectional data and should be used only for assessing size. Although serial measurements may show increasing or decreasing centiles for a fetus over time these charts are not suitable for assessing how unusual such changes are.

Comparison with other published data

The cross-sectional data collected in this study have been compared with the published data selected by the BMUS working party on fetal biometry.[3] Longitudinal data based on serial measurement of 50 fetuses have also been collected. Preliminary analysis of the abdominal circumference data does not reveal any major differences between our longitudinal and cross-sectional data sets; therefore the cross-sectional data are used in the comparisons described below.

Biparietal diameter

The data on the measurement of the BPD collected by Hadlock et al[9] are only slightly different from our data (Fig. 5) with the main difference occurring early in the second trimester when the 50th centile derived from Hadlock's data is greater than ours. This may be a reflection of the very small numbers in the Hadlock study at these gestations – 2 at 12, 3 at 13 and 4 at 14 weeks compared to 10, 18 and 18 respectively in our study. Hadlock's curves show much tighter centiles. This is probably because they unreasonably excluded all fetuses with either head or abdominal circumference outside mean ± 2 SD.

Head circumference

We compared the head circumference data from the same group[10] with our data. The plane used for measurement was the same in both studies. As they used direct measurement around the outer perimeter of the calvarium we have compared their data with our data obtained by direct measurement (Fig. 6). The 50th centile derived from the

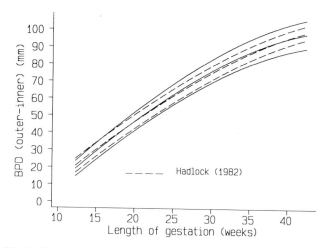

Fig. 5 Comparison of our biparietal diameter chart with that of Hadlock et al.[9]

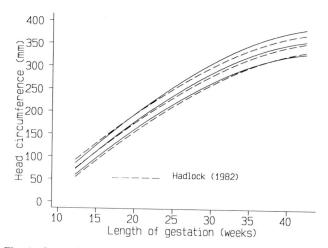

Fig. 6 Comparison of our head circumference (directly measured) chart with that of Hadlock et al.[10]

Hadlock data shows a slightly greater decrease towards term. There are marked differences in the 5th and 95th centiles because of Hadlock's failure to take into account the increase in variability with increasing gestation.

Measurement technique is important as we have found that there is a small but constant difference between the centiles derived from the data obtained by direct measurement around the perimeter of the head circumference and that obtained by derivation from the diameters. The latter is about 1.5% less across all gestations than the direct measurement.

Abdominal circumference

Comparison of our abdominal circumference data with that from Hadlock's group[11] shows that there is no difference between the two 50th centiles (Fig. 7). As with the other

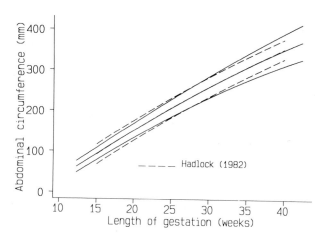

Fig. 7 Comparison of our abdominal circumference (directly measured) chart with that of Hadlock et al.[11]

studies, failure to model the standard deviation results in Hadlock's centiles being wider apart in early pregnancy and much narrower towards term. Deter et al[12] do take the increasing variation into account and the separation between their centiles is very similar to ours (Fig. 8). They used a straight line regression model and therefore their data do not show the customary decrease in abdominal circumference towards term seen in both our data and that reported by Hadlock et al.[11]

Technique is also important in the measurement of the abdominal circumference. The value derived from the measurement of the diameters is about 3.5% smaller than that obtained by direct measurement at all gestations. Jeanty et al[13] derived their data from measurement of the abdominal diameters and so we have compared their data with ours obtained using the same technique (Fig. 9). Jeanty et al excluded fetuses who were below the third cen-

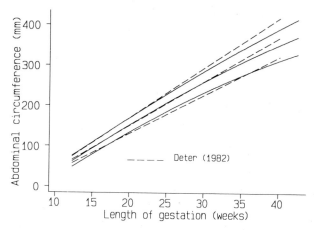

Fig. 8 Comparison of our abdominal circumference (directly measured) with that of Deter et al.[12]

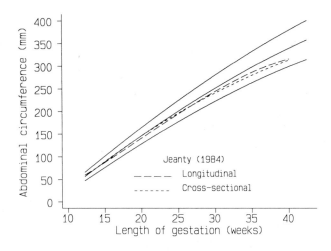

Fig. 9   Comparison of our abdominal circumference (derived from the measurement of the abdominal diameters) chart with the cross-sectional and longitudinal data of Jeanty et al.[13]

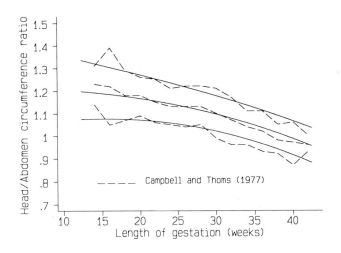

Fig. 10   Comparison of our head/abdominal circumference ratio chart with that of Campbell and Thoms.[8]

tile for birth weight. If these babies were structurally normal we do not consider this to be a reasonable exclusion criterion. However, it does not account for the unusually marked fall in circumference from 30 weeks seen in their data. Difference in study design (i.e. longitudinal rather than cross-sectional) is unlikely to be the cause since this fall is seen in both Jeanty's longitudinal and cross-sectional curves.

HC/AC ratio

The HC/AC chart from our data has been compared with that of Campbell and Thoms (Fig. 10).[8] Although Campbell and Thoms did not apply any mathematical smoothing, the two data sets appear similar overall.

Femur

Femur length has been compared with the data collected by Warda et al.[14] There is a minimal difference in the 50th centiles (Fig. 11). Warda's derived line is straighter than ours. It is noteworthy that the authors state that all examinations in their study were performed because of a clinical indication unrelated to the study. Warda et al modelled the standard deviation as a constant percentage of the mean, resulting in very narrow separation earlier in pregnancy and much wider separation at term.

Centile charts

Centile charts and tabulated values for various fetal measurements are presented. Dating charts shown on pages 557–567 give the best estimate of gestation with a 95%

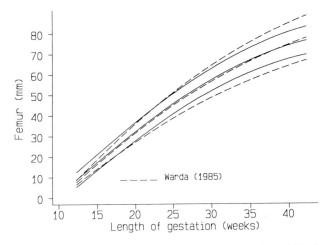

Fig. 11   Comparison of our femur length chart with that of Warda et al.[14]

prediction interval. We did not study fetuses in the first trimester and so have included a dating chart of crown-rump length using the data from Robinson and Fleming.[7] Charts of fetal size shown on pages 523–555 give 5th, 50th and 95th centiles. For both dating and size charts the accompanying tables show the smoothed values rather than the raw data.

Acknowledgements

LSC was supported by a Medical Research Council Training Fellowship. Thanks are due to Trish Chudleigh and Annabel Henderson for their help in scanning the fetuses included in the study described here.

REFERENCES

1 Deter R L, Harrist R B, Birnholz J C, Hadlock F P. Quantitative obstetrical ultrasonography. New York: Wiley. 1986
2 Kurtz A B, Goldberg B B. Obstetrical measurements in ultrasound. A reference manual. New York: Year Book. 1988
3 British Medical Ultrasound Society Fetal Measurements Working Party Report. Clinical applications of ultrasonic fetal measurements. London: British Institute of Radiology. 1990
4 Royston J P. Constructing time-specific reference ranges. Statistics in Medicine 1991; 10: 675–690
5 Altman D G. Construction of age-related reference centiles using absolute residuals. Submitted.
6 Geirsson R T. Ultrasound instead of last menstrual period as the basis of gestational age assignment. Ultrasound Obstet Gynecol 1991; 1: 212–219
7 Robinson H P, Fleming J E E. A critical evaluation of sonar crown-rump length measurements. Br J Obstet Gynaecol 1975; 82: 702–710
8 Campbell S, Thoms A. Ultrasound measurement of the fetal head to abdominal circumference ratio in the assessment of growth retardation. Br J Obstet Gynaecol 1977; 84: 165–174
9 Hadlock F P, Deter R L, Harrist R B, Park K P. Fetal biparietal diameter: a critical re-evaluation to menstrual age by means of real-time ultrasound. J Ultrasound Med 1982; 1: 97–104
10 Hadlock F P, Deter R L, Harrist R B, Park K P. Fetal head circumference: relation to menstrual age. AJR 1982; 138: 647–653
11 Hadlock F P, Deter R L, Harrist R B, Park S K. Fetal abdominal circumference as a predictor of menstrual age. AJR 1982; 139: 367–370
12 Deter R L, Harrist R B, Hadlock F P, Carpenter R J. Fetal head and abdominal circumferences: II. A critical re-evaluation of the relationship to menstrual age. JCU 1982; 10: 365–372
13 Jeanty P, Cousaert E, Cantraine F. Normal growth of the fetal abdominal perimeter. Am J Perinatology 1984; 1: 127–135
14 Warda A H, Deter R L, Rossavik I K, Carpenter R J, Hadlock F P. Fetal femur length: a critical re-evaluation of the relationship to menstrual age. Obstet Gynecol 1985; 66: 69–75

Biparietal diameter (outer-outer) (mm)

Gestation (weeks)	c5	c50	c95
13	19.9	23.3	26.8
14	23.5	27.2	30.8
15	27.1	30.9	34.8
16	30.6	34.6	38.7
17	34.1	38.3	42.5
18	37.5	41.9	46.3
19	40.8	45.4	49.9
20	44.1	48.8	53.5
21	47.3	52.2	57.1
22	50.5	55.5	60.5
23	53.6	58.7	63.8
24	56.6	61.9	67.1
25	59.5	64.9	70.3
26	62.4	67.8	73.3
27	65.2	70.7	76.3
28	67.8	73.5	79.1
29	70.4	76.1	81.8
30	72.9	78.7	84.4
31	75.3	81.1	86.9
32	77.5	83.4	89.3
33	79.7	85.6	91.5
34	81.7	87.7	93.6
35	83.7	89.6	95.6
36	85.5	91.5	97.4
37	87.2	93.1	99.1
38	88.7	94.7	100.7
39	90.1	96.1	102.1
40	91.4	97.4	103.3
41	92.6	98.5	104.4
42	93.6	99.5	105.3

BIPARIETAL DIAMETER (outer-outer)
5th, 50th and 95th centiles

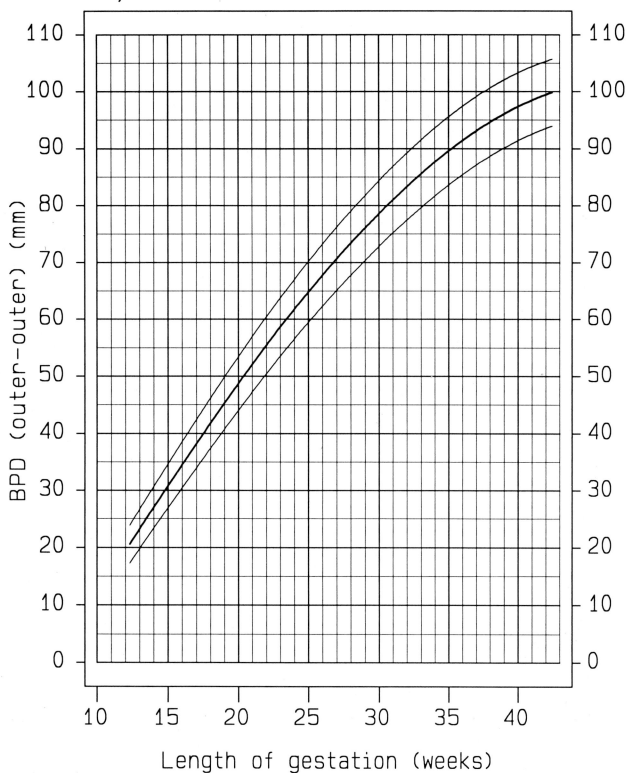

Biparietal diameter (outer-inner) (mm)

Gestation (weeks)	c5	c50	c95
13	18.1	21.8	25.5
14	21.7	25.5	29.3
15	25.2	29.1	33.0
16	28.7	32.7	36.7
17	32.2	36.3	40.4
18	35.6	39.8	44.0
19	38.9	43.2	47.5
20	42.1	46.5	50.9
21	45.3	49.8	54.3
22	48.4	53.1	57.7
23	51.5	56.2	60.9
24	54.4	59.3	64.1
25	57.3	62.2	67.1
26	60.1	65.1	70.1
27	62.8	67.9	73.0
28	65.4	70.6	75.9
29	68.0	73.3	78.6
30	70.4	75.8	81.2
31	72.7	78.2	83.7
32	74.9	80.5	86.1
33	77.0	82.7	88.4
34	79.0	84.8	90.6
35	80.8	86.7	92.6
36	82.6	88.6	94.6
37	84.2	90.3	96.4
38	85.7	91.9	98.1
39	87.0	93.3	99.7
40	88.3	94.7	101.1
41	89.4	95.9	102.4
42	90.3	96.9	103.5

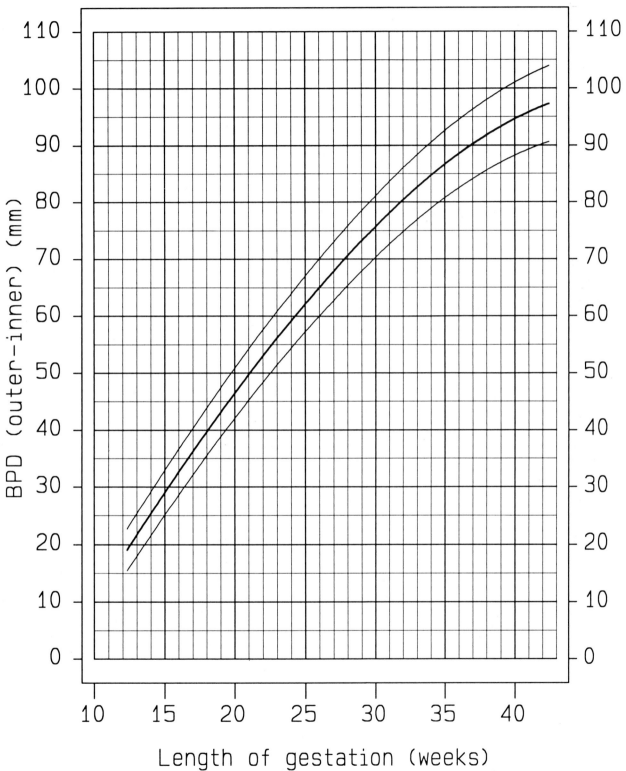

BIPARIETAL DIAMETER (outer-inner)
5th, 50th and 95th centiles

Head circumference (plotted) (mm)

Gestation (weeks)	c5	c50	c95
13	71.9	82.7	93.6
14	85.7	96.9	108.1
15	99.3	110.9	122.5
16	112.6	124.6	136.6
17	125.7	138.1	150.5
18	138.6	151.4	164.1
19	151.2	164.4	177.5
20	163.5	177.1	190.6
21	175.6	189.5	203.4
22	187.3	201.6	215.9
23	198.6	213.3	228.0
24	209.7	224.8	239.8
25	220.4	235.8	251.3
26	230.7	246.5	262.4
27	240.6	256.8	273.1
28	250.1	266.7	283.4
29	259.2	276.2	293.2
30	267.9	285.3	302.7
31	276.1	293.9	311.7
32	283.9	302.1	320.2
33	291.2	309.8	328.3
34	298.0	316.9	335.9
35	304.3	323.6	343.0
36	310.1	329.8	349.5
37	315.3	335.4	355.5
38	320.0	340.5	361.0
39	324.2	345.0	365.9
40	327.7	349.0	370.2
41	330.7	352.3	373.9
42	333.0	355.0	377.1

HEAD CIRCUMFERENCE (plotted)
5th, 50th and 95th centiles

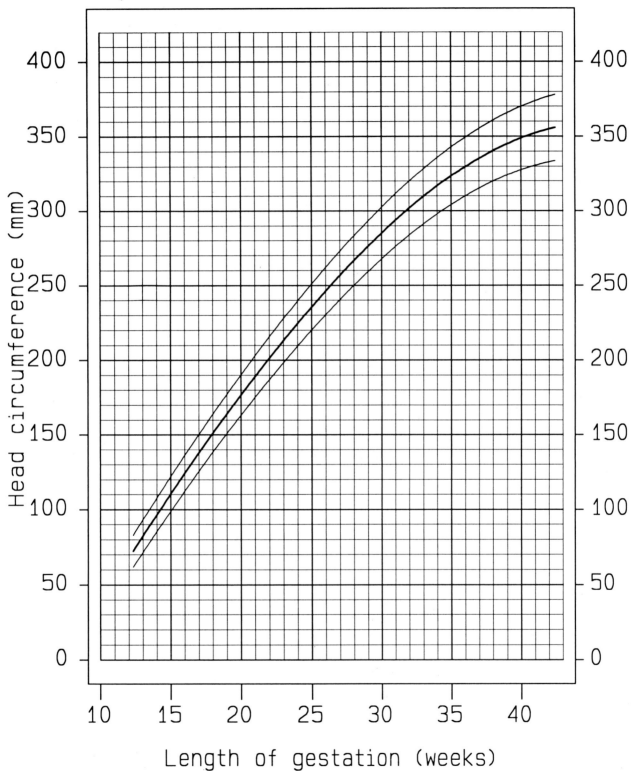

Head circumference (mm)

Length of gestation (weeks)

Head circumference (derived) (mm)

Gestation (weeks)	c5	c50	c95
13	69.3	81.0	92.6
14	83.0	95.0	107.1
15	96.5	108.9	121.3
16	109.8	122.6	135.3
17	122.8	136.0	149.1
18	135.5	149.1	162.6
19	148.0	162.0	175.9
20	160.2	174.6	188.9
21	172.1	186.8	201.5
22	183.7	198.8	213.9
23	195.0	210.4	225.9
24	205.9	221.7	237.6
25	216.4	232.7	248.9
26	226.6	243.2	259.8
27	236.4	253.4	270.4
28	245.8	263.1	280.5
29	254.7	272.5	290.2
30	263.2	281.4	299.5
31	271.3	289.8	308.4
32	278.9	297.8	316.7
33	286.0	305.3	324.6
34	292.6	312.3	332.0
35	298.8	318.8	338.9
36	304.3	324.8	345.2
37	309.4	330.2	351.0
38	313.9	335.1	356.3
39	317.8	339.4	360.9
40	321.1	343.1	365.0
41	323.8	346.2	368.5
42	325.9	348.7	371.4

HEAD CIRCUMFERENCE (derived)
5th, 50th and 95th centiles

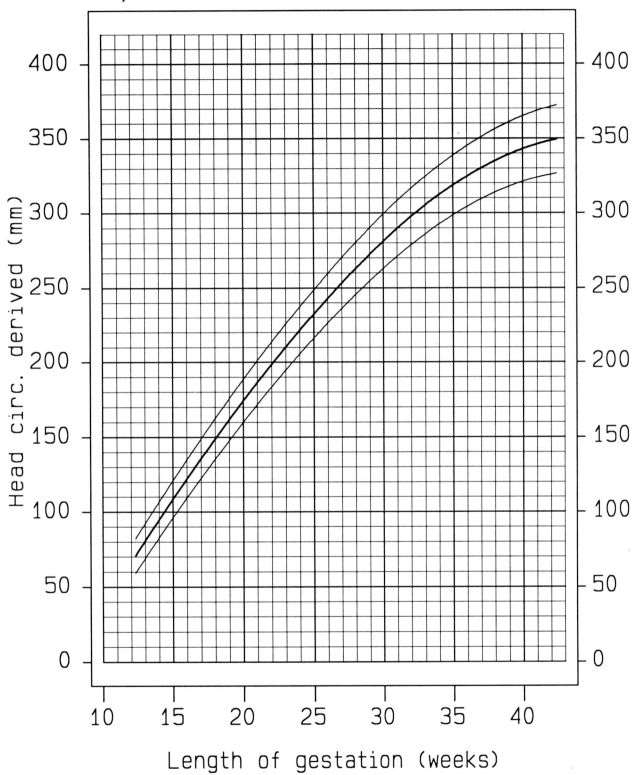

Abdominal circumference (plotted) (mm)

Gestation (weeks)	c5	c50	c95
13	58.9	70.7	82.5
14	70.4	82.6	94.7
15	81.9	94.4	106.8
16	93.2	106.1	118.9
17	104.5	117.7	131.0
18	115.6	129.3	143.0
19	126.6	140.8	155.0
20	137.4	152.1	166.9
21	148.1	163.4	178.7
22	158.7	174.6	190.5
23	169.1	185.6	202.2
24	179.4	196.6	213.8
25	189.5	207.4	225.3
26	199.5	218.1	236.8
27	209.3	228.7	248.2
28	218.9	239.2	259.4
29	228.4	249.5	270.6
30	237.7	259.7	281.7
31	246.8	269.7	292.6
32	255.7	279.6	303.5
33	264.4	289.3	314.2
34	272.9	298.8	324.8
35	281.2	308.2	335.2
36	289.3	317.4	345.6
37	297.2	326.4	355.7
38	304.8	335.3	365.8
39	312.3	344.0	375.7
40	319.5	352.4	385.4
41	326.5	360.7	395.0
42	333.2	368.8	404.4

ABDOMINAL CIRCUMFERENCE (plotted)
5th, 50th and 95th centiles

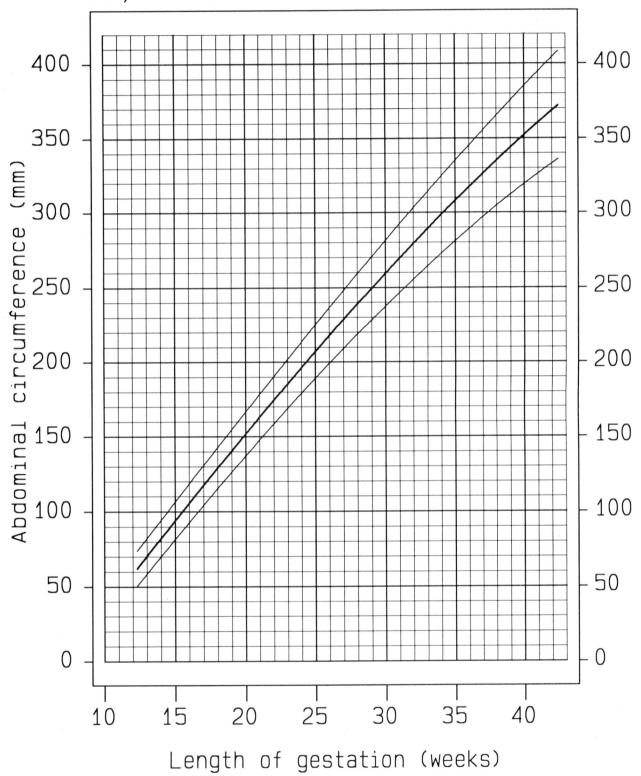

Abdominal circumference (derived) (mm)

Gestation (weeks)	c5	c50	c95
13	57.1	65.5	73.9
14	68.0	77.3	86.6
15	78.8	89.1	99.3
16	89.6	100.7	111.9
17	100.2	112.3	124.3
18	110.8	123.8	136.7
19	121.3	135.1	149.0
20	131.6	146.4	161.2
21	141.8	157.5	173.2
22	151.9	168.5	185.2
23	161.9	179.4	197.0
24	171.7	190.2	208.6
25	181.4	200.8	220.2
26	191.0	211.3	231.5
27	200.4	221.6	242.8
28	209.7	231.7	253.8
29	218.7	241.7	264.7
30	227.6	251.6	275.5
31	236.4	261.2	286.0
32	244.9	270.7	296.4
33	253.3	280.0	306.6
34	261.5	289.1	316.6
35	269.5	297.9	326.4
36	277.2	306.6	336.0
37	284.8	315.1	345.4
38	292.2	323.4	354.6
39	299.3	331.4	363.5
40	306.2	339.2	372.3
41	312.9	346.8	380.8
42	319.3	354.1	389.0

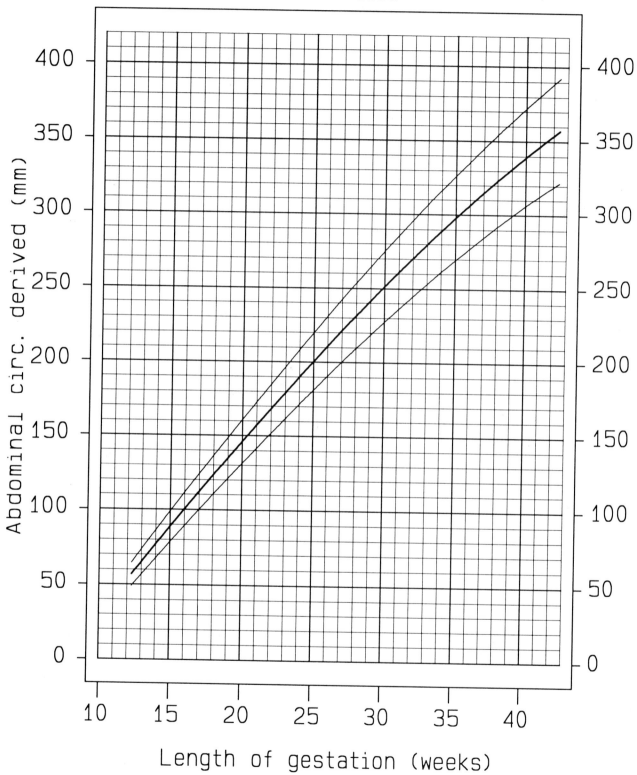

ABDOMINAL CIRCUMFERENCE (derived)
5th, 50th and 95th centiles

Head/abdomen circumference ratio

Gestation (weeks)	c5	c50	c95
13	1.08	1.20	1.33
14	1.08	1.19	1.32
15	1.08	1.19	1.31
16	1.08	1.19	1.30
17	1.08	1.18	1.30
18	1.08	1.18	1.29
19	1.07	1.17	1.28
20	1.07	1.17	1.27
21	1.07	1.16	1.26
22	1.07	1.16	1.25
23	1.06	1.15	1.24
24	1.06	1.14	1.23
25	1.05	1.14	1.23
26	1.05	1.13	1.22
27	1.04	1.12	1.21
28	1.04	1.11	1.20
29	1.03	1.11	1.19
30	1.02	1.10	1.18
31	1.01	1.09	1.17
32	1.00	1.08	1.16
33	0.99	1.07	1.15
34	0.99	1.06	1.14
35	0.97	1.05	1.12
36	0.96	1.04	1.11
37	0.95	1.02	1.10
38	0.94	1.01	1.09
39	0.93	1.00	1.08
40	0.91	0.99	1.07
41	0.90	0.97	1.05
42	0.89	0.96	1.04

HEAD/ABDOMEN CIRCUMFERENCE RATIO
5th, 50th and 95th centiles

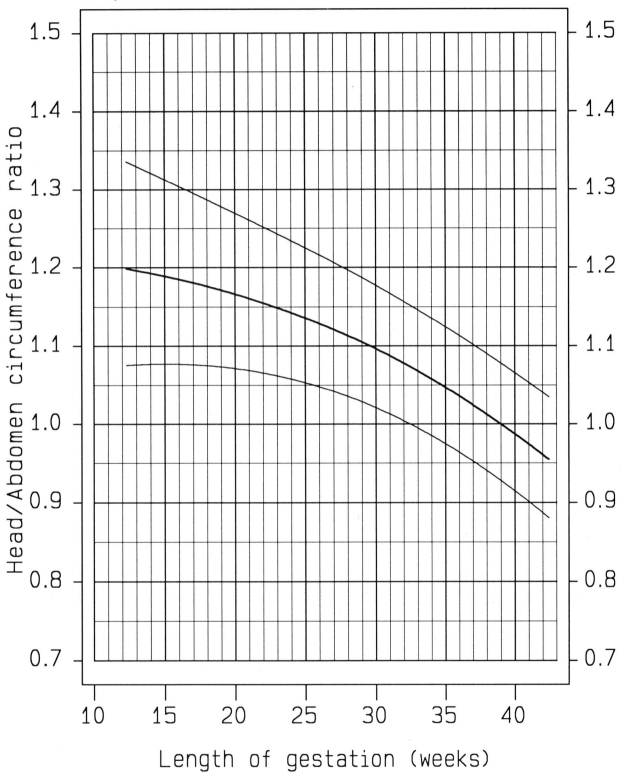

Length of gestation (weeks)

Femur (mm)

Gestation (weeks)	c5	c50	c95
13	8.1	11.1	14.1
14	11.1	14.2	17.3
15	14.1	17.3	20.5
16	17.1	20.3	23.6
17	20.0	23.3	26.7
18	22.9	26.3	29.7
19	25.7	29.2	32.7
20	28.4	32.1	35.7
21	31.2	34.9	38.6
22	33.8	37.6	41.4
23	36.4	40.3	44.2
24	38.9	42.9	46.9
25	41.4	45.4	49.5
26	43.8	47.9	52.1
27	46.1	50.3	54.5
28	48.3	52.6	57.0
29	50.5	54.9	59.3
30	52.6	57.1	61.5
31	54.6	59.1	63.7
32	56.5	61.1	65.8
33	58.3	63.0	67.8
34	60.0	64.9	69.7
35	61.7	66.6	71.5
36	63.2	68.2	73.2
37	64.6	69.7	74.8
38	66.0	71.1	76.3
39	67.2	72.4	77.7
40	68.3	73.6	79.0
41	69.3	74.7	80.2
42	70.2	75.7	81.2

FEMUR
5th, 50th and 95th centiles

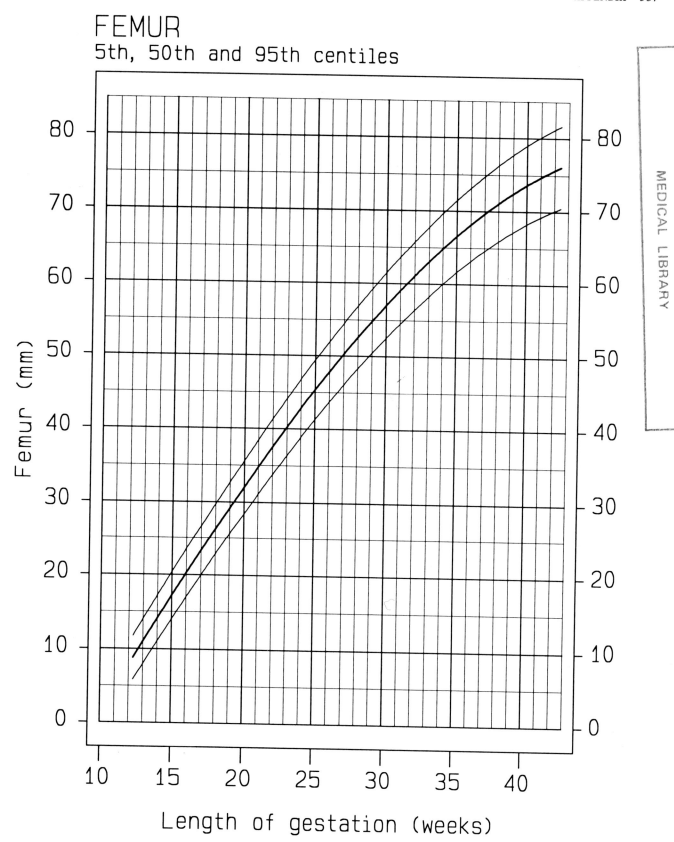

Radius (mm)

Gestation (weeks)	c5	c50	c95
13	6.4	9.7	13.0
14	8.8	12.2	15.5
15	11.2	14.6	18.0
16	13.5	17.0	20.5
17	15.8	19.3	22.9
18	18.0	21.6	25.2
19	20.2	23.9	27.5
20	22.3	26.0	29.7
21	24.4	28.2	31.9
22	26.4	30.2	34.1
23	28.3	32.2	36.1
24	30.2	34.2	38.1
25	32.0	36.0	40.0
26	33.8	37.8	41.9
27	35.4	39.5	43.7
28	37.0	41.2	45.4
29	38.5	42.7	47.0
30	39.9	44.2	48.5
31	41.2	45.6	50.0
32	42.5	46.9	51.4
33	43.6	48.1	52.6
34	44.7	49.2	53.8
35	45.7	50.3	54.9
36	46.5	51.2	55.9
37	47.3	52.0	56.7
38	47.9	52.7	57.5
39	48.5	53.3	58.2
40	48.9	53.8	58.7
41	49.2	54.2	59.1
42	49.4	54.4	59.5

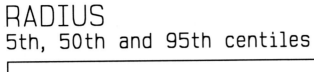

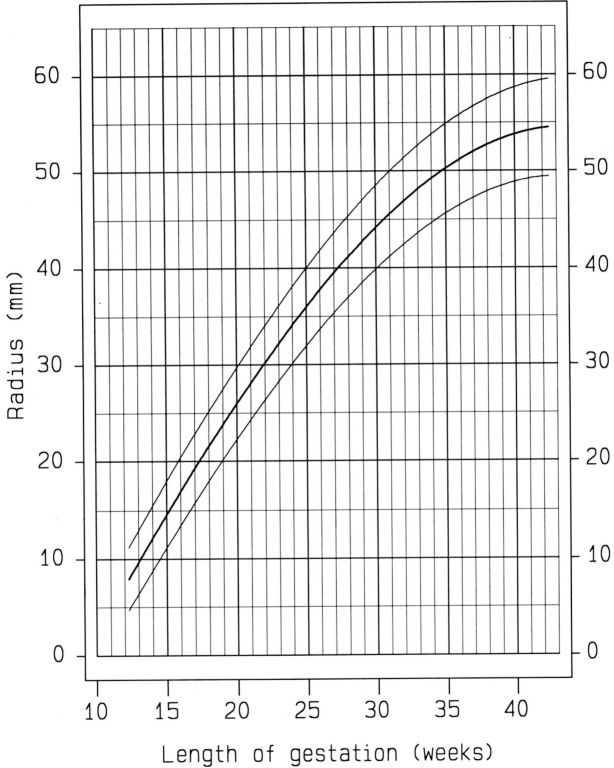

Ulna (mm)

Gestation (weeks)	c5	c50	c95
13	7.1	10.6	14.0
14	9.9	13.3	16.8
15	12.5	16.0	10.6
16	15.1	18.7	22.3
17	17.7	21.4	25.0
18	20.2	23.9	27.7
19	22.7	26.5	30.3
20	25.1	28.9	32.8
21	27.4	31.3	35.3
22	29.7	33.7	37.7
23	31.9	36.0	40.0
24	34.1	38.2	42.3
25	36.2	40.3	44.5
26	38.2	42.4	46.7
27	40.1	44.4	48.7
28	42.0	46.3	50.7
29	43.7	48.2	52.6
30	45.4	49.9	54.4
31	47.0	51.6	56.1
32	48.5	53.2	57.8
33	50.0	54.6	59.3
34	51.3	56.0	60.8
35	52.5	57.3	62.1
36	53.6	58.5	63.4
37	54.6	59.6	64.5
38	55.5	60.5	65.5
39	56.3	61.4	66.4
40	57.0	62.1	67.3
41	57.6	62.8	67.9
42	58.0	63.3	68.5

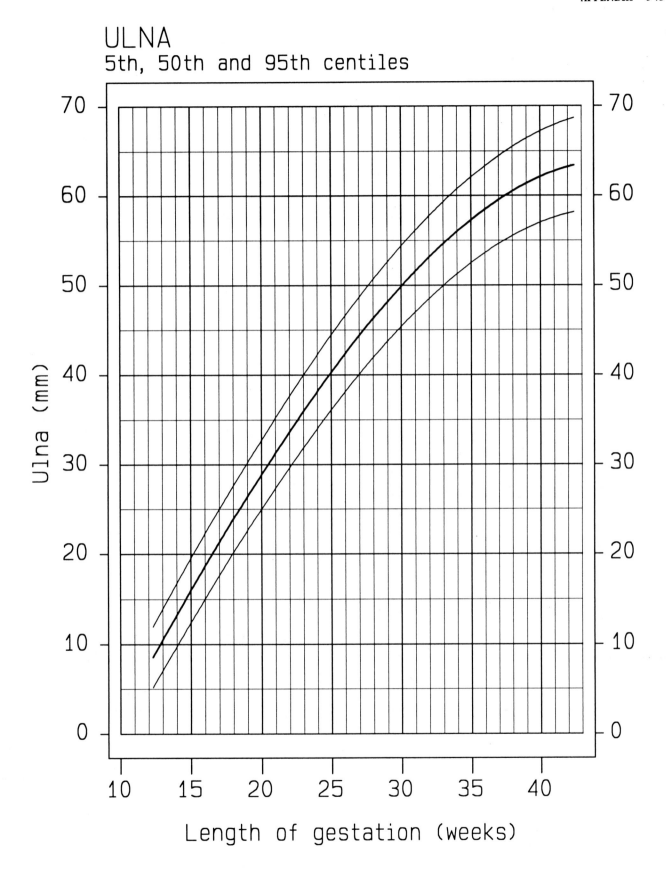

ULNA
5th, 50th and 95th centiles

Fibula (mm)

Gestation (weeks)	c5	c50	c95
13	5.7	8.6	11.5
14	8.4	11.4	14.4
15	11.2	14.2	17.3
16	13.8	17.0	20.2
17	16.5	19.7	23.0
18	19.1	22.4	25.8
19	21.6	25.0	28.5
20	24.1	27.6	31.1
21	26.5	30.1	33.7
22	28.9	32.6	36.3
23	31.2	35.0	38.8
24	33.5	37.3	41.2
25	35.7	39.6	43.6
26	37.8	41.8	45.8
27	39.8	43.9	48.1
28	41.8	46.0	50.2
29	43.7	47.9	52.2
30	45.5	49.8	54.2
31	47.2	51.6	56.1
32	48.8	53.4	57.9
33	50.3	55.0	59.6
34	51.8	56.5	61.3
35	53.2	58.0	62.8
36	54.4	59.3	64.2
37	55.6	60.6	65.5
38	56.6	61.7	66.8
39	57.6	62.7	67.9
40	58.4	63.6	68.9
41	59.1	64.5	69.8
42	59.7	65.1	70.6

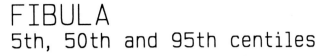

FIBULA
5th, 50th and 95th centiles

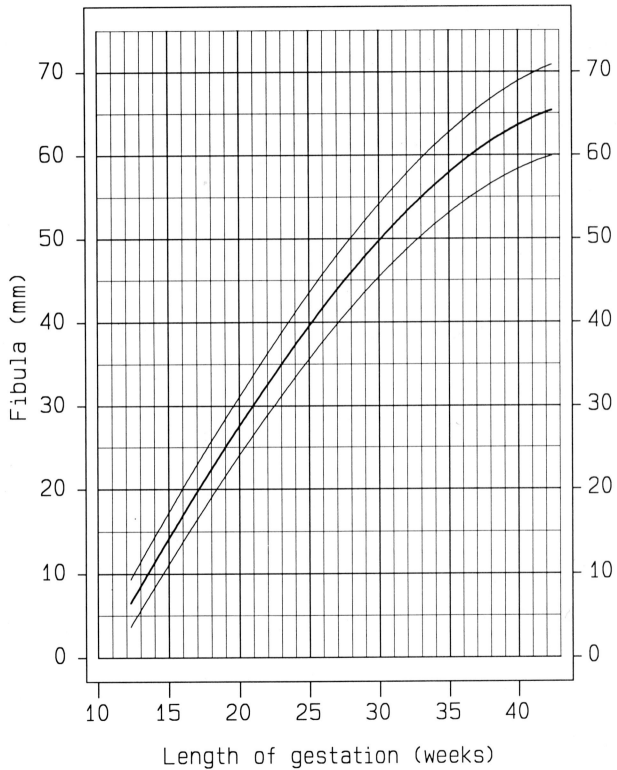

Fibula (mm)

Length of gestation (weeks)

Tibia (mm)

Gestation (weeks)	c5	c50	c95
13	6.1	8.9	11.7
14	8.9	11.8	14.7
15	11.7	14.7	17.7
16	14.4	17.5	20.6
17	17.1	20.3	23.5
18	19.8	23.0	26.3
19	22.4	25.7	29.0
20	24.9	28.3	31.7
21	27.4	30.9	34.4
22	29.8	33.4	37.0
23	32.2	35.9	39.5
24	34.5	38.2	42.0
25	36.7	40.6	44.4
26	38.9	42.8	46.7
27	41.0	45.0	49.0
28	43.0	47.1	51.2
29	44.9	49.1	53.3
30	46.7	51.0	55.3
31	48.5	52.9	57.2
32	50.2	54.6	59.1
33	51.8	56.3	60.8
34	53.3	57.9	62.5
35	54.7	59.4	64.1
36	56.0	60.8	65.6
37	57.2	62.1	66.9
38	58.3	63.2	68.2
39	59.3	64.3	69.4
40	60.2	65.3	70.4
41	60.9	66.1	71.4
42	61.6	66.9	72.2

TIBIA
5th, 50th and 95th centiles

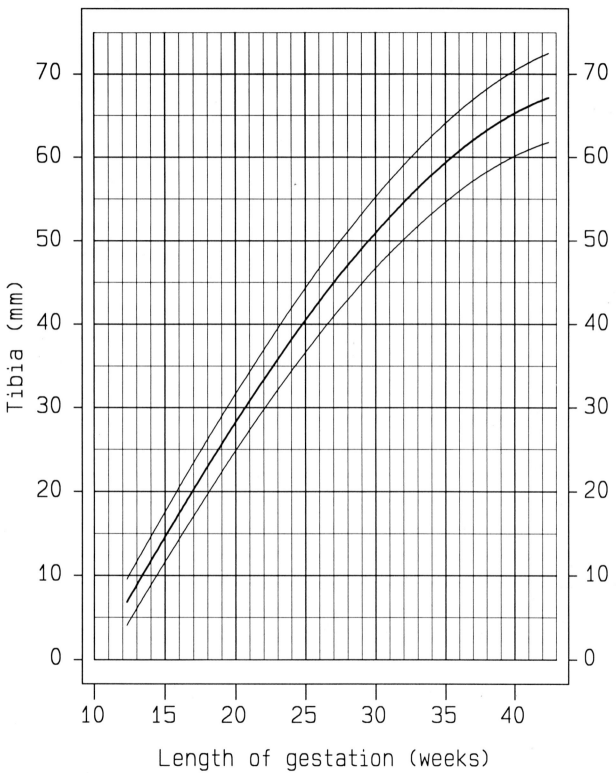

Tibia (mm)

Length of gestation (weeks)

Foot (mm)

Gestation (weeks)	c5	c50	c95
13	7.3	10.4	13.5
14	10.5	13.8	17.0
15	13.6	17.0	20.5
16	16.7	20.3	23.9
17	19.8	23.5	27.3
18	22.8	26.7	30.6
19	25.7	29.8	33.9
20	28.6	32.9	37.1
21	31.5	35.9	40.3
22	34.3	38.9	43.4
23	37.0	41.8	46.5
24	39.7	44.6	49.5
25	42.4	47.4	52.4
26	44.9	50.1	55.3
27	47.4	52.8	58.1
28	49.8	55.3	60.8
29	52.2	57.8	63.5
30	54.4	60.2	66.1
31	56.6	62.6	68.6
32	58.7	64.9	71.0
33	60.7	67.0	73.3
34	62.7	69.1	75.6
35	64.5	71.1	77.7
36	66.3	73.0	79.8
37	67.9	74.8	81.8
38	69.5	76.6	83.7
39	70.9	78.2	85.4
40	72.3	79.7	87.1
41	73.5	81.1	88.7
42	74.7	82.4	90.1

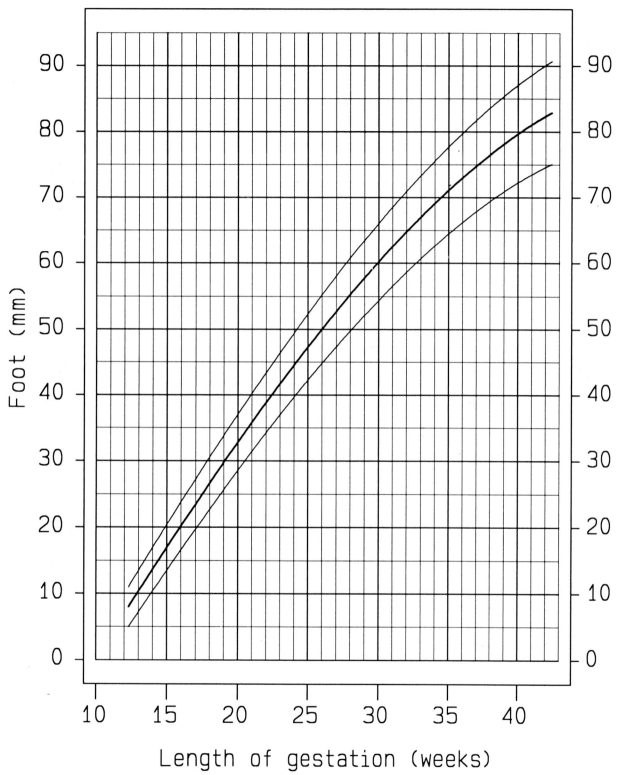

FOOT
5th, 50th and 95th centiles

Foot (mm)

Length of gestation (weeks)

Kidney length (mm)

Gestation (weeks)	c5	c50	c95
14	8.0	9.8	11.8
15	9.3	11.4	13.7
16	10.6	13.1	15.8
17	12.0	14.8	17.9
18	13.4	16.5	20.0
19	14.8	18.3	22.2
20	16.2	20.1	24.4
21	17.6	21.8	26.5
22	19.0	23.6	28.7
23	20.4	25.3	30.8
24	21.8	27.0	32.8
25	23.2	28.7	34.8
26	24.5	30.3	36.8
27	25.8	31.9	38.6
28	27.0	33.4	40.4
29	28.2	34.8	42.1
30	29.4	36.2	43.6
31	30.5	37.4	45.1
32	31.5	38.6	46.4
33	32.4	39.7	47.6
34	33.3	40.6	48.7
35	34.1	41.5	49.7
36	34.9	42.3	50.5
37	35.5	43.0	51.1
38	36.1	43.5	51.6
39	36.6	43.9	52.0
40	36.9	44.2	52.2
41	37.3	44.4	52.3
42	37.5	44.5	52.2

KIDNEY LENGTH
5th, 50th and 95th centiles

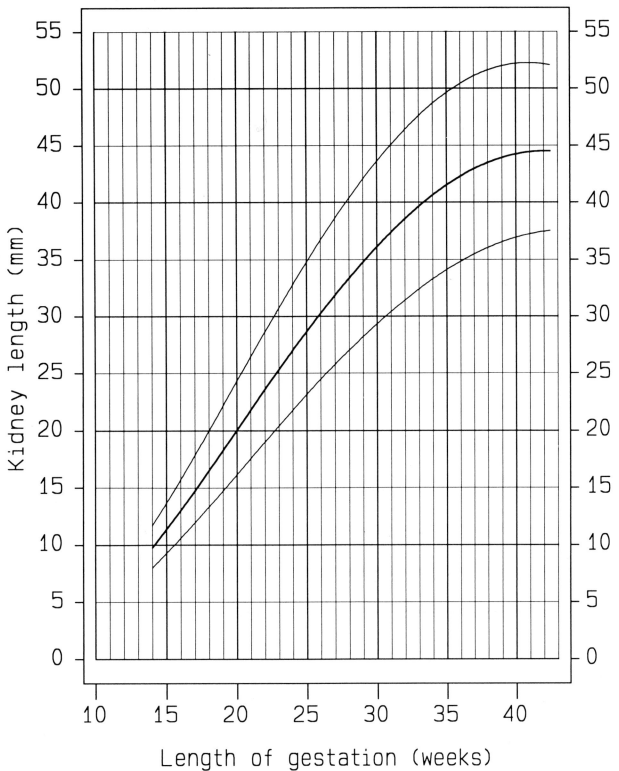

Kidney length (mm)

Length of gestation (weeks)

Kidney antero-posterior diameter (mm)

Gestation (weeks)	c5	c50	c95
14	4.4	7.1	10.4
15	5.1	8.0	11.6
16	6.0	9.0	12.8
17	6.8	10.0	14.0
18	7.6	11.1	15.2
19	8.5	12.1	16.4
20	9.3	13.1	17.5
21	10.2	14.1	18.7
22	11.0	15.1	19.9
23	11.9	16.1	21.0
24	12.7	17.1	22.1
25	13.5	18.0	23.1
26	14.3	18.9	24.1
27	15.0	19.7	25.1
28	15.7	20.5	26.0
29	16.4	21.3	26.8
30	17.0	22.0	27.6
31	17.6	22.7	28.4
32	18.1	23.3	29.0
33	18.6	23.8	29.6
34	19.0	24.3	30.2
35	19.4	24.7	30.7
36	19.7	25.1	31.1
37	20.0	25.4	31.4
38	20.2	25.6	31.6
39	20.3	25.8	31.8
40	20.4	25.8	31.9
41	20.4	25.9	31.9
42	20.4	25.8	31.9

KIDNEY ANTERO-POSTERIOR DIAMETER
5th, 50th and 95th centiles

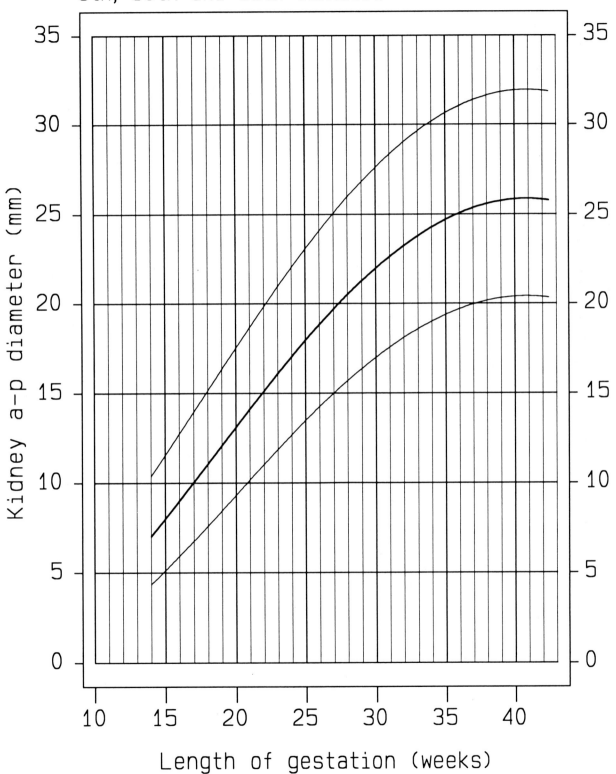

Kidney a-p diameter (mm)

Length of gestation (weeks)

Kidney transverse diameter (mm)

Gestation (weeks)	c5	c50	c95
14	4.1	6.7	9.8
15	4.8	7.6	10.9
16	5.6	8.5	12.0
17	6.4	9.5	13.2
18	7.2	10.4	14.3
19	8.0	11.4	15.5
20	8.8	12.4	16.6
21	9.6	13.4	17.7
22	10.5	14.3	18.8
23	11.3	15.3	19.9
24	12.1	16.2	21.0
25	12.9	17.1	22.0
26	13.6	18.0	23.0
27	14.4	18.9	24.0
28	15.1	19.7	24.9
29	15.8	20.5	25.8
30	16.5	21.3	26.7
31	17.1	22.0	27.5
32	17.7	22.7	28.2
33	18.2	23.3	28.9
34	18.8	23.8	29.5
35	19.2	24.4	30.1
36	19.6	24.8	30.6
37	20.0	25.2	31.1
38	20.3	25.6	31.5
39	20.6	25.9	31.8
40	20.8	26.1	32.1
41	21.0	26.3	32.3
42	21.1	26.4	32.4

KIDNEY TRANSVERSE DIAMETER
5th, 50th and 95th centiles

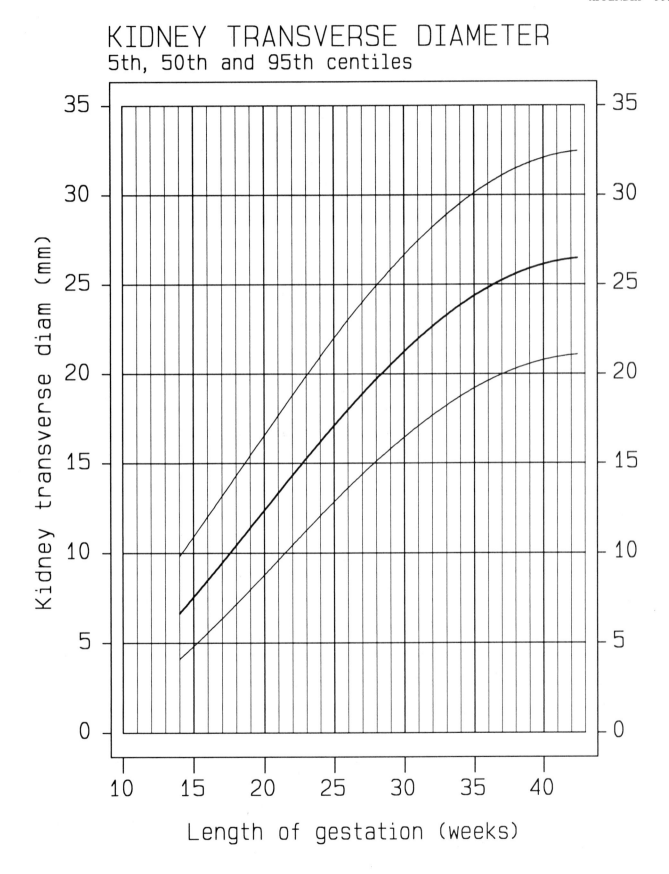

Kidney transverse diam (mm) vs Length of gestation (weeks)

Crown-rump length – Dating table

CRL (mm)	Gestation wks days	95% interval wks days	wks days
4	6 + 0	5 + 2	6 + 5
6	6 + 3	5 + 6	7 + 1
8	6 + 6	6 + 2	7 + 4
10	7 + 2	6 + 4	8 + 0
12	7 + 4	7 + 0	8 + 2
14	7 + 6	7 + 2	8 + 4
16	8 + 2	7 + 4	8 + 6
18	8 + 3	7 + 6	9 + 1
20	8 + 5	8 + 1	9 + 3
22	9 + 0	8 + 2	9 + 5
24	9 + 2	8 + 4	9 + 6
26	9 + 3	8 + 6	10 + 1
28	9 + 5	9 + 0	10 + 3
30	9 + 6	9 + 2	10 + 4
32	10 + 1	9 + 3	10 + 6
34	10 + 2	9 + 5	11 + 0
36	10 + 4	9 + 6	11 + 1
38	10 + 5	10 + 0	11 + 3
40	10 + 6	10 + 2	11 + 4
42	11 + 0	10 + 3	11 + 5
44	11 + 2	10 + 4	11 + 6
46	11 + 3	10 + 5	12 + 1
48	11 + 4	10 + 6	12 + 2
50	11 + 5	11 + 1	12 + 3
52	11 + 6	11 + 2	12 + 4
54	12 + 1	11 + 3	12 + 5
56	12 + 2	11 + 4	12 + 6
58	12 + 3	11 + 5	13 + 0
60	12 + 4	11 + 6	13 + 1
62	12 + 5	12 + 0	13 + 3
64	12 + 6	12 + 1	13 + 4
66	13 + 0	12 + 2	13 + 5
68	13 + 1	12 + 3	13 + 6
70	13 + 2	12 + 4	14 + 0
72	13 + 3	12 + 5	14 + 0
74	13 + 4	12 + 6	14 + 1
76	13 + 5	13 + 0	14 + 2
78	13 + 6	13 + 1	14 + 3
80	14 + 0	13 + 2	14 + 4

Based on formula given by Robinson and Fleming (1975) with CRL adjusted by adding 1 mm and 3.7% as recommended by them

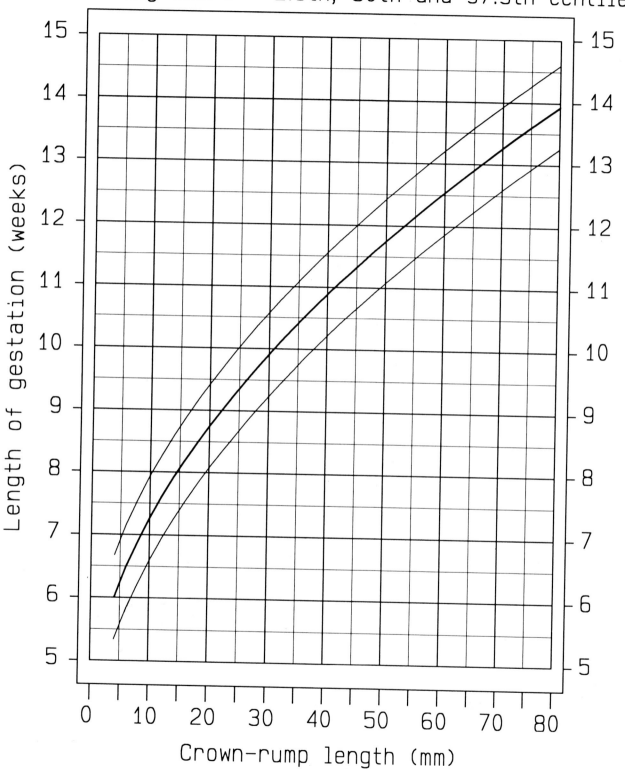

CROWN-RUMP LENGTH
Dating chart – 2.5th, 50th and 97.5th centiles

Length of gestation (weeks)

Crown-rump length (mm)

From Robinson and Fleming (1975)

Biparietal diameter (outer–outer) – Dating table

BPD (mm)	Gestation wks days	95% interval wks days	wks days	Range wks
19	12 + 0	11 + 0	13 + 0	1.9
20	12 + 2	11 + 2	13 + 2	2.0
21	12 + 3	11 + 3	13 + 3	2.0
22	12 + 5	11 + 5	13 + 5	2.0
23	12 + 6	11 + 6	14 + 0	2.1
24	13 + 1	12 + 1	14 + 2	2.1
25	13 + 3	12 + 3	14 + 4	2.2
26	13 + 5	12 + 4	14 + 6	2.2
27	13 + 6	12 + 6	15 + 1	2.2
28	14 + 1	13 + 1	15 + 3	2.3
29	14 + 3	13 + 2	15 + 5	2.3
30	14 + 5	13 + 4	16 + 0	2.4
31	15 + 0	13 + 6	16 + 2	2.4
32	15 + 2	14 + 0	16 + 4	2.5
33	15 + 4	14 + 2	16 + 6	2.5
34	15 + 6	14 + 4	17 + 1	2.5
35	16 + 0	14 + 6	17 + 3	2.6
36	16 + 2	15 + 1	17 + 5	2.6
37	16 + 4	15 + 2	18 + 0	2.7
38	16 + 6	15 + 4	18 + 2	2.7
39	17 + 2	15 + 6	18 + 5	2.8
40	17 + 4	16 + 1	19 + 0	2.8
41	17 + 6	16 + 3	19 + 2	2.9
42	18 + 1	16 + 5	19 + 4	2.9
43	18 + 3	17 + 0	20 + 0	3.0
44	18 + 5	17 + 2	20 + 2	3.0
45	19 + 0	17 + 4	20 + 4	3.1
46	19 + 2	17 + 6	21 + 0	3.1
47	19 + 4	18 + 1	21 + 2	3.2
48	20 + 0	18 + 3	21 + 4	3.2
49	20 + 2	18 + 5	22 + 0	3.3
50	20 + 4	19 + 0	22 + 2	3.3
51	20 + 6	19 + 2	22 + 5	3.4
52	21 + 1	19 + 4	23 + 0	3.4
53	21 + 4	19 + 6	23 + 2	3.5
54	21 + 6	20 + 1	23 + 5	3.5
55	22 + 1	20 + 3	24 + 0	3.6
56	22 + 3	20 + 5	24 + 3	3.6
57	22 + 6	21 + 0	24 + 5	3.7
58	23 + 1	21 + 2	25 + 0	3.7
59	23 + 3	21 + 4	25 + 3	3.8
60	23 + 5	21 + 6	25 + 5	3.8
61	24 + 1	22 + 1	26 + 1	3.9
62	24 + 3	22 + 4	26 + 3	3.9
63	24 + 5	22 + 6	26 + 5	4.0
64	25 + 0	23 + 1	27 + 1	4.0
65	25 + 2	23 + 3	27 + 3	4.1
66	25 + 5	23 + 5	27 + 6	4.1
67	26 + 0	24 + 0	28 + 1	4.2
68	26 + 2	24 + 2	28 + 3	4.2
69	26 + 4	24 + 4	28 + 6	4.3
70	26 + 6	24 + 5	29 + 1	4.3
71	27 + 1	25 + 0	29 + 3	4.4
72	27 + 3	25 + 2	29 + 5	4.4
73	27 + 5	25 + 4	30 + 1	4.5
74	28 + 0	25 + 6	30 + 3	4.5
75	28 + 2	26 + 1	30 + 5	4.6

BIPARIETAL DIAMETER (outer-outer)
Dating chart - 2.5th, 50th and 97.5th centiles

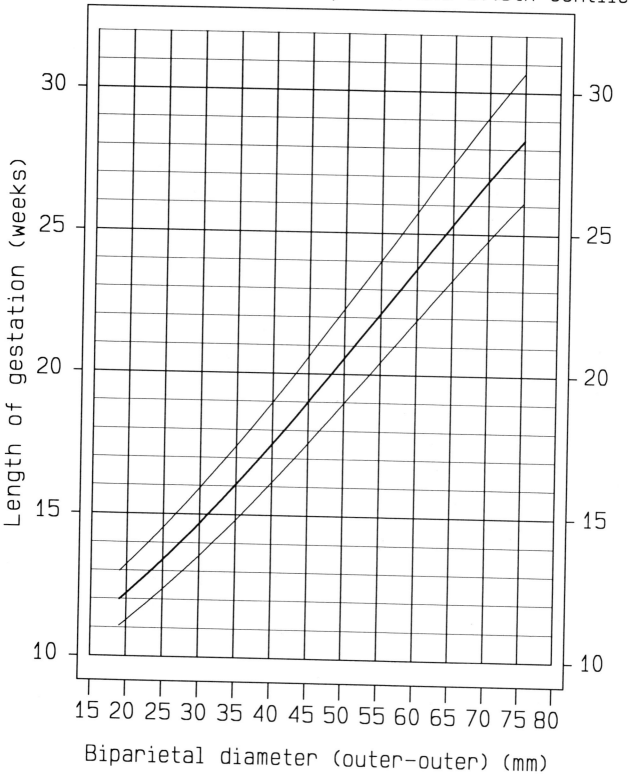

Length of gestation (weeks)

Biparietal diameter (outer-outer) (mm)

Biparietal diameter (outer–inner) – Dating table

BPD (mm)	Gestation wks days	95% interval wks days	wks days	Range wks
18	12 + 1	11 + 2	13 + 1	1.9
19	12 + 3	11 + 3	13 + 3	2.0
20	12 + 4	11 + 5	13 + 5	2.0
21	12 + 6	11 + 6	13 + 6	2.0
22	13 + 1	12 + 1	14 + 1	2.1
23	13 + 2	12 + 2	14 + 3	2.1
24	13 + 4	12 + 4	14 + 5	2.2
25	13 + 6	12 + 6	15 + 0	2.2
26	14 + 1	13 + 0	15 + 2	2.2
27	14 + 3	13 + 2	15 + 4	2.3
28	14 + 5	13 + 4	15 + 6	2.3
29	14 + 6	13 + 6	16 + 1	2.4
30	15 + 1	14 + 0	16 + 3	2.4
31	15 + 3	14 + 2	16 + 5	2.4
32	15 + 5	14 + 4	17 + 0	2.5
33	16 + 0	14 + 6	17 + 3	2.5
34	16 + 2	15 + 1	17 + 5	2.6
35	16 + 4	15 + 2	18 + 0	2.6
36	16 + 6	15 + 4	18 + 2	2.7
37	17 + 1	15 + 6	18 + 4	2.7
38	17 + 4	16 + 1	19 + 0	2.8
39	17 + 6	16 + 3	19 + 2	2.8
40	18 + 1	16 + 5	19 + 4	2.9
41	18 + 3	17 + 0	20 + 0	2.9
42	18 + 5	17 + 2	20 + 2	3.0
43	19 + 0	17 + 4	20 + 4	3.0
44	19 + 3	17 + 6	21 + 0	3.1
45	19 + 5	18 + 1	21 + 2	3.1
46	20 + 0	18 + 3	21 + 4	3.2
47	20 + 2	18 + 5	22 + 0	3.2
48	20 + 4	19 + 1	22 + 2	3.3
49	21 + 0	19 + 3	22 + 5	3.3
50	21 + 2	19 + 5	23 + 0	3.4
51	21 + 4	20 + 0	23 + 3	3.4
52	22 + 0	20 + 2	23 + 5	3.5
53	22 + 2	20 + 4	24 + 1	3.5
54	22 + 4	20 + 6	24 + 3	3.6
55	23 + 0	21 + 1	24 + 6	3.6
56	23 + 2	21 + 3	25 + 1	3.7
57	23 + 4	21 + 6	25 + 4	3.7
58	23 + 6	22 + 1	25 + 6	3.8
59	24 + 2	22 + 3	26 + 2	3.8
60	24 + 4	22 + 5	26 + 4	3.9
61	24 + 6	23 + 0	27 + 0	3.9
62	25 + 2	23 + 2	27 + 2	4.0
63	25 + 4	23 + 4	27 + 5	4.0
64	25 + 6	23 + 6	28 + 0	4.1
65	26 + 2	24 + 2	28 + 3	4.1
66	26 + 4	24 + 4	28 + 5	4.2
67	26 + 6	24 + 6	29 + 0	4.2
68	27 + 1	25 + 1	29 + 3	4.3
69	27 + 3	25 + 3	29 + 5	4.3
70	27 + 6	25 + 5	30 + 1	4.4
71	28 + 1	26 + 0	30 + 3	4.4
72	28 + 3	26 + 2	30 + 5	4.5
73	28 + 5	26 + 4	31 + 0	4.5
74	29 + 0	26 + 6	31 + 3	4.6
75	29 + 2	27 + 0	31 + 5	4.6

BIPARIETAL DIAMETER (outer-inner)
Dating chart - 2.5th, 50th and 97.5th centiles

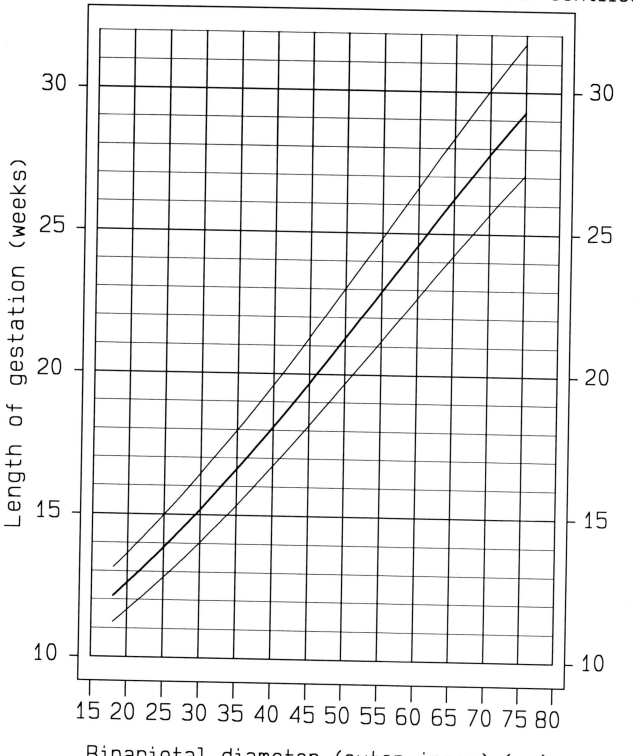

Length of gestation (weeks)

Biparietal diameter (outer-inner) (mm)

Head circumference (plotted) – Dating table

Head circ (mm)	Gestation wks days	95% interval wks days	wks days	Range wks
70	12 + 1	11 + 2	13 + 1	1.9
75	12 + 3	11 + 4	13 + 3	1.9
80	12 + 6	11 + 6	13 + 6	2.0
85	13 + 1	12 + 1	14 + 1	2.0
90	13 + 3	12 + 3	14 + 4	2.0
95	13 + 6	12 + 6	14 + 6	2.1
100	14 + 1	13 + 1	15 + 2	2.1
105	14 + 4	13 + 3	15 + 4	2.1
110	14 + 6	13 + 6	16 + 0	2.2
115	15 + 2	14 + 1	16 + 3	2.2
120	15 + 4	14 + 4	16 + 5	2.2
125	16 + 0	14 + 6	17 + 1	2.3
130	16 + 3	15 + 2	17 + 4	2.3
135	16 + 5	15 + 4	18 + 0	2.3
140	17 + 1	16 + 0	18 + 3	2.4
145	17 + 4	16 + 3	18 + 5	2.4
150	18 + 0	16 + 5	19 + 1	2.4
155	18 + 2	17 + 1	19 + 4	2.5
160	18 + 5	17 + 4	20 + 0	2.5
165	19 + 1	18 + 0	20 + 3	2.5
170	19 + 4	18 + 2	20 + 6	2.6
175	20 + 0	18 + 5	21 + 2	2.6
180	20 + 3	19 + 1	21 + 5	2.6
185	20 + 6	19 + 4	22 + 1	2.6
190	21 + 2	20 + 0	22 + 5	2.7
195	21 + 5	20 + 3	23 + 1	2.7
200	22 + 1	20 + 6	23 + 4	2.7
205	22 + 4	21 + 2	24 + 0	2.7
210	23 + 0	21 + 5	24 + 3	2.8
215	23 + 3	22 + 1	24 + 6	2.8
220	23 + 6	22 + 3	25 + 2	2.8
225	24 + 2	22 + 6	25 + 5	2.8
230	24 + 5	23 + 2	26 + 1	2.9
235	25 + 1	23 + 5	26 + 4	2.9
240	25 + 4	24 + 1	27 + 0	2.9
245	26 + 0	24 + 4	27 + 3	2.9
250	26 + 3	25 + 0	27 + 6	2.9
255	26 + 6	25 + 3	28 + 2	2.9
260	27 + 1	25 + 5	28 + 5	2.9
265	27 + 4	26 + 1	29 + 1	3.0
270	28 + 0	26 + 4	29 + 4	3.0
275	28 + 3	27 + 0	29 + 6	3.0
280	28 + 5	27 + 2	30 + 2	3.0

HEAD CIRCUMFERENCE (plotted)
Dating chart – 2.5th, 50th and 97.5th centiles

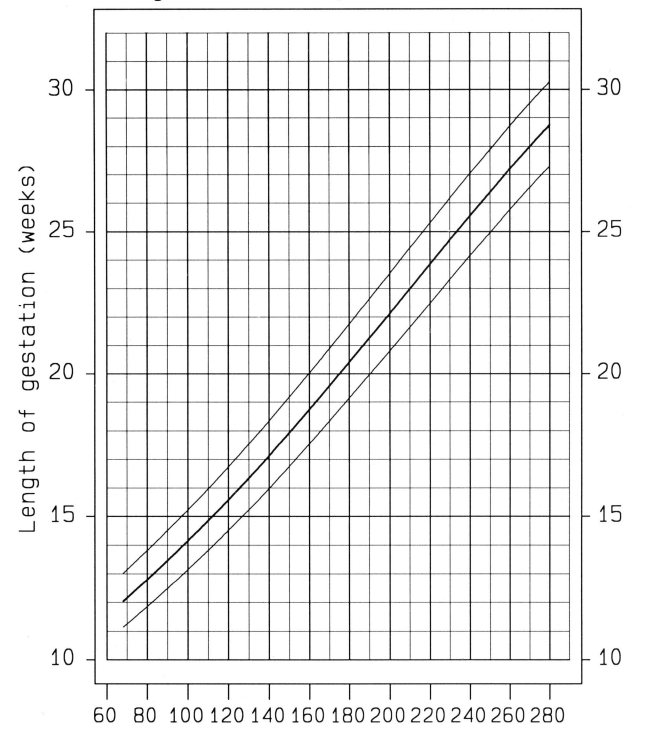

Head circumference (plotted) (mm)

Head circumference (derived) – Dating table

Head circ (mm)	Gestation wks days	95% interval wks days	wks days	Range wks
70	12 + 2	11 + 2	13 + 2	2.0
75	12 + 4	11 + 4	13 + 4	2.0
80	12 + 6	11 + 6	14 + 0	2.0
85	13 + 2	12 + 1	14 + 2	2.1
90	13 + 4	12 + 4	14 + 5	2.1
95	13 + 6	12 + 6	15 + 0	2.2
100	14 + 2	13 + 1	15 + 3	2.2
105	14 + 4	13 + 4	15 + 5	2.2
110	15 + 0	13 + 6	16 + 1	2.3
115	15 + 3	14 + 2	16 + 4	2.3
120	15 + 5	14 + 4	17 + 0	2.3
125	16 + 1	15 + 0	17 + 3	2.4
130	16 + 4	15 + 3	17 + 5	2.4
135	16 + 6	15 + 5	18 + 1	2.4
140	17 + 2	16 + 1	18 + 4	2.5
145	17 + 5	16 + 4	19 + 0	2.5
150	18 + 1	16 + 6	19 + 3	2.5
155	18 + 4	17 + 2	19 + 6	2.6
160	19 + 0	17 + 5	20 + 2	2.6
165	19 + 3	18 + 1	20 + 5	2.6
170	19 + 6	18 + 4	21 + 1	2.7
175	20 + 2	19 + 0	21 + 5	2.7
180	20 + 5	19 + 2	22 + 1	2.7
185	21 + 1	19 + 5	22 + 4	2.8
190	21 + 4	20 + 1	23 + 0	2.8
195	22 + 0	20 + 4	23 + 3	2.8
200	22 + 3	21 + 0	23 + 6	2.9
205	22 + 6	21 + 3	24 + 2	2.9
210	23 + 2	21 + 6	24 + 6	2.9
215	23 + 5	22 + 2	25 + 2	2.9
220	24 + 1	22 + 5	25 + 5	3.0
225	24 + 4	23 + 1	26 + 1	3.0
230	25 + 0	23 + 4	26 + 4	3.0
235	25 + 3	24 + 0	27 + 0	3.0
240	25 + 6	24 + 3	27 + 3	3.0
245	26 + 2	24 + 6	27 + 6	3.0
250	26 + 5	25 + 2	28 + 2	3.1
255	27 + 1	25 + 5	28 + 5	3.1
260	27 + 4	26 + 0	29 + 1	3.1
265	28 + 0	26 + 3	29 + 4	3.1
270	28 + 2	26 + 6	29 + 6	3.1
275	28 + 5	27 + 1	30 + 2	3.1
280	29 + 0	27 + 4	30 + 5	3.1

HEAD CIRCUMFERENCE (derived)
Dating chart – 2.5th, 50th and 97.5th centiles

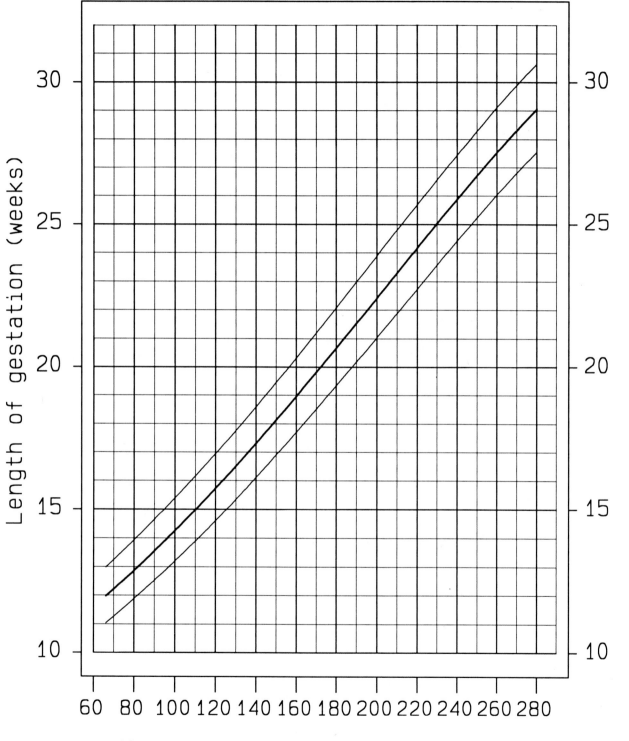

Length of gestation (weeks)

Head circumference (derived) (mm)

Femur – Dating table

Femur (mm)	Gestation wks days	95% interval wks days	wks days	Range wks
8	12 + 4	11 + 5	13 + 4	1.9
9	12 + 6	11 + 6	13 + 6	2.0
10	13 + 1	12 + 1	14 + 1	2.0
11	13 + 2	12 + 3	14 + 3	2.0
12	13 + 4	12 + 4	14 + 5	2.1
13	13 + 6	12 + 6	15 + 0	2.1
14	14 + 1	13 + 1	15 + 2	2.2
15	14 + 3	13 + 3	15 + 4	2.2
16	14 + 5	13 + 4	15 + 6	2.2
17	15 + 0	13 + 6	16 + 1	2.3
18	15 + 2	14 + 1	16 + 4	2.3
19	15 + 4	14 + 3	16 + 6	2.4
20	15 + 6	14 + 5	17 + 1	2.4
21	16 + 1	15 + 0	17 + 3	2.5
22	16 + 4	15 + 2	17 + 6	2.5
23	16 + 6	15 + 4	18 + 1	2.6
24	17 + 1	15 + 6	18 + 4	2.6
25	17 + 3	16 + 1	18 + 6	2.7
26	17 + 6	16 + 4	19 + 2	2.7
27	18 + 1	16 + 6	19 + 4	2.8
28	18 + 3	17 + 1	20 + 0	2.8
29	18 + 6	17 + 3	20 + 2	2.9
30	19 + 1	17 + 5	20 + 5	2.9
31	19 + 4	18 + 1	21 + 1	3.0
32	19 + 6	18 + 3	21 + 3	3.0
33	20 + 2	18 + 5	21 + 6	3.1
34	20 + 4	19 + 1	22 + 2	3.2
35	21 + 0	19 + 3	22 + 5	3.2
36	21 + 3	19 + 6	23 + 1	3.3
37	21 + 5	20 + 1	23 + 3	3.3
38	22 + 1	20 + 4	23 + 6	3.4
39	22 + 4	20 + 6	24 + 2	3.4
40	23 + 0	21 + 2	24 + 5	3.5
41	23 + 2	21 + 4	25 + 1	3.6
42	23 + 5	22 + 0	25 + 4	3.6
43	24 + 1	22 + 2	26 + 0	3.7
44	24 + 4	22 + 5	26 + 3	3.7
45	25 + 0	23 + 1	26 + 6	3.8
46	25 + 2	23 + 3	27 + 3	3.9
47	25 + 5	23 + 6	27 + 6	3.9
48	26 + 1	24 + 2	28 + 2	4.0
49	26 + 4	24 + 5	28 + 5	4.1
50	27 + 0	25 + 0	29 + 1	4.1
51	27 + 3	25 + 3	29 + 4	4.2
52	27 + 6	25 + 6	30 + 1	4.3
53	28 + 2	26 + 2	30 + 4	4.3
54	28 + 5	26 + 4	31 + 0	4.4
55	29 + 1	27 + 0	31 + 3	4.5

FEMUR
Dating chart – 2.5th, 50th and 97.5th centiles

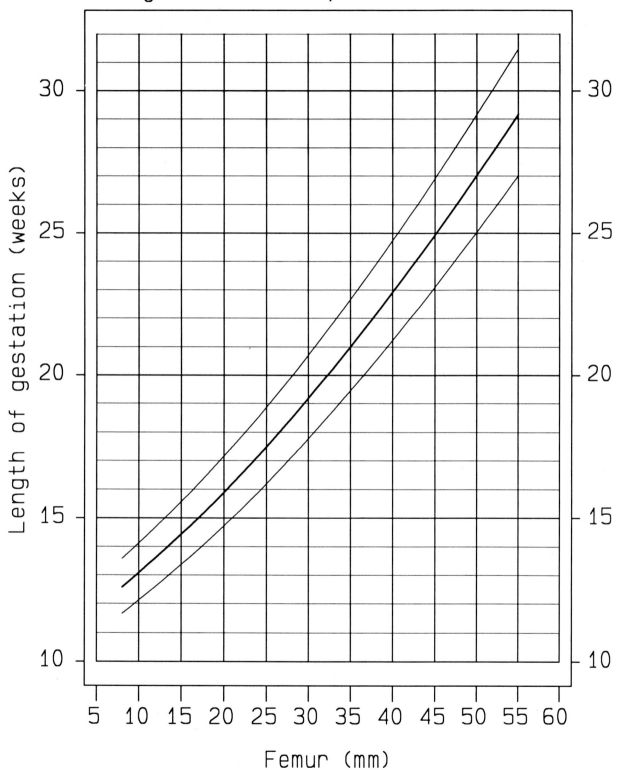

Gestation sac diameter

Sac diameter (cm)	Gestational age (weeks)
1.0	5.0
1.1	5.2
1.2	5.3
1.3	5.5
1.4	5.6
1.5	5.8
1.6	5.9
1.7	6.0
1.8	6.2
1.9	6.3
2.0	6.5
2.1	6.6
2.2	6.8
2.3	6.9
2.4	7.0
2.5	7.2
2.6	7.3
2.7	7.5
2.8	7.6
2.9	7.8
3.0	7.9
3.1	8.0
3.2	8.2
3.3	8.3
3.4	8.5
3.5	8.6
3.6	8.8
3.7	8.9
3.8	9.0
3.9	9.2
4.0	9.3
4.1	9.5
4.2	9.6
4.3	9.7
4.4	9.9
4.5	10.0
4.6	10.2
4.7	10.3
4.8	10.5
4.9	10.6
5.0	10.7
5.1	10.9
5.2	11.0
5.3	11.2
5.4	11.3
5.5	11.5
5.6	11.6
5.7	11.7
5.8	11.9
5.9	12.0
6.0	12.2

Modified from:
Hellman L M, Kobayashi M, Fillisti L, et al.
Growth and development of the human fetus prior to the twentieth
week of gestation. Am J Obstet Gynecol 1969; 103: 789

Gestation sac diameter

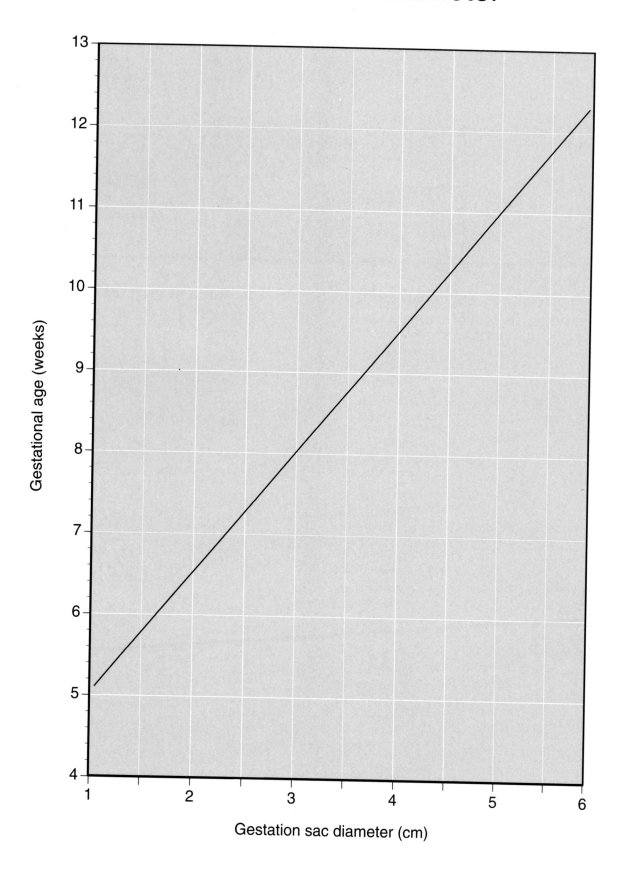

Gestation sac volume

Gestational age (weeks and days)		Volume (ml)		
		−2SD	mean	+2SD
7	6	0.0	23.8	53.6
8	4	5.0	31.8	58.6
9	2	3.0	44.9	86.8
9	6	10.0	64.6	119.2
10	3	16.5	78.1	139.7
10	6	13.6	91.0	168.4
11	3	61.5	127.4	193.3
11	6	85.1	148.7	212.3
12	2	78.7	168.3	257.6
12	4	167.3	253.8	339.0

Modified from:
Golstein S R, Subramanyam B R, Snyder J R. Ratio of gestational sac volume to crown-rump length in early pregnancy. J Reprod Med 1986;31: 320–321

Gestation sac volume (ml)

mean ± 2SD

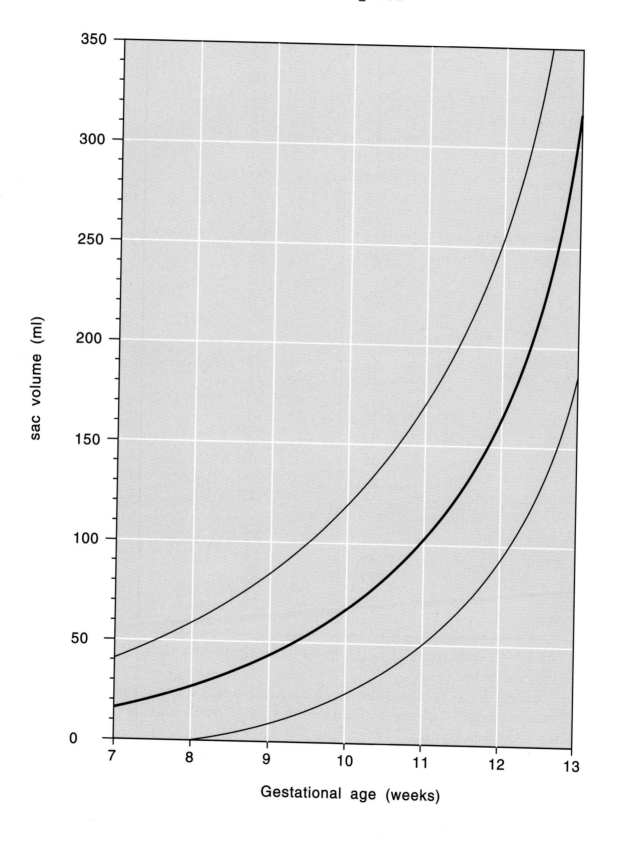

sac volume (ml)

Gestational age (weeks)

Cerebellar diameter

Gestational age (weeks)	Cerebellar diameter (mm)		
	10th	50th centiles	90th
15	10	14	16
16	14	16	17
17	16	17	18
18	17	18	19
19	18	19	22
20	18	20	22
21	19	22	24
22	21	23	24
23	22	24	26
24	22	25	28
25	23	28	29
26	25	29	32
27	26	30	32
28	27	31	34
29	29	34	38
30	31	35	40
31	32	38	43
32	33	38	42
33	32	40	44
34	33	40	44
35	31	40.5	47
36	36	43	55
37	37	45	55
38	40	48.5	55
39	42	52	55

The graph opposite is a polynomial fit to these raw data.
Modified from:
Goldstein I, Reece A, Pilu G, et al. Cerebellar measurements with ultrasonography in the evaluation of fetal growth and development. Am J Obstet Gynecol 1987; 156: 1065

Cerebellar diameter

10th, 50th and 90th centiles

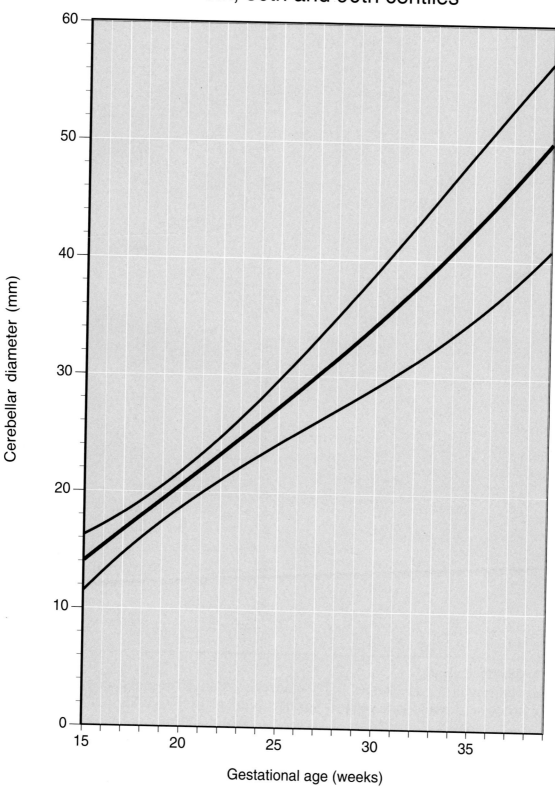

Cerebellar diameter (mm)

Gestational age (weeks)

Lateral ventricle/hemisphere width ratio

Gestational age (weeks)	5th	ratio (%) 50th centiles	95th
11	83	95	107
12	75	87	98
13	68	79	91
14	62	73	83
15	56	66	77
16	51	61	71
17	46	56	66
18	42	52	61
19	39	48	57
20	36	45	54
21	33	42	50
22	31	39	48
23	29	37	45
24	28	36	44
25	27	35	42
26	26	34	41
27	26	33	40
28	26	32	39
29	26	32	38
30	26	32	38
31	26	32	37
32	26	32	37
33	27	32	37
34	27	32	36
35	28	32	36
36	28	32	36
37	28	32	35
38	28	32	35
39	28	31	34
40	28	31	33

Modified from:
Hansmann M, Hackeloer B J, Staudach A. eds. Ultrasound diagnosis in obstetrics and gynecology. Springer Verlag: Berlin. 1985: p 465

Lateral ventricle:hemisphere width ratio

5th, 50th and 95th centiles

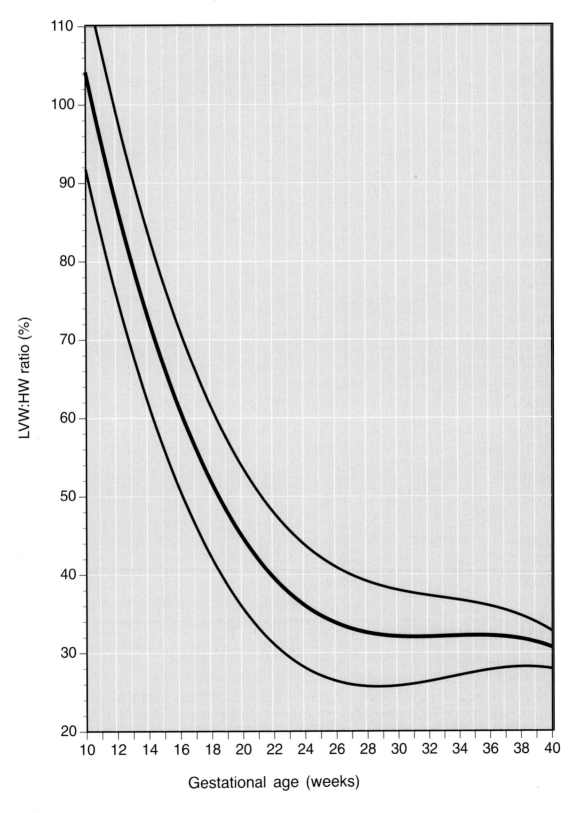

Orbital dimensions

Gestational age (weeks)	IOD (cm)	OOD (cm)
11.6	0.5	1.3
12.6	0.6	1.6
13.6	0.7	1.8
14.6	0.8	2.1
15.5	0.9	2.3
16.5	1.0	2.5
17.5	1.1	2.7
18.4	1.2	3.0
19.4	1.2	3.2
20.4	1.3	3.4
21.3	1.4	3.6
22.3	1.4	3.8
23.3	1.3	4.0
24.3	1.6	4.1
25.2	1.6	4.3
26.2	1.7	4.5
27.2	1.7	4.6
28.1	1.7	4.7
29.1	1.8	4.8
30.0	1.8	5.0
31.0	1.8	5.1
32.0	1.8	5.2
33.0	1.9	5.3
34.0	1.9	5.4
35.0	1.9	5.5
35.9	1.9	5.6
36.9	1.9	5.7
37.8	1.9	5.8
38.8	1.9	5.8
39.8	1.9	5.9

IOD – interorbital distance (inner)
OOD – distance between lateral orbital walls (outer)
Modified from:
Mayden K L, Tortora M, Berkowitz R L, et al. Orbital diameters: a new parameter for prenatal diagnosis and dating. Am J Obstet Gynecol 1982; 144: 289

Interorbital distance

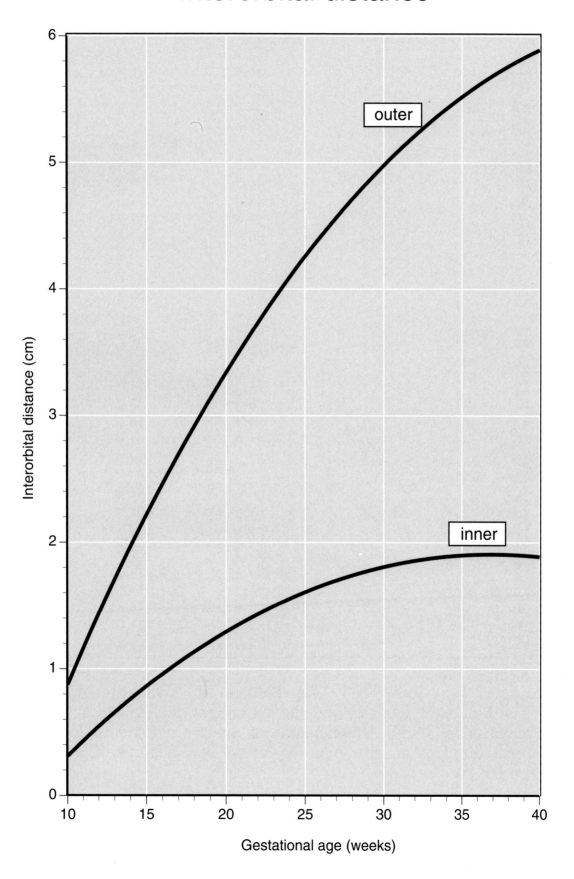

Abdominal diameter

Gestational age (weeks)	Mean abdominal diameter (mm) 5th	50th centiles	95th
13	18.2	22.7	27.2
14	21.7	26.4	31.1
15	25.3	30.1	34.9
16	28.6	33.7	38.8
17	32.0	37.3	42.7
18	35.4	40.9	46.5
19	38.7	44.5	50.3
20	41.9	48.0	54.0
21	45.2	51.4	57.7
22	48.3	54.9	61.5
23	51.4	58.3	65.2
24	54.5	61.7	68.9
25	57.5	65.0	72.6
26	60.5	68.4	76.2
27	63.4	71.7	79.9
28	66.3	74.9	83.6
29	69.1	78.2	87.2
30	71.9	81.4	90.9
31	74.6	84.6	94.5
32	77.2	87.7	98.2
33	79.8	90.8	101.8
34	82.4	93.9	105.5
35	84.8	97.0	109.2
36	87.3	100.1	112.9
37	89.5	103.1	116.5
38	91.9	106.1	120.3
39	94.1	109.0	124.0
40	96.2	112.0	127.8

Modified from:
Eriksen P S, Secher N J, Weis-Bentzon M. Normal growth of the fetal biparietal diameter and the abdominal diameter in a longitudinal study. An evaluation of the two parameters in predicting fetal weight. Acta Obstet Gynecol Scand 1985; 64: 65–70

Abdominal diameter

5th, 50th and 95th centiles

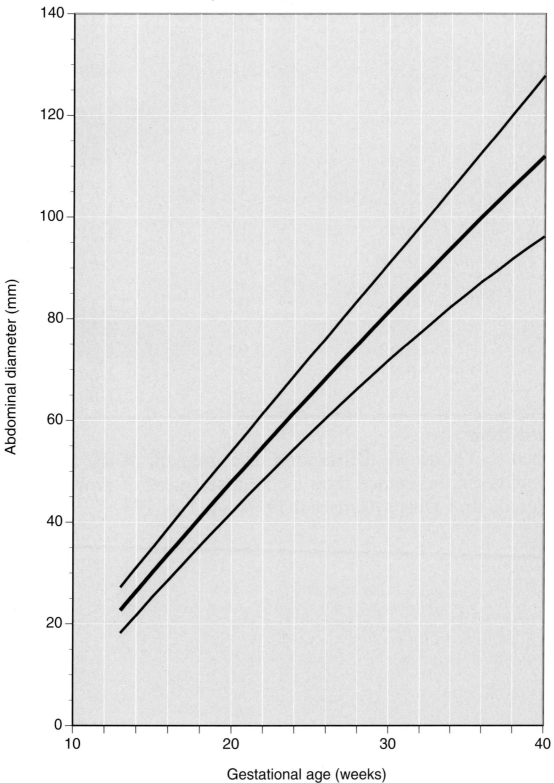

Abdominal diameter (mm)

Gestational age (weeks)

Head/abdomen circumference ratio

Gestational age (weeks)	5th	50th centiles	95th
13–14	1.14	1.23	1.31
15–16	1.05	1.22	1.39
17–18	1.07	1.18	1.29
19–20	1.09	1.18	1.39
21–22	1.06	1.15	1.25
23–24	1.05	1.13	1.21
25–26	1.04	1.13	1.22
27–28	1.05	1.13	1.21
29–30	0.99	1.10	1.21
31–32	0.96	1.07	1.17
33–34	0.96	1.04	1.11
35–36	0.93	1.02	1.11
37–38	0.92	0.98	1.05
39–40	0.87	0.97	1.06
41–42	0.93	0.96	1.00

Modified from:
Campbell S, Thoms, A. Ultrasound measurement of the fetal head to abdomen circumference ratio in the assessment of growth retardation. Br J Obstet Gynaecol 1977; 84: 165–174

Head:abdomen circumference ratio

5th, 50th and 95th centiles

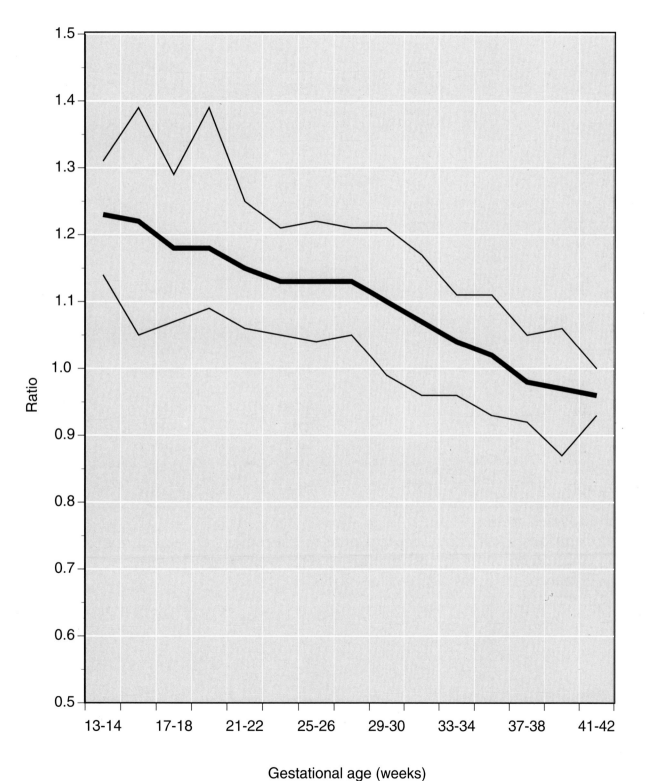

Gestational age (weeks)

Weight estimation from abdominal circumference

Abdominal circumference (mm)	Estimated birth weight (gms)		
	5th	50th centiles	95th
210	780	900	1040
220	900	1030	1190
230	1030	1180	1360
240	1170	1340	1540
250	1320	1510	1730
260	1470	1690	1940
270	1640	1880	2150
280	1810	2090	2380
290	1990	2280	2610
300	2170	2490	2850
310	2350	2690	3080
320	2530	2900	3320
330	2710	3100	3550
340	2880	3290	3760
350	3030	3470	3970
360	3180	3640	4160
370	3310	3790	4330
380	3420	3920	4490
390	3510	4020	4610
400	3570	4100	4720

Modified from:
Campbell S, Wilkin D. Ultrasonic measurement of fetal abdomen circumference in the estimation of fetal weight. Br J Obstet Gynaecol 1975; 82: 689–697

Weight:abdominal circumference

5th, 50th and 95th centiles

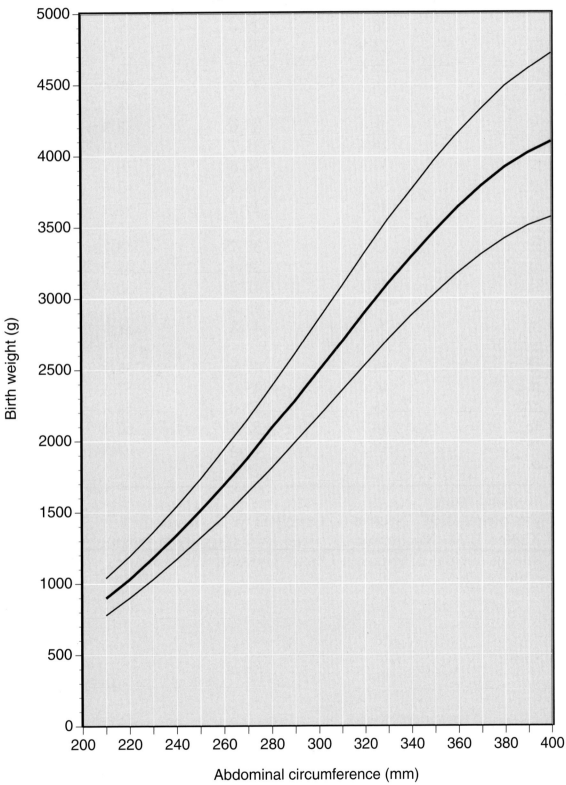

Liver length

Gestational age (weeks)	Liver length (mm) −2SD	mean	+2SD
20	20.9	27.3	33.7
21	26.5	28.0	29.5
22	23.9	30.6	37.3
23	26.4	30.9	35.4
24	26.2	32.9	39.6
25	28.3	33.6	38.9
26	29.4	35.7	42.0
27	33.3	36.6	39.9
28	34.4	38.4	42.4
29	34.1	39.1	44.1
30	33.7	38.7	43.7
31	33.9	39.6	45.3
32	35.2	42.7	50.2
33	37.2	43.8	50.4
34	37.7	44.8	51.9
35	38.7	47.8	56.9
36	41.4	49.0	57.4
37	45.2	52.0	58.8
38	48.7	52.9	57.1
39	48.7	55.4	62.1
40		59.0	

Modified from:
Vintzileous A M, Neckles S, Campbell W A, Andreoli J W Jnr, Kaplan B M, Nochimson D. Fetal liver ultrasound measurements during normal pregnancy. Obstet Gynecol 1985; 66: 477–480

Liver length

5th, 50th and 95th centiles

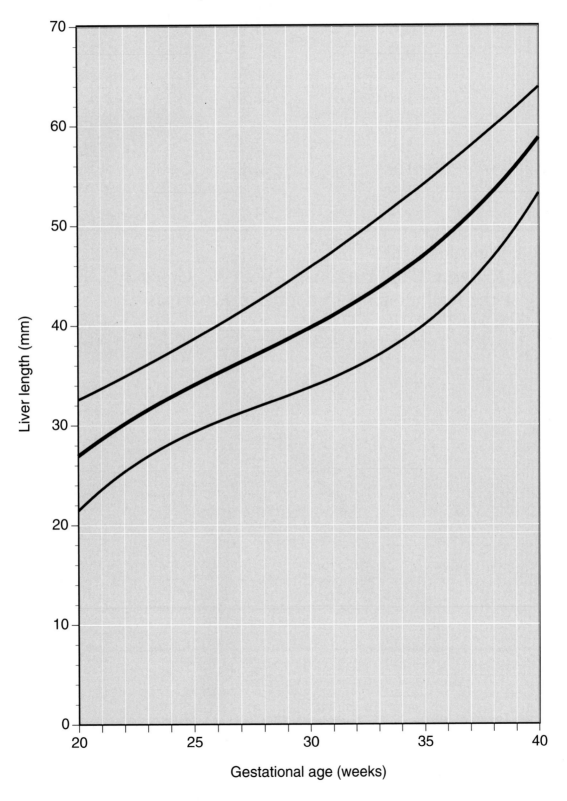

Stomach diameters

Gestational age (weeks)	Longitudinal diameter (cm) −2SD	mean	+2SD
13–15	0.6	0.9	1.2
16–18	0.9	1.3	1.7
19–21	1.1	1.6	2.1
22–24	1.3	1.9	2.5
25–27	1.3	2.3	3.3
28–30	1.8	2.3	2.8
31–33	1.9	2.8	3.7
34–36	1.9	2.8	3.7
37–39	2.3	3.2	4.1

Modified from:
Goldstein I, Reece E A, Yarkoni S, Wan M, Green J C, Hobbins J C.
Growth of the fetal stomach in normal pregnancies.
Obstet Gynecol 1987; 70: 641–644

Stomach longitudinal diameter

mean ± 2SD

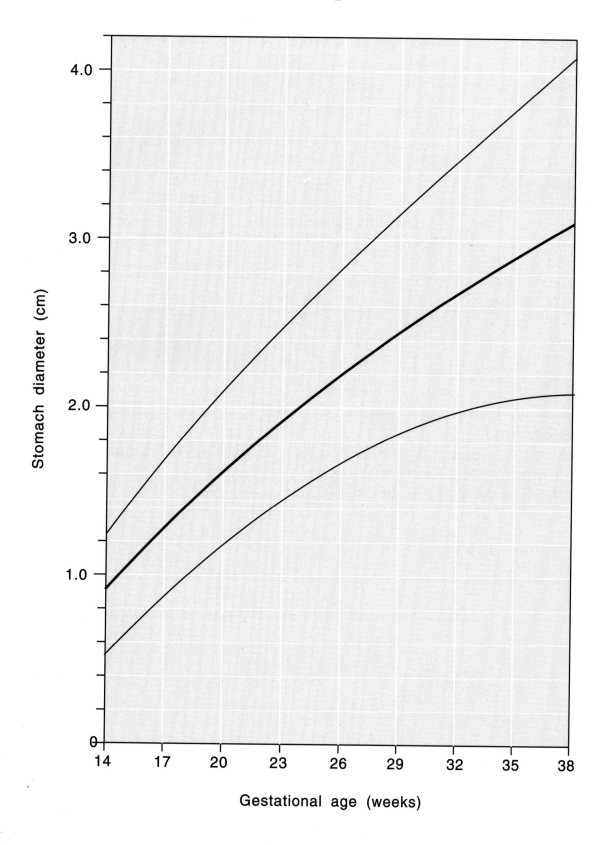

Stomach diameters

Gestational age (weeks)	AP diameter (cm)		
	−2SD	mean	+2SD
13–15	0.3	0.4	0.5
16–18	0.4	0.6	0.8
19–21	0.6	0.8	1.0
22–24	0.6	0.9	1.2
25–27	0.5	1.0	1.5
28–30	0.9	1.2	1.5
31–33	1.1	1.4	1.7
34–36	1.0	1.4	1.8
37–39	1.2	1.6	2.0
	Transverse diameter (cm)		
13–15	0.4	0.6	0.8
16–18	0.6	0.8	1.0
19–21	0.7	0.9	1.1
22–24	1.5	1.8	2.1
25–27	1.4	1.9	2.4
28–30	1.2	1.6	2.0
31–33	1.2	1.6	2.0
34–36	1.2	1.6	2.0
37–39	1.6	2.0	2.4

Modified from:
Goldstein I, Reece E A, Yarkoni S, Wan M, Green J C, Hobbins J C.
Growth of the fetal stomach in normal pregnancies.
Obstet Gynecol 1987; 70: 641–644

Stomach AP and transverse diameters

mean ± 2SD

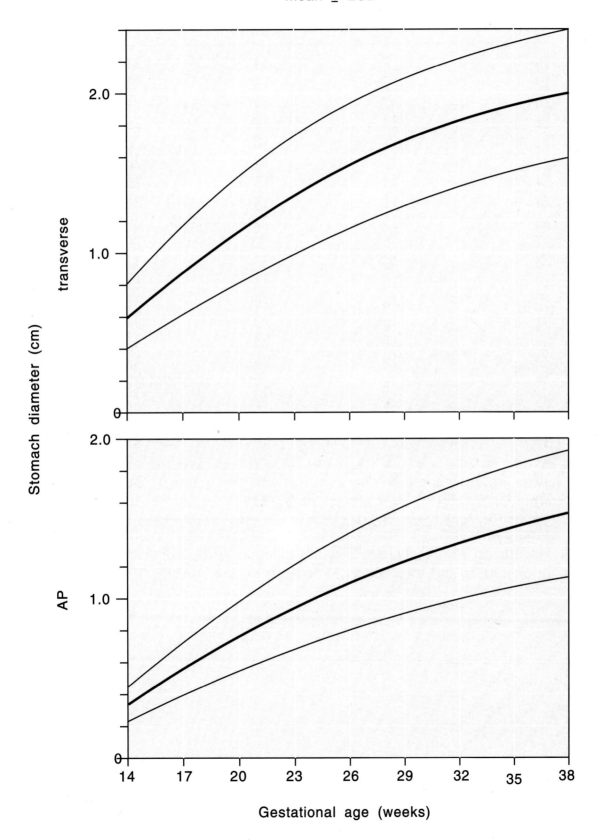

Stomach diameter (cm)

transverse

2.0

1.0

0

AP

2.0

1.0

0

Gestational age (weeks)

14 17 20 23 26 29 32 35 38

Spleen length

gestational age (weeks)	5th	length (mm) 50th centiles	95th
18	7	14	21
19	7	14	21
20	7	14	21
21	11	18	26
22	11	18	26
23	11	18	26
24	11	18	26
25	11	18	26
26	15	22	29
27	15	22	29
28	16	23	31
29	16	23	31
30	16	23	31
31	16	23	31
32	18	25	32
33	18	25	32
34	22	29	37
35	22	29	37
36	22	29	37
37	22	29	37
38	22	29	37
39	24	31	38
40	25	33	40

Modified from:
Hansmann M, Hackeloer B J, Staudach A. Eds. Ultrasound diagnosis in obstetrics and gynecology. Springer Verlag: Berlin; 1985: p 181

Spleen length (mm)

5th 50th and 95th centiles

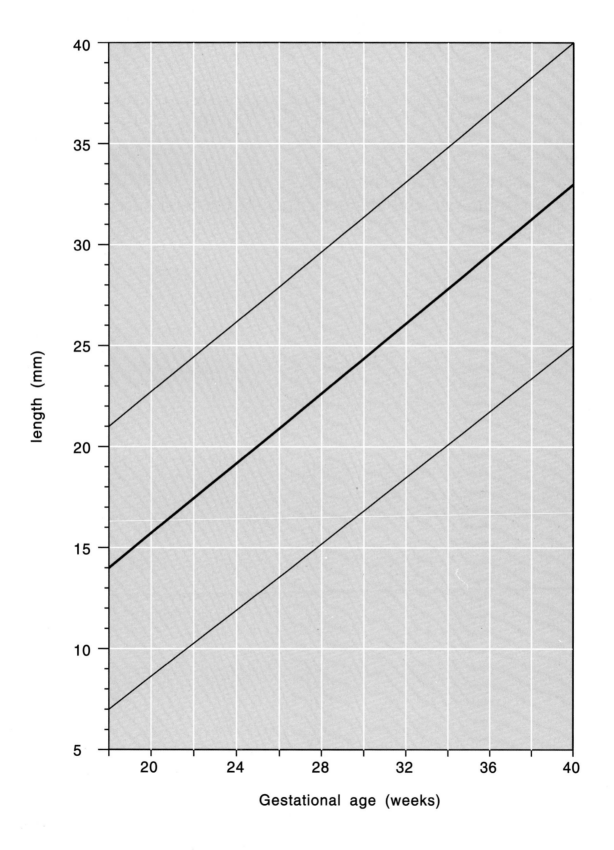

Adrenal glands

Gestational age (weeks)	Thickness (mm)			Width (mm)		
	min	mean	max	min	mean	max
20–25	2	3	5	7	10	12
26–30	2	5	8	12	13	17
31–35	3	5	7	14	16	18
36–40	4	6	9	16	19	24

Modified from:
Jeanty P, Chervenak F, Grannum P, et al.
Normal ultrasonic size and characteristics of the fetal adrenal glands.
Prenat Diagn 1984; 4: 21–28

Adrenal glands

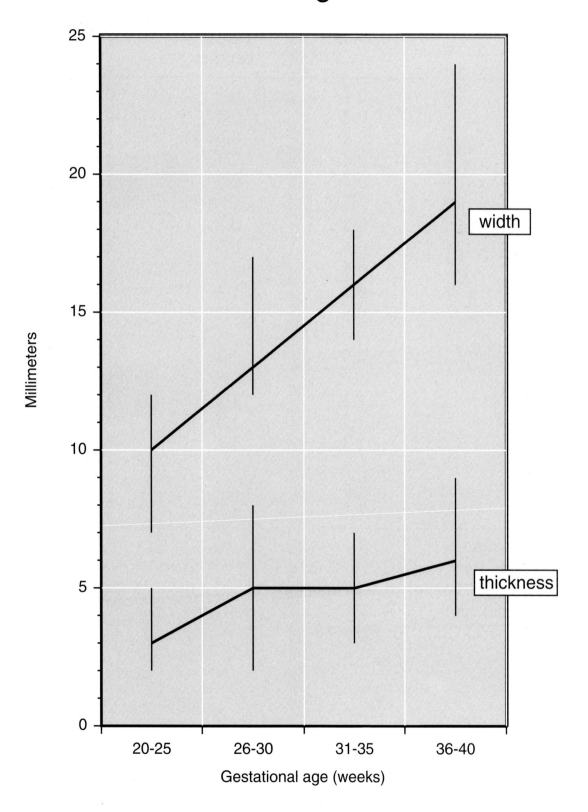

Transverse colon diameter

Gestational age (weeks)	Colon diameter (cm)		
	10th	50th centiles	90th
26	0.1	0.5	0.9
27	0.2	0.5	0.9
28	0.3	0.6	1.0
29	0.4	0.7	1.1
30	0.4	0.8	1.1
31	0.5	0.8	1.2
32	0.6	0.9	1.3
33	0.6	1.0	1.3
34	0.7	1.1	1.4
35	0.8	1.1	1.5
36	0.9	1.2	1.6
37	1.0	1.3	1.7
38	1.1	1.4	1.8
39	1.2	1.5	1.9
40	1.3	1.6	2.0
41	1.4	1.7	2.1
42	1.5	1.9	2.2

Modified from:
Goldstein I, Lockwood C, Hobbins J C.
Ultrasound assessment of fetal intestinal development in the evaluation of gestational age.
Obstet Gynecol 1987; 70: 682–686

Transverse colon diameter

10th, 50th and 90th centiles

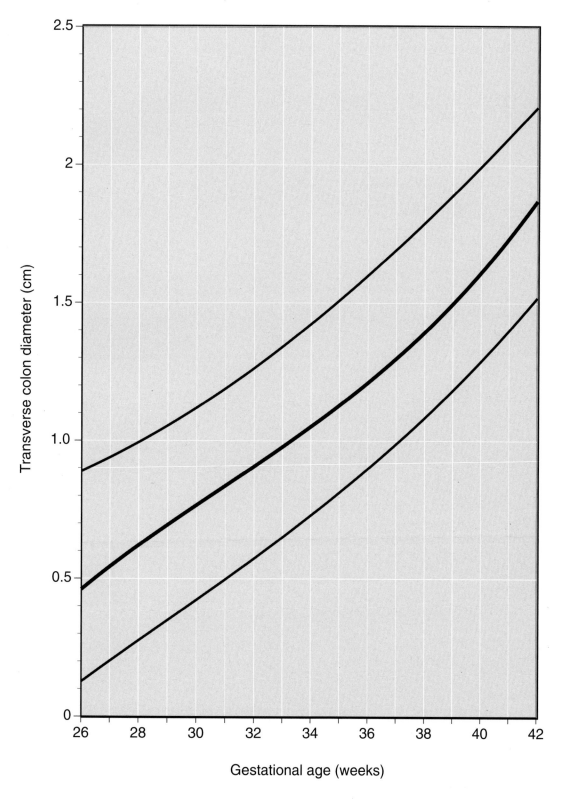

Index